ALLE·ZEIT·WACH
1842

Carcinoma of the Esophagus and Gastric Cardia

Edited by
Guo Jun Huang and Wu Ying K'ai

With 295 Figures in 429 Separate Illustrations,
Some in Color and 59 Tables

Springer-Verlag
Berlin Heidelberg New York Tokyo 1984

Guo Jun (Kuo Chun) Huang, BS, MD, FCCP

Professor and Chairman, Department of Surgical Oncology, Cancer Institute and Hospital, Chinese Academy of Medical Sciences, Panjiayiao, Beijing, P.R. China

Wu Ying K'ai (Y. K. Wu), MB, ChB, FACS (Hon)

Professor of Cardiothoracic Surgery, Director of Beijing Heart, Lung, and Blood Vessel Medical Center, Beijing, P. R. China

ISBN-13:978-3-642-69185-0 e-ISBN-13:978-3-642-69183-6
DOI: 10.1007/978-3-642-69183-6

Library of Congress Cataloging in Publication Data
Main entry under title: Carcinoma of the esophagus and gastric cardia. Bibliography: p. Includes index. 1. Esophagus-Cancer. 2. Cardia-Cancer. 3. Esophagus-Cancer-China. 4. Stomach-Cancer-China. I. Huang, Guo Jun, 1920-. II. Wu, Ying-K'ai, 1910-. [DNLM: 1. Esophageal neoplasms. 2. Stomach neoplasms. WI 250 C2645] RC280.E8C37 1984 616.99'432 84-5308

Softcover reprint of the hardcover 1st edition 1984

2124/3140-543210

Preface

This book has its roots in a monograph on cancer of the esophagus and gastric cardia edited by us in 1965 and published in Chinese only. Along with a number of colleagues in various fields, we summarized our work in the epidemiology, pathology, diagnosis, radiotherapy, and surgery of carcinoma of the esophagus and gastric cardia, carried out chiefly at Peking Union Medical College Hospital, Fuwai Hospital, and the Cancer Institute of the Chinese Academy of Medical Sciences during the 25 years from 1939 to 1964. In the 18 years since the publication of that monograph, further progress has been made in China in various aspects of research and surgical treatment. Abundant material has been accumulated on the long-term results of surgery, and a number of newer principles and methods for diagnosis and management have been evolved. In order to meet the need for the exchange of scientific and technical information, both domestically and internationally, we have invited a group of our current colleagues working on the different aspects of carcinoma of the esophagus and gastric cardia to contribute to the present volume, which is being printed in both Chinese and English. The Chinese edition, like the original monograph, is being published by Shanghai Science and Technology Publishers. Through the kind invitation of Dr. Heinz Götze, the English text is being published for international circulation by Springer-Verlag. We wish to express our heartfelt appreciation to both publishers, whose encouragement and assistance have made the completion of this new monograph possible at this time.

We also want to express our thanks to all the contributors, who have done a splendid job in summarizing the scientific achievements to date in their own particular fields. No attempt has been made to go into the voluminous international literature, in order to keep the volume to a moderate size. We hope the book will serve its purpose as an introduction to our experience and achievements in carcinoma of the esophagus and gastric cardia in China. We believe that the progress in early diagnosis and the prospect of being able to prevent cancer altogether should encourage future work.

Guo Jun Huang
Wu Ying K'ai

Contents

Contributors

Cheng, Shu Jun, MD
Chief, Division of Genetic Toxicology, Department of Chemical Etiology and Carcinogenesis, Cancer Institute and Hospital, Chinese Academy of Medical Sciences, Beijing, P. R. China
Gu, Xian Zhi (Ku, Hsien-chih), BS, MD
Professor and Chairman, Department of Radiation Oncology, Cancer Institute and Hospital, Chinese Academy of Medical Sciences, Beijing, P. R. China
Huang, Guo Jun (Huang, Kuo-chun), BS, MD, FCCP
Professor and Chairman, Department of Surgical Oncology, Cancer Institute and Hospital, Chinese Academy of Medical Sciences, Beijing, P. R. China
Li, Bing (Li, Ping), MD
Vice-Director, Cancer Institute and Hospital, Chinese Academy of Medical Sciences, Beijing, P. R. China
Li, Ling, MD
Department of Pathology, Cancer Institute and Hospital, Chinese Academy of Medical Sciences, Beijing, P. R. China
Li, Ming Xin (Li, Min-hsin), MS, PhD
Professor and Chairman, Department of Chemical Etiology and Carcinogenesis, Cancer Institute and Hospital, Chinese Academy of Medical Sciences, Beijing, P. R. China
Liu, Bo Qi, MD
Department of Epidemiology, Cancer Institute and Hospital, Chinese Academy of Medical Sciences, Beijing, P. R. China
Liu, Fu Sheng, MD
Vice-Chairman, Department of Pathology, Cancer Institute and Hospital, Chinese Academy of Medical Sciences, Beijing, P. R. China
Pan, Guo Li, MD
Department of Pathology, Cancer Institute and Hospital, Chinese Academy of Medical Sciences, Beijing, P. R. China
Shen, Qiong (Shen, Chuin), MD
Professor of Pathoanatomy, Department of Pathoanatomy, Henan Medical College, Henan, P. R. China
Su, Ji Hao, MD
Associate Professor and Chairman, Department of Diagnostic Radiology and Computed Tomography, Henan Cancer Research Institute, Henan, P. R. China

Sun, Yan (Sun, Yen), MD
Associate Professor and Vice-Chairman, Department of Medical Oncology, Cancer Institute and Hospital, Chinese Academy of Medical Sciences, Beijing, P. R. China

Wang, Zheng Yan (Wang, Cheng-yen), MD
Associate Professor and Vice-Chairwoman, Department of Diagnostic Radiology, Cancer Institute and Hospital, Chinese Academy of Medical Sciences, Beijing, P. R. China

Wu, Ying K'ai (Y. K. Wu), MB, ChB, FACS (Hon)
Professor of Cardiothoracic Surgery, Director of Beijing Heart, Lung, and Blood Vessel Medical Center, Beijing, P. R. China

Xia, Qiu Jie (Hsia, Chu-chieh), MD
Associate Professor and Chairwoman, Department of Pathology, Cancer Institute and Hospital, Chinese Academy of Medical Sciences, Beijing, P. R. China

Zhang, Da Wei (Chang, Da-wei), MD
Associate Professor and Vice-Chairman, Department of Surgical Oncology, Cancer Institute and Hospital, Chinese Academy of Medical Sciences, Beijing, P. R. China

Zhou, Chuan Nong, MD
Central Laboratory, Cancer Institute and Hospital, Chinese Academy of Medical Sciences, Beijing, P. R. China

Chapter 1
Epidemiology of Carcinoma of the Esophagus in China

Bo Qi Liu and Bing Li

1 Introduction

Cancer of the esophagus, a common malignancy in various parts of the world, was first recorded in China over 2000 years ago, under the name of *"Ye Ge"* (噎嗝), meaning dysphagia and belching. Descriptions of this disease are found in a number of traditional Chinese medical texts, some authors attributing it to "heavy indulgence in heated liquors" [1]. It is also stated in the text of Yi-Guan as "commonly seen in the elderly and rarely developing in young people."

Ever since the founding of the new China, medical researchers have carried out extensive investigations into the epidemiology of esophageal cancer. In 1969, cancer registration was initiated in order to obtain data on incidence and mortality. From 1973 to 1975, a 3-year retrospective survey of cancer mortality covering a total population of 850 million people was undertaken, with analysis of the geographic distribution and mortality of esophageal cancer. In 1974, a multidisciplinary group of scientists started work in north China, the northwestern part of Sichuan, and parts of Guangdong, Xinjiang, and Jiangsu provinces on the etiology and genesis of esophageal carcinoma. Since 1970, six field stations devoted to the treatment and prevention of esophageal carcinoma have been established in the high-risk areas, greatly facilitating the research into this malignancy.

2 Mortality

The rate of death from esophageal cancer varies greatly between different countries and regions. Data obtained by WHO and published in 1977 show that mortality, standardized to the world population, was highest in both sexes in China, with Puerto Rico coming second and Singapore third. Cumulative mortality up to 74 years of age was 4.05% for Chinese men and 1.96% for Chinese women. The incidence in Chinese men is double that in Singapore, and mortality in Chinese women is 5 times as high as that in Puerto Rican women (Table 1.1, Fig. 1.1). Among the 29 provinces, municipalities, and autonomous regions in China (mortality information from Taiwan is not available), 20 have a higher mortality standardized to the world population for men, and 23 for women, than those of Puerto Rico and Singapore (Fig. 1.2). Linxian county in Henan province has the highest incidence of all (Figs. 1.3, 1.4). Among the five continents, the highest incidence is in Asia and Africa.

Relative Mortality by Site

In China, deaths from cancer of the esophagus constitute 26.46% of all cancer deaths in men and 19.74% in women, both figures surpassing those in all other countries (Table 1.1). Esophageal cancer ranks second only to cancer of the stomach (Table 1.2). However, the position of esophageal cancer among all malignancies varies greatly in different parts of China. It can be as high as 70% in the high-risk areas, taking the first place in the table, and as low as a few percent in the low-risk areas. Among the 29 provinces, municipalities, and autonomous regions, it occupies the first place for male cancer deaths in nine, the second place in eight, the third or fourth place in ten, and the fifth place in two. Female mortality occupies one of the first five places in 23 and one of the first eight in the other six [2].

Table 1.1. Mortality for esophageal cancer in selected countries

Country	Total			Male			Female			Sex ratio (M:F)
	World--adjusted rate (per 100000)	Cumulative rate (%)	Proportion of total malignancy (%)	World--adjusted rate (per 100000)	Cumulative rate (%)	Proportion of total malignancy (%)	World--adjusted rate (per 100000)	Cumulative rate (%)	Proportion of total malignancy (%)	
Asia										
China	23.40	2.96	23.53	31.66	4.05	26.46	15.93	1.96	19.74	1.99
Singapore	8.44	1.14	5.72	14.41	1.94	7.13	2.27	0.38	2.25	6.35
Hong Kong	7.62	0.96	5.55	12.59	1.67	6.84	3.41	9.39	3.37	3.69
Japan	4.01	0.49	3.43	7.09	0.88	4.74	1.56	0.17	1.71	4.54
Africa										
Mauritius	1.90	0.13	2.89	3.75	0.19	4.39	0.60	0.07	1.15	6.25
Europe										
Scotland	5.17	0.58	3.13	7.08	0.81	3.40	3.73	0.40	4.97	1.90
Ireland	4.72	0.50	3.18	5.76	0.60	3.45	3.78	0.40	2.86	1.52
England and Wales	3.97	0.45	2.64	5.47	0.62	2.88	2.85	0.31	2.30	1.78
Iceland	3.90	0.56	3.49	3.70	0.52	3.13	4.14	0.59	3.84	0.89
Switzerland	3.58	0.41	2.60	7.23	0.83	3.98	0.79	0.07	0.75	9.15
Belgium	2.15	0.24	1.38	3.85	0.44	1.87	0.87	0.08	0.73	4.43
Netherlands	2.04	0.22	1.34	3.18	0.36	1.58	1.17	0.12	1.03	2.72
Denmark	1.98	0.23	1.30	2.99	0.34	1.76	1.12	0.13	0.80	2.67
West Germany	1.95	0.22	1.27	3.79	0.44	1.95	0.72	0.06	0.56	5.26
Sweden	1.91	0.22	1.50	3.14	0.38	2.12	0.85	-.08	0.77	3.69
Austria	1.77	0.21	1.18	3.77	0.43	1.95	0.46	0.05	0.37	8.19
East Germany	1.38	0.17	1.05	2.78	0.34	1.64	0.54	0.06	0.49	5.14
Romania	1.11	0.13	1.02	1.85	0.23	1.37	0.51	0.06	0.57	3.63
America										
Puerto Rico	9.31	1.09	9.27	13.60	1.64	11.16	5.17	0.54	6.49	2.62
Chile	7.08	0.86	5.16	9.84	1.18	6.34	4.95	0.59	3.99	1.99
Costa Rica	3.62	0.40	3.01	5.29	0.59	3.89	1.97	0.22	1.87	2.96
Paraguay	3.22	0.33	3.38	5.26	0.54	6.19	1.44	0.13	1.38	3.65
United States	2.55	0.31	1.93	4.28	0.52	2.63	1.15	0.13	1.06	3.72
Oceania										
New Zealand	3.48	0.39	2.42	5.18	0.62	3.52	2.02	0.18	1.66	2.56
Australia	2.97	0.34	2.35	4.42	0.51	2.77	1.77	0.18	1.76	2.50

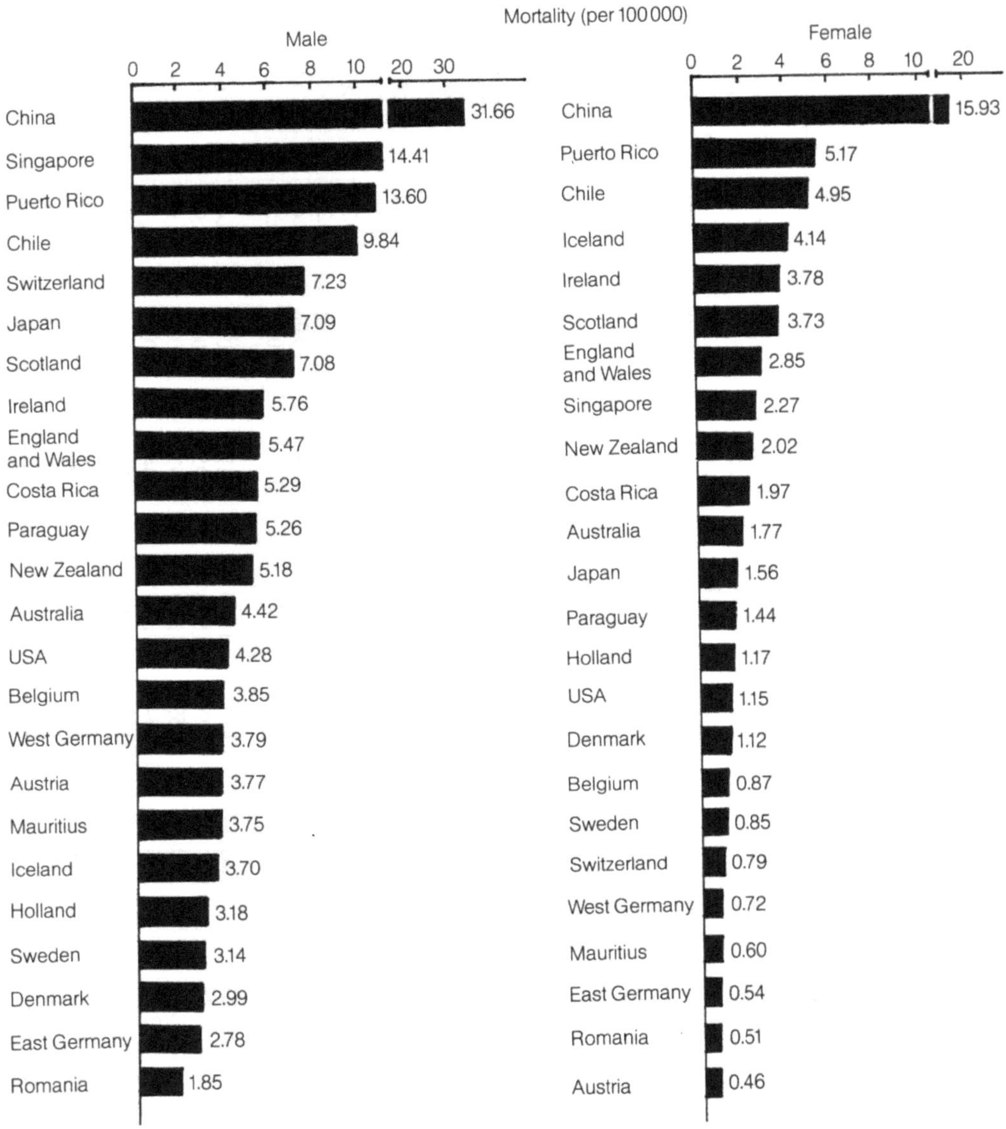

Fig. 1.1. Age-adjusted mortality for esophageal cancer in selected countries

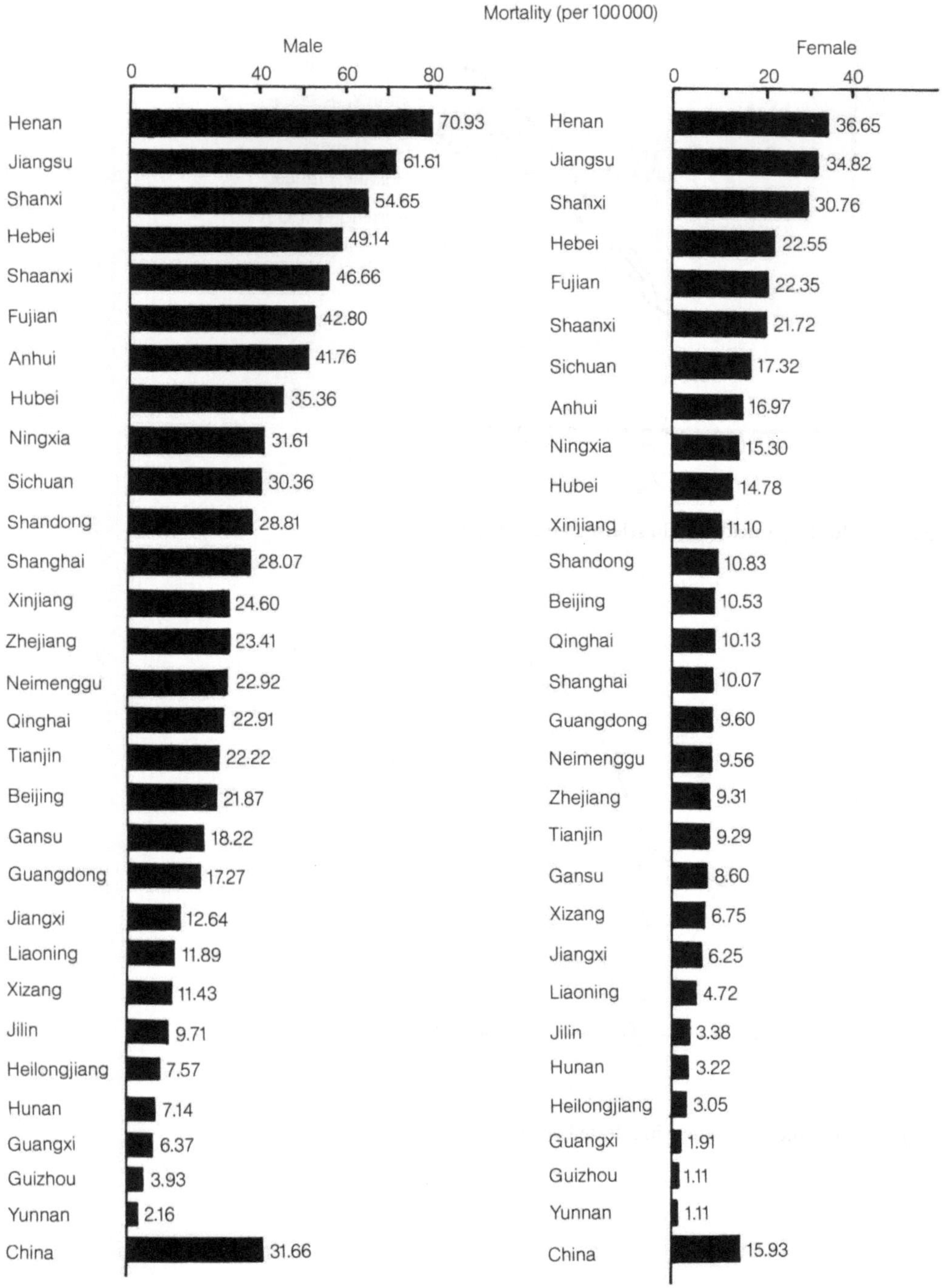

Fig. 1.2. Age-adjusted [to World Population Standard (1960)] mortality in the 29 provinces, municipalities, and autonomous regions of China

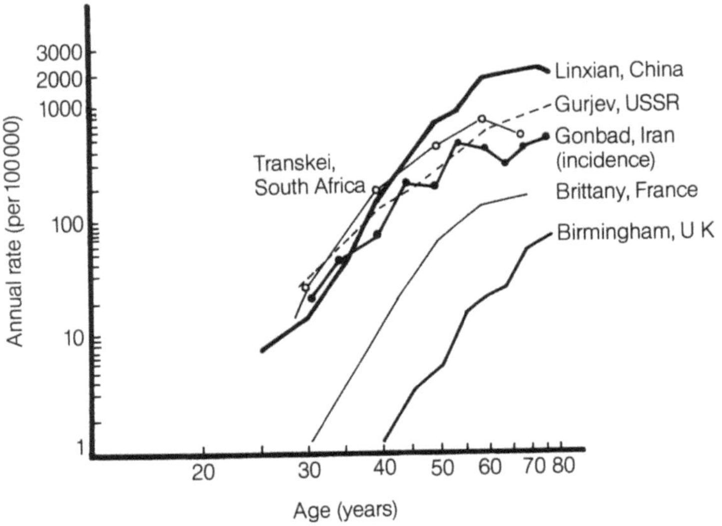

Fig. 1.3. Mortality (incidence) in selected areas (male)

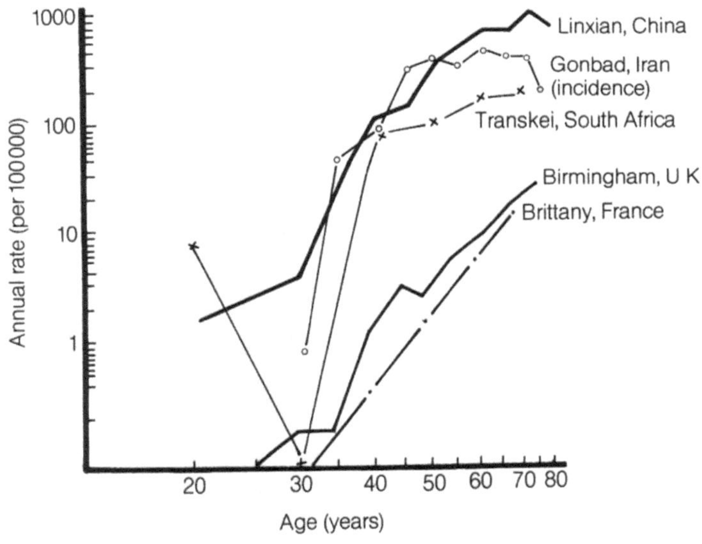

Fig. 1.4. Mortality (incidence) in selected areas (female)

Table 1.2. Cancer mortality by site and sex in China (1973–1975)[a]

Male			Female		
Site/type	Rate	(%)	Site/type	Rate	(%)
Stomach	20.93	26.11	Stomach	10.16	18.72
Esophagus	19.68	24.55	Cervix uteri	9.98	18.39
Liver	14.52	18.11	Esophagus	9.85	18.15
Lung	6.82	8.51	Liver	5.61	10.34
Colon/rectum	4.08	5.09	Lung	3.20	5.90
Leukemia	2.79	3.48	Colon/rectum	3.03	5.58
Nasopharynx	2.49	3.11	Breast	2.61	4.81
Brain	1.43	1.78	Leukemia	2.23	4.11
Lymphoma	1.35	1.68	Nasopharynx	1.27	2.34
Bladder	0.80	1.00	Brain	1.07	1.97
Penis	0.39	0.49	Lymphoma	0.96	1.77
Breast	0.06	0.07	Bladder	0.27	0.50
Other	4.83	6.03	Choriocarcinoma	0.23	0.42
			Other	3.80	7.00
Total	80.17	100.00	Total	54.27	100.00

[a] Age-adjusted to 1964 population

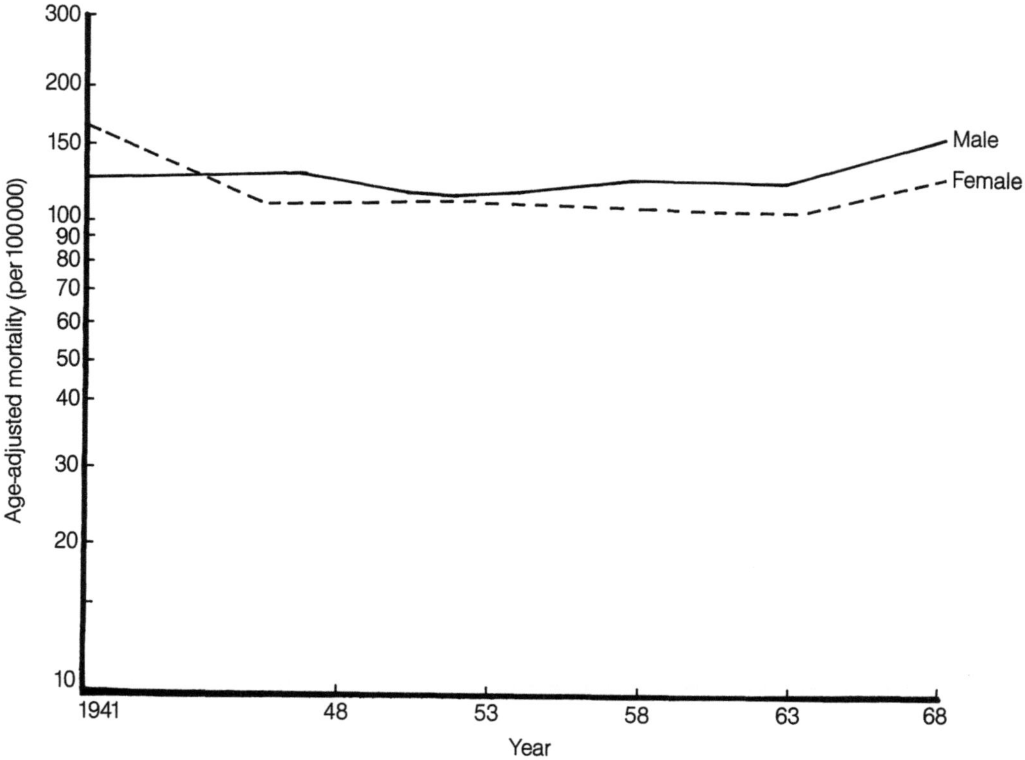

Fig. 1.5. Mortality in 76 districts of Linxian county, Henan province

3 Trends of Incidence

In 1971, a retrospective study was made of mortality during 27 years (1941–1968) among 110,000 people over 28 years of age in Linxian county, Henan province. It was found that age-adjusted mortality in that area was fairly constant throughout that period, fluctuating between 100 and $150/10^5$. There was no significant rise or fall in the mortality curve (Fig. 1.5) [3]. Cancer registration and mortality reports showed that the incidence of esophageal carcinoma had not changed since 1959, mortality from esophageal carcinoma and overall morbidity remaining more or less parallel. It must be noted that during this period, there have been conspicuous improvements both in standard of living and in general evironmental conditions. Esophageal cancer registration and mortality reports in the city of Shanghai and in Haimen county of Jiangsu province also showed a more or less constant incidence (Fig. 1.6).

Mortality among Caucasian Americans during the period 1950–1967 fluctuated between 3.82 and $4.23/10^5$ for men and between 0.93 and $1.08/10^5$ for women. The fluctuations in both the male and female populations were very slight. The incidence among non-Caucasian Americans, black South Africans, and Puerto Ricans, on the other hand, has tended to increase during recent years. In Denmark, Finland, and Switzerland the opposite is true [4–6].

Due to the multiplicity of methods adopted and the variation in the statistical parameters used, the significance of these discrepancies can hardly be evaluated. However, it is still important to assess the validity of changing trends in epidemiology.

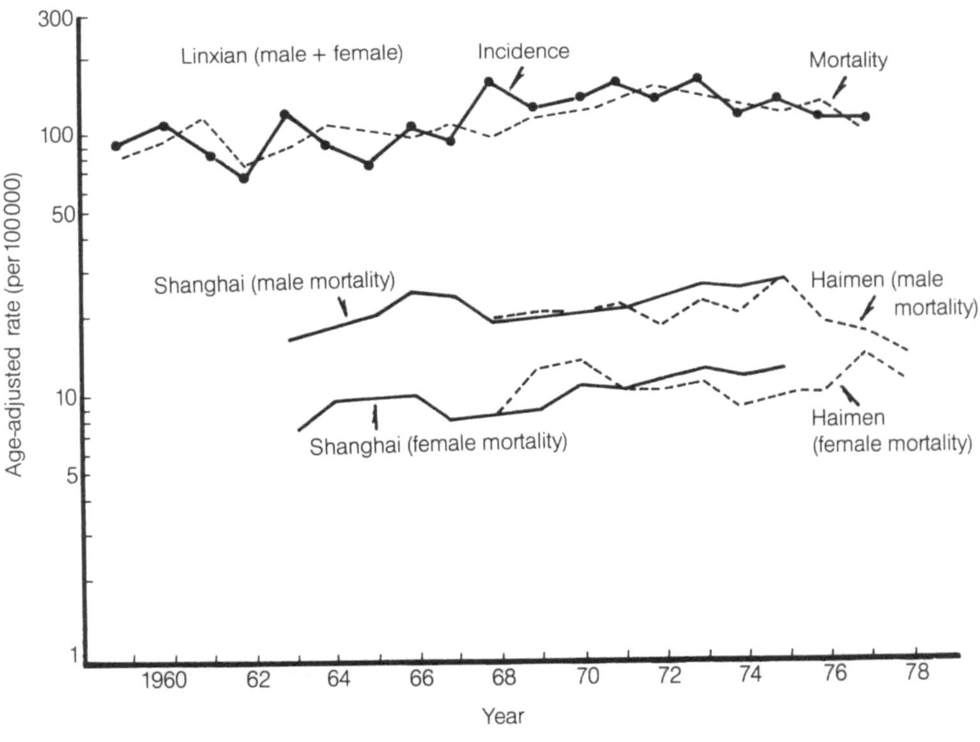

Fig. 1.6. Mortality/incidence in selected areas of China

4 Geographic Distribution

4.1 Clustering Phenomenon

From the study of the epidemiology of esophageal cancer in China, it is clear that there are certain characteristics peculiar to this disease in the geographic distribution of the high-risk regions. Those districts with mortality higher than the average constitute a band-like zone extending from the port of Lian Yun in the east to Mian Yang county of Sichuan province in the west. The northern boundary of this zone extends up to the suburbs of Beijing and its southern boundary reaches Jiujiang city in Jiangxi province. This grouping or clustering of high-risk regions could be subdivided into the Taihang mountain range, the Qinling mountain range, the Dabie mountain range, and the Huai river system, all linked in a vast confluent geographic area. There are further high-risk areas along the coastline of Guangdong and Fujian provinces and in the parts of Xinjiang autonomous regions inhabited by the Kazakh minorities (Fig. 1.7).

4.2 Variation Between Districts

There is great variation in the geographic distribution of esophageal carcinoma, more than in any other malignancy in China. On the county level, the difference between maximum and minimum mortality can be as high as $161.08/10^5$ in men and $102.75/10^5$ in women. The maximum mortality for men is 645 times as high as the minimum, and for women 791 times as high. These differences far exceed those in other malignancies (Tables 1.3, 1.4). Furthermore, there are obvious step-like differences in the geographic distribution of mortality, which can differ greatly between adjacent areas (Table 1.5).

Table 1.3. Mortality by county for some common cancers in China (male)[a]

Site/type	High-mortality areas		Low-mortality areas		
	County	Mortality (per 100000)	County	Mortality (per 100000)	Ratio (high : low)
All sites	Yangzhong (Jiangsu)	279.33	Daguan (Yunnan)	9.75	28
Esophagus	Linxian (Henan)	161.33	Lancang (Yunnan)	0.25	645
Stomach	Changle (Fujian)	120.47	Chongyi (Jiangxi)	0.22	547
Liver	Fusui (Guangxi)	96.99	Yengisar (Xinjiang)	0.65	149
Lung	Gejiu (Yunnan)	70.62	Yongshan (Yunnan)	0.18	392
Nasopharynx	Sihui (Guangdong)	24.88	Feixiang (Hebei)	0.09	276
Colon/rectum	Jiashan (Zhejiang)	23.62	Huaiji (Guangdong)	0.24	98
Leukemia	Jiangpu (Jiangsu)	11.12	Qianjiang (Sichuan)	0.15	74
Brain	Yinchuanshi (Ningxia)	3.21	Hotandiqu (Xinjiang)	0.01	312
Lymphoma	Jiaozuoshi (Henan)	3.06	Andashi (Heilonjiang)	0.26	11
Bladder	Shanghai Shiqu	2.62	Wenshanzhou (Yunnan)	0.07	37
Penis	Tongren (Guizhou)	1.21	Fuxin (Liaoning)	0.03	40

[a] Age-adjusted to 1964 population

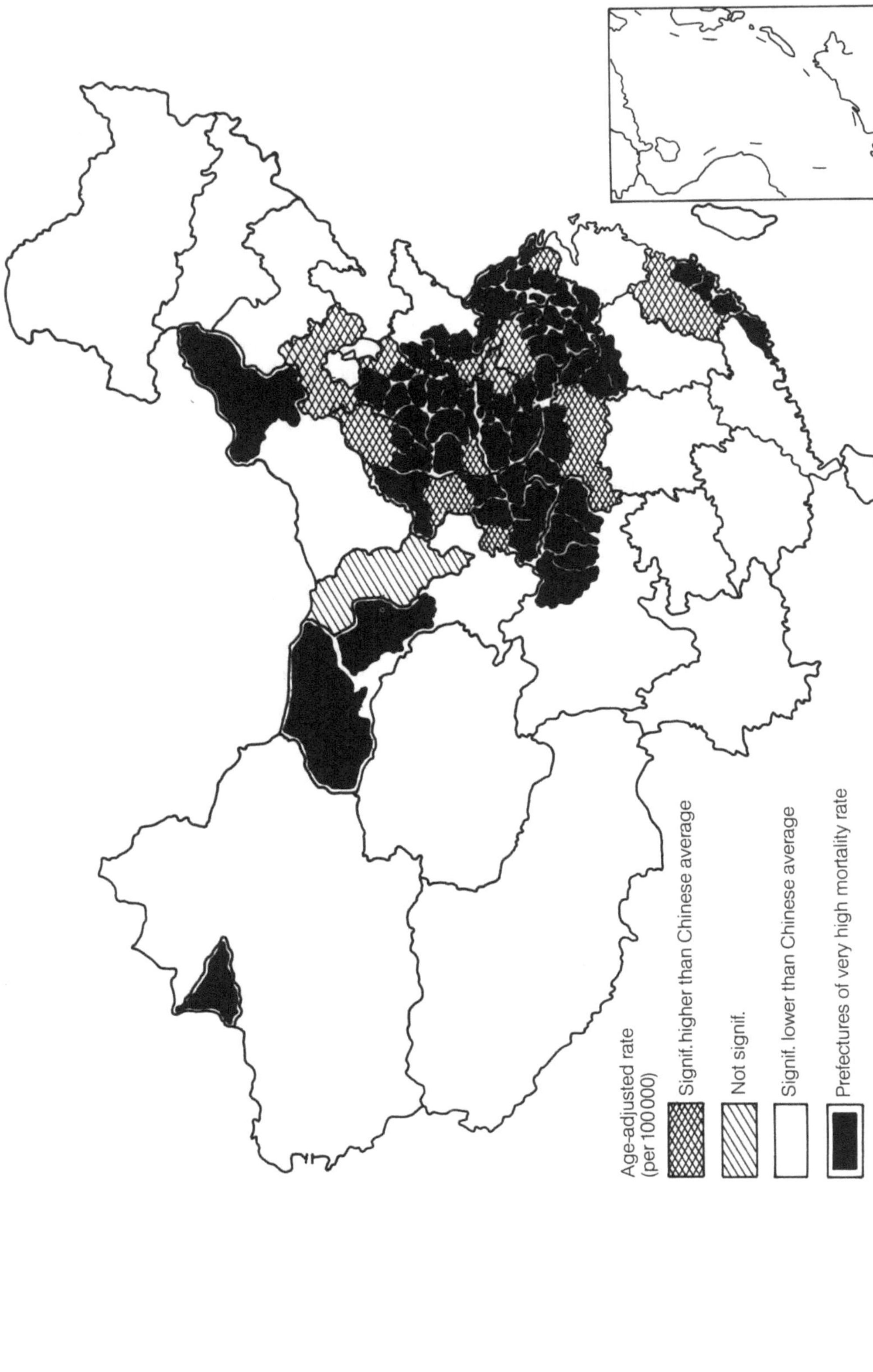

Fig. 1.7. Distribution of mortality in China

Table 1.4. Mortality by county for some common cancers in China (female)[a]

Site/type	High-mortality areas		Low-mortality areas		
	County	Mortality (per 100000)	County	Mortality (per 100000)	Ratio (high:low)
All sites	Xiangyuan (Shanxi)	213.64	Daguan (Yunnan)	6.90	30
Esophagus	Linxian (Henan)	102.88	Xundian (Yunnan)	0.13	791
Cervix uteri	Wufeng (Hubei)	66.30	Luodian (Guizhou)	0.20	330
Stomach	Yangzhong (Jiangsu)	51.13	Xichou (Yunnan)	0.37	138
Lung	Xuanwei (Yunnan)	24.50	Rongxian (Guangxi)	0.08	306
Liver	Tong'an (Fujian)	23.13	Yangjiang (Guangdong)	0.31	74
Colon/rectum	Jianshan (Zhejiang)	22.70	Jinping (Yunnan)	0.21	108
Leukemia	Jiangxian (Shanxi)	9.02	Yutai (Shangdong)	0.12	75
Nasopharynx	Sihui (Guangdong)	8.65	Haidianqu (Beijing)	0.07	123
Breast	Wudu (Gansu)	8.22	Yengisar (Xinjiang)	0.19	43
Brain	Shizuishanshi (Ningxia)	2.88	Wenshanzhou (Yunnan)	0.11	26
Lymphoma	Jiaozuoshi (Henan)	2.37	Baoji (Shanxi)	0.13	18
Bladder	Yinnan Diqu (Ningxia)	0.83	Wenshanzhou (Yunnan)	0.03	27
Choriocarcinoma	Yueyang (Henan)	0.76	Anshanshi (Liaoning)	0.02	38

[a] Age-adjusted to 1964 population

Table 1.5. Regional gradients in the mortality for esophageal cancer in China

County	Age-adjusted mortality (35–64 years)		Ratio	Range of mortality	Distance
	Male	Female	(M:F)	(high–low)	(km)[a]
Linxian (Henan)	435.45	285.84	1.5	7(M)– 3(F)	200
Fanxian (Henan)	60.13	113.55	4.4		
Yangchengxian (Shanxi)	403.01	253.63	1.6	30(M)–49(F)	450
Hunyuanxian (Shanxi)	13.55	5.13	2.6		
Huai'anxian (Jiangsu)	300.56	222.54	1.4	26(M)–37(F)	200
Qidongxian (Jiangsu)	11.62	5.98	1.9		
Langzhongxian (Sichuan)	255.57	143.21	1.8	23(M)–17(F)	250
Rongchangxian (Sichuan)	11.23	8.33	1.3		

[a] Distance between the centers of the counties

4.3 *Irregular Concentric Distribution Pattern*

The peculiar distribution characteristics are shown clearly by standardized mortality statistics at county (or commune) level. The districts with high mortality are: (a) the Taihang mountain district bordering the provinces of Hebei, Henan, and Shanxi; (b) the northern part of Sichuan province; (c) the northern part of Jiangsu province; (d) the Dabie mountain area situated along the border between Hubei and Anhuei provinces; (e) the area where Fujian and Guangdong provinces meet; and (f) the Kazakh minority district in Xinjiang autonomous region. There is usually a center of highest incidence, going outward from which mortality gradually decreases, forming irregular concentric circles on a

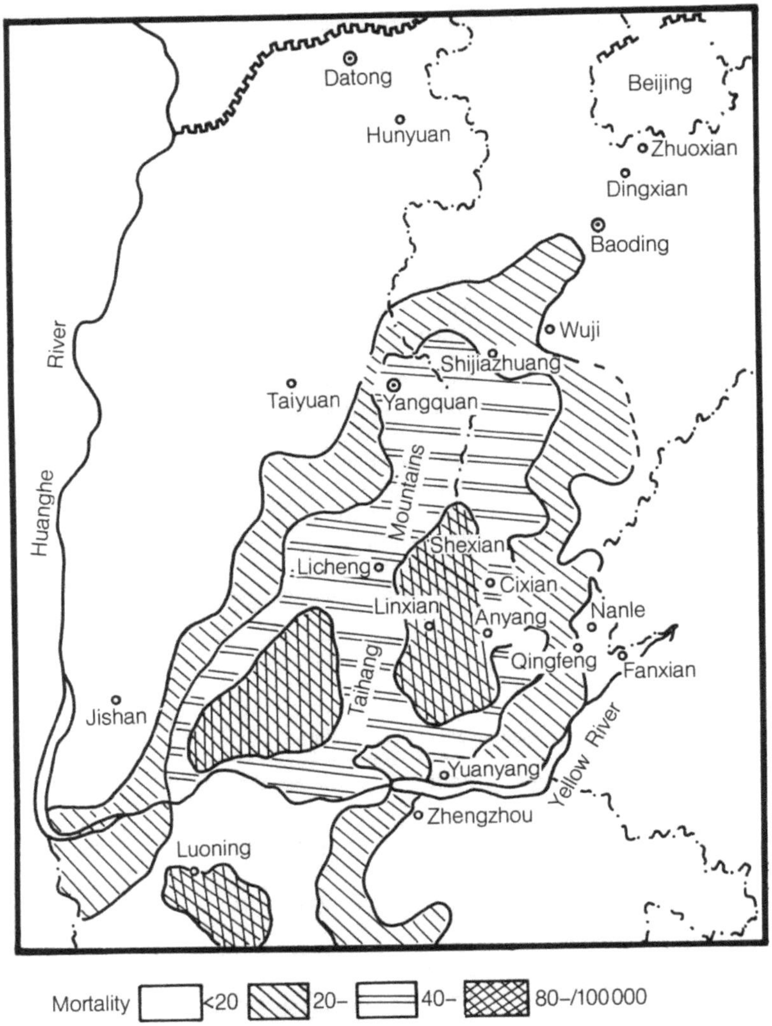

Fig. 1.8. Distribution of mortality along the Taihang mountains

distribution map. This phenomenon is present in all the districts just listed except the Kazakh district (Figs. 1.8–1.10).

Geographically concentric distribution of carcinoma of the esophagus has never been reported from other countries. However, decline in incidence from one region to another has recently been observed. In an area about 400 km long on the coastline of the Caspian Sea in Iran, for example, the incidence of esophageal cancer tends to decline from east to west, with a 130-fold decrease in men and a 58-fold decrease in women (Fig. 1.11) [7]. In the Transkei, western Kenya, and Uganda, the incidence varies so greatly that clearly defined localities with scarcely any distance between them show 10- to 20-fold differences.

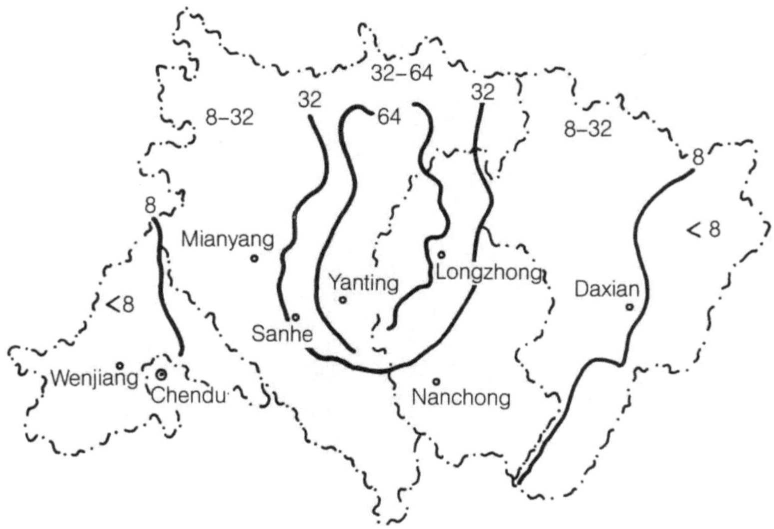

Fig. 1.9. Distribution of mortality in the northern part of Sichuan province

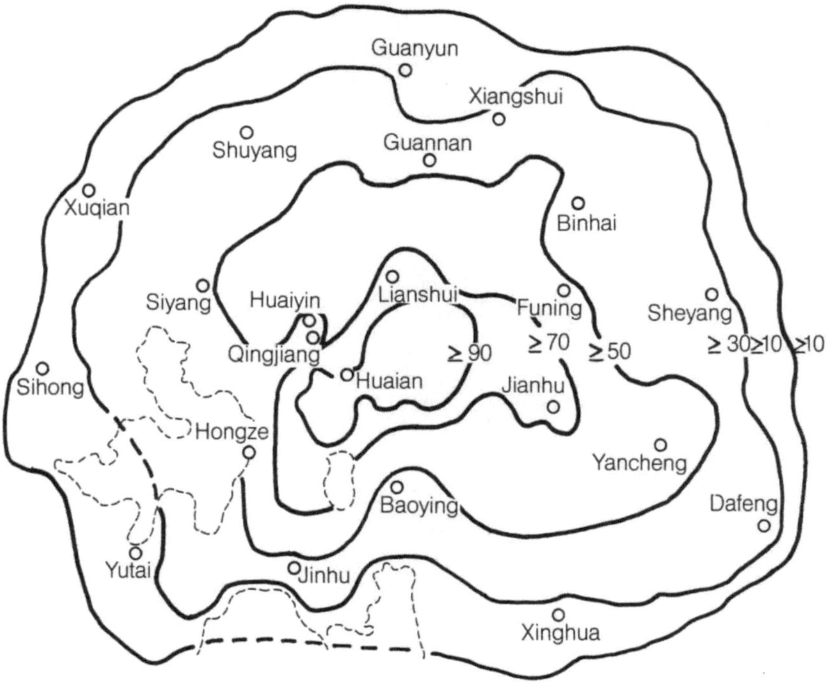

Fig. 1.10. Distribution of mortality in the northern part of Jiangsu province

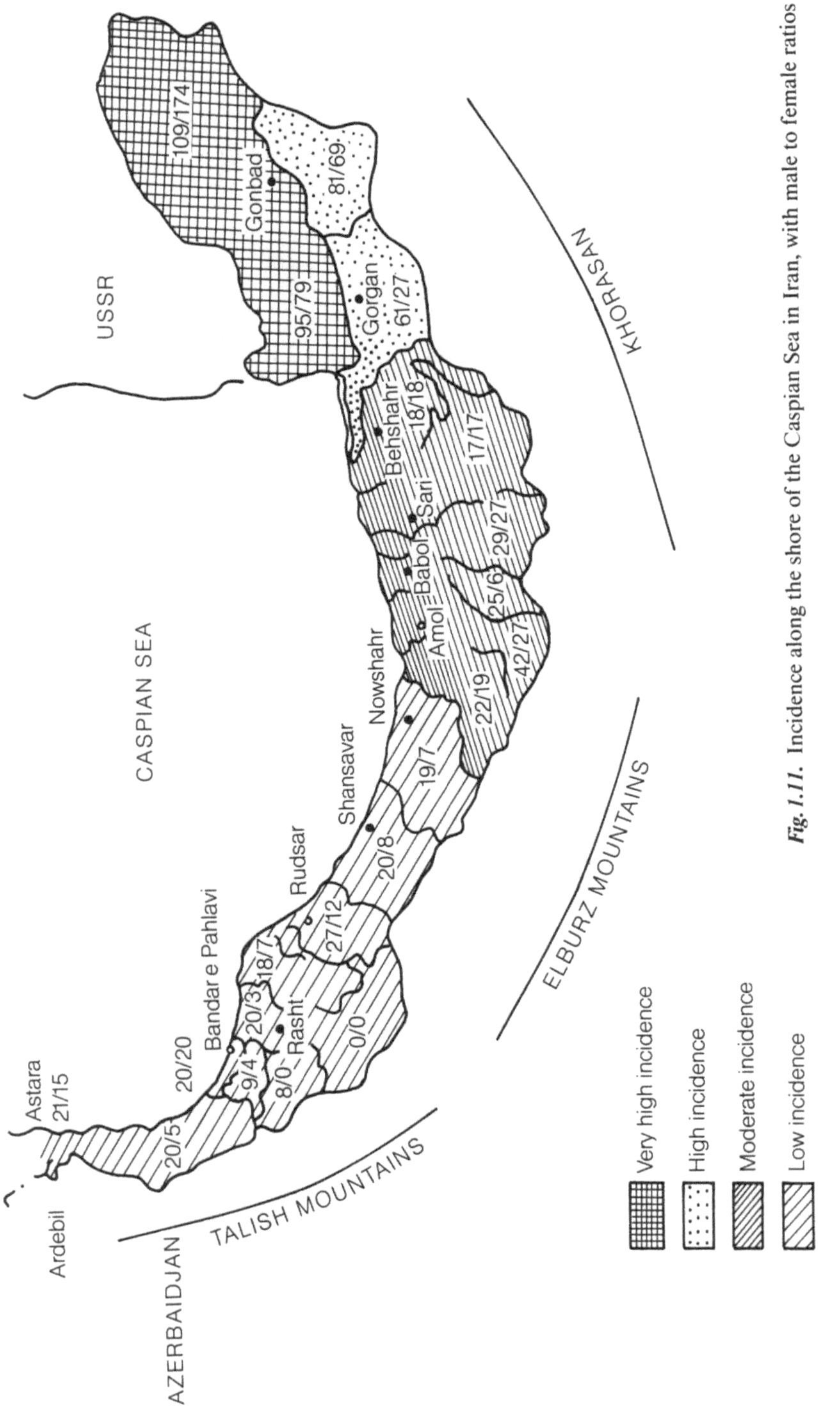

Fig. 1.11. Incidence along the shore of the Caspian Sea in Iran, with male to female ratios

5 Distribution by Population Group

5.1 *Sex*

In China there is a general preponderance of men among esophageal cancer patients, with a male to female ratio of about 2:1, but this varies across the country. In high-risk areas men and women tend to have about the same incidence, but in low-risk areas the proportion of men tends to be greater than women (Table 1.6). The Chinese sex ratio is similar to those reported elsewhere. Most European countries, however, show greater sex ratios than those observed in other nations (Table 1.1), with the exception of Finland, where the 1953–1956 registration statistics reported 630 male and 647 female patients, with no apparent variations between the sexes. The Turkoman tribe in the Gonbad district of northern Iran shows a preponderance of female victims [7].

Table 1.6. Sex ratio at different levels of mortality for esophageal cancer in counties and cities in northern China

Mortality level (per 100000)	No. of counties and cities	Crude mortality (per 100000)				Age-adjusted rate (per 100000)			
		Male	Female	Total	M:F	Male	Female	Total	M:F
0–	12	12.69	4.70	8.92	2.70	7.63	3.38	5.56	2.26
8–	36	28.00	11.53	19.80	2.43	15.95	8.16	12.16	1.95
16–	50	50.24	22.31	36.26	2.25	30.44	15.96	23.40	1.91
32–	50	85.51	47.41	66.47	1.80	58.06	36.67	47.65	1.58
64–	31	128.56	82.24	110.28	1.68	103.83	68.69	86.73	1.51
128–	2	211.54	111.60	161.12	1.90	169.83	103.97	137.78	1.63
Total	181	70.22	37.62	53.96	1.87	45.77	28.55	37.39	1.60

5.2 *Age*

There is also great variation between age-groups. Usually, patients dying from esophageal cancer are from the upper end of the age spectrum. Very few are below 35, but above 35 incidence increases with age, reaching a peak of 17.95% of total esophageal cancer deaths (male 18.67%, female 16.63%) in the 60–64 age-group. Next comes the 65–69 age-group, with 17.34% (male 17.66%, female 16.75%), and from then on the proportion gradually decreases. Of the total mortality, 74.99% (male 76.62%, female 71.7%) occurs between the ages of 50 and 74.

Counting both sexes together, the greatest increase from one age-group to the next occurs in the 35–39 group, and the rate of increase with age noticeably slackens after 55. It can be seen from the mortality curves through the age-groups that there is always a majority of men (Fig. 1.12). Mortality curves from different localities always show a similar pattern. Death from cancer of the esophagus tends to occur at an earlier age in high-risk areas than in low-risk areas. Patients in populations with a mortality of over $128/10^5$ die about 10 years earlier than those in populations with a mortality of $0–8/10^5$ (Fig. 1.13). From this we could speculate that carcinogens might be present in concentration in the environment of high-risk areas.

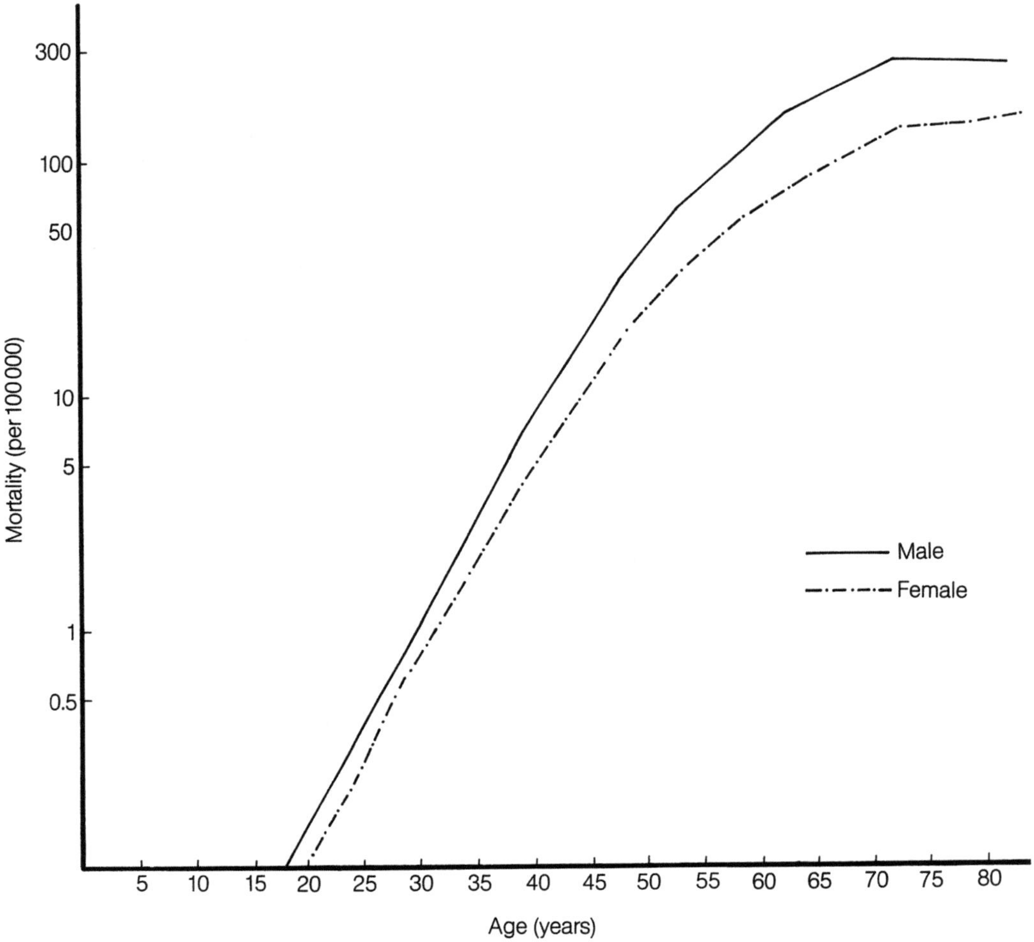

Fig. 1.12. Mortality in China by sex and age

Table 1.7. Mortality for esophageal cancer in various minority groups in China[a]

Minority	Mortality (per 100000)	
	Male	Female
Kazakh	39.27	27.08
Hui	17.89	6.32
Mongol	15.24	5.73
Uygur	14.17	7.93
Zang	8.00	5.34
Korean	6.30	1.62
Yi	1.64	0.91
Miao	1.63	0.63

[a] Age-adjusted to 1964 population

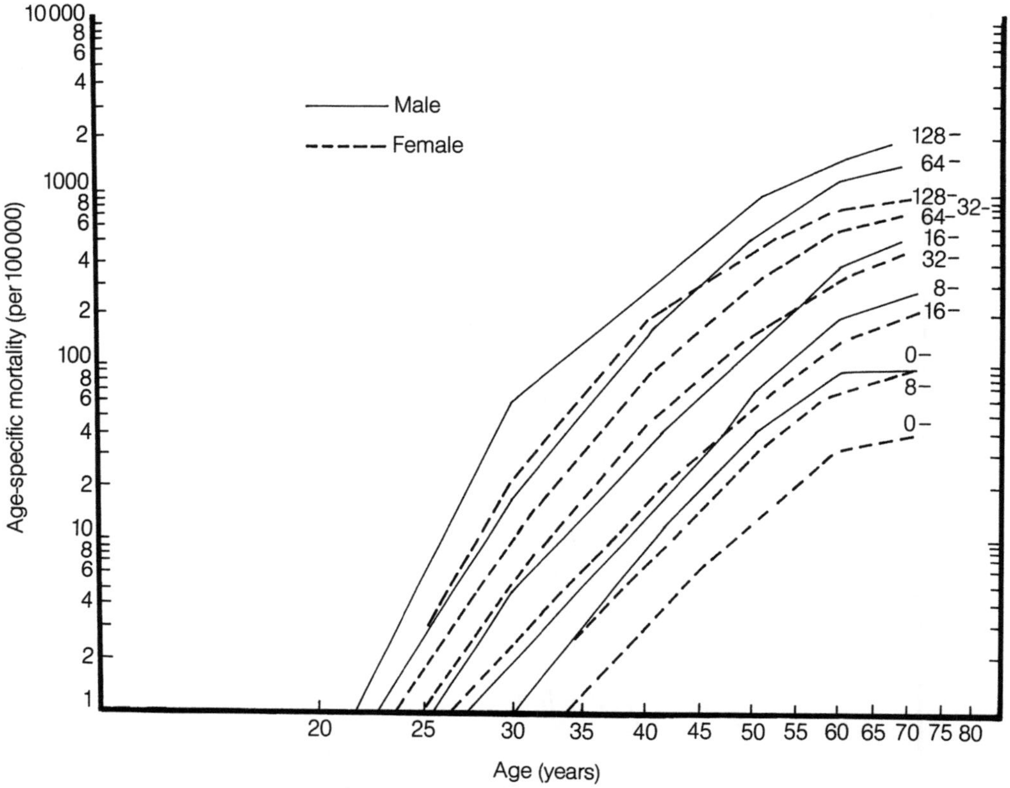

Fig. 1.13. Age- and sex-specific mortality curves for different mortality levels in China

5.3 Ethnicity and Immigration

Comparative statistics from various ethnic minorities in China show that cancer of the esophagus is common among the Uygur people of Xinjiang autonomous region (Table 1.7), whose rate of death from this disease is 2–31 times as high as that among other minority groups and 2,3 times higher than the average for the whole country. The mortality statistics of different age-groups, however, show patterns similar to the national statistics (Fig. 1.14).

Living in the same county (Jingho), Kazakhs, Uygurs, and Mongolians have totally different mortalities. As far as the Kazakhs are concerned, this might be related to their particular eating habits.

According to Doll [5], there is a high incidence among the Turkomans and Kazakhs in the Soviet Union. In America, the incidence among blacks exceeds that among Caucasians and that among immigrant Chinese is higher than that among native-born Chinese [8]. The incidence among overseas Chinese is highest in those speaking Chaozhou and Fujian dialects; that among those speaking Hakka rank next, while that among those speaking Cantonese is the lowest [9]. This is in accordance with our findings in China.

From 1967 to 1969, about 60 000 people migrated to Zhongxiang and Jinmen counties of Hubei province from Zhechuan county of Henan province. The original standardized

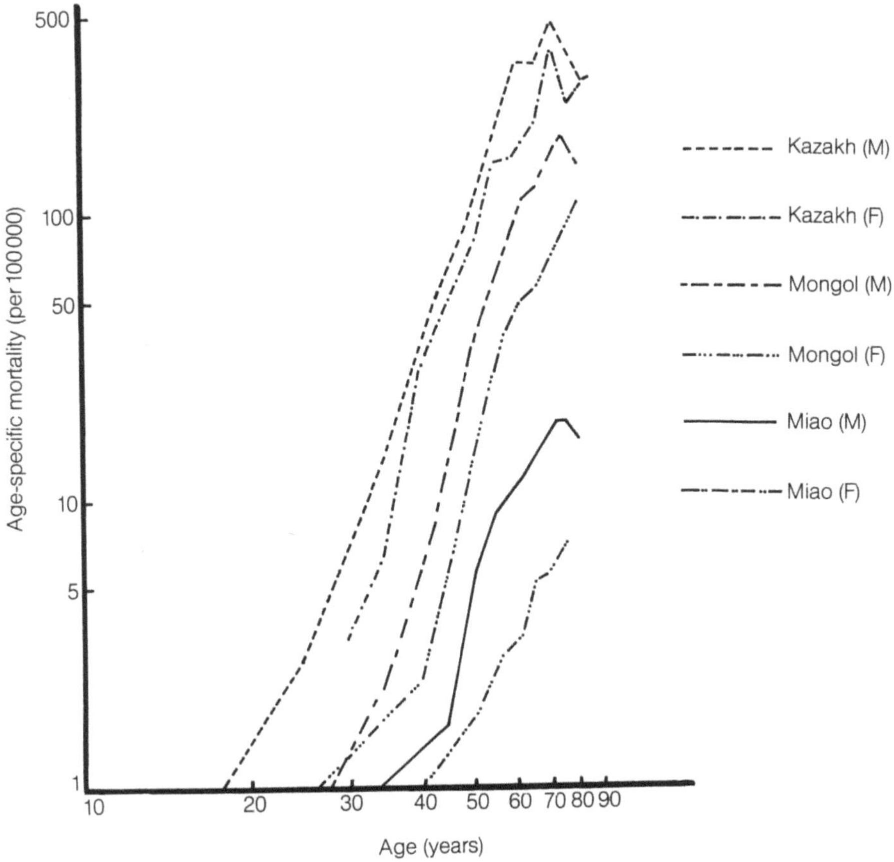

Fig. 1.14. Age- and sex-specific mortality curves for three minority groups in China

esophageal carcinoma death rates in Zhongxiang and Jinmen were $15.39/10^5$ and $7.13/10^5$ respectively (1968–1978); the immigrants, however, still have rates of $75.81/10^5$ and $98.30/10^5$ (1968–1978), i.e., 5–13 times as high as the local people. The mortality in Zhechuan is $55.40/10^5$ (1970–1972). Comparative study of mortality among immigrants and the local population, and of subsequent changes, may well help us to discriminate environmental factors from genetic ones in the etiology of carcinoma of the esophagus.

6 Distribution in Rural and Urban Communities

Rural and urban communities, when arranged according to rates of death from esophageal cancer (male and female combined), appear in the following decreasing order: village > small city > town > large city. Mortality in rural areas is 1.63 times as high as that in large cities; the cumulative mortality up to 74 years of age is 3.45% in villages and 2.21% in large cities. When going by deaths from cancer of the esophagus as a proportion of deaths from all malignancies combined, the order is for men, village > town > small

Table 1.8. Adjusted and cumulative mortality for esophageal cancer in urban and rural communities in China

Community	Total			Male			Female			
	Adjusted mortality	Cumulative mortality	Proportion of total malignancy (%)	Adjusted mortality	Cumulative mortality	Proportion of total malignancy (%)	Adjusted mortality	Cumulative mortality	Proportion of total malignancy (%)	Sex ratio (M:F)
Large city	10.78	2.21	13.49	16.42	3.14	15.43	8.02	1.31	10.28	2.05
Small city	16.73	3.50	21.16	21.60	4.66	23.08	13.17	2.38	18.63	1.64
Town	13.56	2.73	18.87	16.99	3.65	27.50	10.00	1.82	16.19	1.70
Village	17.51	3.45	24.78	24.73	4.72	27.97	15.19	2.46	22.45	1.63

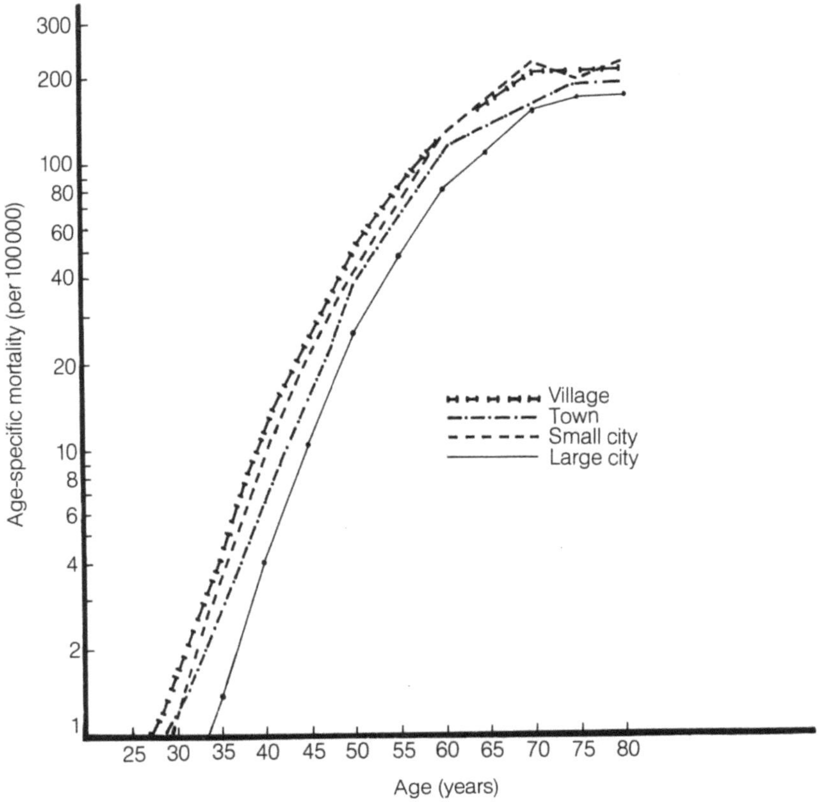

Fig. 1.15. Age-specific mortality in urban and rural areas in China

city > large city; and for women, village > small city > town > large city. The ratio of men to women is greatest in large cities and smallest in the villages (Table 1.8). Mortality curves by age and sex in the countryside and the city are similar in shape and pattern. The age at death among the rural population is lower than in people living in large and small cities and towns (Fig. 1.15). The higher incidence of cancer of the esophagus in rural than in urban areas is also reported in other countries.

7 Hyperplastic Changes of the Esophageal Epithelium

Mass screening of the population by cytology has shown that in high-risk areas, not only is cancer of the esophagus prevalent, but so are hyperplastic changes of the esophageal epithelial cells (Table 1.9). These changes develop with time. It has been observed in cytologic smears obtained in high-risk areas that some normal cells changed via mild and severe hyperplasia into frank squamous cell carcinoma. Another observation was that some of the severely hyperplastic cells could return to normal after proper treatment [10, 11]. Study of this phenomenon is continuing. Pathological and cytologic findings during the induction of cancer of the esophagus by nitrosamines in the rat are very much similar

Table 1.9. Findings of esophageal cytologic screening in selected areas in China

Area	Age-adjusted mortality (per 100000)	No. of people screened	Findings			
			Carcinoma		Severe dysplasia	
			(*n*)	(%)	(*n*)	(%)
Manasxian (Xinjiang)	240.70	579	11	1.90	33	5.70
Linxian (Henan)	169.28	14002	221	1.58	460	3.29
Yangchengxian (Shanxi)	161.90	3316	48	1.45	39	1.18
Yantingxian (Sichuan)	79.00	5714	52	0.91	78	1.37
Zhongxiangxian: immigrants (Hubei)	74.04	13613	60	0.44	136	1.00
Anyang prefecture (Henan)	71.12	17471	88	0.50	48	0.27
Langzhongxian (Sichuan)	68.34	5169	27	0.52	16	0.31
Shanghai	10.69	878	–	–	3	0.34
Zhongxiangxian: natives (Hubei)	7.68	6909	3	0.04	16	0.23

to findings in mass screening of the human population and in autopsy specimens obtained from smokers as compared with those from nonsmokers. Similar hyperplastic changes are observed when there is deficiency of trace substances, e.g., zinc, manganese, and vitamin B complex [12]. Identifying the conditions leading to this deficiency and the causes of it could help materially in the study of the etiology, treatment, and prevention of cancer of the esophagus.

8 Incidence in Animals

Study of incidence of tumors of the upper alimentary tract in animals shows that in the high-risk areas for human esophageal carcinoma, cancers have also been found in the upper gullet of domestic animals and fowls (Table 1.10, Figs. 1.16, 17). Tumors in chickens are found mainly in the pharynx and the upper part of the esophagus (58.55% in the esophagus). The largest lesion found had a diameter of more than 5 cm. Clinically, the tumors may be grossly classified into cauliflower, nodular, and infiltrating types. Patho-

Table 1.10. Prevalence of pharyngeal and esophageal carcinoma in domestic fowls from Linxian and Fanxian counties, Henan province

Age (years)	Linxian			Fanxian		
	No. of chickens	No. of carcinomas	Prevalence (per 100000)	No. of chickens	No. of carcinomas	Prevalence (per 100000)
0–	3460	–	–	3911	–	–
2–	11563	6	52	6087	2	32
5–	2617	20	764	518	–	–
7–	941	6	638	62	–	–
10–	193	1	518	10	–	–
Total	18774	33	175.78	10588[a]	2	18.89

[a] Including 819 chickens of uncertain age

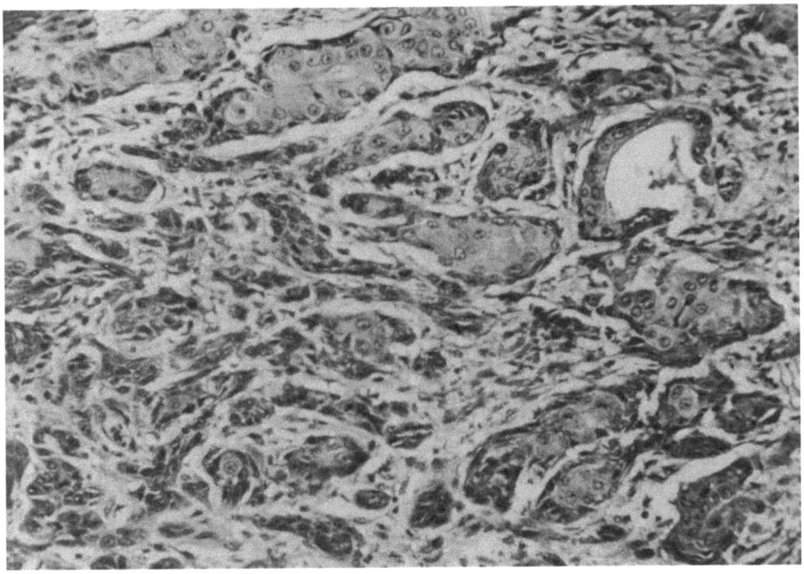

Fig. 1.16. Section of esophageal carcinoma in a chicken

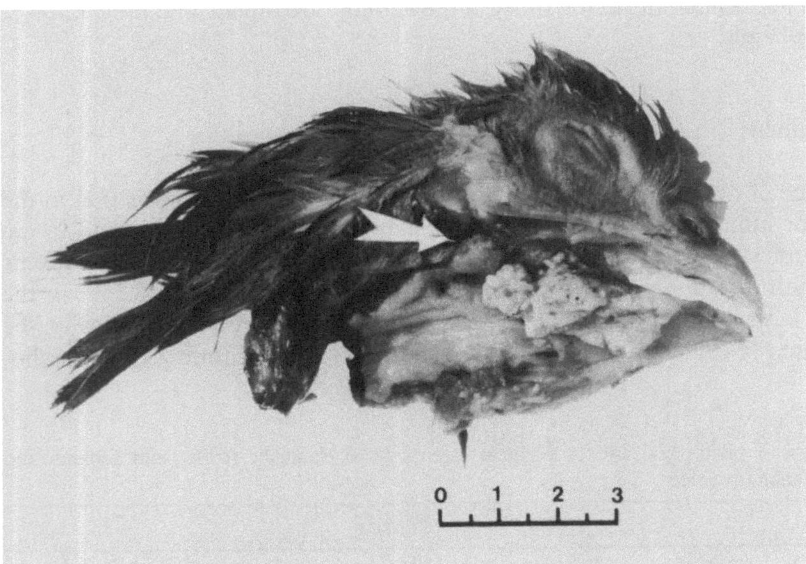

Fig. 1.17. Carcinoma of the hypopharynx *(arrow)* in a chicken

logically, 96.6% of the lesions are squamous cell carcinomas, while adenoacanthoma and adenocarcinoma are relatively rare. Cancers of the esophagus in animals closely resemble those in man in clinicopathological morphology [13]. Carcinoma of the esophagus in the goat is found in Linxian county of Henan province. Particularly interesting is the observation of a higher incidence of tumors in chickens raised by the immigrants from Henan province to Zhongxiang county of Hubei province. Whether this is related to the traditional way of life which the immigrants insist on retaining is subject to investigation.

9 Summary

The rate of death from esophageal carcinoma in China is high. Mortality standardized to world population is $23.40/10^5$; cumulative mortality up to 74 years of age is 2.96%. Cancer of the esophagus is responsible for 23.53% of all deaths from malignancy, being second only to cancer of the stomach. The mortality in 18 provinces, municipalities, and autonomous districts surpasses that in Puerto Rico, the highest-risk area elsewhere in the world. To our knowledge, Linxian county has a rate of death from esophageal carcinoma unsurpassed in the world.

Retrospective study of the incidence of cancer of the esophagus in various parts of China has shown that there has been no significant increase or decrease in morbidity or mortality during recent decades. Nor has there been any change in the mortality by age-group.

Occurrence of cancer of the esophagus is higher than average within a band-like zone bounded in the north by the suburbs of Beijing, in the south by Jiujiang city of Jiangxi province, in the east by Lianyun seaport, and in the west by Mianyang county of Sichuan province. The high-incidence localities therein are more or less contiguous but vary greatly in mortality.

From standardized death rates at county or commune level, it is observed that the incidence of cancer of the esophagus is very high at the center of a high-risk area, but decreases going outwards, forming irregular concentric circles around the center on a distribution map.

The ratio of male to female victims of cancer of the esophagus is 2:1. In areas of very high risk this ratio is much lower, but in areas of low incidence it tends to be higher.

The rate of death from cancer of the esophagus increases with age. Mortality among patients over 35 years of age makes up 99.04% of the total, and that among those between 50 and 74 years of age accounts for 74.99%. Mortality among men is constantly higher in women, as shown by the mortality curves through the age-groups. Age at death is on average about 10 years lower in high-risk areas than in low-risk areas.

The population of China is made up of many minorities, which exhibit great variety in esophageal cancer mortality. Mortality among the Kazakh people in Xinjiang province is 2–31 times higher than among other minorities. There are great differences in mortality among different tribes living near to each other, e.g., Kazakhs, Mongolians, and Uygurs. The Henan immigrants in Hubei province have a mortality 5–13 times higher than that of the local Hubei residents. The existence of marked variations in mortality among the many minority groups may greatly facilitate the study of esophageal cancer.

Esophageal carcinoma mortality in China by size of community is in the following decreasing order: village > small city > town > large city. There is a high predilection for the countryside in which the population has little tendency to migrate.

Hyperplastic changes of the esophageal epithelium are more commonly seen in the populations of high-risk areas than in those of low-risk areas. Extensive cytologic study has shown that the normal cells of the epithelium can change into mild hyperplasia and then into severe hyperplasia, which in some instances can finally give rise to cancer. On the other hand, severe hyperplasia can also revert back through mild hyperplasia into normal epithelium. This phenomenon is still under investigation.

It was found that cancer of the pharyngoesophagus was more common in chickens raised by people in high-risk areas than in their counterparts raised in low-risk areas. Histopathologically, the tumors closely resembled human esophageal carcinoma. It was also observed that in goats and rats, papilloma of the foregut and cancer of the esophagus, as well as hyperplastic changes of the esophageal epithelium, were more common in high-risk areas than in low-risk areas.

It is speculated that thorough, extensive study of the epidemiology of esophageal carcinoma could eventually lead to fruitful understanding of the fundamental causes of this disease and to the development of specific preventive measures.

References

1. Qian ZX (1961) Investigation on esophageal cancer in the province of Xinjiang (in Chinese). Collected Paper of the Second Symposium on Esophageal Carcinoma, Chinese Academy of Medical Sciences, pp 74–78
2. Office of Prevention and Treatment of Malignant Tumors (1979) Study of mortality due to malignant tumors in China (in Chinese). People's Medical Publishing House, Beijing, pp 73–103
3. Collaboration Group of North China for the Investigation of Epidemiology and Carcinogenesis of Cancer of the Esophagus (1974) Preliminary study on the epidemiology and carcinogenesis of esophageal carcinoma in North China (in Chinese). Cancer Res Prev Treat 4: 1–11
4. Rose EF (1973) Esophageal cancer in the Transkei. J Natl Cancer Inst 51: 7–16
5. Doll R (1969) The geographic distribution of cancer. Br J Cancer 23: 1–8
6. Clemmesen J (1965) Statistical studies in malignant neoplasm, vol 1. Munksgaard, Copenhagen, pp 104–106
7. Mahboubi E (1971) Epidemiologic study of esophageal carcinoma in Iran. Int Surg 56: 68–71
8. King HT, Haenszel W (1973) Cancer mortality among foreign and nativeborn Chinese in the United States. J Chronic Dis 26: 623–646
9. De Hong UW, Breslow N, Hong JGE, Sridharan M, Shanmugaratnam K (1974) Etiological factors in esophageal cancer in Singapore Chinese. Int J Cancer 13/3: 291–303
10. Team of Prevention and Treatment for Esophageal Cancer, Linxian County, Chinese Academy of Medical Sciences (1974) The fate of hyperplastic changes in the esophageal epithelium: a follow-up study by cytology (in Chinese). Cancer Res Prev Treat 1: 42–46
11. Cooperative Group of Research on Esophageal Cancer, Henan Province (1974) Study of hyperplastic changes in the esophageal epithelium (in Chinese). Cancer Res Prev Treat 4: 28–31
12. Zeng GY (1980) Epidemiology, vol 2. Carcinoma of esophagus (in Chinese). The People's Medical Publishing House, Beijing, pp 614–625
13. Department of Pathology, Cancer Institute, Chinese Academy of Medical Sciences (1976) Epidemiology and pathology of cancer of the pharynx and esophagus in the chicken (in Chinese). Cancer Res Prev Treat 3: 6–12

Chapter 2
Etiology of Carcinoma of the Esophagus

Ming Xin Li (Min-Hsin Li) and Shu Jun Cheng

---

1 Introduction

In recent years considerable progress has been made in research into the etiologic factors of esophageal cancer. The most striking feature of the distribution of this cancer is the existence of high-risk areas. These areas are usually rather limited in size with mortality highest at the center and gradually decreasing toward the periphery. During the past decade, some clinicians and researchers have visited or stayed in the high-incidence areas, e.g., along the eastern part of the shore of the Caspian Sea in Iran and in Linxian county and surrounding districts in China, to study the problem at first hand and work collaboratively [1–3]. Through intensive investigation, several environmental and endogenous factors have been incriminated as causative or contributory in the genesis of esophageal carcinoma. We review and discuss some of the results in this chapter.

2 Tobacco, Alcohol, and Opium

2.1 Tobacco

Excessive exposure to tobacco and alcohol has repeatedly been implicated as a principal factor in carcinoma of the esophagus [4, 5]. It is known that smoking also increases the risk for cancer of the oropharynx, larynx, lung, kidney, and bladder. The presence in tobacco tars and cigarette smoke of chemical carcinogens such as polycyclic aromatic hydrocarbons (PAHs), *N*-nitroso compounds, epoxides, lactones, peroxy compounds, and halo ethers has been demonstrated (Table 2.1), [6–9]. The tumor-promoting action of phenol and related compounds in cigarette smoke condensate has also been identified [8].

Table 2.1. Carcinogens in cigarette smoke and tars[a]

Aromatic hydrocarbons	
Benzo[*a*]pyrene	Dibenz[*a, j*]acridine
Benz[*a*]anthracene	Dibenzo[*a,i*]pyrene
Benzo[*b*]fluoranthene	Dibenzo[*a,h*]anthracene
Benzo[*j*]fluoranthene	7-H-Dibenzo[*c,g*]carbazole
Chrysene	Indeno[1,2,3-cd]pyrene
Dibenzo[*a,h*]acridine	
Nitroso compounds	
N-nitrosodimethylamine	*N*-nitrosopyrrolidine
N-nitrosodiethylamine	*N*-nitrosopiperidine
N-nitrosoethylmethylamine	*N*-nitrosonornicotine
N-nitrosodiethanolamine	*N*-nitrosodi-*n*-propylamine
N-nitrosodi-*n*-butylamine	*N*-nitrosomorpholine
4-(methylnitrosamino)-1-(3-pyridyl)-1-butanone	
N-nitrosanatabine	*N*-nitrosoanabasine
Epoxides, lactones, peroxy compounds, and halo-ethers	
β-Propiolactone	1,2,5,6-Diepoxyhexane
β-Butyrolactone	1,2,6,7-Diepoxyheptane
1,2,4,5-Diepoxybutane	1,2,7,8-Diepoxyoctane
1,2,4,5-Diepoxypentane	Vinylcyclohexene hydroperoxide
Glycidaldehyde	Bis(chloromethyl)ether

[a] From Hoffmann and Hecht [6]; Brunnemann and Hoffmann [7]; Van Duuren [8]; McCormick et al. [9]

Perhaps the most suggestive evidence for the role of tobacco as a carcinogen in the esophagus is that from Auerbach et al. [10]. Autopsies in 1202 American men whose smoking history was known were the source of esophageal specimens for histologic examination. Of the nonsmokers, only 6.6% showed some atypical nuclei in the basal layer and none had carcinoma in situ. In the smokers, some atypical nuclei were found in 79.8% of cases and carcinoma in situ was found in the epithelium of 15 patients (1.9%). The epithelium tended to be thick in those who had been cigarette smokers at the time of death, reflecting a hyperplastic response. Thus the histologic changes in the esophagus in smokers are strikingly similar to those in the trachea and bronchi.

The habit of chewing – tobacco, betel, or combinations of these with lime – is very common in some parts of the world, especially in Ceylon, India, Burma, and other South and Southeast Asian countries, and is probably responsible for the relatively high incidence of cancer in the oral cavity and esophagus. The chronic irritation of the mucosa by constituents of tobacco, betel, or lime damages the epithelium and stimulates hyperplastic and neoplastic changes of the epithelial cells [5, 11].

2.2 Alcohol

Consumption of tobacco and alcohol by the same individual is common, and the relative importance of each is difficult to assess. In the United States, Wynder and Bross have asserted that the risk of developing esophageal cancer is increased in heavy drinkers (10-fold for beer, about 25-fold for whisky) compared to smoking-matched nondrinkers [4]. Wynder and Bross suggest that alcohol and tobacco may act synergistically; in the absence of smoking and heavy alcohol consumption, the incidence of esophageal cancer in the United States would be reduced by at least 80%. In Japan, Hirayama estimated that for persons who both smoked and drank daily the rate of cancer of the esophagus was 3 times higher than normal; the risk was lowest with beer but increased with saki, whisky, and shochu according to alcohol content [12]. There is strong epidemiologic evidence that esophageal cancer in northeast France is related to excessive consumption of homemade alcoholic beverages and to smoking. Samples of apple cider and its distillates (Calvados) consumed in Brittany were collected from retail outlets and from farms, and some distillates produced under experimental conditions in the laboratory were also examined. Mutagenicity tests on the cider-based drinks and on other commercially available alcoholic beverages have shown a weak response; that for most farm distillates can be attributed neither to nitrosamines nor to PAHs but is due to other as yet unidentified compounds [13]. The high risk for esophageal cancer in Brittany and Normandy may be ascribed to the combined effect of drinking and smoking [14]. High incidence has been associated with certain workers whose exposure to alcohol and/or tobacco tends to be excessive, such as brewery employees, bartenders, waiters, and hotel keepers [15].

A high frequency of esophageal cancer occurs in parts of eastern Africa and in South Africa. Epidemiologic studies by Cook [16] have shown a strong correlation between the regional consumption of home-brewed maize beer and the geographic distribution of esophageal cancer in Africa. Areas such as the Transkei and western Kenya, where corn is extensively produced and used to make maize beer, have a high incidence of esophageal carcinoma; regions where little or no maize beer is brewed, notably Uganda and west Africa, show a very low incidence of the disease. Since maize is not an indigenous African crop, its introduction to some areas is comparatively recent and the traditional kafir beer made from sorghum is increasingly being replaced by maize beer. Cook's theory tallies with the striking increase of esophageal cancer noted in the Transkei and other areas in the past 30 years. Recently, Marasas et al. [17] reported that the highest known esophageal cancer rate in Africa occurred in the southwestern districts of the Transkei; the level of natural contamination of maize kernels with *Fusarium* mycotoxins is higher there than in the low-incidence areas, and in making maize beer many Transkeians preferred the moldy ears because of the allegedly improved flavor. Maize is most frequently contaminated with *Fusarium* fungi and their toxic metabolites have been shown to induce hyperplastic and papillomatous growths in the esophageal epithelium and squamous forestomach (lower extension of the esophagus) of rats [18, 19]. Moreover, squamous cell carcinoma of the forestomach developed in rats after prolonged feeding of *Fusarium moniliforme*-inoculated cornbread [20]. The results give strong evidence for the production of carcinogenic mycotoxins in the moldy maize which may also be present in the maize beers.

In contrast, studies in Linxian and northeastern Iran have shown that the high incidence of esophageal cancer is not associated with alcohol or tobacco [2, 3]. According to hospital records from north China [21], the highest proportion of habitual drinkers among esophageal cancer patients was about 50%, most of whom drank white spirit distilled from sorghum. Statistical data from large numbers of clinical cases and from surveys in high-incidence areas do not indicate alcohol as an important etiologic factor, with the possible exception of fishermen on Nan'ao Island, Guangdong province. In the rural areas of north China, cut tobacco is more popular for smoking than cigarettes, and there are very few women smokers in the countryside. Alcohol and tobacco thus play only a negligible part in the development of esophageal cancer in most high-risk areas in China [22].

2.3 Opium

Hewer et al. [23] have reported that opium addiction is widespread in northeast Iran; both crude opium and opium dross *(sukhteh)* are eaten in considerable quantities. In part of the Transkei, various tobacco residues from the bowl or stem of the pipe are eaten or chewed. Hewer et al. showed that these pyrolyzed substances displayed mutagenic activity in *Salmonella typhimurium* strains TA_{98} and TA_{100} in the presence of rat liver microsomes. Further investigation on the isolation and characterization of the mutagenic compounds formed during opium pyrolysis, smoke condensates from pyrolysis of the major alkaloid constituents of opium, was undertaken at the International Agency for Research on Cancer. Their tests on the microsome-mediated bacterial mutagenicity of opium dross samples [24] have indicated the presence of potent mutagens. Crude opium itself is not mutagenic, but its pyrolysates, or those of certain opium alkaloids such as morphine, are highly mutagenic, being many times more active than tobacco-smoke condensate. At least two compounds (cycloartenol and 10-oxomorphine) have been identified in opium. As opium intake appears to be rather common in Iran, it seems unlikely to be responsible for the marked regional gradient in esophageal cancer distribution [2].

3 Local Lesions of the Esophagus

3.1 Stricture

The esophagus may be damaged by various ingested materials, possibly leading to the development of cancer. For example, esophageal carcinoma has been linked with stricture, especially caustic stricture, and an average latency time between lye corrosion and cancer in 63 cases was 41 years [25, 26]. Experimentally, Dunham and Sheets [27] studied the effects of esophageal constriction on benzo[*a*]pyrene carcinogenesis in hamster esophagus by implantation of a polyethylene cuff around the esophagus. The result showed that more severe and earlier development of papillomatous and carcinomatous lesions occurred at the level proximal to the constricture.

3.2 Hot Tea and Food

The possible role of hot tea in the etiology of esophageal cancer has attracted much speculation. The majority of people in the Guryev region and Aktubinsk province of Kazakhstan consume large amounts of hot tea daily [28]. However, in a case-control study of 301 Kazakhs with esophageal cancer the difference was too small to establish hot tea as the main factor responsible for the local high incidence [29]. The drinking of hot tea is also habitual among inhabitants of northeastern Iran, Puerto Rico, Chaoshan region in Guangdong province, and other high-incidence areas.

In Linxian county, where cancer of the esophagus is prevalent, it was first thought that dietary habits such as consumption of hard and coarse food in the form of hot and hastily taken meals might be related to the development of esophageal cancer. However, comparative surveys undertaken in high- and low-incidence areas and preliminary laboratory investigations revealed that although poor food and bad eating habits might well damage the mucosal epithelium of the esophagus and facilitate carcinogenesis, they could not be the principal carcinogenic factors. For instance, corn meal or millet gruel, which usually has a temperature of 51 °C, is sometimes as hot as 69 °C, but 65 °C is comfortable and food at a temperature of 75 °C only causes minor scalds [3].

In Japan, Nara, Wakayama, and Mie prefectures form a high-risk area for esophageal cancer. The local people are known by their custom of taking *chagayu,* very hot tea-cooked rice gruel. Segi [30] suggested that chronic thermal irritation, high levels of tannin in the heated state, and the use of iron pots in preparation of *chagayu* may play a role in carcinogenesis. Hirayama [12] conducted a case-control study in these three prefectures, showing that men and women who consume *chagayu* and bracken daily have an increased risk of developing esophageal carcinoma, especially when also suffering from nutritional deficiencies. Bracken is widely eaten in Japan, and Hirayama showed that the greater the intake of bracken, the higher the risk. He considered *chagayu,* bracken, and cigarettes as initiators or promoters and daily meat and fruit as protective factors, and asserted that this could explain 80% of the cases of esophageal cancer in this area of relatively high incidence.

3.3 Bracken and Tannin

Bracken is associated with chronic enzootic hematuria and bladder cancer in cattle [31]. Its induction of intestinal, bladder, and other tumors in experimental animals suggests that it contains chemical carcinogens [32]. The carcinogenic activity of bracken has been attributed to its content of favanoid compounds such as quercetin and kaempferol [33] and to tannin [34]. However, Morino et al. [35] failed to confirm the carcinogenicity of quercetin or rutin in animal experiments. Tannins are a class of heterogeneous polymeric substances differing chemically from plant to plant [36]; their chemical nature and their carcinogenicity via the oral route remain to be determined.

Tumors have been induced in rats and mice by repeated subcutaneous injection of various tannin extracts. Condensed tannins evoked sarcomas at the site of injection and induced liver tumors [36]. Tannins of plants commonly used in teas and remedies by the natives of the Caribbean island of Curacao, where esophageal cancer is frequent, have recently been suggested as the causative agents of the cancer in this population [37]. Extracts of tannins of these plants, e.g., *Krameria ixina, Acacia villosa, Melochia tomentosa,* and *Heliotropium angiospermum,* induced sarcomas in rats after repeated subcutaneous administration. After removal of tannins by precipitation with caffeine, the aqueous extract did not induce sarcoma [37–39].

Dunham et al. [40] tested in hamster cheek pouch the carcinogenicity of plant extracts, with the addition of calcium hydroxide (lime) and arecoline from betel, both from Curacao. They found that cancer developed in pouch epithelium following topical application of the plant extracts and that esophageal papillomas were also induced, whereas no neoplasia was seen after ingestion of a concentrated tea *(Acacia villosa)* or when *Annona muricate* and arecoline were administered in the diet. They assumed that there are weak carcinogens present in the plant extracts.

3.4 Plant Irritants

Plant irritants in foods, such as phytoliths, thorns, and spicules, have been considered as a possible causative factor in esophageal cancer in the Transkei, where 89% of high-incidence areas are found on Beaufort sediment soil containing much silica and quartz [41]. Most plants can absorb silica from the soil, depositing it as opal in the epidermis of the leaves and using it to reinforce stems and thorns. These siliceous bodies have definite shapes and are called phytoliths, with a diameter of 15–20 μm. It is assumed that these sharp objects in a bolus of food could scarify a narrow gullet. Furthermore, maize is ground on a stone, and the ground mixture contains innumerable particles of quartz. Maize is also prepared by stamping, and the air is filled with the chaff. Both these circumstances have been incriminated in the silicosis found in young women in the Transkei. Rose [41] suggested that these irritants exerted chronic "esophageal insults", a possible contributory factor in Transkeian patients.

Recently, O'Neill et al. [42] found contamination by a fine fibrous silica in wheat flour in the high esophageal cancer area of northeast Iran. The fibers have a smoothly tapering shape and are between 50 and 150 μm long with a diameter of between 1 and 10 μm. They consist almost entirely of silica and originate mostly from the seeds of a common Mediterranean grass, *Phalaris minor,* and other related species. They are broken off from the seed when the wheat is milled but persist in the flour, where up to 3000 are found in each gram.

It was suggested that these plant mineral fibers are possible etiologic factors in esophageal cancer in Iran and other high-incidence areas.

In the past, a form of sweet cake prepared from a mixture of millet bran and persimmon peel flour was served as a delicacy during the autumn in Linxian county. O'Neill et al. [43] examined the millet bran, which consists of bracts and the outer coating of the grain, and found it to contain up to 20% of silica by weight. The silica occurs as friable sheets or sharply pointed fibers with an average diameter of 10 μm (range 1–70 μm). The same investigators found large amounts of these fragments (100 ppm by weight) in the esophageal mucosa surrounding tumors in Linxian patients, not only on the surface but also in the body of the mucosa. It was suggested that such fragments may be able to stimulate the epithelial proliferation by trauma and may be involved in the development of esophageal cancer.

3.5 Fungal Infection

Fungal infection and invasion in esophageal tissue have been considered as another type of local irritation which may contribute to the focal inflammation, epithelial hyperplasia, dysplasia, and neoplastic changes of the esophagus. Xia and Zhan [44] examined 155 biopsy samples of human esophagus, including 30 cases of early carcinoma and adenocarcinoma of the cardia, from Linxian and other areas and found various degrees of fungal infection in hyperplastic epithelium (30%), early carcinoma tissue (15%), and hyperplastic epithelium near the early carcinoma lesion (50%); however, the rate of infection in normal esophageal mucosa was rather low. Fungal infection, especially with *Candida albicans,* may be associated with the hyperplastic growth of esophageal epithelium. Xia and Zhan postulated a relationship of fungal infection and invasion in esophageal tissue to cancer development of the gullet (see also Chap. 3, Sect. 4).

4 Nitrosamines and Their Precursors

4.1 Nitrosamines Formed In Food

Of all the groups of known chemical carcinogens, the *N*-nitroso compounds possess characteristics which make them the most likely agents in the induction of human cancer. Although the levels of preformed *N*-nitroso compounds in food are usually less than 10 ppb, their precursors, i. e., nitrates, nitrites, and secondary or tertiary amines, are widely distributed in foodstuffs and in the environment. Under acidic conditions, *N*-nitroso compounds can easily be formed in the stomach by the reaction of nitrites and amines, becoming the principal source of these carcinogens [45, 46]. More than 100 of the 130 different *N*-nitroso compounds tested in rats have been shown to be carcinogenic [47], and it is probably that no animal species is refractory to these compounds. Some nitrosamines such as methylbenzylnitrosamine (MBNA), nitrososarcosine ethyl ester, and methyl amylnitrosamine have been used as model substances for the induction of esophageal cancer. In small rodents, they induce tumors of the esophagus and forestomach selectively and frequently.

The in vitro metabolism of dimethylnitrosamine (DMNA) is similar in human and rat liver [48]. Furthermore, the rate of metabolism and the levels of nucleic acid methylation are comparable in the two species [49]. Using an explant culture system developed for rat and human esophagus, Harris et al. reported that cultured human esophagus activates DMNA, but not nitrosopyrrolidine (NPY), into DNA-binding metabolites [50]. In further studies, Autrup and Stoner [51] noted that the highest level of metabolite binding was seen with MBNA, an organotropic carcinogen for rat esophagus. The binding level was about 100 times higher than in human esophagus. This compound methylated rat esophageal DNA at positions 7 and 0^6 of guanine. *N*-Nitrosoethylmethylamine showed the highest binding level to DNA with the methyl group. However, no binding was detected to human esophagus. NPY was oxidized by both rat and human esophagus, but binding of its metabolites to DNA was detected only in rat esophagus. DMNA was metabolized by both human and rat esophagus, and methylation of the guanine positions 7 and 0^6 was detected by chromatography of hydrolyzed rat DNA. The results indicated significant quantitative and qualitative differences between cultured rat and human esophagus in their ability to activate nitrosamines, and suggested that some unknown physiologic differences after culture may contribute to this.

In Linxian county some foodstuffs are frequently tainted by fungi due to dietary habits and improper storage and preservation. We demonstrated the formation of DMNA, diethylnitrosamine (DENA), MBNA, and a new *N*-nitroso compound, *N*-1-methylacetonyl-*N*-3-methylbutylnitrosamine (MAMBNA) in cornbread following inoculation of *Fusarium monoliforme* (a common species of fungi found in Linxian) or with other fungi, with an addition of a small amount of $NaNO_2$ after an 8-day incubation. MAMBNA was obtained more often from cornbread inoculated with *F. moniliforme,* with levels in moldy cornbread estimated at 0.2–0.3 ppm. The 3-methylbutylamine radical of MAMBNA is derived from leucine, which is abundant in maize meal. This new nitrosamine was synthesized and confirmed by gas chromatography and mass spectrometry (GC-MS), with a molecular weight of 186.1 [45, 52, 53].

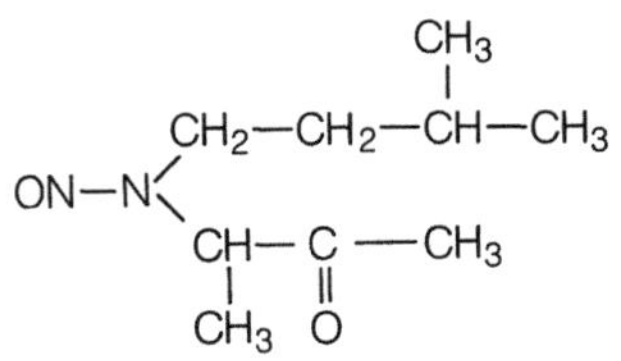

The carcinogenicity of MAMBNA was shown by the induction of forestomach papillomas and carcinomas and liver tumors in mice and rats following the gastric intubation of this compound [54, 55]. Among 42 mice treated with MAMBNA (20 mg/week), 22 showed epithelial hyperplasia of the esophagus, 29 papillomas and four squamous carcinomas developed in the forestomach, and there were six adenomas and three carcinomas in the liver (Table 2.2). Most tumors developed in mice receiving the treatment for 136–317 days (Fig. 2.1). Another group of 26 mice received the secondary amine of MAMBNA together with $NaNO_2$. These precursors synthesized MAMBNA in vivo and induced esophageal hyperplasia, forestomach papillomas (17 cases) and carcinoma (one case), liver cell hyperplasia, and other tumors (Table 2.3).

In an experiment with 29 rats, administration of MAMBNA by gastric intubation resulted in the development of 11 epithelial hyperplasias in the lower portion of the esophagus, and 14 atypical hyperplasias and papillomas and 11 squamous carcinomas in the forestomach. All carcinomas developed in rats receiving MAMBNA treatment for

Table 2.2. MAMBNA-induced forestomach and liver carcinomas in mice

Duration in days (total dosage in mg)	No. of mice	Esophageal hyperplasia	Forestomach		Liver		
			Papilloma	Carcinoma	Hyperplasia	Adenoma	Carcinoma
28–83 (45–125)	7	1	1	–	–	–	–
136–192 (210–370)	25	21	20	2	8	2	–
227–317 (490–670)	10	–	8	2	3	4	3
Total	42	22	29	4	11	6	3

Table 2.3. Induction of forestomach and liver lesions in mice by in vivo formation of MAMBNA from its precursors

Duration in days (MAMBamine/$NaNO_2$ in mg)	No. of mice	Esophageal hyperplasia	Forestomach		Liver cell hyperplasia
			Papilloma	Carcinoma	
117–297 (470–1230/47–115)	14	11	9	–	–
450–591 (3050–4060/197–298)	7	1	4	–	2
658–742 (4230–5120/315–404)	5	2	4[a]	1	4
Total	26	14	17	1	6

[a] Three cases showed atypical hyperplasia

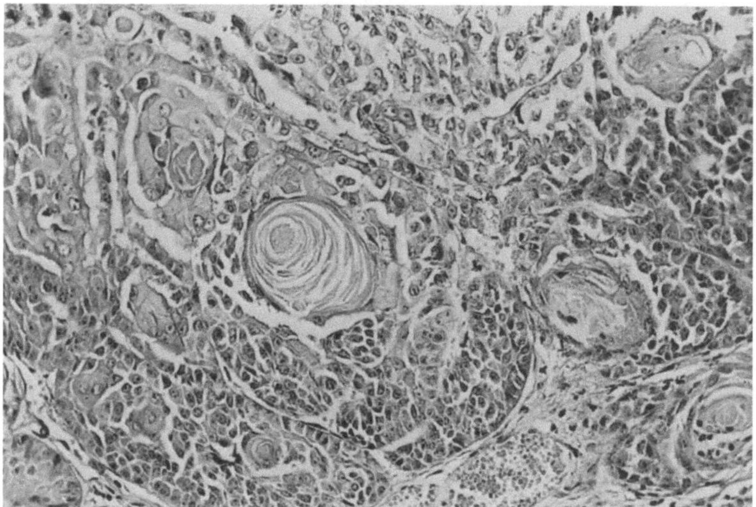

Fig. 2.1. Carcinoma of the forestomach in a mouse treated by gastric intubation of 10 mg MAMBNA twice weekly for 153 days. × 200

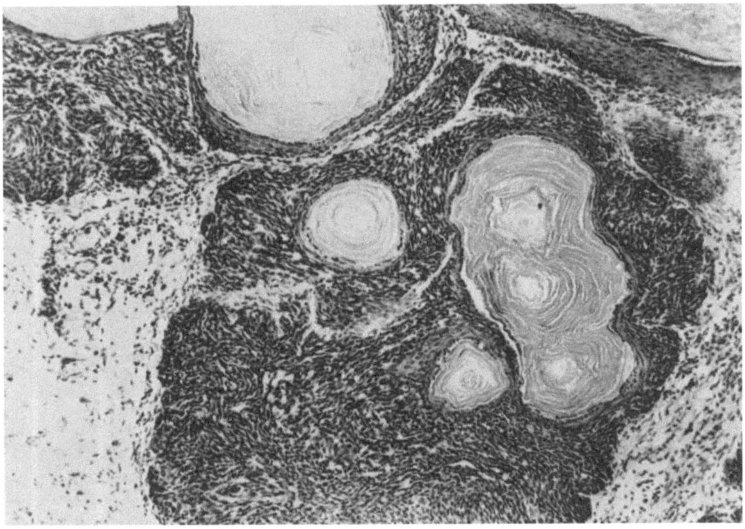

Fig. 2.2. Carcinoma of the forestomach in a rat which received a total dosage of 5940 mg MAMBNA in 581 days. × 100

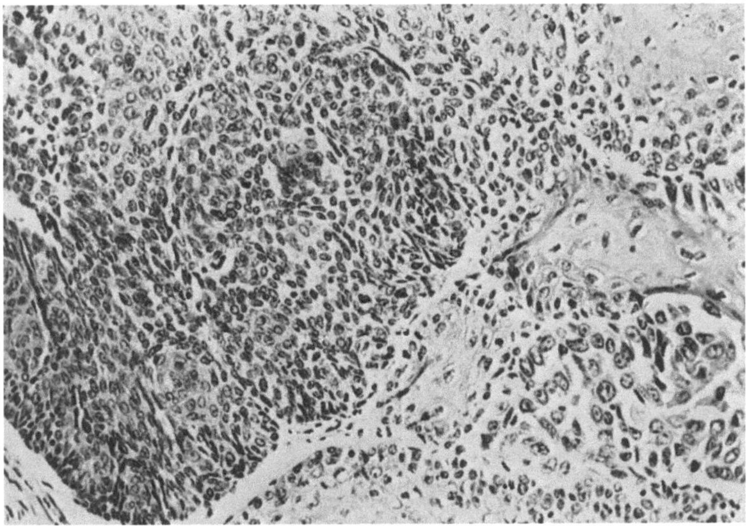

Fig. 2.3. Carcinoma of the forestomach in a rat which received a total dosage of 6600 mg MAMBNA in 640 days. × 200

454–640 days with a total dosage of 4480–6600 mg (Figs. 2.2, 2.3). Hyperplasia of liver cells was noted in three rats, liver adenoma in seven, and liver carcinoma in eight (Table 2.4) [54].

In vitro experiments showed that MAMBNA exerted a mutagenic effect on *Salmonella typhimurium* (TA_{98} and TA_{100}) after activation by S-9 mix according to the Ames system

Table 2.4. MAMBNA-induced forestomach and liver carcinomas in rats

Duration in days (total dosage in mg)	No. of rats	Esophageal hyperplasia	Forestomach			Liver	
			Atypical hyperplasia	Papil-loma	Carci-noma	Adenoma	Carcinoma
46–178 (150–760)	6	4	1	3	–	–	–
292–365 (1560–1940)	4	2	–	3	–	2	–
404–484 (3700–4780)	6	3	3	2	1	2	1
518–584 (5400–5940)	7	1	–	2	5	1	4
606–640 (5992–6600)	6	1	–	–	5	2	3
Total	29	11	4	10	11	7	8

[56], induced forward gene mutation in V_{79} cells [57], and transformed foci in the culture of Syrian hamster lung cells [58].

We recently found that Linxian cornmeal naturally contains trace amounts of DMNA and DENA, and that the content increases after the addition of $NaNO_2$ [59]. It has been reported from eastern Africa and South Africa that the incidence of esophageal cancer is high in areas where corn is a common food, and the consumption of alcoholic drinks made from corn was thought to be a possible etiologic factor [16]. Our results might provide evidence for such a relationship.

Another new nitrosamine, namely *N*-1-methylacetonyl-*N*-2-methylpropylnitrosamine (MAMPNA), was recently isolated in *F. moniliforme*-inoculated millet and wheat flour after addition of $NaNO_2$. MAMPNA was synthesized and identified with GC-MS, and its secondary amine can be derived from the valine. The molecular weight of MAMPNA is 172 (Fig. 2.4) [61].

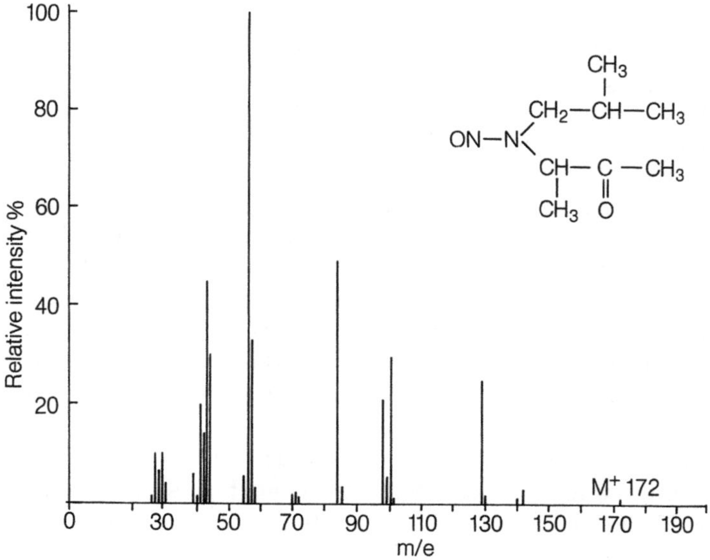

Fig. 2.4. Mass spectroscopy of MAMPNA formed in millet inoculated with *Fusarium moniliforme* with addition of $NaNO_2$

Table 2.5. Formation of nitrosamines in *Fusarium moniliforme*-inoculated foodstuffs (preliminary results)[a]

Foodstuff	DMNA	DENA	MBNA	MAMBNA	MAMPNA	NPEE
Cornmeal	+	+	+	+	−	−
Millet	−	−	−	+	+	+
Wheat flour	−	−	−	+	+	−

[a] After 8 days incubation, 1 mg $NaNO_2$ was added to 1 g foodstuff. Nitrosamines were determined with GC-MS; + designates positive response of nitrosamine. NPEE, *N*-nitrosoproline ethyl ester

Table 2.6. Nitrate and nitrite levels in drinking water from four counties in Anyang prefecture[a]

	Linxian	Anyangxian	Huaxian	Fanxian
Esophageal cancer age-adjusted death rate	199.7	133.2	35.0	18.2
Population (1971)	188588	119194	128718	129828
Nitrates (mg/l)	16.4	18.1	14.4	3.2
Nitrites (mg/l)	0.053	0.016	0.055	0.017
No. of water samples assayed	59	57	54	52

[a] The four counties are given in west-to-east order [62]

The carcinogenicity of MAMPNA remains to be studied. Our work indicated that more *N*-nitroso compounds are present in moldy foodstuffs. The discovery of chemical carcinogens other than mycotoxins formed in such foodstuffs opens a new research field in cancer etiology (Table 2.5).

4.2 *Nitrates and Nitrites*

In Anyang prefecture, Henan province, the mortality rate of esophageal cancer diminishes progressively from west to east [3]. In order to study the causal relationship between the endogenous formation of carcinogenic nitrosamines from their precursors and esophageal cancer, nitrate and nitrite levels in drinking water were determined. A preliminary analysis of 222 samples of drinking water taken from Anyang prefecture revealed that the nitrate content and its detection rate also decreased markedly from west to east (Table 2.6). In contrast, the concentrations of chemical elements such as Br, Cl, Cu, I, Fe^{3+}, K, Hg, Mg, Mn, Mo and Na and of the NH_4^+, HPO_4^{2-}, HCO_3^-, and SO_4^{2-} ions in samples of water and food were lower in the west and gradually increased toward the east [62]. A more elaborate investigation of the concentration of nitrates and nitrites has been carried out on water from 495 wells in 49 production brigades of Yaocun commune, Linxian county, a high-risk area for esophageal cancer in the western part of Anyang prefecture. Nitrates and nitrites were in evidence in most wells, nitrates ranging from 0 to 75 mg/liter (average 10.55 mg/liter) and nitrites from 0 to 2.63 mg/liter (average 0.039 mg/liter) over the whole year concentrations being highest in the summer (averages of 12.65 and 0.052 mg/liter respectively). A positive correlation was found between the average incidence of esophageal cancer in the 49 brigades (1969–1976) and the level of nitrates in the well water in the summer ($r=0.233$; $P<0.05$). A positive correlation was also noted between nitrate level and incidence of marked epithelial dysplasia. Nitrite concentrations in warm water in pots (0.512 mg/liter) and liquid gruel (0.696 mg/liter) were 10–20 times higher than those in water stored in jars [63].

Nitrates and nitrites were recovered from the gastric juice of most Linxian peasants, with average levels of 31.67 and 1.37 mg/liter respectively. A comparative study of nitrites in saliva among peasants in Linxian and Xinyangxian, a low-risk area for esophageal cancer, revealed averages of 4.5 mg/liter (216 samples) and 5.74 mg/liter (51 samples) respectively. A significant difference in content of salivary nitrites was observed in Linxian, however, between patients with marked epithelial hyperplasia (6.00 mg/liter) or carcinoma (5.06 mg/liter) of the esophagus and normal controls (3.17 mg/liter) [45, 46]. Lowenfels et al. [64] studied salivary nitrite levels in French patients (20 males) with esophageal cancer and volunteer adult controls (six males and nine females) before and after administrating 100 ml beet juice containing 160 mg sodium nitrate. Initial salivary nitrite levels were slightly lower in the cancer patients, but in both groups there was a marked increase 90 min after ingestion of the beet juice, and the levels attained were similar. These results implied that the formation of salivary nitrite was highly dependent on exogenous dietary nitrate and that there was no difference in the capacity to form nitrites between esophageal cancer patients and healthy adult subjects.

The level of urinary ascorbic acid among natives of Linxian (av. 10.71 mg/liter) was only one-eighth or one-ninth of that among Xinyanxian inhabitants, and the amount of nitrite excreted in the urine was markedly diminished following the administration of vitamin C, indicating that a low intake of vitamin C in Linxian might have provided favorable conditions for the formation of nitrosamine from nitrites [65].

A series of experiments demonstrated that nitrosamines can be synthesized under endogenous conditions from their precursors. Nitrosamines formed rapidly in the stomachs of rats and pigs fed suitable amounts of secondary amines extracted from Linxian foodstuffs together with $NaNO_2$ [3]. The synthesis of nitrosamines from secondary amines and $NaNO_2$ could be prevented by simultaneous administration of ascorbic acid [65]. A similar inhibitory effect on nitrosamine formation was demonstrated with tannins, gallic acid, and some other antioxidants, resulting from a competitive interaction for nitrite [66–68].

5 Moldy Foods and Mycotoxins

5.1 Carcinogenicity of Moldy Foods

Cornbread and millet are the staple foods in Linxian, though the consumption of wheat has increased in recent years. The dietary habits and improper preservation of food frequently cause contamination of foodstuffs by fungi in the same area. The commonly occurring fungi are *Fusarium moniliforme* Sheldon, *Geotrichum candidum* Link, *Penicillium cyclopium* Westling, *Aspergillus flavus* Link, and *P. chrysogenum* Thom [22]. In *F. moniliforme*-inoculated cornbread, we have demonstrated the formation of carcinogenic nitrosamines, e.g., DMNA, DENA, MBNA, and MAMBNA, following 8-day incubation with the addition of a small amount of $NaNO_2$. DENA, MAMBNA, and MAMPNA are found in moldy millet and wheat flour subsequent to similar treatment.

Further studies showed that some common species of fungus belonging to *Fusarium, Geotrichum, Aspergillus,* and other genera could not only reduce nitrates to nitrites, as observed with certain bacteria, but also decompose proteins and increase the amount of amines in foods, promoting the formation of introsamines. After inoculation of cornbread with fungi common in Linxian county, the content of secondary amines increased after a 4-day incubation, and a 17-fold increase in secondary amines was noted in *F. moniliforme*-inoculated cornbread. In *G. candidum*-inoculated Sabouraud's culture, the addition of $NaNO_3$ and diethylamine or methylphenylamine after a few days incubation resulted in the formation of nitrosamine [20, 69].

The carcinogenicity of moldy cornbread was substantiated further in another experiment. In one group, female Wistar rats were fed *F. moniliforme*-inoculated cornbread and water ad libitum. The cornbread was disinfected before inoculation of the fungus and to each 400-g sample was added 400 mg $NaNO_2$ after 8 days of incubation. The presence of MAMBNA in cornbread was determined regularly by thin-layer chromatography during the course of the experiment. Eleven papillomas, four early carcinomas, and one squamous cell carcinoma developed in the forestomachs of 35 rats fed the moldy cornbread for 238–883 days. Most carcinoma lesions were observed after 775 days of treatment. In addition, there were papillary hyperplastic growth and other lesions in the forestomach of treated rats. In some experimental animals, simple epithelial hyperplasia was observed in the lower portion of the esophagus and in the glandular stomach. One adenoma and three fibroadenomas of the mammary glands were noted in four females. A second group of female rats was fed the fungus-inoculated cornbread alone. Four papillomas and two early carcinomas developed in the forestomach of 31 rats after 554–701 days. Epithelial hyperplasia of the esophagus, forestomach, and glandular stomach was observed in some animals of this group, and two fibroadenomas and two adenomas of the mammary glands were also noted. It is known that certain mycotoxins, such as zearalenone, produced by *Fusarium* fungi, can exert an estrogenic activity in target organs. Another group of ten females, serving as controls, were fed with conventional cornbread; no epithelial lesions were noted in their forestomachs (Table 2.7) [70, 71]. The experimental results indicated the presence of carcinogenic mycotoxins in the *F. moniliforme*-contaminated cornbread, and the MAMBNA was formed following the addition of $NaNO_2$, which produced more papillomas and carcinomas in the forestomach. Thus at least two kinds of chemical carcinogens, nitrosamines and mycotoxins, are formed in the fungal metabolites.

Extracts of cornbread inoculated with fungi isolated from Linxian – *Fusarium moniliforme* alone or a combination of *F. moniliforme, Aspergillus flavus, Geotrichum candidum,* and *Penicillium cyclopium* (FAGP) – significantly increased the frequency of sister chromatid exchange in V_{79} cells and in bone marrow cells in Chinese hamsters. The FAGP ex-

Table 2.7. Forestomach carcinomas in rats fed with *Fusarium moniliforme*-contaminated cornbread[a]

Food	No. of rats	No. of rats developing lesions[b]		
		Forestomach papilloma	Forestomach carcinoma	Mammary tumors
F. moniliforme-inoculated cornbread	31	4 (554–679)	2 (621–701)	4 (454–774)
F. moniliforme-inoculated cornbread plus $NaNO_2$	35	11 (238–768)	5 (664–885)	4 (360–838)
Uninoculated cornbread[c]	10	–	–	–

[a] Epithelial hyperplasia was observed in the lower portion of the esophagus and in the glandular stomach of some rats

[b] Figures in parentheses show number of days after initiation of feeding when lesions were detected

[c] Duration of experiment 330–700 days

tract also induced 6-thioguanine-resistant (6-TG^r) mutants in V_{79} cells in the presence of microsomal preparations. Both extracts increased the recovery of 6-TG^r V_{79} cells when wild-type V_{79} cells (6-TG sensitive) and 6-TG^r V_{79} cells were cultured together. The results indicate the possible presence of mutagen(s) and promoter(s) in the moldy foods [72].

A preliminary study of the potential causative factors of esophageal and forestomach tumors contained in the moldy food was carried out by Zhang and He [73], who reported for the first time the induction of forestomach papilloma in rats fed with *Fusarium*-inoculated food. Researchers at Hebei Medical College (1972–1974) noted the development of hyperplasia and papillomatous lesions in the esophagus and forestomach of mice after prolonged feeding with fungi-contaminated dried sweet potato, dried radish, and pickled vegetable juice. Later, Wang and Zhang [19] reported two papillomas in the esophagus and three papillomas in the forestomach of 13 rats fed with F. *moniliforme*-inoculated cornbread for 168–467 days, though no carcinomas were formed. The research group in Henan Medical College found that two papillomas and three carcinomas developed in the esophagus of 16 rats fed or 445–649 days with cornbread naturally contaminated by fungi in Linxian [74]. Recently, Liu et al. [75] reported that the lifelong feeding of rats with cornbread containing an alcohol extract of *F. moniliforme*-contaminated cornmeal induced only epithelial hyperplasia of the forestomach. However, in a group of 23 rats fed with $NaNO_2$- and alcohol-extract-added cornbread, three papillomas and one early carcinoma were induced in the forestomach, indicating that the presence of nitrosamines in fungal metabolites may play a principal role in carcinogenesis. In addition, Liu et al. [75] observed the development of papilloma and atypical hyperplasia of the forestomach in rats subsequent to experimental feeding with *Stemphylium ilicis*-contaminated cornbread. This fungus was isolated from the grains in Huixian county, another high-incidence area for esophageal cancer neighboring Linxian in Henan province. All these experimental results are further evidence that prolonged feeding with foods inoculated with certain species of fungi from high-risk areas can induce cancer of the upper digestive tract in rats and mice.

A comparative survey of cereal fungi in five high- and three low-incidence counties in Henan province was undertaken recently by Zhen et al. [76], who examined 1121 samples taken from wheat, maize, dried sweet potato, rice, and beans and isolated 1970 strains of fungi, including *Aspergillus* (472), *Penicillium* (358), *Fusarium* (467), *Alternaria* (447), and *Stemphylium* (93), with 133 strains from other genera. No significant difference was noted between the high- and low-incidence counties. The most common species in high-incidence counties was *Penicillium cyclopium*. The following fungi have high cereal contamination rates in high-incidence areas: *P. cyclopium* (0.39%), *Asp. flavus* (1.32%), *Asp. nidulans* (0.23%), *Asp. fumigatus* (0.18%), *F. moniliforme* (6.80%), *Alt. alternata* (6.53%), *Rhizopus* and *Mucor* spp. (23.7%). The rates were significantly higher than those in the low-incidence counties. It was postulated that the metabolites of *P. cyclopium, Alt. alternata,* and *F. moniliforme* may be related to the development of esophageal cancer.

Another similar investigation on the distribution of cereal fungi was carried out in esophageal cancer high-incidence areas in Sichuan province, western China, by researchers at Sichuan Sanitary Cadre Postgraduate College (1980) [77]. They isolated and identified 1099 samples, and the strains with highest contamination levels were as follows: Asp. flavus (284), *Asp. niger* (221), *Rhizopus* spp. (184), and *F. moniliforme* (107) for maize; *Asp. niger* (93), *Asp. flavus* (90), *Rhizopus* spp. (63), and *Alt. alternata* (28) for dry sweet potato; *Asp. flavus* (244), *Rhizopus* spp. (225), *Asp. niger* (167), and *Alt. alternata* (122) for wheat; *P. cyclopium* (116), *Asp. versicolor* (109) and *Geotrichum candidum* (59) for pickled vegetables; and *Asp. versicolor* (171), *P. chrysogenum* (69), and *Cladosporium herbarum* (54) for sour pickles.

5.2 *Carcinogenicity of Myocotoxins*

According to Marasas et al. [17], the highest known esophageal cancer rate in Africa occurs in the southwestern districts of the Transkei, while the incidence in the northeastern region is relatively low. Corn is the main dietary staple in both areas. *Fusarium graminearum, F. moniliforme* and *F. moniliforme* var. *subglutinans* were isolated from corn kernels in both areas, and two *Fusarium* mycotoxins, deoxynivalenol and zearalenone, were detected at biologically significant levels in kernels. Preleminary work showed that the level of natural infection of corn kernels with both mycotoxins was considerably higher in the high-incidence area than in the low-incidence area. However, there is no evidence that deoxynivalenol and zearalenone are carcinogenic.

It is known that some mycotoxins, such as aflatoxins, sterigmatocystin, penicillic acid, luteoskyrin, cyclothlorotin, and patulin, are carcinogenic in experimental animals [78, 79]. With regard to *Fusarium* fungi, a group of metabolites known as trichothecenes, e.g., T-2 toxin, diacetoxyscirpenol, neosoleniol, nivalenol, and fusarenone, are produced. Schoental and Joffe [18] reported that crude alcoholic extracts from culture of *F. poae* and *F. sporotrichioides,* which were responsible for the alimentary toxic aleukia during World War II in certain parts of the USSR, were tested by various routes in rodents. The small doses of crude extracts induced only epithelial hyperplasia of the esophagus in rats. Gastric intubation of T-2 toxin in rats resulted in cardiovascular lesions of various degrees of severity and/or tumors, benign and malignant, of the forestomach, glandular stomach, duodenum, pancreas, and brain [80]. T-2 toxin appears to be a versatile carcinogen for the rat, showing no organ specificity. The role of T-2 toxin and other metabolites of *Fusarium* species in the etiology of certain idiopathic chronic disorders and cancer in man and animals deserves further study.

5.3 *Pickled Vegetables*

Pickled vegetables are eaten daily in several esophageal cancer high-incidence areas, e.g., Linxian county in Henan province, Yangcheng county in Shanxi province, Yanting county in Sichuan province, and Yangzhong county in Jiangsu province, and mortality appears to be correlated with the time span of consumption and the amount consumed [22]. *Geotrichum candidum* is the predominant species of fungi occurring in Linxian pickles. We observed the development of glandular stomach adenocarcinoma and other tumors in rats subsequent to prolonged feeding of the extract or concentrated fluid, evidence for the presence of potential carcinogens in pickled vegetables from Linxian county [81]. Recently, mice fed by gastric intubation with concentrated pickle fluid, equivalent to about 50 ml of original fluid weekly for each animal, developed papillomas in the forestomach after 143 days of treatment [20]. A series of short-term tests showed that extracts of Linxian pickles gave positive mutagenic effects as shown by the sister chromatid exchange test, V_{79} cell mutation, the Ames test, and induced transformed foci in culture of Syrian hamster embryo cells. Moreover, the pickles also exerted a promoting effect in carcinogenic action, as revealed in C3H/10T½ cell culture (Table 2.8) [82, 83].

Table 2.8. Mutagenic, transforming, and promoting effects of pickled vegetables from Linxian county

Pickled vegetables	Ames test (+S-9)		Sister chromatid exchanges		Forward gene mutation (+S-9) V_{79}	Transformed foci in Syrian hamster embryo cells	Transformed foci in C3H/10T½ cells initiated with 3-MC
	TA_{100}	TA_{98}	V_{79}	Chinese hamster embryo cells			
Dichloromethane extract	−	±	+	+	+	+	+
Ether extract	+	+	+	+	+	Not done	Not done

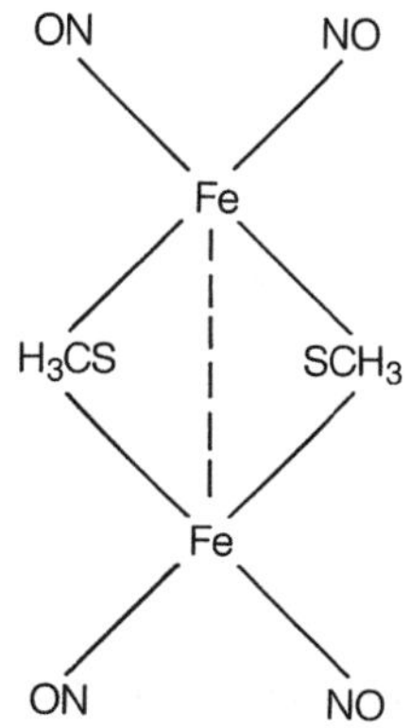

Fig. 2.5. Chemical structure of Roussin red methyl ester: molecular weight 326

The dichloromethane or ether extract of pickled vegetables from Linxian was found to contain a nitroso compound, Roussin red methyl ester (di-μ-methanethiolatotetranitroso-diiron), which was first synthesized by Roussin in 1858, although it has not so far been reported to exist in natural products (Fig. 2.5) [84, 85]. Among 69 samples of Linxian pickles the positive rate for Roussin red was 55%, and its concentration was estimated at 1–5 ppm. Roussin red showed neither a mutagenic nor a transforming effect in Syrian hamster embryo cells. However, it induced foci type 3 in C3H/10T½ cells initiated with 3-methyl-cholanthrene (3-MC) and has shown a positive action in short-term skin tests in mice, leading to a significant decrease in the number of sebaceous glands and a significant increase of epidermal thickness, as induced by 12-O-tetradecanoyl-phorbol-13-acetate (TPA) [86]. Roussin red is therefore one of the possible natural promoters present in pickled vegetables.

Roussin red may provide (NO_2) ions, which would react readily with secondary amines to form nitrosamines. In experiments with mice, the gastric intubation of this compound alone or with sarcosin ethyl ester induced epithelial hyperplasia of the upper digestive tract and papilloma of the forestomach after administration for more than 200 days [20].

In addition, our preliminary studies showed that cyclohexane extract from Linxian pickled vegetables contained benzo[*a*]-pyrene (B*a*P) and other PAHs [97]. The concentration of B*a*P is much higher in pickles (0.55–7.6 μg/kg) than in the fresh vegetables (0–1.3 μg/kg; $P<0.001$) (Figs. 2.6, 2.7). It is known that some microorganisms (e.g., *Escherichia coli, Clostridium putride*), *Chlorella vulgaris*, vegetables, and other plants can synthesize B*a*P and other PAHs endogenously [88–90].

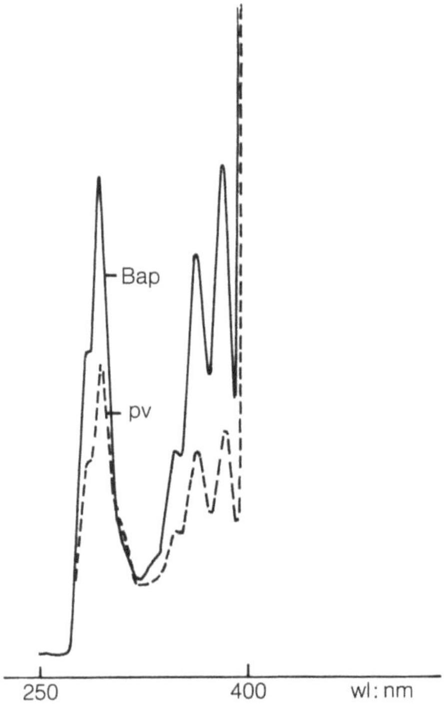

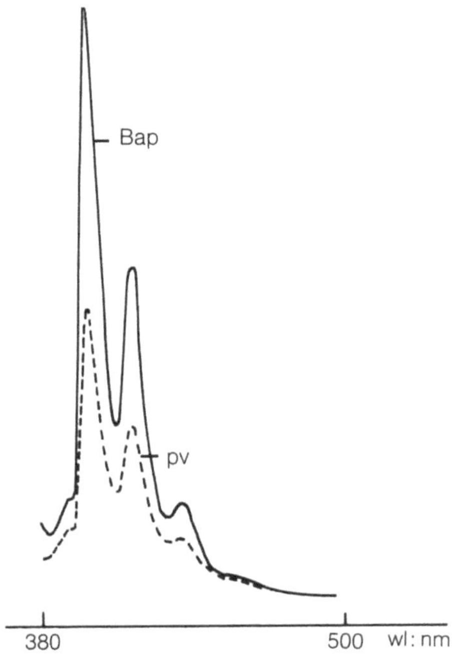

Fig. 2.6 (left). Spectrofluorometric determination of B*a*P in pickled vegetable extract *(pv)*: excitation spectrum. *wl*, wavelength

Fig. 2.7 (right). Spectrofluorometric determination of B*a*P in pickled vegetable extract *(pv)*: emission spectrum. *wl*, wavelength

6 Dietary Factors and Trace Elements

Poor diet, a common feature of most esophageal cancer high-incidence areas, might play a role in the development of the disease. In the past, cornbread and millet were the staple foods in Linxian, though the consumption of wheat has increased in recent years. There is a low intake of vitamins A and C, riboflavin, animal protein, fat, fresh vegetables, and fruit. Preliminary surveys show that the caloric intake of Linxian peasants is generally sufficient, but protein intake from vegetable sources is mostly inadequate. Riboflavin deficiency, with symptoms of cheilosis, glossitis, and a burning sensation of the tongue, was frequently encountered. Zheng et al. [91] studied the urinary excretion of a test dose (5 mg) of riboflavin in peasants of Linxian county during the four seasons of the year (Table 2.9). It was revealed that the majority of the test subjects excreted under 1000 μg riboflavin in 4-h urine, indicating the dietary intake of riboflavin is below the adequate level; 38.8% excreted less than 400 μg. During winter the riboflavin inadequacy was severe; only 4.5% of subjects excreted over 1000 μg, and 52.3% below 400 μg. In an experiment with rats, riboflavin deficiency significantly increased the incidence of esophageal tumors induced by methylbenzylnitrosamine and shortened the latent period for tumor development [92].

Table 2.9. Urinary excretion of a test dose of 5 mg riboflavin in peasants of Linxian county[a]

Season	Total no. of samples	Deficient (<400 μg)		Inadequate (400–1000 μg)		Adequate (>1000 μg)	
		(*n*)	(%)	(*n*)	(%)	(*n*)	(%)
Spring	43	13	30.2	20	46.5	10	23.3
Summer	42	17	40.5	14	33.3	11	26.2
Autumn	41	13	31.7	23	56.1	5	12.2
Winter	44	23	52.3	19	43.2	2	4.5
Total	170	66	38.8	76	44.7	28	16.5

[a] From Zheng et al. [91]

Comparative studies on geographic conditions, including geologic and geomorphologic features, climate, soil, and vegetation of high- and low-risk areas in China did not reveal any definite and distinct factors associated with the etiology of esophageal cancer. The DCEC and collaborators [62] carried out a preliminary analysis of chemical elements in drinking water (222 samples) and in grains and vegetables (216 samples) from Anyang prefecture. The levels of most chemical elements, e.g., Mn, Mg, Fe^{2+}, Fe^{3+}, Mo, Na, K, I, Br, and Cl and of HCO_3^- ions, decreased gradually from the east to Anyang and Linxian counties in the west of the prefecture. Trace elements such as Mo, Zn, Cu, Mg, Mn, and Co were low in the drinking water of high-risk areas. However, Plummer-Vinson syndrome, a long-standing iron deficiency disease occurring in northern Sweden, was not noted in people of the Anyang prefecture. Burrell et al. [93] reported a relative deficiency of Mo, Cu, Zn, Mg, and B in the soil of the Transkei, in South Africa, where cancer of the esophagus is prevalent. Nemenko et al. [94] noted a low content of molybdenum in the Guryev region of Kazakhstan, USSR.

It is known that the trace element molybdenum is an important constituent of certain enzymes, such as nitrate reductase and other oxidases, and deficiency of molybdenum may lead to the accumulation of nitrates in plants. Emission spectrometric analysis of samples from seven counties in Henan province showed that the foodstuffs from Linxian and other areas with a high incidence of esophageal cancer contained low amounts of molybdenum [45, 46, 95]. Furthermore, molybdenum concentrations in 360 hair, 126 serum, and 276 overnight urine samples from inhabitants of Linxian (high incidence) and Yuxian and Xinyangxian (low incidence) have been analyzed using catalytic polarography, the results demonstrating that molybdenum levels in the human body are also much lower in Linxian than in low-risk areas. There was, in addition, a marked difference between the ratios of copper to molybdenum in the hair of Linxian and Yuxian residents; 161–194 and 89–101 respectively. Since copper can counteract the physiologic action of molybdenum, the high ratio of these trace elements in Linxian residents may have intensified the effect of molybdenum deficiency [45, 46, 95]. Concentrations of Cu, Mg, and Zn in 200 serum samples were determined by atomic absorption spectrophotometry. The average level of zinc was reduced in esophageal and cardiac cancer patients from Henan province, while that of copper was increased. The investigation revealed that serum zinc levels in both normal subjects and cancer patients, as well as hair copper and zinc concentrations, were lower in both high- and low-risk areas than reported previously by other workers [96]. In another survey, Mo, Mg, and Zn concentrations in overnight urine samples from 67 male esophageal cancer patients and 72 normal subjects were estimated. Magnesium levels

Table 2.10. Copper, iron, magnesium, and zinc concentrations in the hair of peasants in Linxian and Yuxian counties[a]

Element	Age-group (years)	Linxian		Yuxian		P	
		No. of cases	Mean ± SE	No. of cases	Mean ± SE	Counties	Age-groups
Cu	7–15	51	8.31 ± 0.12	56	7.73 ± 0.12	< 0.05	< 0.25
	30+	113	8.41 ± 0.12	101	8.02 ± 0.12		
Fe	7–15	48	27.8 ± 1.1	53	23.1 ± 1.1	< 0.001	< 0.001
	30+	103	18.0 ± 0.6	97	15.3 ± 0.5		
Mg	7–15	48	21.3 ± 0.8	49	21.2 ± 1.0	> 0.25	< 0.001
	30+	109	30.9 ± 1.0	97	31.8 ± 1.0		
Zn	7–15	51	120 ± 4.0	54	127 ± 3.0	< 0.005	< 0.001
	30+	111	144 ± 2.0	101	151 ± 1.0		

[a] From Zheng et al. [101]

were lower in the urine of cancer patients than in the control group. In contrast, zinc levels were significantly higher in the urine of cancer patients than that of controls ($P<0.01$). This increase of zinc in urine might explain the observed decrease of serum zinc concentration in esophageal cancer patients [95]. Lin et al. [98] reported that lower levels of zinc were found in the blood, hair, and esophageal tissue of esophageal cancer patients than in matched control subjects or matched patients with other forms of cancer. The reduced level of zinc was associated with an increased serum level of copper. Dietary zinc deficiency has been shown to induce parakeratosis in the esophagus of rats [99].

Furthermore, Fong et al. [100] showed that dietary zinc deficiency increased the incidence and shortened the latent time for induction of esophageal cancer in rats by methylbenzylnitrosamine.

In another study, Cu, Mg, Fe, and Zn concentrations in 323 hair samples from male subjects were likewise determined (Table 2.10).

In Linxian the average levels of zinc and magnesium were slightly lower than in Yuxian, a low-incidence county, whereas that of copper was slightly higher. The average level of iron in Linxian males was much higher in the 7–15 age-group than in the adult group, but average levels of magnesium and zinc were much lower. Recent investigations reveal that both zinc and copper contents were lower than reported previously by other workers [101]. Sichuan Medical College [102] reported the emission spectrometric analysis of 18 trace elements in hair samples from Yangting county, Sichuan province. Examination of 63 patients with esophageal cancer and 63 controls showed that only Mo, Fe, and Ba were significantly lower in the hair of the cancer patients.

Formation of carcinogenic nitrosamines in the stomach can be induced by ingestion of nitrates, nitrites, and secondary and tertiary amines. Since molybdenum deficiency could lead to the accumulation of nitrates in crops, the application of ammonium molybdate as a trace element fertilizer might reduce the amount of nitrates and nitrites in food. Following the experimental utilization of ammonium molybdate in Linxian, it was found that the molybdenum concentrations in millet, wheat, maize, and rice increased from 0.33–0.48 mg/kg to 0.50–1.49 mg/kg, along with a 25.8%–47.8% decrease in nitrite concentration. In vegetables, nitrate and nitrite levels decreased by 18.0% and 27.5% respectively, and the amount of vitamin C increased on average by 24.8%. Incidentally, the crop yield also increased as a result of using molybdenum fertilizer, but no change was noted in Cu, Fe, Mg, Mn, and Zn levels in grains [45].

7 Hereditary Factors

According to several epidemiologic surveys undertaken in north China, about 25%–60% of patients with cancer of the esophagus had a family history, but in most cases had lived with the other patients in their families for more than 20 years. Common exposure to extraneous carcinogens therefore appears more feasible as a causative factor than genetic susceptibility.

In 1958, Howell, Evans et al. [103] reported 18 cases of esophageal carcinoma in three generations of two families in Liverpool. In 17 cases there was unequivocal evidence of associated tylosis (keratosis) palmaris et plantaris, and tylosis may have been present in the remaining case. Of the other 86 family members in whom tylosis was not identified, only one had carcinoma of the esophagus. Follow-up of these families has shown a continued high rate of esophageal cancer in the tylotic family members and no cases among their nontylotic relatives. It was suggested that the tylosis is inherited as an autosomal dominant and that the tendency for the carcinoma may also be genetically related. In recent years, case reports of esophageal cancer with tylosis have increased in frequency, and hyperkeratosis and oral leukoplakia may also be associated with laryngeal, gastric, and bronchial carcinomas [104–106]. However, not all patients with tylosis develop esophageal cancer; in high-incidence areas in China no association was noted, although oral leukoplakia occurred frequently.

Pour and Ghadirian [107] reported on a family in a small isolated village in the eastern part of Khorasan, Iran, with 13 cancer patients in three generations, of whom nine had carcinoma of the esophagus. Six of the patients were in the age-group of 23–40 years, as compared with the other esophageal cancer patients in the community who were aged 50–54 years. Consanguineous marriages might have aggravated susceptibility to cancer development in members of this family, but none had tylosis palmaris et plantaris.

Pan et al. [108] studied the genealogical history of esophageal cancer in seven Linxian families, and reinterviewed the members in 1980. In a few large families the history could be traced for more than ten generations. However, the causes of death in earlier generations could not be positively identified, and in addition, most members of the last two generations did not reach the age at which esophageal cancer is most likely to occur. Definite information can therefore only be obtained for three or four generations. With regard to consanguinity, some families displayed close blood relationships between the victims, while in others many patients were more distantly related or had no blood ties at all. The latter pattern was predominant when considering the seven families together. In two families, for instance, the esophageal cancer patients were mainly daughters-in-law. Hence, this survey of family history does not lend support to the importance of heredity in the etiology of cancer of the esophagus.

The distribution of AB0 blood groups among 1055 patients with cancer of the esophagus and gastric cardia in Linxian County Hospital has been compared with that of 12,005 normal subjects in north China. The results showed no significant association of these cancerous lesions with an AB0 antigen [109].

In a cytogenetic study of chromosome aberrations, Wu and Ruan [110] examined 5500 metaphase plates of lymphocytes from 103 members of five high-risk families and 1567 metaphase plates from 30 members of four low-risk families who lived in close proximity in Linxian county. Although the model number and karyotype were normal diploid (2n = 46), many more cells from members of high-risk families showed aneuploidy and various types of structural aberrations than from members of low-risk families. The 101 chromatid breaks found in the high-risk families were mostly distributed among chromosomes of A, B, and C groups and occurred more frequently in long arms than in short arms. During karyotyping it was found that the A_2 chromosomes could not be matched with each other in ten of 300 cells. Wu and Ruan [111] made a further study of the chromosomal aberrations of cultured lymphocytes from 23 untreated esophageal cancer patients and 20 untreated epithelial dysplasia patients with positive family history and made a comparison with 31 samples from controls. They found that both the numerical and structural aberration rates were higher in the patients than in the controls, and the results seemed to indicate the probability of a relationship between hereditary predisposed chromosomal aberration and the development of esophageal cancer in the high-risk families.

A preliminary study on the possible association of esophageal cancer with HLA phenotype was undertaken among 35 people from high-incidence families (HIF) and 31 members of low-incidence families (LIF) in Linxian, using 62 HLA typing sera [112]. It was observed that on the A locus, the frequency of HLA-A_2 antigen was high in both HIF and LIF, especially in the former. On the B locus, the frequency of HLA-B_{40} was higher in HIF than in LIF. No definite findings were noted with C and DR loci. The delta values showed that HLA-A_{10} and B_{40} in HIF were in linkage disequilibrium. Similar studies on HLA profile had previously been carried out in patients from different ethnic groups residing on the shore of the Caspian Sea in Iran by Hashemi et al. [113]. A total of 151 esophageal cancer patients and 214 controls were typed for 24 antigens. No statistically significant differences were found between patients and controls with regard to HLA antigens.

More date concerning the hereditary factor in the etiology of esophageal cancer in high-incidence areas are needed in order to elucidate this intricate problem.

8 Summary

The epidemiology of cancer of the esophagus shows the following salient features:

1. There are high-incidence areas which are separated geographically from each other and are characterized by sharp gradients of incidence.
2. The high-incidence areas are usually in economically poor regions where there are dietary deficiencies and/or consumption of moldy foods containing chemical carcinogens or their precursors and promoting substances.
3. Epithelial hyperplasia of the esophagus is also prevalent in high-incidence areas and if severe may become malignant. On average, the precancerous lesions appear about 10 years prior to diagnosis of a squamous carcinoma.
4. Incidence and mortality usually increase progressively with age, indicating the cumulative effects of environmental agents.

Some environmental factors have been implicated in the etiology of esophageal cancer. For example, alcohol abuse and smoking may be responsible for the few cases of esophageal cancer which occur in the low-incidence areas with more male victims, as noted in Europe and North America. Local lesions of the esophagus such as caustic stricture are known to cause some cases of carcinoma after long latency. In Linxian county of Henan province in China, the formation of carcinogenic nitrosamines, such as dimethylnitrosamine, diethylnitrosamine, methylbenzylnitrosamine, *N*-1-methylacetonyl-*N*-3-methylbutylnitrosamine, and *N*-1-methylacetonyl-*N*-2-methylpropylnitrosamine in moldy foods has been demonstrated, and the administration of precursors of these compounds induced carcinoma in experimental animals, indicating in vivo formation of nitrosamines. Prolonged feeding of rats with moldy cornbread alone produced forestomach cancer; the carcinogenicity of *Fusarium moniliforme* and other fungi metabolites remains to be determined. Pickled vegetables are heavily contaminated by *Geotrichum candidum* and other molds which contains a nitroso compound, Roussin red methyl ester, and trace amounts of B*a*P and other PAHs. Extracts of Linxian pickles induced hyperplasia of esophageal epithelium as well as papilloma of the forestomach in mice. In vitro experiments showed the presence of mutagen and/or carcinogen and promoter in the pickled vegetable extracts. Thus the moldy foods may provide carcinogens and promoters, e.g., nitrosamines, mycotoxins, Roussin red, and B*a*P and other PAHs. The etiologic agents appear to be many, and may act together or successively upon the esophagus in carcinogenesis.

Other contributory environmental factors include dietary deficiencies of animal proteins, fat, and vitamins A, B_2, and C; high levels of nitrates and nitrites in water and foods; low molybdenum and zinc levels and imbalances of trace elements; and indoor air pollution during the winter months. The importance of hereditary predisposition should be studied further. It has been suggested that the combined action of dietary potential carcinogens and other contributory factors may account for the high frequency of esophageal cancer in Linxian. It seems important, therefore, first to identify the potential carcinogens and promoters in each high-risk area and then to investigate the exact role played by each causal agent in carcinogenesis.

References

1. Coordinating Group for Research on Etiology of Esophageal Cancer in China (1975) The epidemiology and etiology of esophageal cancer in North China. Sci Sin 18: 131–148
2. Joint Iran-IARC Study Group (1977) Esophageal cancer studies in the Caspian littoral of Iran: results of population studies – a prodrome. J Natl Cancer Inst 59: 1127–1138
3. Li MH, Li P, Li BR (1980) Recent progress in research on esophageal cancer in China. Adv Cancer Res 33: 173–249
4. Wynder EL, Bross IJ (1961) A study of etiological factors in cancer of the esophagus. Cancer 14: 389–413
5. Warwick GP, Harington JS (1973) Some aspects of the epidemiology and etiology of esophageal cancer with particular emphasis on the Transkei, South Africa. Adv Cancer Res 17: 82–230
6. Hoffmann D, Hecht SS (1983) Tobacco and tobaccosmoke, general aspect, IARC Sci Publ 45: 63–65
7. Brunnemann KD, Hoffmann D (1978) Chemical studies on tobacco smoke. LIX. Analysis of nitrosamines in tobacco smoke and polluted indoor environments. IARC Sci Publ 19: 343–356
8. Van Duuren BL (1968) Tobacco carcinogenesis. Cancer Res 28: 2357–2362
9. McCormick A, Nicholson MJ, Baylis MA, Underwood JG (1973) Nitrosamines in cigarette smoke condensate. Nature 244: 237–238
10. Auerbach O, Stout AP, Hammond EC, Garfinkel L (1965) Histologic changes in esophagus in relation to smoking habits. Arch Environ Health 11: 4–15
11. Malhotra SL (1967) Geographical distribution of gastrointestinal cancers in India with special reference to causation. Gut 8: 361–372
12. Hirayama T (1979) Diet and cancer. Nutr Cancer 1: 67–81
13. Tuyns AJ (1980) Recherches concernant les facteurs étiologiques du cancer de l'oesophage dans l'Ouest de la France. Bull Cancer (Paris) 67: 15–28

14. Cook-Mozaffrai P (1979) The epidemiology of the esophagus. Nutr Cancer 1: 51–60
15. Mosbech J, Videbaek A (1955) On the etiology of esophageal carcinoma. J Natl Cancer Inst 15: 1665–1675
16. Cook P (1971) Cancer of the esophagus in Africa: a summary evaluation of the evidence for the frequency of occurrence and a preliminary indication of the possible association with the consumption of alcoholic drinks made from maize. Br J Cancer 25: 853–880
17. Marasas WFO, van Renbhurg SJ, Mirocha CJ (1979) Incidence of *Fusarium* species and the mycotoxins, deoxynivalenol and zearalenone, in corn produced in esophageal cancer areas in Transkei. Agric Food Chem 27: 1108–1112
18. Schoental R, Joffe AZ (1974) Lesions induced in rodents by extracts from cultures of *Fusarium poae* and *F. sporotrichioides*. J Pathol 112: 37–42
19. Wang FR, Zhang ZD (1979) Investigation on the induction of esophageal tumor in rats by *Fusarium moniliforme* (in Chinese). Cancer Res Prev Treat 3: 12–15
20. Li MH, Lu SH, Ji C, Wang YL, Wang MY, Cheng SH, Tian GZ (1980) Experimental studies on the carcinogenicity of fungus-contaminated food from Linxian county. Proc 10th Int Symp Princess Takamatsu Cancer Res Fund, Tokyo, pp 139–148
21. Wu YK, Loucks HH (1951) Carcinoma of esophagus or cardia of stomach: analysis of 172 cases with 81 resections. Ann Surg 134: 946–956
22. Department of Epidemiology, Cancer Institute, Department of Statistics, Medical Information Institute, and Institute of Microbiology, Academia Sinica (1977) Preliminary investigation of the epidemiological factors of esophageal cancer in China (in Chinese). Cancer Res Prev Treat 2: 1–8
23. Hewer T, Rose E, Ghadirian P, Castegnaro M, Bartsch H, Malaveill C, Day N (1978) Ingested mutagens from opium and tobacco pyrolysis products and cancer of the esophagus. Lancet 2: 494–496
24. International Agency for Research on Cancer (1981) Environmental carcinogenesis. IARC Annu Rep 101–102
25. Appelquist P, Salmo M (1980) Lye corrosion carcinoma of the esophagus: a review of 63 cases. Cancer 45: 2655–2658
26. Tokunaga M, Sato E, Imakyure K (1979) Carcinoma of the esophagus developing in lye stricture: a case report. Jpn J Clin Oncol 9: 145–152
27. Dunham LJ, Sheets RH (1974) Effects of esophageal constriction on benzo(a)pyrene carcinogenesis in hamster esophagus and forestomach. J Natl Cancer Inst 53: 875–881
28. Kramchaninor NF (1968) The mortality from esophageal cancer in the population of Guryev (in Russian). Vopr Onkol 14: 38–42
29. Brunning DA (1974) Oesophageal cancer and hot tea. Lancet 1: 272
30. Segi M (1975) Tea gruel as a possible factor for cancer of the esophagus. Gan 66: 199–202
31. Price JM, Pamukcu AM (1968) The induction of neoplasms of the urinary bladder of the cow and the small intestine of the rat by feeding bracken fern *(Pteris aquilina)*. Cancer Res 28: 2247
32. Hirono I, Fushimi K, Mori H, Miwa T, Haga M (1973) Comparative study of carcinogenic activity in each part of bracken. J Natl Cancer Inst 50: 1367–1371
33. Pamukcu AM, Hatcher J, Tagcachi H, Bryan GT (1980) Quercetin: an intestinal and bladder carcinogen present in bracken fern. AACR Annu Meet 71: 296
34. Wang CY, Chiu CW, Pamukcu AM, Bryan GT (1976) Identification of carcinogenic tannin isolated from bracken fern *(Pteridium aquilinum)*. J Natl Cancer Inst 56: 33–36
35. Morino K, Matsukura N, Kawachi T, Ohgnki H, Sugimura T, Hirono I (1982) Carcinogenicity of quercetin and rutin in golden hamsters by oral administration. Carcinogenesis 3: 93–97
36. Kirby KS (1960) Induction of tumors by tannin extracts. Br J Cancer 14: 147–150
37. Pradhan SN, Chung EB, Ghosh B, Paul BD, Kapadia GJ (1974) Potential carcinogens. 1. Carcinogenicity of some plant extracts and their tannin-containing fractions in rats. J Natl Cancer Inst 52: 1579–1582
38. O'Gara RW, Lee C, Morton JF (1971) Carcinogenicity of extracts of selected plants from Curacao after oral and subcutaneous administration to rodents. J Natl Cancer Inst 46: 1131–1137
39. O'Gara RW, Lee CW, Morton JF, Kapadia GJ, Dunham LJ (1974) Sarcoma induced in rats by extracts of plants and by fractionated extracts of *Krameria ixina*. J Natl Cancer Inst 52: 445–448
40. Dunham LJ, Sheets RH, Morton ZF (1974) Proliferative lesions in cheek pouch and esophagus of hamsters treated with plants from Curacao, Netherlands Antilles. J Natl Cancer Inst 53: 1259–1269
41. Rose EF (1968) The effects of soil and diet on disease. Cancer Res 28: 2390–2392
42. O'Neill CH, Hodges GM, Riddle PN, Jordan PW, Newman PH, Flood SJ, Toulson EC (1980) A fine

fibrous silica contaminant of flour in the high esophageal cancer area of north-east Iran. Int J Cancer 26: 617–628
43. O'Neill CH, Clarke G, Hodges GM, Jordan PW, Newman RH, Pan QQ, Liu FS, Ge M, Cheng YM, Toulson EC (1982) Silica fragments from millet bran in mucosa surrounding oesophageal tumors in patients in northern China. Lancet 1: 1202–1206
44. Xia SH, Zhan Y (1978) Fungal invasion in esophageal tissue and its possible relation to esophageal carcinoma (in Chinese). Chin Med J 58: 392–396
45. Department of Chemical Etiology and Carcinogenesis, Cancer Institute, Chinese Academy of Medical Sciences (1978) Recent studies on the etiology of esophageal cancer (in Chinese). Chin J Med 58: 593–597
46. Department of Chemical Etiology and Carcinogenesis, Cancer Institute, Chinese Academy of Medical Sciences (1978) Further studies on the etiology of esophageal cancer. In: Birch JM (ed) Advances in medical oncology research and education, vol 3. Pergamon, London, pp 39–44
47. Druckrey H, Preussmann R, Ivankovic S, Schmähl D (1967) Organotrope carcinogene Wirkungen bei 65 verschiedenen *N*-Nitroso-Verbindungen an BD-Ratten. Z Kresbforsch 69: 103–201
48. Montesano R, Magee PN (1970) Metabolism of DMN by human liver slices *in vitro*. Nature 228: 173–174
49. Preussmann R (1972) On the significance of *N*-nitroso compounds as carcinogens and on problems related to their chemical analysis. IARC Sci Publ 3: 6–9
50. Harris CC, Autrup H, Stoner GD, Trump BF, Hillman E, Schofer PW, Jeffrey AM (1979) Metabolism of benzo(a)pyrene, *N*-nitrosodimethylamine, and *N*-nitrosopyrrolidine and identification of the major carcinogen-DNA adducts formed in cultured human esophagus. Cancer Res 39: 4401–4406
51. Autrup H, Stoner GD (1982) Metabolism of *N*-nitrosamines by cultured human and rat esophagus. Cancer Res 42: 1037–1311
52. Li MH, Lu SH, Ji C, Wang MY, Cheng SJ, Jin CL (1979) Formation of carcinogenic *N*-nitroso compounds in cornbread inoculated with fungi. Sci Sin 22: 471–477
53. Lu SH, Li MH, Ji C, Wang YL, Huang L (1979) A new nitroso compound, *N*-3-methylbutyl-*N*-1-methylacetonylnitrosamine, in corn bread inoculated with fungi. Sci Sin 22: 601–608
54. Li MH, Guo SP, Fan WG, Zhao XJ, Jiang YZ, Li GY, Han NJ (to be published) Induction of forestomach and liver cancer in mice and rats by MAMBNA (in Chinese).
55. Li MH, Tian GZ, Guo SP, Ji C, Jiang YZ, Li GY, Lu SH (to be published) Forestomach carcinoma induced in mice by in vivo formation of MAMBNA (in Chinese).
56. Lu SH, Camus AM, Li C, Wang YL, Wang MY, Bartsch H (1980) Mutagenicity in *Salmonella typhimurium* of *N*-3-methylbutyl-*N*-1-methylacetonylnitrosamine and *N*-methylbenzylnitrosamine, N-nitrosation products isolated from corn bread contaminated with commonly occurring moulds in Linxian county. Carcinogenesis 1: 867–870
57. Cheng H, Zao JJ, Wang XQ, Wu M, Lu SH (1981) Mutagenic effect of a new nitrosamine, *N*-3-methylbutyl-*N*-1-methylacetonylnitrosamine, on V_{79} cells (in Chinese). Chin Med J 61: 736–739
58. Wu DF, Wu M, Wang XQ, Li SD, Lu SH, Wang YL, Ji C (1982) Malignant transformation of golden hamster lung fibroblasts induced by MAMBNA (in Chinese). Sci Sin [B] 5: 427–435
59. Ji C, Li MH (1983) The occurrence of natural nitrosamines in pickled vegetables and cornbread from Linxian county (in Chinese). Chin J Oncol 5: 73
60. Ji C, Li MH, Singer GM, Lijinsky W (1982) Factors determining the formation of nitroso compounds in moldy corn bread. Acta Acad Med Sin 4: 224–228
61. Ji C, Xu GZ, Li MH, Li KY, Li GL (1984) A new *N*-nitroso compound: *N*-2-methylpropyl-*N*-1-methylacetonylnitrosamine isolated from moldy millet and wheat flour (in Chinese). Sci Sin [B] 2: 143–149
62. Department of Chemical Etiology and Carcinogenesis, Cancer Institute, Chinese Academy of Medical Sciences and Henan Province Cooperative Groups (1980) Preliminary analyses of the distribution of esophageal cancer mortality rate, the geographical environment, and the chemical elements in food and drinking water in Anyang district, Henan Province (in Chinese). Chin J Oncol 2: 29–37
63. Wang YL, Lu SH, Li MH (1979) Determination of nitrates and nitrites in well water from Yaocun Commune, Linxian County, Henan Province (in Chinese). Chin J Oncol 1: 201–205
64. Lowenfels AB, Tuyns AJ, Walker EA, Roussel A (1978) Nitrite in esophageal cancer. Gut 19: 199–201
65. Department of Chemical Etiology and Carcinogenesis, Cancer Institute, Chinese Academy of Medical Sciences (1974) Inhibitory effect of vitamin C on the *in vivo* synthesis of nitrosamine (in Chinese). Cancer Res Prev Treat 3: 29–33

66. Bogovski P, Castegnaro M, Pignatelli B, Walker EA (1972) The inhibiting effect of tannins on the formation of nitrosamines. IARC Sci Publ 3: 127–129
67. Mirvish SS, Wallcave L, Eagen M, Shubik P (1972) Ascorbate nitrite reaction: possible means of blocking the formation of carcinogenic *N*-nitroso compounds. Science 177: 65–68
68. Pignatelli B, Castegnaro M, Walker EA (1976) Effects of gallic acid and of ethanol on formation of nitrosodiethylamine. IARC Sci Publ 14: 173–178
69. Lu SH, Wang YL, Li MH (1980) Effects of fungi on the formation of carcinogenic *N*-nitrosamines and their precursors in food (in Chinese). Acta Acad Med Sin 1: 24–27
70. Li MH (1980) Studies on potential carcinogens on the diet of individuals at high risk for esophageal cancer. In: Marks PA (ed) Cancer research in the People's Republic of China and the United States of America. Grund & Stratton, New York pp 131–136
71. Li MH, Tian GZ, Lu SH, Guo SP, Jin CL, Wang YC (1982) Forestomach carcinoma induced in rats by cornbread inoculated with *Fusarium moniliforme* (in Chinese). Chin J Oncol 4: 241–244
72. Cheng SJ, Li MH, Wang YL (1982) A preliminary study on mutagenic effect of extracts prepared from moldy cornbread (in Chinese). Acta Biol Exp Sin 15: 25–30
73. Zhang BG, He MZ (1965) Pathology of forestomach papillomas induced by prolonged feeding of *Fusarium*-inoculated food in rats (in Chinese). Chin J Pathol 9: 51–53
74. Cancer Prevention, Treatment and Research Group, Henan Province, Etiology Research Group of Esophageal Cancer, Henan Province (1975) Studies on esophageal cancer and fungus: 1. Preliminary result of induction of esophageal cancer in rats by moldy food. 2. Synergic carcinogenesis of nitrosamine and moldy food (in Chinese). Cancer Res Prev Treat 3: 19–25
75. Liu GT, Zhen YZ, Yu GJ, Liu ZP, Miao J, Zhao CY, Chang JZ, Hao HL (to be published) Experimental study on the papillomas of the forestomach induced by *Stemphylium ilicis* in rats (in Chinese). Cancer Res Prev Treat
76. Zhen YZ, Yang SL, Ting LP, Fan TX, Han HM, Chu PQ (to be published) Molds in some foodstuffs collected from a few high and low incidence counties of esophageal cancer in Henan province (in Chinese).
77. Sichuan Sanitary Cadre Postgraduate College (to be published) Molds in some foodstuffs collected from the high-middle, and low incidence areas of esophageal cancer in Sichuan province (in Chinese)
78. Yen IC (1978) Etiology and pathogenesis: mycotoxins (in Chinese), People's Hygiene Publisher, Beijing (Applied oncology vol 1, pp 100–104)
79. Mirocha CJ, Pathre SV, Christensen CM (1978) Chemistry of *Fusarium* and *Stachybotrys* mycotoxins. In Wyllie TD, Morehouse LG (eds): Mycotoxic fungi, mycotoxins, mycotoxicoses. An encyclopedic handbook, vol 1. Dekker, New York, pp 365–520
80. Schoental R, Joffe AZ, Yagen B (1979) Cardiovascular lesions and various tumors found in rats given T-2 toxin, a trichothecine metabolite of *Fusarium*. Cancer Res 39: 2179–2189
81. Department of Chemical Etiology and Carcinogenesis, Cancer Institute, Chinese Academy of Medical Sciences (1977) Preliminary observation on the carcinogenicity of pickled vegetables from Linxian county (in Chinese). Cancer Res Prev Treat 2: 46–49
82. Cheng SJ, Sala M, Li MH, Wang MY, Pot-Deprun J, Chroulinkov I (1980) Mutagenic, transforming and promoting effect of pickled vegetables from Linxian county, China. Carcinogenesis 1: 685–692
83. Lu SH, Camus AM, Tomatis L, Bartsch H (1981) Mutagenicity studies of extracts of pickled vegetables collected in Linxian county, a high-incidence area for esophageal cancer in northern China. J Natl Cancer Inst 66: 33–36
84. Wang GH, Zheng WX, Chia WG (1980) The identification of natural Roussin red methyl ester (in Chinese). Acta Chem Sin 38: 95–102
85. Wang MY, Lu SH, Ji C, Wang YL, Li MH (1983) The occurrence of a nitroso compound, Roussin red, and its precursor in pickled vegetables from Lin county (in Chinese). Cancer Res Prev Treat 10: 12–15
86. Cheng SJ, Sala M, Li MH, Courtois I, Chouroulinkov I (1981) Promoting effect of Roussin's red identified in pickled vegetables from Linxian, China. Carcinogenesis 2: 313–319
87. Wang MY, Li MH, Jiang YZ, Sun YH, Li GY, Zheng WX, Chai WG, Wang GH (1983) Nitrosation of secondary amines with Roussin red methyl ester (in Chinese). Cancer Res Prev Treat 10: 144–147
88. Borneff J, Slenka F, Kunte H, Maximos A (1968) The studies of BP and PAH in plants. Arch Hyg Bakteriol 152: 279–282
89. Knorr M, Schenk D (1968) Zur Frage der Synthese polyzyklischer Aromate durch Bakterien. Arch Hyg Bakteriol 152: 282–285
90. Suess MJ (1976) The environmental load and cycle of polycyclic aromatic hydrocarbons. Sci Total Environ 6: 239–250

91. Zheng SF, Qin QS, Li QL, Liu XF (1981) A study on urinary excretion of test-dose riboflavin in peasants of Linxian county (in Chinese). Chin J Prev Med 15: 300
92. Lin PZ (to be published) Effect of riboflavin deficiency and high dose of vitamin C on tumor development in the esophagus and liver in rats (in Chinese)
93. Burrel RJW, Roach WA, Schadwell A (1966) Esophageal cancer in the Bantu of the Transkei associated with mineral deficiency in garden plants. J Natl Cancer Inst 36: 204–214
94. Nemenko BA, Moldakuloba MM, Zorina SN (1976) Esophageal cancer incidence in Guryev province depending on mineral water content (in Russian). Vopr Onkol 9: 75–76
95. Department of Chemical Etiology and Carcinogenesis, Cancer Institute, Chinese Academy of Medical Sciences (1978) Analysis of molybdenum in serum, urine and hair samples of the inhabitants in high- and low-incidence areas of esophageal cancer (in Chinese). Cancer Res Prev Treat 4: 19–25
96. Zheng SF, Liu XF, Li QL (1980) Preliminary analysis of serum copper, zinc and magnesium contents in esophageal and cardiac cancer patients and in normal men (in Chinese). Cancer Res Prev Treat 6: 4–7
97. Li MH, Ji C, Sun YH, Jiang YZ (1981) Preliminary analysis of benzo[*a*]pyrene in Linxian pickled vegetables (in Chinese). Chin J Oncol 3: 303–304
98. Lin HJ, Chan WC, Fong YY, Newberne PM (1977) Zinc levels in serum, hair and tumors from patients with esophageal cancer. Nutr Rep Int 15: 635–643
99. Follis RH Jr, Day HG, McCollum EV (1941) Histological studies of rats fed a diet extremely low in zinc. J Nutr 22: 223–237
100. Fong LYY, Sivak A, Newberne PM (1978) Zinc deficiency and methylbenzylnitrosamine-induced oesophageal cancer in rats. J Natl Cancer Inst 61: 145–150
101. Zheng SF, Wei HJ, Lou HM, Hu KG, Shang AL (1982) Copper, iron, magnesium and zinc contents in the hair of peasants in high and low incidence areas of esophageal cancer (in Chinese). Chin J Oncol 4: 174–177
102. Sichuan Medical College (1978) Comparative analysis of trace element content in hair ash of esophageal cancer patients and normal subjects (in Chinese). Cancer Res Prev Treat 2: 5–9
103. Howell-Evans AW, McConnell RB, Clarke CA, Sheppard PM (1958) Carcinoma of the esophagus with keratosis palmaris et plantaris (tylosis). Q J Med 27: 413–429
104. DeAngelis PD, Johnson S (1969) Tylosis palmaris et plantaris, its occurrence with internal malignancy. Arch Dermatol 100: 7–9
105. Harper PS, Harper RMJ, Howel-Evans AW (1970) Carcinoma of the esophagus with tylosis. Q J Med 39: 317–333
106. Ritter SB, Petersen G (1976) Esophageal cancer, hyperkeratosis, and oral leukoplakia: follow-up family study. JAMA 236: 1844–1845
107. Pour P, Ghadirian P (1974) Familial cancer of the esophagus in Iran. Cancer 33: 1649–1652
108. Pan HC, Ning AL (to be published) Studies on the genealogical history of esophageal cancer in seven Linxian families (in Chinese)
109. Wu M, Wang XG, Zhu QL, Shao LF (1981) Distribution of AB0 blood groups among patients with carcinoma of esophagus and gastric cardia in Linxian People's Hospital (in Chinese). Chin J Oncol 3: 16–18
110. Wu YQ, Ruan XZ (1979) Genetic etiology of esophageal cancer: cytogenetic study of individuals in five "cancer families" in Linxian (in Chinese). Acta Genet Sin 6: 3–7
111. Wu YQ, Ruan XZ (1981) Genetic etiology of esophageal cancer: II. Cytogenetic studies on peripheral blood cells of esophageal cancer and epithelial dysplasia patients with positive family history in Linxian county (in Chinese). Chin J Oncol 3: 12–15
112. Zhu XK, Li GS, He QQ, Hu, ZC, Cao MH (1982) A preliminary report on the possible association of esophageal cancer and HLA (in Chinese). Chin J Oncol 4: 257–261
113. Hashmi S, Dowlatshahi K, Day NE, Kmet J, Takasugi M, Mohagheghpour N, Modabber FZ (1979) Esophageal cancer studies in the Caspian littoral of Iran: introductive assessment of the HLA profile in patients and controls. Tissue Antigens 14: 422–425

Chapter 3
Carcinogenesis in the Esophagus

Qiu Jie Xia

1 Introduction

Approaches to carcinogenesis are of supreme importance in the strategy of prevention and treatment of esophageal cancer. Our understanding of this process is still limited, but there has been encouraging progress during recent years. Investigations in high-incidence areas, improvements in the technology used in detection of carcinogens and their adducts, advances in organ and cell culture of epithelial cells, studies on the metabolism of carcinogens in tissues, etc. have afforded a lot of valuable data on different aspects. Much evidence suggests that esophageal carcinogenesis is most likely a multifactorial and multistage process.

2 Background Diseases

Pathological studies have revealed that the noncancerous parts of the esophageal mucosa of patients with esophageal carcinoma always show various degrees of chronic inflammation. Studies in Linxian county of Henan province, a high-incidence area in China, have shown that chronic esophagitis is also common there [1]. A relative incidence of 13.5% of esophagitis was found in a series of 1635 adults examined by means of cytologic smears

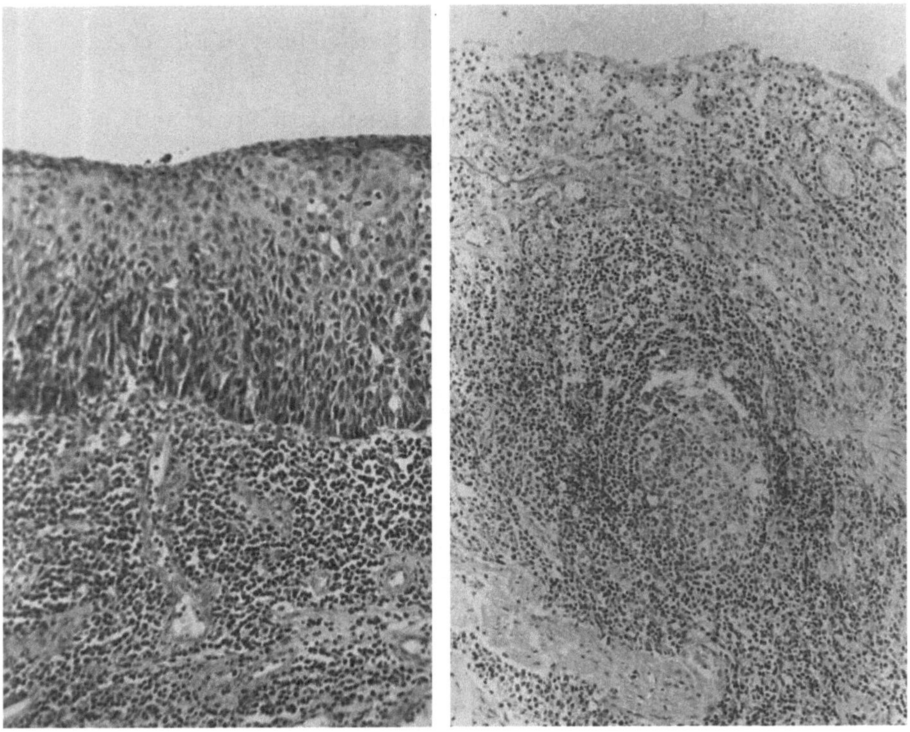

Fig. 3.1. Background lesion of early esophageal carcinoma. *Left:* Marked lymphocytic infiltration in the lamina propria. The epithelium is thickened with basal cell dysplasia. H & E, ×100. *Right:* Same case, showing erosion of the epithelium and marked chronic inflammation with lymph follicle formation in the lamina propria. H & E, ×100

[2]. A high level of esophagitis has also been found in the esophageal carcinoma high-incidence area in northern Iran [3]. In chronic esophagitis the epithelium displays erosion, atrophy, or hyperplasia and there is very prominent lymphocytic infiltration and lymph follicle formation in the lamina propria (Fig. 3.1). The esophageal glands are usually seriously affected, with lymphocytic infiltration and decrease of mucinous acini. The muscularis mucosae is interrupted and replaced in some parts by fibrous tissue.

The inhabitants of Linxian county mostly have maize, which is deficient in vitamins B_2 and C, as a staple food stuff. Their food is usually coarse and often contaminated by fungi of *Fusarium, Aspergillus, Penicillium,* and other genera. These might be causative factors for the development of esophagitis in this area, and there are reasons to suggest that chronic esophagitis might be the associated background disease in most cases of esophageal carcinoma.

Other chronic irritations to the esophagus, such as alcoholism, heavy smoking, poor oral hygiene, carious teeth, consumption of hot food, chronic peptic esophageal reflux, upper GI or respiratory tract infections, caustic strictures, achalasia of the cardia, acanthotic hyperplasia, or persistent unhealed ulcers or erosions, may also give rise to chronic inflammation of the esophagus (Fig. 3.2). On fiberoptic esophagoscopy the mucosa of such patients may show various changes, e.g., multifocal hyperplasia of epithelium, leukoplakia, impaired secretory function, small diverticula, impairment of esophageal mobility, retention cyst, or roughness. Patients with these lesions run a much higher risk of esophageal carcinoma than normal subjects [4, 5]. Chronic inflammation of the esophagus may result in decreased effectiveness of defence mechanisms against carcinogens, increased susceptibility of the epithelial cells to carcinogens, or both.

3 Precancerous Lesions of Esophageal Epithelium

The results of studies in Linxian have suggested that severe dysplasia of the epithelium (Fig. 3.3) might be the major precancerous change in the esophagus. Follow-up cytologic studies have indicated that severe dysplasia of the esophageal epithelium is an unstable intermediate state. After 5–8 years follow-up in a series of over 500 patients with severe dysplasia, about 40% displayed a regression to mild dysplasia or normal epithelium, about 20% showed persistence of severe dysplasia, another 20% fluctuated between severe and mild dysplasia, and the remaining 15%–20% progressed to carcinoma. In a group of 11011 individuals with normal epithelium, only 13 (0.12%) developed cancer during the same period. Thus the risk of esophageal carcinoma in patients with severe dysplasia was much greater than in subjects with normal epithelium [6].

Many lesions of the esophagus have been considered in the literature [5] as precancerous, e.g., chronic peptic esophagitis with Barrett's esophagus, peptic esophagitis with columnar metaplasia, caustic stricture and scar formation after X-ray exposure or tuberculosis, iron deficiency dysphagia (Plummer-Vinson syndrome), epiphrenic diverticulum, megaesophagus, and familial keratosis (tylosis) palmaris et plantaris. Howell-Evans et al. [7] reported two families in which the incidence of esophageal carcinoma was as high as 30% in the members with tylosis. Naef et al. [8] reported that of 140 patients with Barrett's esophagus, 12 developed adenocarinoma. However, tylosis and Barrett's esophagus are very rare in China, and therefore cannot be the major precancerous changes.

Patients with precancerous lesions should be considered high-risk for esophageal cancer, and detection, prevention, and treatment of these lesions is of great importance.

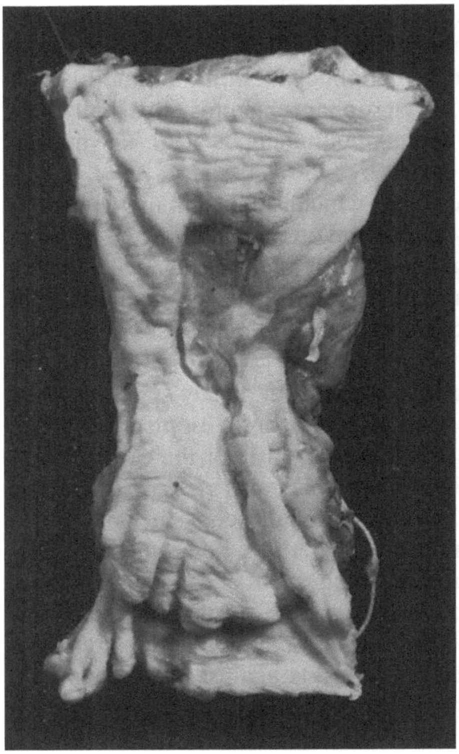

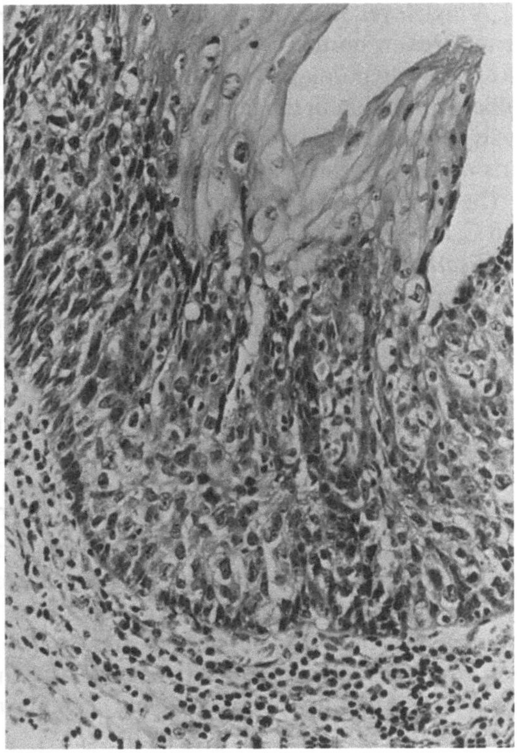

Fig. 3.2 (left). Chronic unhealed ulcer with severe stricture of the esophagus. The patient, a 26 year-old male, had severe dysphagia mimicking advanced esophageal carcinoma

Fig. 3.3 (right). Severe dysplasia in the noncancerous esophageal epithelium of early esophageal carcinoma. H & E, ×200

4 Possible Role of Fungal Esophagitis

Further investigation of the nature of the esophagitis in Linxian has revealed that esophagitis in many patients is caused by combined fungal and bacterial infection. The symptoms, gross features, and site distribution of fungal esophagitis are very similar to those of early esophageal carcinoma; the patients usually have complaints such as dysphagia and retrosternal pains. On fiberoptic esophagoscopy the lesions present as focal plaques, roughness, or erosions of the mucosa. About 60%–70% of the lesions are located in the middle third of the esophagus. The average age of patients with fungal esophagitis is 7–10 years lower than in early esophageal carcinoma [1] and 20 years lower than in advanced esophageal carcinoma.

Pathological studies in a series of 155 esophageal biopsies that was later extended revealed that fungal invasions of the mucosa were present in about 40%–50% of patients with severe dysplasia and early esophageal carcinoma. In fungal esophagitis, there were varying amounts of fungal mycelia and spores growing in the thickened epithelium, with marked inflammatory reactions in the corresponding lamina propria. Lymphocytic infiltrations of the epithelium were mild. Sometimes the epithelium was markedly thickened,

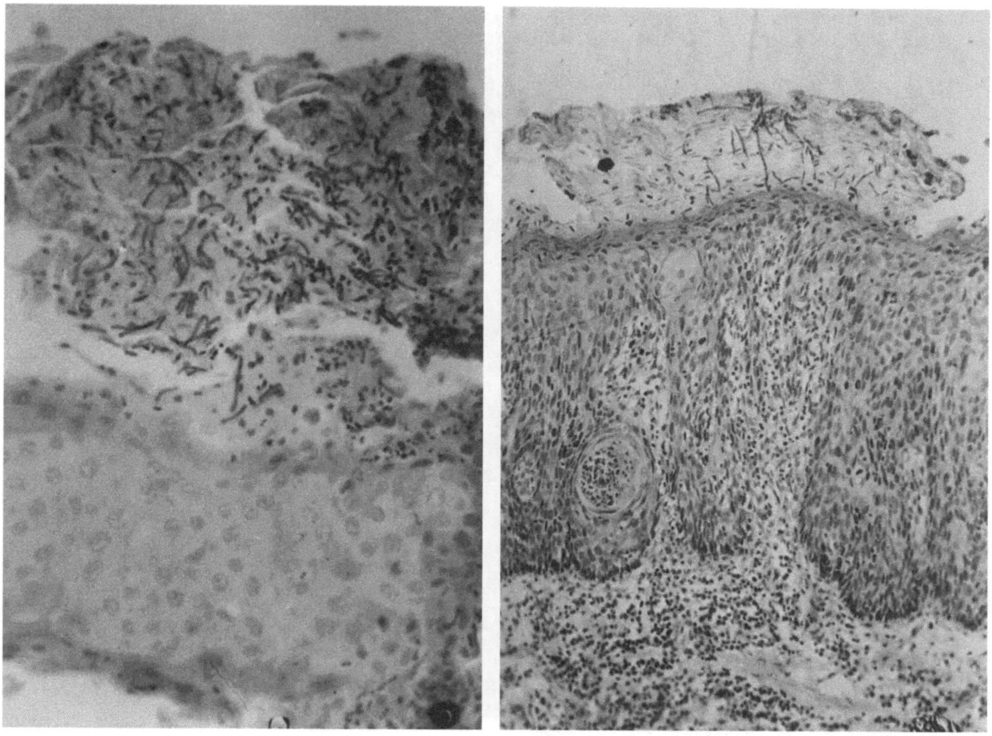

Fig. 3.4. Left: Candida esophagitis in the noncancerous epithelium of early esophageal carcinoma. The superficial layers of the epithelium are highly thickened, with numerous *Candida* pseudohyphae and spores invading. The deeper epithelium shows mild dysplastic change. H & E, ×200. *Right: Candida* infection in the superficial layers of epithelium. The deeper layers show severe dysplasia. Inflammatory cell infiltration is seen in the lamina propria. H & E, ×110

with numerous mycelia and spores invading the epithelial tissues (Figs. 3.4, 3.5). More than half of the invading fungi were *Candida* species. Sometimes there were more than one species of fungi invading the epithelium of the same patient. Fungal esophagitis was associated with various degrees of epithelial dysplasia, i. e., mild, moderate, and severe up to early carcinomatous changes (Figs. 3.4, 3.6, 3.7). The epithelial cells adjacent to the foci of fungal invasion usually showed dysplastic changes, with irregular and hyperchromatic nuclei and prominent nucleoli (Fig. 3.8). Pathological studies of surgical specimens of early esophageal carcinoma have revealed that the noncancerous epithelium often has lesions of fungal esophagitis.

Electron microscopic observations of *Candida* esophagitis showed that most of the *Candida* organisms are seen to invade the intercellular spaces of esophageal epithelium, few to invade the cytoplasm of epithelial cells (Figs. 3.9, 3.10). Some species of fungal mycelia invade several layers of epithelial cells (Fig. 3.11). Bacterial invasions occur together with the fungi in the intercellular spaces of esophageal epithelium (Figs. 3.9, 3.10) [9].

A pure strain of *Candida albicans* has been isolated from a surgical specimen of carcinoma in situ of esophagus (Fig. 3.12). *Candida* species were isolated from about 23% of surgical specimes of esophageal carcinoma, and more than 90% were identified as C. *albicans*.

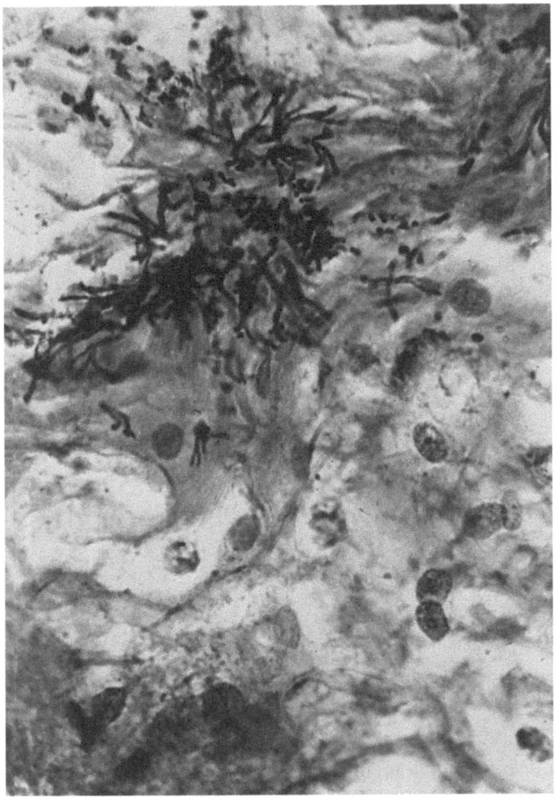

Fig. 3.5. Esophageal biopsy of a patient with fungal esophagitis. There are several foci of fungal invasion in the thickened epithelium. The nuclei of the epithelium are enlarged and there is a cell with double nuclei. H & E, ×400

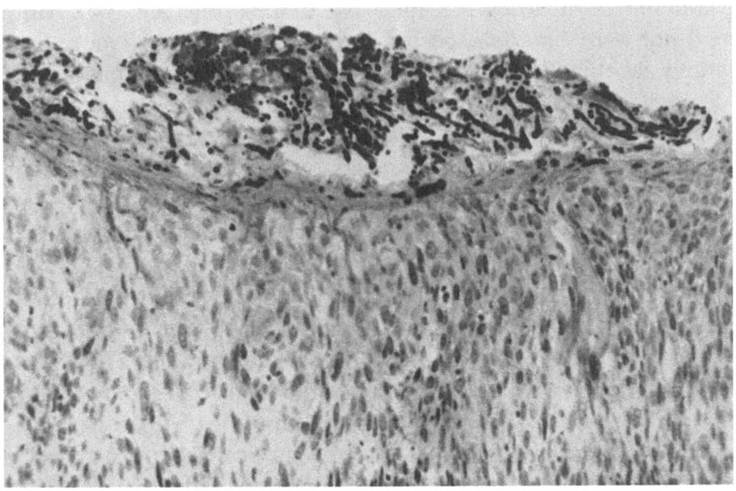

Fig. 3.6. Candida infection in the superficial layers of the noncancerous epithelium of early esophageal carcinoma, the deeper layers showing severe dysplasia. H & E, ×200

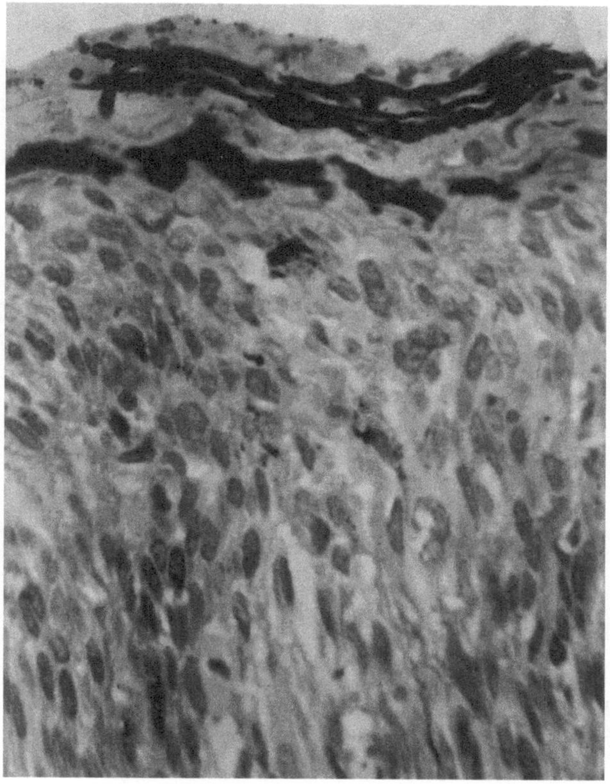

Fig. 3.7. Carcinoma in situ of the esophagus, showing a few *Candida* pseudohyphae and spores in the superficial layers of the epithelium. H & E, ×500

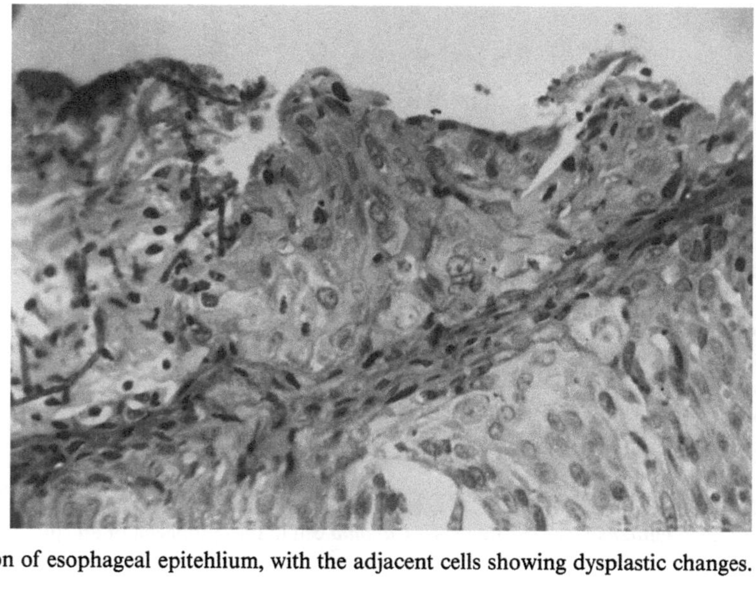

Fig. 3.8. *Candida* infection of esophageal epitehlium, with the adjacent cells showing dysplastic changes. H & E, ×400

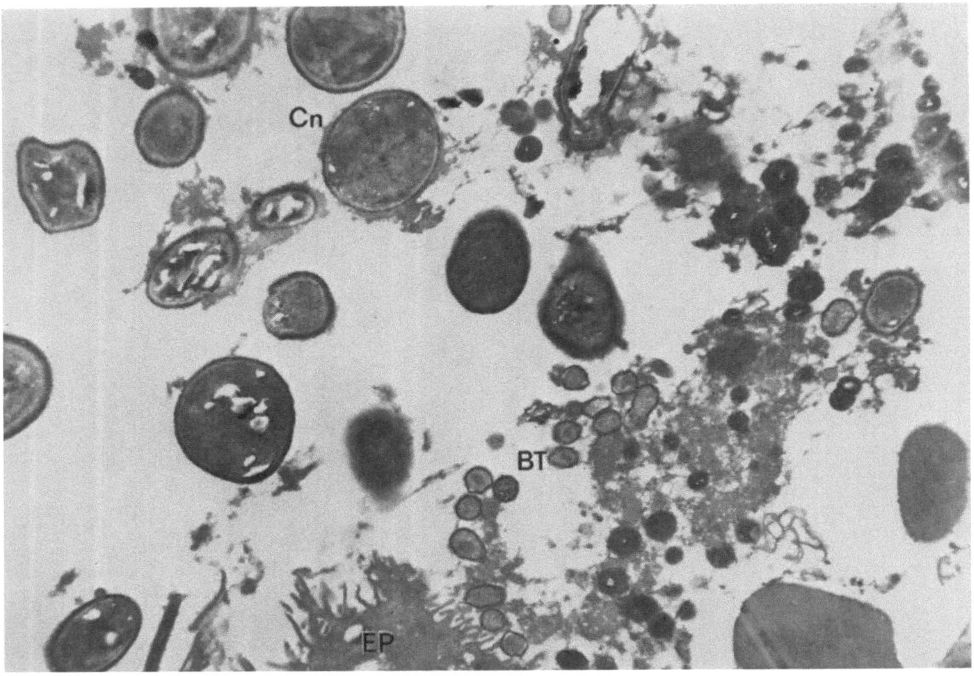

Fig. 3.9. Electron micrograph of *Candida* esophagitis. There are numerous *Candida* cells *(Cn)* and bacteria *(BT)* in the intercellular spaces of epithelial cells *(EP)*. × 8000

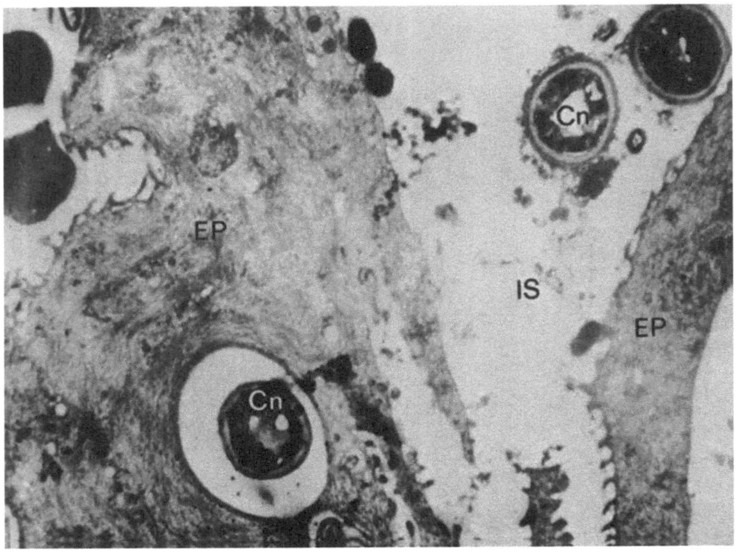

Fig. 3.10. Electron micrograph of *Candida* esophagitis. As well as *Candida* cells *(Cn)* and bacteria *(BT)* in the intercellular space *(IS)*, there is a *Candida* cell in the cytoplasm of an epithelial cell *(EP)*. × 7200

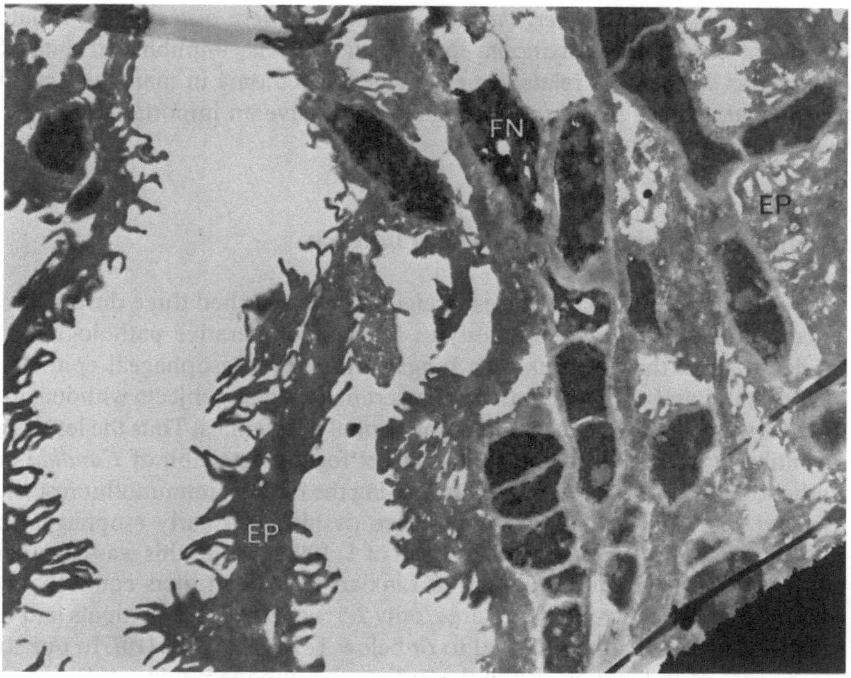

Fig. 3.11. Electron micrograph of a biopsy specimen of fungal esophagitis, showing fungi *(FN)* traversing the epithelial cells *(EP)*. ×8000

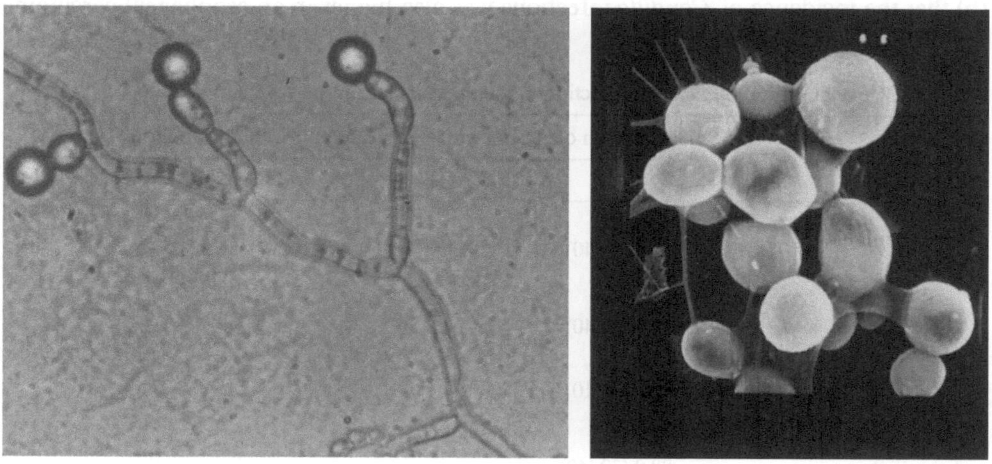

Fig. 3.12. A pure strain of *Candida albicans* isolated from epithelial tissues from a carcinoma in situ of the esophagus in Linxian county. *Left:* Chlamydospores are seen at tops and sides of pseudohyphae in cornmeal agar culture. *Right:* Scanning electromicrograph of *Candida albicans*

Other species, e.g., *Aspergillus* and *Penicillium,* were occasionally isolated from specimens of esophageal carcinoma in Linxian (QJ Xia, unpublished data). Since fungal esophagitis was closely related to esophageal carcinoma in many aspects, we suspected that fungal, mainly *Candida* esophagitis might have an important etiologic relationship with esophageal carcinoma.

5 Seroepidemiologic Studies of Candida Infection

For further studies on *Candida* esophagitis, we established three different techniques for detection of anti-*Candida* antibody in serum. Comparative pathological and serologic studies showed that patients with fungal invasions in esophageal epithelium also have high titers of anti-*Candida* antibody in serum, whereas subjects without fungal invasion have very low titers, like the majority of normal individuals. Thus the levels of anti-*Candida* antibody may be used as a good marker for the detection of *Candida* infection. Our studies on one series of 130 individuals, using the indirect immunofluorescence technique, revealed that 80% of patients with severe dysplasia or early esophageal carcinoma in Linxian had anti-*Candida* antibody titers of 1:100 or more; this was considered to be significant. In the normal population in Linxian 17.5% had titers equal to or above 1:100 while in Beijing, a low-incidence area, only 2.5% of normal individuals had titers of 1:100 or more and 95% had titers equal to or below 1:10 (Fig. 3.13) [10]. In our studies on two other series of individuals, using the indirect immunoperoxidase [11] and cell agglutination [12] techniques, we obtained results similar to those in first series (Table 3.1). A total of 979 subjects were examined in the three series.

These results suggested (a) that in patienst with severe dysplasia or early esophageal carcinoma there are many more *Candida* infections than that in normal individuals, and (b) that the incidence of *Candida* infections was also higher in an esophageal carcinoma

Table 3.1. The relationship of *Candida* infection to esophageal cancer and severe dysplasia

Group	(*n*)	Proportion of subjets with significant anti-*Candida* antibody titers (%)		
		IF[a]	IP[a]	Aggl.[a]
Normal Beijing inhabitants	317	2.5 (1/40)	0 (0/40)	Age: 20–30: 8.2 (6/73); over 30: 3.8 (2/53); unknown: 7.2 (8/111)
Normal Linxian inhabitants	501	17.5 (7/40)	11.5 (3/26)	Age: 20–30: 30.8 (4/13); over 30: 24.2 (102/422)
Severe dysplasia, Linxian	29	80.0 (8/10)	-	57.9 (11/19)
Esophageal cancer, early and intermediate stages	83	80.0 (32/40) (early stage)	70.8 (17/24)	68.4 (13/19)
Esophageal cancer, advanced stage after therapy	49	-	48.0 (12/25) (Linxian)	45.8 (11/24) (Ritan Hospital)
Total	979	130	115	734

[a] *IF,* indirect immunofluorescence; *IP,* indirect immunoperoxidase; *Aggl.,* cell agglutination test

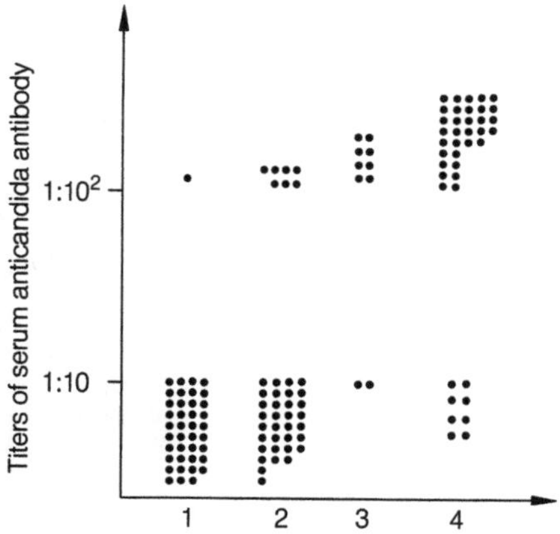

Fig. 3.13. Comparison of levels of anti-*Candida* antibody titers found in sera of different groups of individuals using the indirect immunofluorescence technique. *1* Beijing controls; *2* Linxian controls; *3* Linxian severe dysplasia patients; *4* Linxian early esophageal carcinoma patients

high-incidence area (Linxian) than in a low-incidence area (Beijing). Since patients with severe dysplasia, which is a premalignant lesion, have a very high proportion of *Candida* infections, we suspect that the infection is an etiologic factor rather than a secondary complication. The high incidence of esophageal carcinoma in Linxian might be related in part to the higher incidence of *Candida* infections. There is some evidence that chronic *Candida* infection might induce dysplastic, even malignant changes of the infected epithelial cells. Kugelman et al. [13] followed up a patient with cutaneous candidiasis complicated with esophageal candidiasis from the age of 14 until the patient died of esophageal cancer at 38. They suspected that the cancer had developed from the chronic candidiasis. Cawson [14] followed up ten patients with chronic oral candidiasis and found that no less than six of them developed oral cancer. Preliminary experiments [15] showed that when extracts of *C. albicans* was injected into mice, the incidence of leukemia, lung tumor, breast cancer, and sarcoma were higher than in the control group.

Studies of the possible role of the pathogenic fungi which invade the esophagus may be a new and important approach to carcinogenesis.

6 Prospective Studies of Etiologic Relationship of Candida Infection to Dysplasia and Cancer of the Esophagus

In order to investigate whether *Candida* infection of esophagus has etiologic importance or not, we carried out a preliminary prospective study in two production brigades with high incidences of esophageal cancer in Linxian county [12]. Anti-*Candida* antibody titers of sera from 300 randomly selected inhabitants above the age of 26 were determined by the cell agglutination technique. Seventy-two (24%) had titers of 1:16 or more, which was considered to be significant under our experimental conditions. Of These 72 subjects, 48 permitted further cytologic examinations of the esophagus, X-ray examinations also being done when necessary. All 48 proved to have esophagitis, mostly moderate or severe. Four had squamous esophageal carcinoma; two were in the early stage (Figs. 3.14, 3.15), one in the intermediate stage, and one in the advanced stage (Table 3.2). Another three were suspected to have cancer on cytology but no definite lesions were found on X-ray. Thirty-two subjects had severe dysplasia and seven had mild dysplasia of the esophageal epithelium.

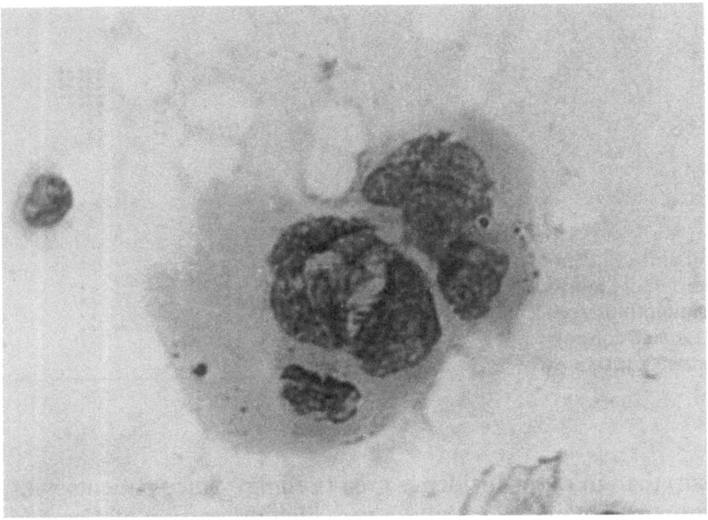

Fig. 3.14. Cancer cells in a cytologic smear from a 44-year-old female patient who had no symptoms but was found to have a significant anti-*Candida* antibody titer during a prospective study

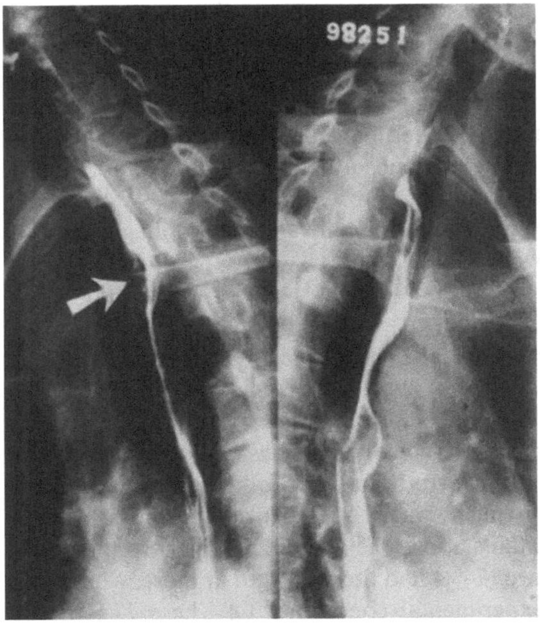

Fig. 3.15. Barium swallow in the same patient as in Fig. 3.14, showing a filling defect about 3 cm long in the upper *segment of the esophagus,* diagnosed as esophageal carcinoma

In the group of patients with *Candida* esophagitis there were 8.3% of newly detected esophageal cancer patients. This incidence was much than that in individuals with normal esophageal epithelium in the high-incidence area. Of the 48 patients with *Candida* esophagitis, 81.3% had cancer or precancerous lesions and 14.6% had mild dysplasia. From this study it is believed that *Candida* esophagitis may be one of the important

Table 3.2. Clinical data from four cases of esophageal carcinoma detected among 48 subjects with high *Candida* agglutinin titers

No.	Sex	Age	X-ray findings	Clinical stage
1	M	63	Irregularities of mucosa	Very early
2	F	44	Filling defect 3 cm long	Early
3	M	71	Filling defect 4 cm long	Intermediate
4	M	59	Filling defect 7–8 cm long	Advanced

Table 3.3. Effect of *Candida albicans* on pH of media and formation of NBMA from its precursors

Exp. No.	pH	Components	Cells ($\times 10^7$)	Incubation (h)	Conc. buffer (*M*)	NBMA (μg/5 ml)
1	6.8	MBA + $NaNO_2$	–	48	0.08	30.7 ± 5.1
		MBA + $NaNO_2$ + living *Candida*	7.4	48	0.08	62.1 ± 3.3
		cells	26	48	0.08	110.2 ± 22.6
		MBA + $NaNO_2$ + conditioned medium	–	48	0.08	34.1 ± 18.9
		MBA + $NaNO_2$ + boiled *Candida* cells	7.4	48	0.08	32.0 ± 4.0
2	7.4	MBA + $NaNO_2$	–	24	0.12	1.9 ± 0.1
	7.4 (decreased to 7.2[a])	MBA + $NaNO_2$	–	48	0.038	8.4 ± 2.7
	7.4 (decreased to 6.1[a])	MBA + $NaNO_2$ + living *Candida* cells	12.0	48	0.038	121.3 ± 19.6
3	8.0 (at end of incubation)	MBA + $NaNO_2$	–	48	without buffer	1.3
	6.8 (at end of incubation)	MBA + $NaNO_2$ + living *Candida* cells	4.5	48	without buffer	75.0

[a] pH change after incubation for 48 h

pathogenic factors in esophageal cancer in Linxian. Besides the etiologic significance, serum anti-*Candida* antibody titer can possibly be used as a simple and acceptable screening test for early detection of esophageal cancer and precancerous lesions in high-incidence areas. Further prospective studies on a larger population are in progress.

7 Interaction of Fungi and Nitrosamines

Three possible roles of fungal esophagitis in esophageal carcinogenesis can be postulated:

1. The esophagitis might induce a chronic persistent inflammation that stimulates the basal cells to become hyperplastic. DNA synthesis is increased during hyperplasia, and so the susceptibility to carcinogens is increased.

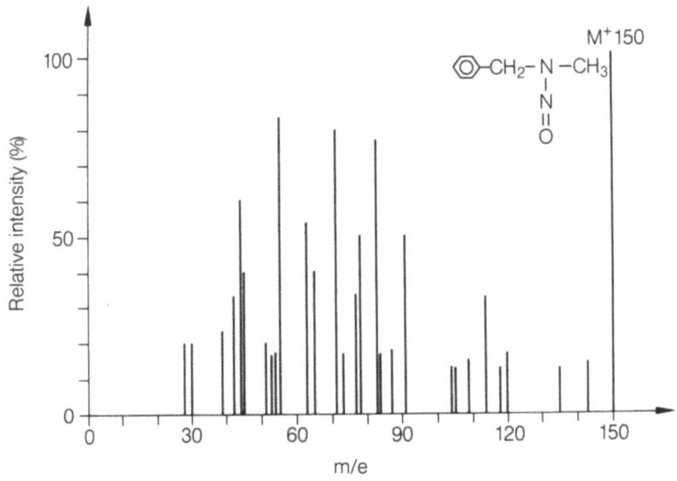

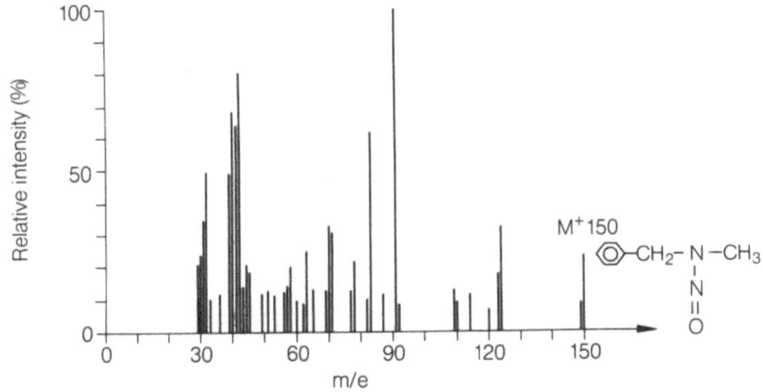

Fig. 3.16. *Above:* Mass spectroscopy of NBMA formed in culture of *Candida albicans* with MBA and $NaNO_2$: m/e fragment ions with 30, 42, 77, 91, 120 and M^+150. *Below:* Mass spectroscopy of standard NBMA

2. The fungi and bacteria that colonize the esophageal epithelium might enhance the endogenous synthesis of nitrosamines or other carcinogens in situ.
3. The metabolites of fungi invading the epithelium might have acted directly on the epithelium, causing necrosis or hyperplasia.

Our recent studies [16] support the second possibility. When *C. albicans* was cultured with benzylmethylamine (MBA) and $NaNO_2$, the *Candida* significantly enhanced the formation of benzylmethylnitrosamine (NBMA) in vitro (Table 3.3). The identity of the NBMA formed in a culture of *Candida* with MBA and nitrite was confirmed by coelution in three HPLC solvent systems with standard NBMA and by mass spectroscopy of the isolated material (Fig. 3.16). NBMA has been proved to be a strong esophageal carcinogen in rodents [17]. *C. albicans* could cause a 30- to 50-fold enhancement of rate of formation of NBMA from its precursors when there was no buffer or only a low concentration of

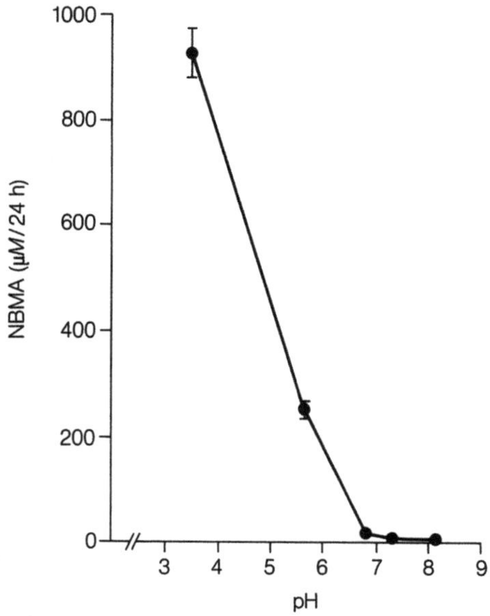

Fig. 3.17. Formation of NBMA from its precursors at different pH levels

buffer in the media. The *Candida* enhanced nitrosation by two separate additive mechanisms: decreases in pH through production of acidic metabolites, and cell-mediated catalysis. *C. albicans* produces various acidic metabolites that cause a decrease of the pH of the media. The nitrosation of NBMA depends significantly on pH (Fig. 3.17). At pH values above 7.4, the amounts of NBMA detected were very low, near the limits of sensitivity of the methods employed. Significantly increasing levels of NBMA formation were found over the pH range of 7.4–3.5 (2.6 μM/24 h at pH 7.4, 928 μM/24 h at pH 3.5). When *Candida* was cultured with MBA and $NaNO_2$, the pH of the media decreased from 7.4 to 6.1 and NBMA formation increased about 30 times more than in precursors-only controls at pH 7.4 (Table 3.3 Exp. 2). With pH controlled at 6.8, the presence of *C. albicans* in either the stationary or the exponential phase of growth enhanced the formation of NBMA two- to fourfold compared with precursors-only control cultures. The amount of NBMA formed depended on the number of cells. The nitrosating activity of the cells was destroyed by boiling them (Table 3.3, Fig. 3.18). The conditioned medium in which *Candida* cells had been cultured for 48–68 h and then removed by filtration did not enhance nitrosation at controlled pH (Fig. 3.18). These experiments suggest that *Candida* may have a cell-mediated nitrosating activity which requires live *Candida* cells. We suggest an enzymatic catalysis. The total enhancement of NBMA formation depends on the combined effects of cell-mediated nitrosation and reduction in pH. The fungi infecting the esophageal epithelium could cause epithelial cell destruction and protein dissociation, thus leading to accumulation of diamines in the esophageal tissue. Many species of bacteria and some fungi may reduce nitrate to nitrite, and some of them may enhance formation of nitrosamines [18, 19]. It is possible that there may be accumulations of precursors of some nitrosamines in foci of infection in esophageal epithelium. The effect of fungal infections on local epithelial pH is not known. Experimental irritative exudates may have a pH of 6.95 [20]. When esophageal mucosa is heavily infected with *Candida,* the epithelium is highly thickened without blood vessels, acidic products may accumulate, and a pH as low as 6.8

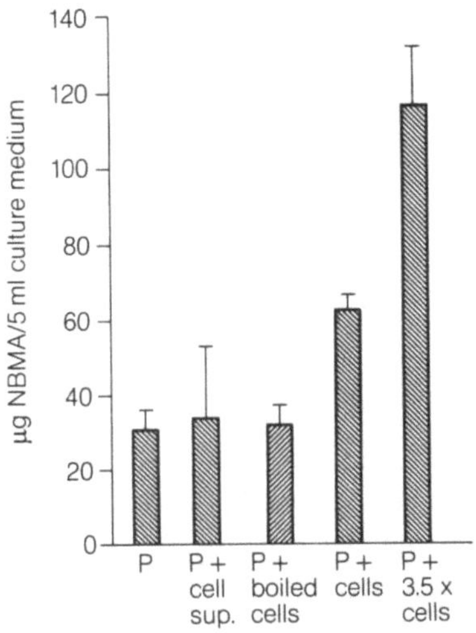

Fig. 3.18. NBMA formation at different conditions with pH controlled at 6.8. *P.* precursors only; *P+cell sup,* precursors + conditioned medium; *P+cells,* precursors + 7.4 × 10^7 *Candida* cells, *P+3.5 × cells,* precursors + 26 × 10^7 *Candida* cells

seems possible. The combined effects of cell-mediated nitrosation and reduction of pH of the epithelial fluid from 7.4 to 6.8 could cause a 30- to 50-fold enhancement of rate of formation of NBMA from its precursors. Generation of nitrosamine in close proximity to the target tissue, especially under conditions of poor fluid circulation, could result in a concentration sufficient to initiate tumorigenesis. Initiation of tumorigenesis by carcinogen in situ is much more efficient than by carcinogens ingested with food or water. We believe that the foci of fungal and bacterial infection in esophageal epithelium might be one of the sites of endogenous synthesis of nitrosamines or other carcinogens. The new approaches to in situ formation of carcinogen and its local action on target cells deserve further study.

8 Organ Culture as a Model for Carcinogenesis Study: Effects of Mycotoxins and Nitrosamines on Esophageal Epithelium

Organ culture is an important recently developed model system for carcinogenesis studies. Whether the extrapolation of data from experimental animals to human beings is reasonable remains to be determined. The organ culture technique offers the possibility of studying the direct effects of chemical carcinogens, fungi, and mycotoxins on the human esophagus, and has also been used in studying the metabolism of carcinogens.

The technique for long-term organ culture of esophageal mucosa has only recently been perfected. Hillman et al. [21] were able to maintain human adult esophageal mucosa for 5 weeks to 6 months. We have succeeded in culturing explants of human fetal esophagus for up to about 3 months (Fig. 3.19) [22]. Stoner et al. [23] cultured rat esophagus for a period of 28 days both in serum-free medium and in medium containing 5% heat-inactivated fetal bovine serum.

We have suggested that infection of the esophagus by pathogenic fungi is one of the modes of action. Another may be the effects of toxic or carcinogenic mycotoxins or metabolites of fungi commonly contaminating food or drinking water in high-incidence areas. *Fusarium* is the most common genus of fungi contaminating cereals in Linxian

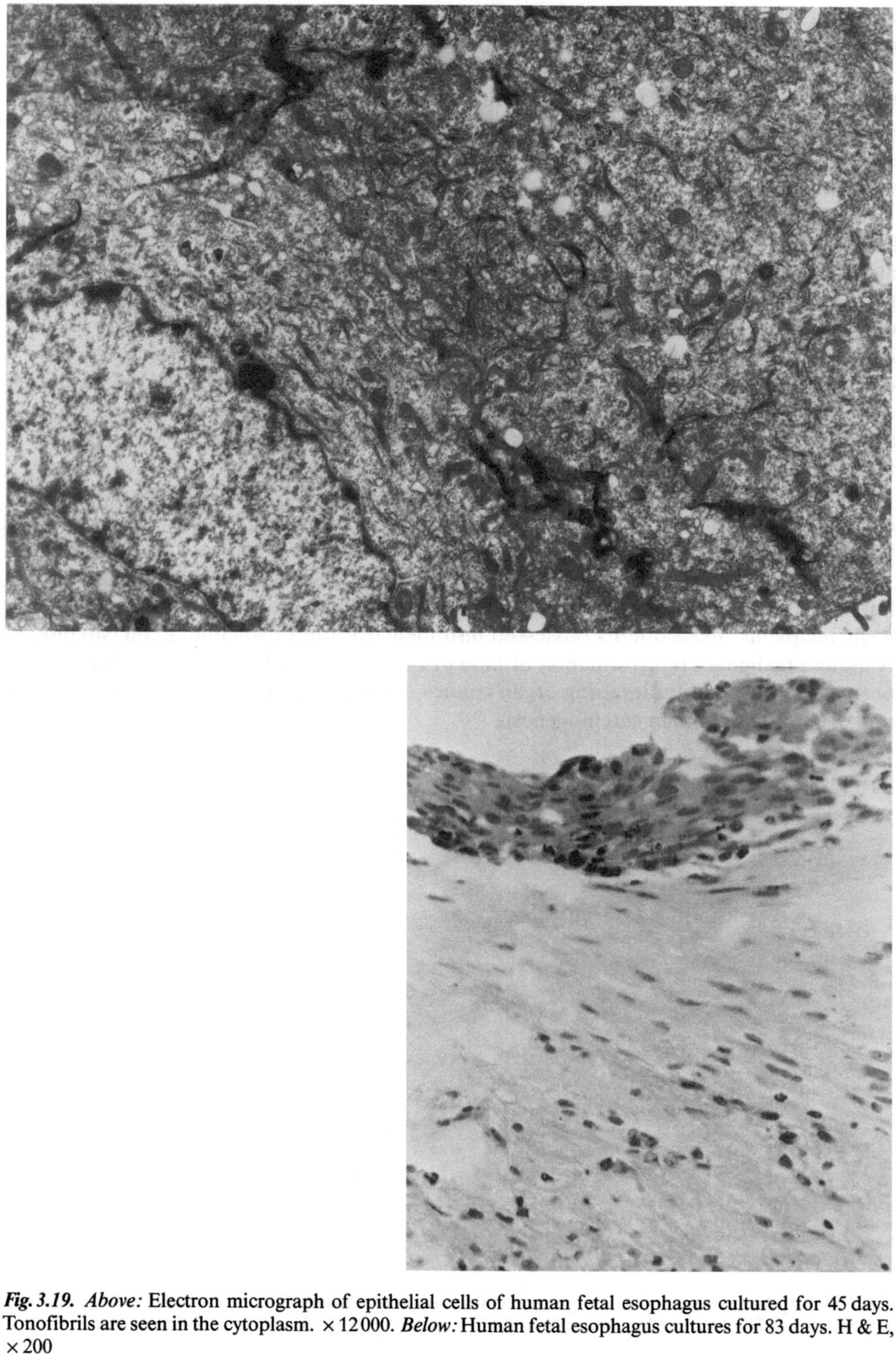

Fig. 3.19. *Above:* Electron micrograph of epithelial cells of human fetal esophagus cultured for 45 days. Tonofibrils are seen in the cytoplasm. × 12000. *Below:* Human fetal esophagus cultures for 83 days. H & E, × 200

county. Ingestion of corn infected with *Fusarium sporotrichiella* induced forestomach papilloma in rats [24]. T-2 toxin, a kind of trichothecene produced by various species of *Fusarium*, caused inflammation and necrosis of the oral mucosa in chickens [25]. Intragastric administration of T-2 toxin induced tumors of various organs and hyperplasia of basal epithelial cells of the esophagus in rats [26]. Recent studies showed that T-2 toxin caused single-strand DNA breaks in lymphocytes [27]. T-2 toxin is suspected to exist in *Fusarium*-contaminated cereals in Linxian.

We tested the effects of T-2 toxin on organ culture of human adult and fetal esophagus [22]. When larger doses (5 ng/ml medium for 4–6 days) were used, necrosis and desquamation of the epithelial cells usually occurred. With smaller doses (0.2–1.2 ng/ml medium for 6 days), proliferative effects could be observed in about 60% of cases. The proliferation of basal cells is impressive; they form papillae or cords extending downward into the lamina propria (Fig. 3.20, 3.21). Dysplasia may be observed in about 50% of the cases. Atypical mitosis (Fig. 3.22), an increase in the number of mitotic figures, enlarged nuclei, hyperchromatism, and prominent nucleoli are often seen in the esophageal epithelium after the application of T-2 toxin. In some cases, superficial desquamation and basal cell proliferation can be observed at the same segment of esophageal epithelium.

Autrup and Stoner [28] observed that NBMA has a very high level of metabolite binding to DNA of rat esophagus. Stoner et al. [29], using an explant/cell culture system, found that rat esophageal epithelial cells were transformed in vitro by exposure to NBMA. Cell lines could only be established from the NBMA-treated explants. Two cell lines were able to grow in soft agar and produce palpable tumors upon injection into syngenic recipients; these tumors possessed histologic features of squamous cell carcinoma. Although malignant transformation of human esophageal epithelium in vitro has not yet been accomplished, studies using organ culture of human tissues promise to increase our understanding of human carcinogenesis.

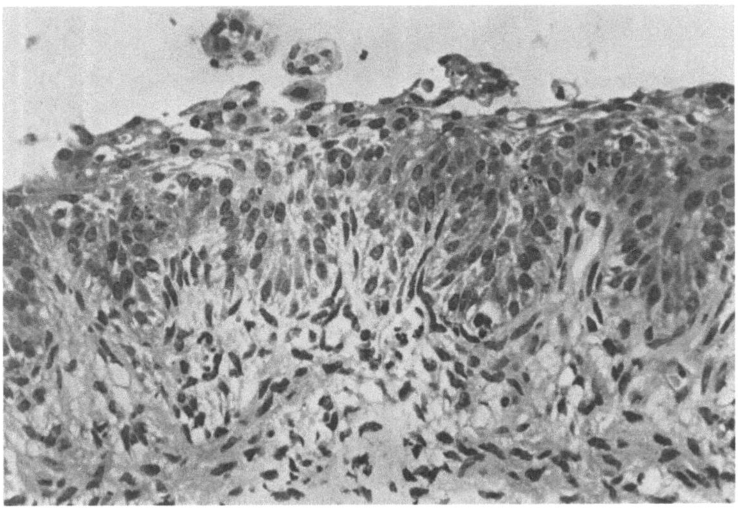

Fig. 3.20. Explants of human fetal esophageal epithelium after action by T-2 toxin (0.4 ng/ml) for 6 days in organ culture. The basal cells proliferate to form papillae growing downwards. 10-day culture. H & E, ×200

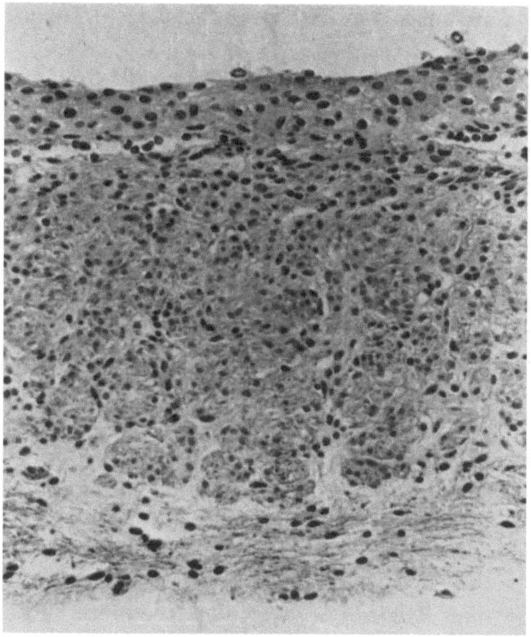

Fig. 3.21. Light micrograph of epithelium of organ culture of human fetal esophagus. Control (10-day culture) for that shown in Fig. 3.20. H & E, ×200

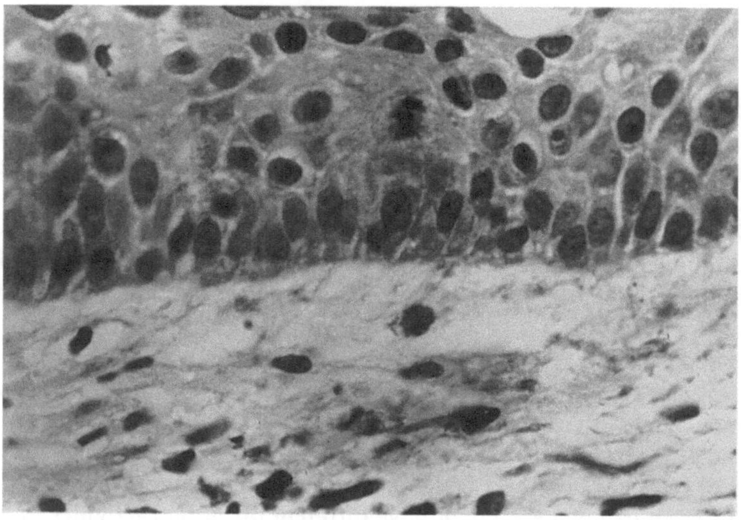

Fig. 3.22. Atypical mytosis seen in fetal esophageal epithelium after action by T-2 toxin. H & E, ×400

9 Carcinogen Metabolism in Esophageal Tissues and Cells

Study of the metabolism of different carcinogens in human esophageal tissues and cells contributes to the understanding of human carcinogenesis. Most chemical carcinogens are inactive per se and require biotransformation in tissues to become active. There are three groups of enzymes related to carcinogen metabolism.

Cytochrome P-450 and Mixed Function Oxidases. Mixed function oxidases are a class of enzymes involved in the biotransformation and oxidative activation of chemical carcinogens and other exogenous compounds. They are located primarily in the endoplasmic reticulum and contain one or more of the various forms of cytochrome P-450 and the associated electron transport enzymes such as NADPH cytochrome P-450 reductase, cytochrome b_5, and NADH cytochrome b_5 reductase.

Epoxide Hydrolase. This enzyme plays an important role in the activation and deactivation of chemical carcinogens and toxic compounds. It catalyzes the formation of *trans*-dihydrodiols from epoxides initially formed by the mixed function oxidases. Epoxide hydrolase activity has been detected in many human tissues.

Enzymes Related to Conjugation Reactions. These enzymes, such as glucuronyl transferase, sulfotransferase, and glutathione transferase, have detoxifying action. They convert the primary metabolites into water-soluble and less toxic metabolites that can be excreted more easily. Conjugation of toxic metabolites is an integral part of the cellular defense mechanism against environmental carcinogens. The activity of the detoxifying enzymes might be related to differences in susceptibility to carcinogens in various animal species, including man.

Until recently, metabolism of only a few carcinogens, including benzo[*a*]pyrene (B*a*P), aflatoxin B_1, and some nitrosamines, had been studied in human esophageal tissues [30, 31]. The range of variation of water-soluble metabolites of B*a*P in different segments of esophagus in the same individual was narrow (twofold), while that among different segments from different donors was very wide (68-fold). The pattern of organic metabolites of B*a*P is similar in the three anatomic segments of the esophagus. The binding level of B*a*P to protein was greater than to DNA; the interindividual variations were 99-fold for binding to DNA and ninefold for binding to protein. The major B*a*P-DNA adducts found in the esophageal mucosa resulted from a *trans* addition of the 2-amino group of guanine to the 10-position of$(\pm)$-$(7\beta,8\alpha)$-dihydroxy-$(9\alpha,10\alpha)$-epoxy-7,8,9,10-tetrahydrobenzo(*a*)-pyrene (BPDE 1) [30, 31].

When either [^{14}C]dimethylnitrosamine (DMNA) or [^{14}C]nitrosopyrrolidine (NPY) was incubated with explants of esophagus, radioactivity was tightly bound to cellular protein, but only metabolites of DMNA were bound to DNA of human esophagus. NPY metabolites were not bound to DNA of human esophageal mucosa [31]. These data suggest that different carcinogens might have different metabolic activities in human esophagus. The electrophilic metabolites (methyl carbonium ions) of DMNA methylate DNA bases. Three methylated bases were identified: 0^6-methylguanine, 3-methyladenine, and 7-methylguanine. The binding levels of DMNA to DNA varied widely and ranged from nondetectable quantities to 1109 pmol/10 mg DNA. The human esophagus has the metabolic ability to activate compounds from three classes of environmental chemical procarcinogens, i.e., polynuclear aromatic hydrocarbons (B*a*P), mycotoxins (aflatoxin B_1) and

N-nitrosamines (DMNA) into electrophilic metabolites that bind to cellular DNA and protein. 0^6-Methylguanine could lead to base mispairing during DNA synthesis and thus may be an important factor in mutagenesis and carcinogenesis. The importance of this methylated base in carcinogenesis of the human esophagus remains to be determined. The major carcinogen-DNA adducts of B*a*P and DMNA are identical to those found on human bronchus and colon. The metabolic pathways are similar to those found in experimental animals susceptible to these carcinogens (B*a*P, aflatoxin B_1, and DMNA).

There are not only interindividual but also interspecies variations in *N*-nitrosamine metabolism. Variations of carcinogen metabolism in various animals are wide, and binding levels of DMNA, diethylnitrosamine (DENA), NBMA with DNA of esophagus are much higher in rats than in human beings [32]. NPY has a very high binding level with DNA of rat esophagus, but binding is almost undetectable in human esophagus,

10 Multifactorial and Multistage Hypothesis

Carcinogenesis is now generally recognized as a multistage process [33, 34]. The first stage, known as initiation, occurs rapidly and is essentially irreversible. The initiated cells cannot be recognized directly. The second stage, called promotion, requires much longer than initiation, and appears to be reversible in the early phase. Some chemicals have essentially only initiating activity and others act primarily as promoters. Under the effect of promoters, initiated cells can develop into tumor cells. Most carcinogens appear to be complete, i.e., have both initiating and promoting activity. The relative amounts of initiating and promoting activity may vary widely for different complete carcinogens.

Most chemical carcinogens are not ultimate carcinogens when they enter the human body, but require metabolic activation [35, 36], which may consist of one or several steps. Proximate carcinogens may be formed as intermediate metabolites, and inactive metabolites may also be generated. Carcinogenicity is related in part to the ratio of active carcinogenic products to inactive metabolites.

The chemical which are active in initiation usually have the characteristic of being strong electrophilic reactants: they are positive or uncharged molecules with electron-deficient atoms which react by sharing electron-pairs of electron-rich atoms such as S, O, and N. These reactants are typified by the alkylating agents.

When electrophils react with DNA, the structure of the DNA may be changed such that mutations will occur. It has been accepted that the initiation step is usually a mutagenic event, and DNA would be the target of the electrophils for initiation. However, mutation may not be the only basis for initiation [37, 38].

On the basis of our studies in Linxian county, we suspect that esophageal carcinogenesis is multifactorial and multistage: esophageal carcinoma may be the end result of the combined effects of several etiologic factors. We suggest a hypothesis for carcinogenesis as diagrammed in Fig. 3.23. There is first a background disease, followed later by the initiation and promotion stages. Due to the presence of the background disease, the basal cells of the epithelium are usually hyperplastic, and the synthesis of DNA may thus increase. When the double chains of DNA dissociate, they are more susceptible to the action of carcinogens and there is a greater danger of mutation.

Initiating agents may come from two sources: (a) foci of fungal infection in the esophageal mucosa, and (b) carcinogens or their precursors in food or drinking water. The initiators may act at the weak point of the esophagus, probably the background lesions, induc-

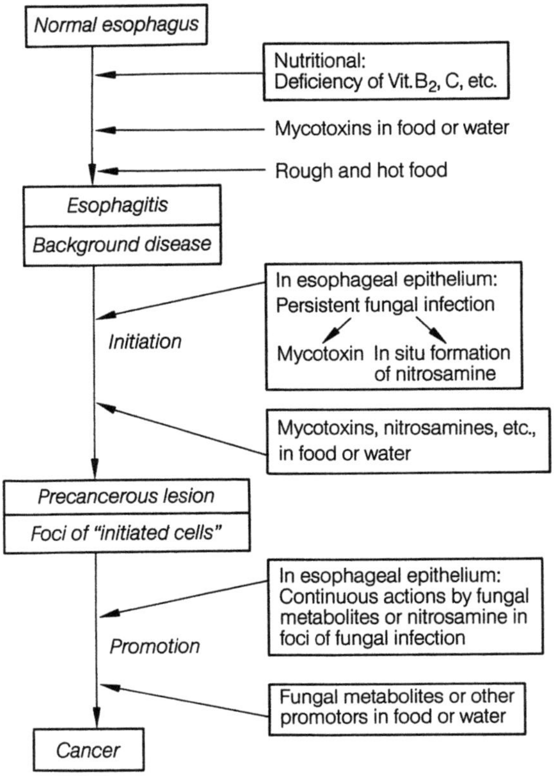

Fig. 3.23. Hypothesis for multifactorial and multistage esophageal carcinogenesis in Linxian county

ing foci of initiated cells. These cells are difficult to identify. They will not develop into a tumor unless stimulated by promoters. We consider initiated cells to be latent cancerous lesions; whether they are identical with the precancerous cells as we see in cytologic smears remains uncertain. Promoters may also come from the two above-mentioned sources.

Nutritional factors probably play a role before initiation, but they may also have some influence on the initiation process. For example, vitamin C might block the endogenous synthesis of nitrosamines, and vitamin A might to some extent protect DNA from the action of chemical carcinogens.

It is plain that esophageal carcinogenesis is extremely complicated, and much work remains to be done.

References

1. Xia QJ, Wang KC, Zue WT, LU SC (1978) Fungal infections of esophagus and esophageal carcinoma. In: Scientific reports from 1958–1978, Cancer Institute, Chinese Academy of Medical Sciences, Beijing, pp 860–867
2. Sheng C, Chiu SL, Liu FY, Lian TS (1964) Preliminary clinicopathological analysis of esophagitis in Linxian county, Henan province (in Chinese). Chin J Pathol [Suppl] 8: 407–409
3. Crespi M, Grassi A, Amiri G, Munoz N, Aramesh B, Mojtabai A (1979) Esophageal lesions in northern Iran: a premalignant condition? Lancet 2: 217–221
4. Kay EB, Cross FS (1956) Chronic esophagitis – a possible factor in the production of carcinoma of the esophagus. Arch Intern Med 98: 475–481
5. Savary M, Miller G (1978) The esophagus. Handbook and atlas of endoscopy. Gassmann, Solothurn
6. The Coordinating Groups for the Research of Esophageal Carcinoma, Henan Province and Chinese Academy of Medical Sciences (1975) Studies on relationship between epithelial dysplasia and carcinoma of the esophagus (in Chinese). Chin Med J 1: 110–116
7. Howell-Evans AW, McConnell RB, Clark CA, Shappard PM (1958) Carcinoma of the esophagus with keratosis palmaris et plantaris (tylosis): a study of two families. Q J Med 27: 413–429
8. Naef AP, Savary M, Ozzello L (1975) Columnar-lined lower esophagus, an acquired lesion with malignant predisposition. Report on 140 cases of Barrett's esophagus with 12 adenocarcinomas. J Thorac Cardiovasc Surg 70: 826–835
9. Xia QJ, Cao IY (1978) Fungal invasions in esophageal tissues and its possible relation to esophageal carcinoma (In Chinese) Natl Med J China 58: 392–396
10. Xia QJ, Sun ZT, Lu SC (1979) Determination of anticandida antibody titer by indirect immuno-fluorescence and its application in studying esophageal carcinoma (in Chinese). Chin J Oncol 1: 190–194
11. Wang YY, Xia QJ, Lu SC, Sun ZT (1982) Determination of the titer and classes of anticandida antibody in serum of esophageal cancer patients by indirect immunoperoxidase technique (in Chinese). Chin J Oncol 4: 86–88
12. Xia QJ, Cao SK, Zing TS, Lu SC (1984) Studies on the relation of *Candida* infection and esophageal carcinoma (in Chinese). Chin J Oncol 6: 168
13. Kugelman TP, Cripps DJ, Harrell ER (1963) *Candida* granuloma with epidermophytosis. Arch Dermatol 88: 150–157
14. Cawson RA (1959) Leukoplakia and oral cancer. Proc R Soc Med 62: 610–614
15. Blank F, Chi O, Just G, Meranze DR, Shimkin MB, Wieder R (1968) Carcinogens from fungi pathogenic for man. Cancer Res 28: 2276–2281
16. Xia QJ, Sun ZT, Wang YY, Anderson LM, Armstrong D, Good RA (1981) Enhancement of formation of the esophageal carcinogen benzylmethylnitrosamine from its precursors by *Candida albicans*. Proc Natl Acad Sci USA 78: 1878–1881
17. Druckrey H, Preussmann, Ivankovic S, Schmähl D (1967) Organotrope carcinogene Wirkungen bei 65 verschiedenen *N*-nitroso-Verbindungen an bd-Ratten. Z Krebsforsch 69: 103–201
18. Ayanaba A, Alexander M (1973) Microbial formation of nitrosamines in vitro. Appl. Microbiol 25: 862–868
19. Uibu J, Bogovsk P, Tauts O (1978) Formation of nitrosodimethylamine by microorganisms used in the baking industry or isolated from the raw materials of bakery products. IARC Sci Publ 19: 247–256
20. Robbins SL (1976) Pathology, 3rd edn. Saunders, Philadelphia
21. Hillman EA, Vocci MJ, Schurch W, Harris CC, Trump BF (1980) Human esophageal organ culture studies. In: Harris CC, Trump BF, Stoner GD (eds) Methods in cell biology, vol. 21. Academic Press, New York London, pp 332–348
22. Xia QJ, Jiang BL, Harris CC (1983) Proliferative and cytotoxic effects of *Fusarium* T-2 toxin on cultured human fetal esophagus. Carcinogenesis 4 (9): 1101–1107
23. Stoner GD, Pettis W, Haugen A, Jackson F, Harris CC (1981) Explant culture of rat esophagus in a chemically defined medium. In Vitro 17: 681–688
24. Chang BG, Heu MC (1965) Observations on papilloma formation in forestomach of rats induced by long-term intubation and feeding cereals inoculated with *Fusarium* (in Chinese). Chin J Pathol 9: 51–53
25. Chi MS, Mirocha CJ (1978) Necrotic oral lesions in chickens fed diacetoxyscirpenol, T-2 toxin and crotocin. Poult Sci 57: 807–808
26. Schoental R, Joffe AZ, Yagen B (1979) Cardiovascular lesions and various tumors found in rats given T-2 toxin, a trichothecene metabolite of *Fusarium*. Cancer Res 39: 2179–2184

27. Lafarge-Frayssinet C, Decloitre F, Mousset S, Martin M, Frayssinet C (1981) Induction of DNA single-strand breaks by T-2 toxin, a trichothecene metabolite of *Fusarium:* effect on lymphoid organs and liver. Mutat Res 88: 115–123
28. Autrup H, Stoner GD (1982) Metabolism of *N*-nitrosamines by cultured human and rat esophagus. Cancer Res 42: 1307–1311
29. Stoner GD, Babcock MS, Cothern GA, Klaunig JE, Gunning WT, Knipe SM (1982) In vitro transformation of rat esophageal epithelial cells with *N*-nitrosobenzylmethylamine. Carcinogenesis 3: 629–634
30. Harris CC, Autrup H, Stoner GD, Trump BF, Hillman E, Schafer PW, Jeffrey AM (1979) Metabolism of benzo[*a*]pyrene, *N*-Nitrosodimethylamine, and *N*-nitrosopyrrolidine and identification of the major carcinogen-DNA adducts formed in cultured human esophagus. Cancer Res 39: 4401–4406
31. Harris CC, Autrup H (1980) Interspecies, interindividual and intertissue variations in benzo[*a*]pyrene metabolism. VDI Ber 358: 293–299
32. Harris CC, Grafstrom RC, Lechner JF, Autrup H (1982) Metabolism of *N*-nitrosamines and repair of DNA damage in cultured human tissues and cells. In: Magee PN (ed) The possible role of *N*-nitrosamines in human cancer. Cold Spring Harbor, New York (Banbury Reports, vol 12, pp 121–139)
33. Berenblum I (1974) Carcinogenesis as a biological problem. North-Holland, Amsterdam Oxford
34. Slaga TJ, Sivak A, Boutwell RK (1978) Mechanisms of tumor promotion and cocarcinogenesis. Raven, New York
35. Miller EC, Miller JA (1976) The mechanism of chemical carcinogens to reactive electrophiles and their possible mechanisms of action in carcinogenesis. In: Searle CE (ed) Chemical carcinogens. American Chemical Society, Washington (American Chemical Society Monograph no 173, pp 737–762)
36. Miller JA, Miller EC (1979) Perspectives on the metabolism of chemical carcinogens. In: Emmelot P, Kriek E (eds) Environmental carcinogenesis. Elsevier Biomedical, Amsterdam, pp 25–50
37. Robin H (1980) Is somatic mutation the major mechanism of malignant transformation? J Natl. Cancer Inst 64: 995–1000
38. Weinstein IB, Yamasaki H, Wigler M, Lee LS, Fisher PB, Jeffrey A, Grunberger D (1978) Molecular and cellular events associated with the action of initiating carcinogens and tumor promoters. In: Griffin AC, Shaw CR (eds) Carcinogens, identidication and mechanisms of action. Raven, New York, pp 399–418

Chapter 4
Pathology of Carcinoma of the Esophagus

Fu Sheng Liu and Chuan Nong Zhou

1 Distribution and Site

1.1 Age

Carcinoma of the esophagus is largely a disease of late middle and old age. It is rare in patients below 30 years, and the incidence gradually increases with age. Postlethwait and Sealy [1] reviewed 9244 cases from the literature and found that 2755 of these patients (29.8%) were aged 50–59 years and 3121 (33.8%) were aged 60–69 years. Li et al. [2] analyzed 1831 esophageal cancer patients from three provinces in northern China and also found the highest incidence in the age-groups 50–59 years (618 cases, 33.8%) and 60–69 years (593 cases, 32.4%).

1.2 Sex

Carcinoma of the esophagus is more common in men, but the male to female ratios reported in the literature vary. Kiviranta [3] surveyed data from various countries totalling over 12000 cases and found that esophageal cancer always occurred more often in males, with ratios ranging from 2:1 to 20:1. In material collected from the literature, Postlethwait and Sealy [1, p 350] found 10519 male cases and 4044 female cases, a ratio of 2.6:1.

A similar situation has been demonstrated in China. According to Li et al. [2] the ratio varies from 1.3:1 to 2.7:1. A recent epidemiologic investigation [4] in an area in northern China covering a population of 50 million showed that the ratios average between 1.6:1 and 1:1 and that the higher the mortality in a locality, the smaller the ratio. These data differ clearly from the literature reports based on clinical and pathological material, presumably reflecting the true situation more closely.

1.3 Site

The site distributions of carcinoma of the esophagus reported in the literature differ greatly due to variation in methods. Palmer [5] collected 11037 cases of esophageal cancer from the literature and found that the lesion was in the upper third of the organ in 2418 cases (21.9%), the middle third in 3861 cases (35.0%), and the lower third in 4758 cases (43.1%). The high incidence in the distal third of the esophagus is probably due to the inclusion of cancer of the gastric cardia by some authors. Postlethwait and Sealy [1, p. 351] recently collected 14181 cases from the literature and found that the lesion was located in the upper third in 2174 cases (15.33%), the middle third in 7299 cases (51.47%), and the lower third in 4708 cases (33.20%). Giuli and Gignoux [6] reported the results of a study based on the records of 22 surgical teams: there were 106 carcinomas (5.8%) of the upper third, 926 (50.9%) of the middle third, and 789 (43.3%) of the lower third.

It has been shown that esophageal cancer in China is most frequently located in the middle third. In a collected group [7] of 4957 cases, the lesion was in the upper third in 699 cases (14.1%), the middle third in 2612 cases (52.7%), and the lower third in 1646 cases (33.2%). Liu [8] analyzed 858 surgical specimens and revealed that the lesion was in the upper third in 24 (2.8%), the middle third in 500 (58.3%), and the lower third in 334 (38.9%). The data obtained from surgical material may not be accurate, as tumors located in the lower third of the esophagus are usually more amenable to surgery than those located higher.

Table 4.1. Site distribution of carcinomas in the esophagus

Authors	Source of material	Total cases	Site		
			Upper third	Middle third	Lower third
Palmer [5]	Literature	11037	2418 (21.9)	3861 (35.0)	4758 (43.1)
Postlethwait and Sealy [1]	Literature	14181	2174 (15.3)	7299 (51.5)	4708 (33.2)
Giuli and Gignoux [6]	Surgery	1821	106 (5.8)	926 (50.9)	789 (43.3)
Sun and Wu [7]	Surgery	4957	699 (14.1)	2612 (52.7)	1646 (33.2)
Liu [8]	Pathology	858	24 (2.8)	500 (58.3)	334 (38.9)
Yin et al. [9]	Radiotherapy	3798	225 (5.9)	825 (21.7)[a] 2370 (62.4)[b]	378 (10.0)
Linxian County Hospital [10]	Balloon cytology, esophagoscopy, and X-ray	3633	426 (11.7)	2301 (63.3)	906 (25.0)

Figures in parentheses are percentages.
[a] Upper thoracic segment
[b] Middle thoracic segment

Some data are based on analysis of patients treated by radiation. For example, in a series of 3798 cases from the Cancer Institute of the Chinese Academy of Medical Sciences [9], the cancer was in the cervical segment in 225 cases (5.9%), the upper thoracic segment in 825 cases (21.7%), the middle thoracic segment in 2370 cases (62.4%), and the lower thoracic segment in 378 cases (10.0%). Such analyses may also be inaccurate, because carcinomas of the cervical and supra-aortic portions of the esophagus are often chosen for radiotherapy, while lesions in the lower third are more often treated by surgery. Besides, most of the radiation-treated patients are in the late stage of the disease, when the tumor can be so large that it is difficult to determine its initial site.

It seems likely that site distribution data obtained from a combination of surgical, pathological, and X-ray examinations will be more accurate.

In recent years, a method combining balloon cytology with esophagoscopy and X-ray examination has been employed in the diagnosis of esophageal cancer in high-incidence areas in China. It is evident that the site distribution is more likely to be determined accurately by this method. In a group of 3633 cases from Linxian County Hospital [10], the tumor was located in the upper third of the esophagus in 426 cases (11.7%), the middle third in 2301 cases (63.4%), and the lower third in 906 cases (24.9%).

Table 4.1 shows some data on the distribution of carcinoma in different segments of the esophagus.

2 Clinicopathological Typing

Several typing and staging classifications of carcinomas of the esophagus are reported in the literature. Schenken and Burns [11] classified carcinomas of the esophagus into ulcerative, fungating, scirrhous, and intraepidermoid types. Palmer [5, p.376–386] suggested that most esophageal cancers fall rather readily into four groups: polypoid, fungating, ulcerative, and infiltrating. Gowing [12] divided carcinomas of the esophagus into crateriform, fungating, and desmoplastic stenosing types. Takahashi [13] classified the lesions into sclerosing, proliferating, and lymphatic infiltrating types, based on the criteria used in gastric cancer typing. Miller [14], referring to the criteria used by Dukes in analyzing the extent of spread of carcinoma of the rectum, divided carcinomas of the esophagus into stages I, II, III (−), III (+), and IV.

2.1 *Gross Types in the Early Stage*

With the advances in diagnostic techniques, more cases of early esophageal carcinoma have been detected [15–17]. Four types can be distinguished: occult, erosive, plaque-like, and papillary.

Occult. The mucosa in the cancerous area is neither protruded nor depressed, corresponding in thickness to the normal esophageal mucosa. In nonfixed specimens, the diseased mucosa appears pink in color and the capillaries are dilated and congested. In fixed speci-

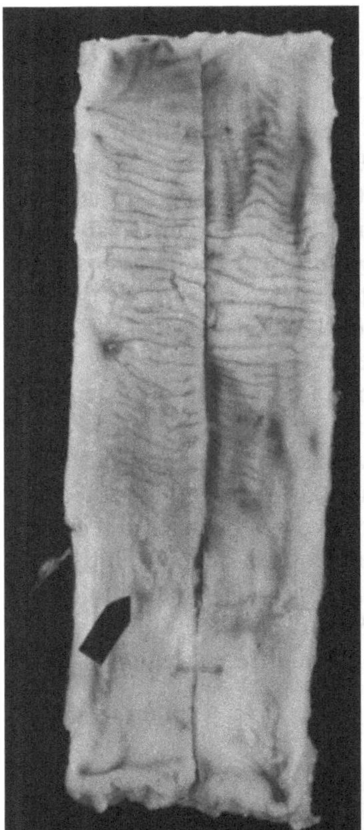

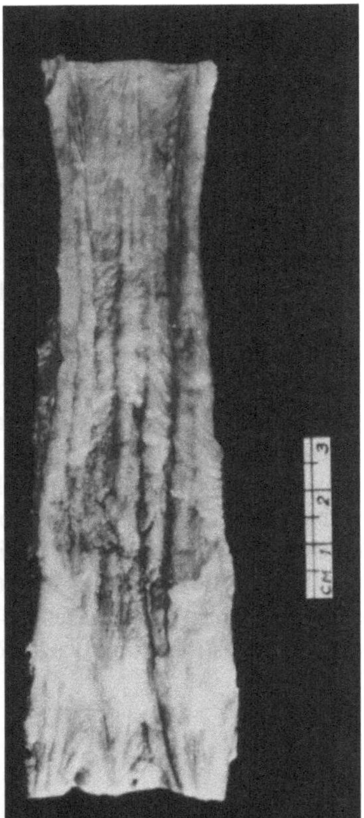

Fig. 4.1 *(left).* Early esophageal carcinoma, occult type. The lesion is small and its boundary is indistinct *(arrow)*

Fig. 4.2 *(right).* Early esophageal carcinoma, erosive type. The lesion is map-like with irregular margins but sharply demarcated from the normal mucosa mens, however, the lesion is hardly perceptible to the naked eye, and its properties and location can only be determined microscopically. Early esophageal carcinoma of this type is rarely seen in surgical material (Fig. 4.1).

Erosive. The esophageal mucosa at the cancer site is slightly depressed or mildly eroded. The lesion is map-like, with irregular margins but sharply demarcated from the normal mucosa. The depressed area of the lesion is finely granular with occasional islets of normal mucosa. Superficial defects of the mucosa may be seen on the cut surface. This type is quite often seen among surgically resected early esophageal carcinomas (Fig. 4.2).

Plaque-Like. The involved esophageal mucosa is slightly elevated and swollen and has a coarse, granular surface which may show small areas of erosions. After fixation, the mucosa becomes pale. Both longitudinal and transverse rugae are interrupted. The lesion is rather extensive and in some cases may involve the whole circumference of the mucosa. On the cut surface the mucosa is markedly thickened in the region of the lesion. Most lesions of this type are located within the lamina propria, but in some cases the submucosa may be involved. Most early esophageal carcinomas removed by surgery are of this type (Fig. 4.3).

Papillary. The lesion presents as a papillary or polypous protrusion, usually 1–3 cm in diameter. There is marked demarcation between the edge of the cancer and the surrounding normal mucosa. Occasionally, small areas of erosion covered with inflammatory exudate can be seen on the surface of the lesion. On the cut surface the lesion protrudes toward the esophageal lumen and infiltrates the wall. Early esophageal carcinoma of this type is rarely seen (Fig. 4.4).

Liu et al [18] made an analysis of 150 surgical specimens of early esophageal carcinoma. The lesions were situated in the middle and lower portions of the esophagus in 148 cases (98.7%), in the upper portion in only two cases (1.3%). In this material, 11 lesions (7.3%), all carcinoma in situ, were occult. In 50 cases (33.3%) the lesions were erosive; 22 (44%) were carcinoma in situ, 20 (40%) were intramucosal carcinoma, and eight (16%) showed cancer cell infiltration of the submucosa. In 77 cases (51.3%) the lesions were plaque-like, including 14 (18.2%) cases of carcinoma in situ, 35 (45.4%) of intramucosal carcinoma, and 28 (36.4%) of infiltration of the submucosa. The remaining 12 cases (8.0%) were papillary; only one case was carcinoma in situ, four were intramucosal carcinoma, and seven were submucosal carcinoma. The smallest of the 150 tumors was 0.4 cm in diameter, the largest 8.5 cm. Of the 11 occult lesions, nine were less than 1 cm in diameter while most lesions of the other three types were larger, ranging from 1 to 4 cm (See also Sects. 3.1.1, 3.1.2)

2.2 Gross Types in the More Advanced Stages

Based upon the experience accumulated in China over the past three decades, a classification of carcinoma of the esophagus has been formulated which is as valuable clinically as it is pathologically [19–23]. We divide the lesions into medullary, fungating, ulcerative, scirrhous, and intraluminal types.

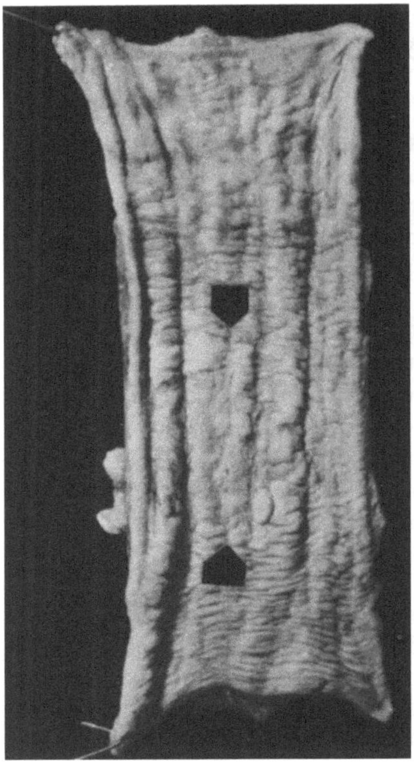

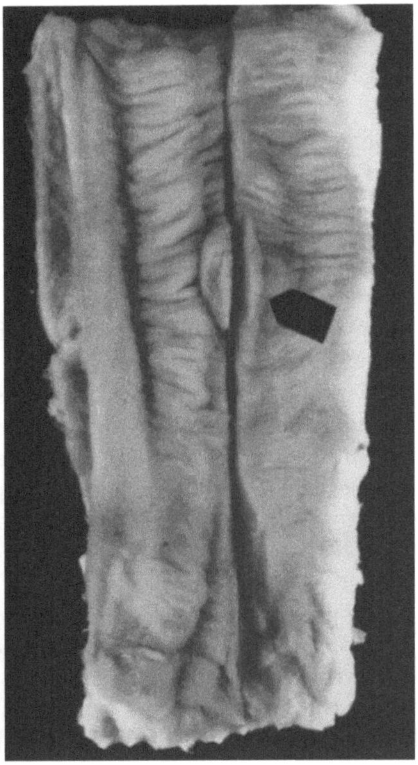

Fig. 4.3 (left). Early esophageal carcinoma, plaque-like type. The lesion *(arrow)* is slightly elevated and swollen, with a coarse, granular surface

Fig. 4.4 (right). Early esophageal carcinoma, papillary type. The lesion *(arrow)* presents as a small papillary mass protruding from the surface of the esophageal mucosa

Medullary. The cancer usually involves the whole thickness of the esophageal wall and most or all of its circumference (Fig. 4.5). The involved segment is markedly thickened. The edges of the tumor are raised and there is ulceration of varying depth on the surface of the solid tumor mass. The cut surface of the cancer is grayish-white in color and has a homogeneous appearance. *Microscopically,* the cancer cells are arranged in clumps and sheets, varying in degree of differentiation, with moderate or scanty connective tissue and mild inflammatory reaction.

Fungating. The cancer is usually oval in shape and protrudes into the lumen of the esophagus like a flat mushroom (Fig. 4.6). The edges are well defined, being raised from the surface of the mucosa and sometimes everted. Some shallow ulcerations may be present on the surface of the tumor. In the majority of the cases the cancer does not involve the entire circumference of the esophagus. The cut surface shows that the cancer may infiltrate the whole thickness of the esophageal wall, but seldom involves neighboring structures. *Microscopically,* the cancer cells are arranged in large patches with moderate inflammatory reaction and connective tissue proliferation.

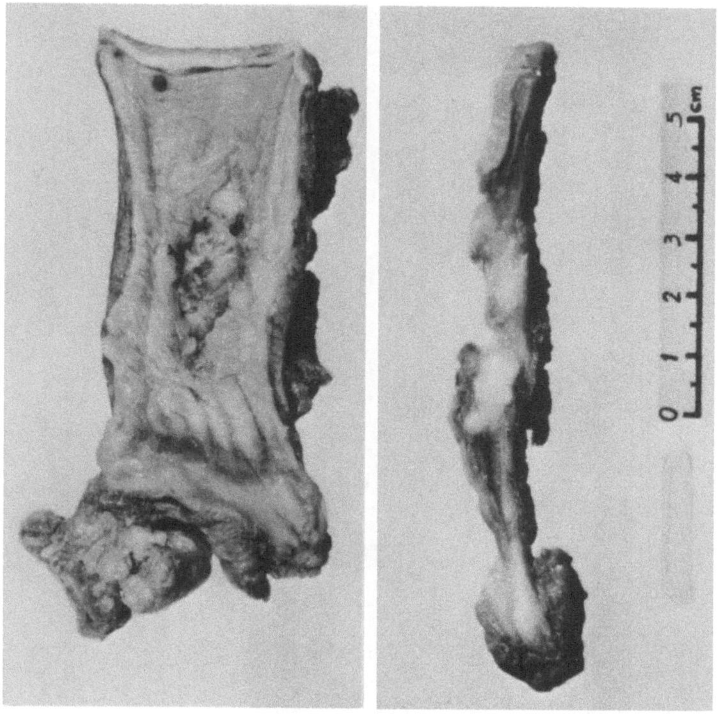

Fig. 4.5 Esophageal carcinoma, medullary type. *Left:* The edges of the tumor are raised and an ulceration is present on the surface. *Right:* The cut surface shows that the segment of esophageal wall occupied by the carcinoma is markedly thickened with an ulceration in the center

Ulcerative. The lesion presents as an undermining ulcer, usually involving only a portion of the circumference of the esophagus (Fig. 4.7). The edges of the ulcer may be slightly raised from the surface of the surrounding mucosa. The base penetrates deep into the muscular layer of the esophagus, often invading the periesophageal fibrous tissue and sometimes causing perforation of the esophagus. The surface of the ulcer may be covered with abundant inflammatory exudate. *Microscopically,* the cancer cells show a moderate degree of differentiation, with relatively more prominent inflammatory infiltration and connective tissue proliferation.

Scirrhous. The cancer forms a short tubular stenosis or obstruction of the esophagus (Fig. 4.8). The lesions almost always involve the whole circumference of the organ, and are usually less than 5 cm in length. The cancerous tissue infiltrates into and gradually merges with the esophageal wall, forming radiating rugae of the mucosa after fixation of the specimen. Usually there is no ulceration, or only a few erosions, on the tumor surface. The stenosis of the esophagus is characteristically concentric and symmetrical, with marked dilatation above the lesion. The cut surface of the cancer shows dense tumor tissue mingled with fibrous tissue. *Microscopically,* the cancer cells are arranged into irregular strands with abundant connective tissue proliferation, infiltrating deep into the muscular layer of the esophagus and sometimes beyond the normal boundary of the organ.

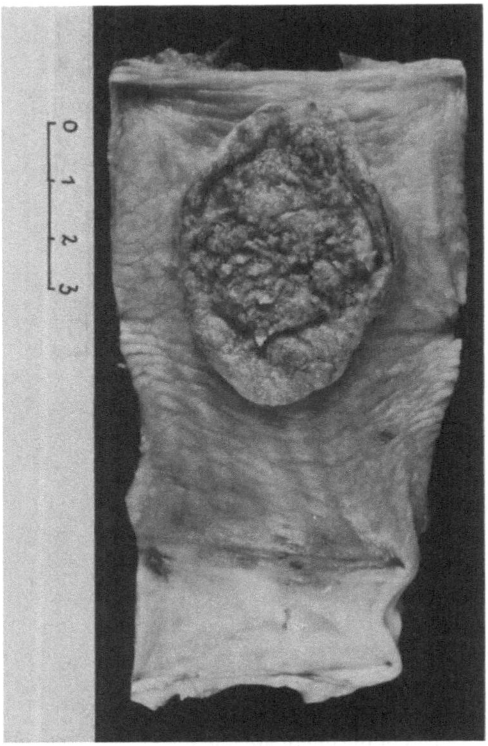

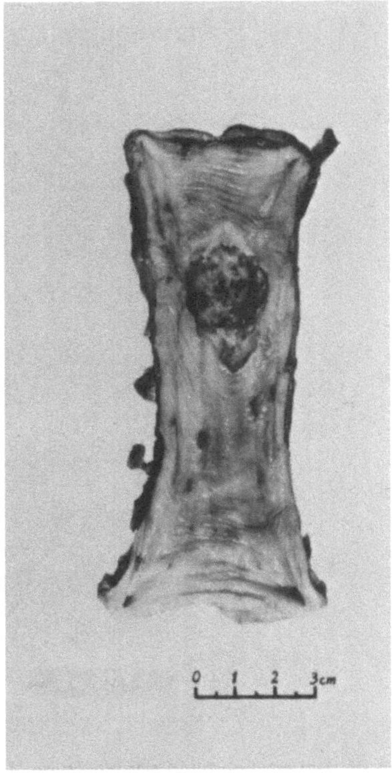

Fig. 4.6 (left). Esophageal carcinoma, fungating type. The tumor is oval and like a flat mushroom, protruding into the lumen of the esophagus

Fig. 4.7 (right). Esophageal carcinoma, ulcerative type. The lesion presents as a deeply penetrating ulcer covered with inflammatory exudate

Intraluminal. The oval or round mass of the tumor protrudes into the markedly dilated lumen of the esophagus (Fig. 4.9). The base is usually broad and there is often an erosion or a shallow, irregular ulceration on the surface of the tumor. *Microscopically,* most cases of this type are squamous cell carcinoma, with occasional adenocarcinoma and adenoacanthoma. In the majority of squamous cell carcinomas, the cancer cells are poorly to moderately differentiated with indistinct keratinization and intercellular bridges. In some cases the cancer cells are diffusely arranged. The tumor sometimes infiltrates only a portion of the thickness of the muscular layer of the esophagus. There are usually numerous blood vessels, with only mild inflammatory reaction in the stroma. Tumor emboli are often seen in both blood and lymph vessels

Sun and Wu [22] analyzed 444 surgical specimens of more advanced esophageal carcinoma: 252 (56.8%) were medullary, 82 (18.5%) fungating, 59 (13.3%) ulcerative, 38 (8.5%) scirrhous, and 13 (2.9%) miscellaneous. In another analysis of the gross types of 397 surgical specimens [8], there were 242 (61.0%) medullary, 48 (12.1%) fungating, 50 (12.6%) ulcerative, 22 (5.5%) scirrhous, 13 (3.3%) intraluminal, and 22 (5.5%) miscellaneous cases.

Huang et al [23] found 27 intraluminal cases (about 2% of the total) among the esophageal carcinomas surgically resected during the past 20 years in the Cancer Institute of the Chinese Academy of Medical Sciences in Beijing. Twenty-three of the patients were male

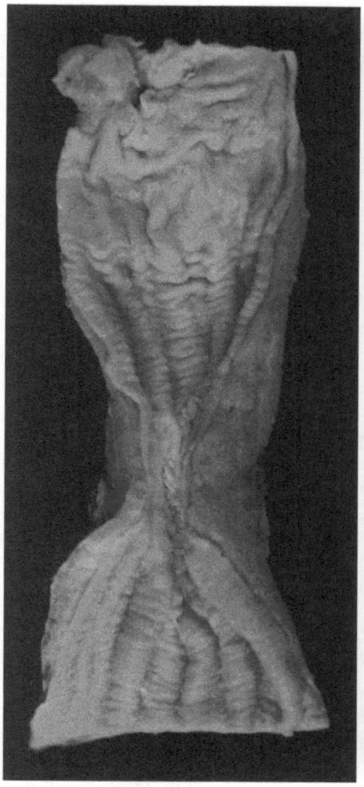

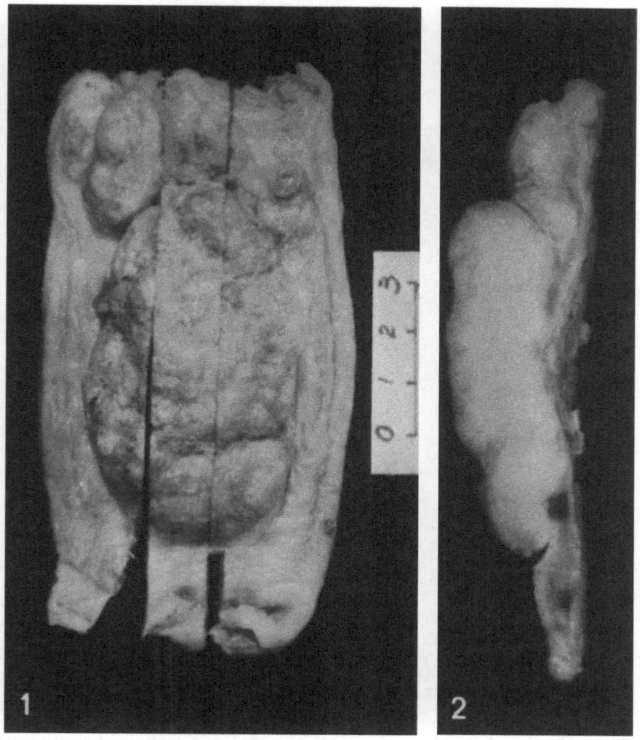

Fig. 4.8 (left). Esophageal carcinoma, scirrhous type. The tumor forms a short tubular stenosis of the esophagus and causes radiating rugae of the esophageal mucosa

Fig. 4.9 (right). Esophageal carcinoma, intraluminar type. Mucosa *(1)* and cut surface *(2)*. The oval mass of the tumor protrudes into the markedly dilated lumen of the esophagus

and only four female. Histologically, there were 24 cases of squamous cell carcinoma, two of adenocarcinoma, and one of adenoacanthoma.

Some characteristic features of the various types can be noted. None of them seem to have a predilection for any particular site. About half of the medullary type carcinomas are more than 5 cm long, whereas the majority of the ulcerative and scirrhous types are under 5 cm. Marked dysphagia is often observed in the scirrhous type, but ulcerative and fungating types usually produce only mild to moderate dysphagia. Scirrhous and medullary types usually infiltrate the entire thickness of the esophageal wall, but the fungating type often infiltrates only part of the muscular layer. The fungating and ulcerative types have a somewhat better prognosis than the others. In intraluminal carcinomas, the resectability rate is usually high but long-term results are often poor.

2.3 Esophageal Carcinosarcoma

We must point out that although esophageal carcinoma of the intraluminal type and esophageal carcinosarcoma are similar in that they both protrude into the lumen, they are clearly different in respect of clinical, X-ray, surgical, and pathological features and bio-

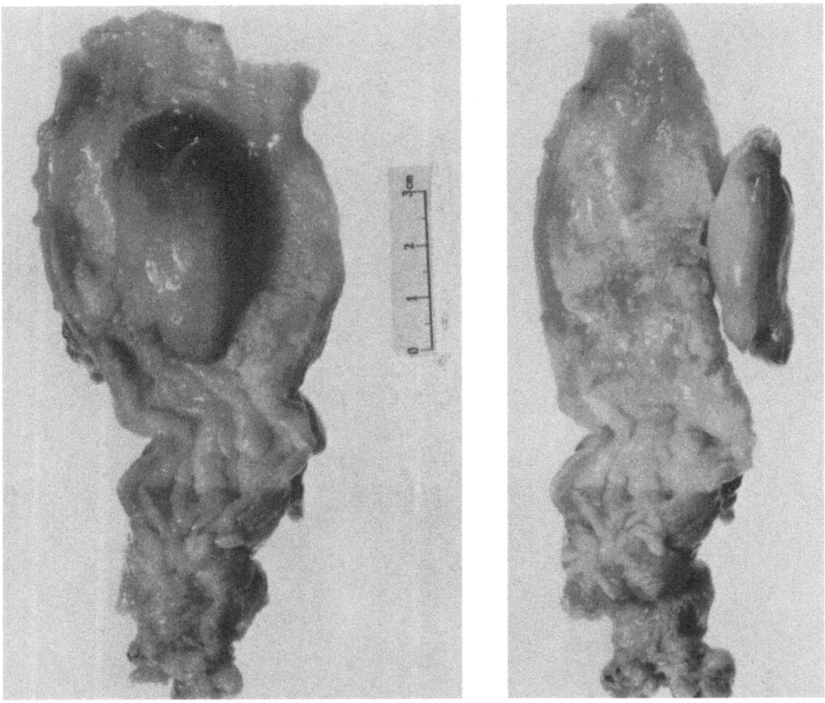

Fig. 4.10. Esophageal carcinosarcoma. A large polypoid tumor mass protruding into the lumen of the esophagus *(left)* is connected to the esophageal wall by a rather slender pedicle *(right)*

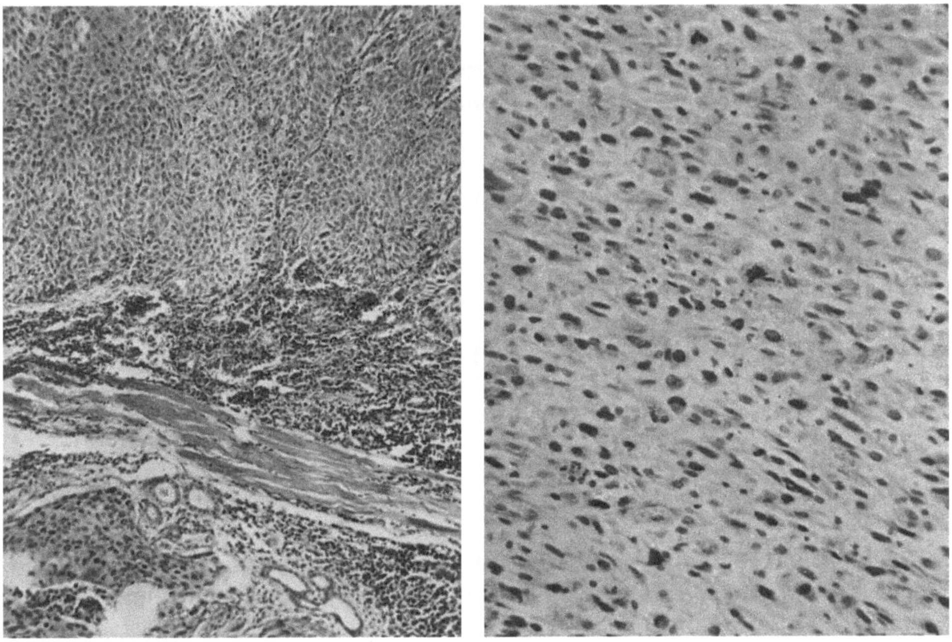

logic behavior. On this basis it is justifiable to classify intraluminal esophageal carcinoma separately, not including esophageal carcinosarcoma.

Esophageal carcinosarcoma is a rare and unusual type of malignant tumor; according to Postlethwait and Sealy [1, p.426], approximately 51 cases have been reported in the literature. The tumor is composed of both epithelial and mesenchymal malignant elements. Huang et al. [23] have carefully analyzed eight cases. *Grossly* (Fig.4.10), most esophageal carcinosarcomas are in the form of a large polypoid mass with a rather long and slender pedicle. The surface of the tumor is either smooth and intact or has only small, scattered, shallow ulcerations. On the cut surface the tumor is grayish-white like fish flesh, distinctly demarcated from the surrounding tissues. *Microscopically* (Fig.4.11), it is composed principally of sarcomatous tissue – of our eight cases, six were fibrosarcoma and two were leiomyosarcoma. The carcinomatous component is usually of the squamous cell type, often preinvasive, and may be found only at the base of the mass or in the adjacent mucosa around the pedicle. The results of surgical treatment in esophageal carcinosarcoma in our series are better than in intraluminal esophageal carcinoma.

3 Histology

3.1 Early Stage

With the improvement of diagnostic techniques and with the advent of mass screening in high-incidence areas, many early cases of esophageal carcinoma have been discovered in China. It is thus desirable to study and characterize the histologic features at this stage.

3.1.1 Morphology of Cancerous Tissue

In the material studied by Liu et al. [18] all 150 cases were squamous cell carcinoma except for one adenoacanthoma. *Microscopically,* they may be divided into intraepithelial, intramucosal, and submucosal carcinomas.

Intraepithelial Carcinoma (Carcinoma In Situ). Cancer cells occupy the entire thickness of the epithelium of the esophageal mucosa, but the basement membrane remains intact (Fig.4.12). This group comprised 48 cases (32.0%). According to the differentiation and morphology of the cancer cells, subdivision into large cell and small cell (spindle cell) carcinoma in situ can be made.

Large Cell Carcinoma In Situ. The carcinomatous mucosa is thickened and the cancer cells are large and well differentiated, evidently pleomorphic, and arranged irregularly. Mitoses are frequently observed. This type of lesion is commonly seen in plaque-like and papillary early esophageal carcinoma.

◁ *Fig.4.11.* The same case of esophageal carcinosarcoma as shown in Fig.4.10 *Left:* Squamous cell carcinoma penetrating into the submucosa. *Right:* Fibrosarcoma with numerous mitoses and abundant blood vessels

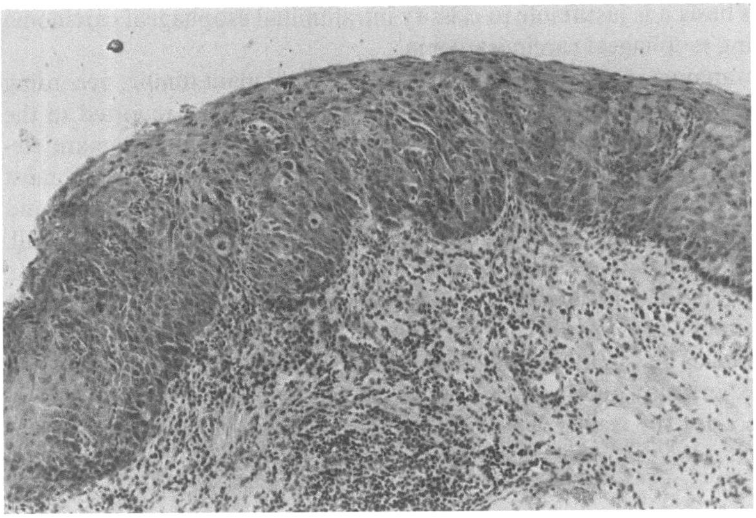

Fig. 4.12. Squamous cell carcinoma in situ of the esophagus. The entire thickness of epithelium is occupied by tumor cells, but the basement membrane is intact

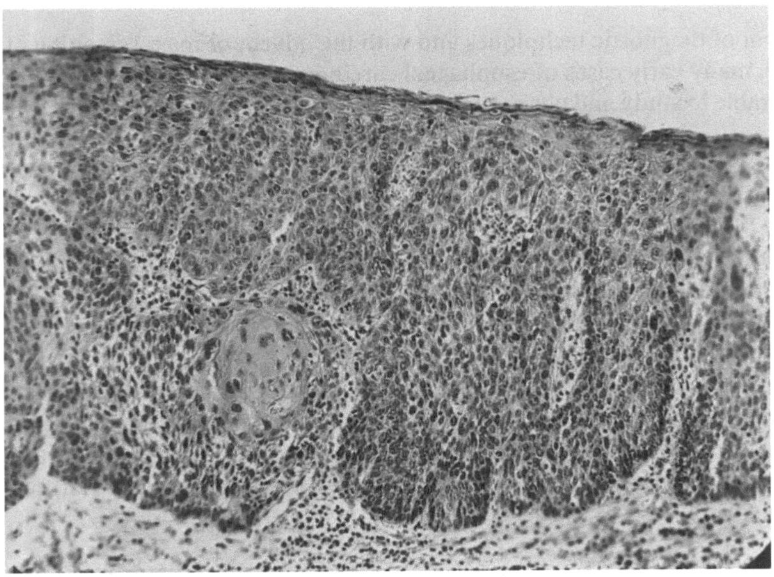

Fig. 4.13. Intramucosal carcinoma of the esophagus. Groups of tumor cells are penetrating into the lamina propria

Small Cell (Spindle Cell) Carcinoma In Situ. The cancerously changed mucosa is thin and cancer cells are poorly differentiated, small, round, or spindle-shaped, and contain scanty cytoplasm. The nuclei are hyperchromatic and mitoses are numerous. This type of lesion is often seen in erosive early esophageal carcinoma.

Table 4.2. Relationship between gross morphology and histology in early esophageal carcinoma

Histology	Gross morphology				
	Occult	Erosive	Plaque-like	Papillary	Total (%)
Intraepithelial (carcinoma in situ)	11	22	14	1	48 (32.0)
Intramucosal	0	20	35	4	59 (39.3)
Submucosal	0	8	28	7	43 (28.7)
Total	11	50	77	12	150 (100.0)

Glandular involvement in intraepithelial esophageal carcinoma is less frequent than in the uterine cervix, and the cancerous lesions are confined to the basement membrane of the glandular ducts in the esophageal mucosa. Of the 150 cases, 11 (7.3%) showed glandular involvement.

Intramucosal (Very Early Invasive) Carcinoma. This carcinoma developes when small groups of cancer cells escape from an intraepithelial carcinoma, penetrate the basement membrane, and infiltrate the lamina propria or part of the muscularis mucosae of the esophagus (Fig. 4.13). The area of invasion is small, usually difficult to distinguish with the naked eye. This category included 59 cases (39.3%).

Submucosal (Early Invasive) Carcinoma. Cancer cells have penetrated through the muscularis mucosae into the submucosa, but have not reached the muscular layer, and there are no metastases into the regional lymph nodes (Fig. 4.14). This type of lesion is rather large, the area of invasion is wide, and there is inflammatory reaction of variable degree around the lesion. Of the 150 cases, 43 (28.7%) were in this group.

Table 4.2 shows the relationship between gross morphology and histologic type in the 150 cases.

3.1.2 The Adjacent Epithelium

Varying alterations can be observed in the epithelium adjacent to carcinoma in most cases of esophageal cancer. Among Liu et al's 150 cases [18] (see also Sects. 2.1, 3.1.1), simple hyperplasia occurred in 142 patients (94.7%), atypical hyperplasia in 100 (66.7%), and epithelial atrophy in only eight (5.3%). Most lesions were contiguous to the main tumors, but in 34 cases they were 0.3–7.5 cm away. Among the 102 cases of early invasive carcinomas, there were 36 with carcinoma in situ in the adjacent epithelium. Multicentric carcinomas in situ can sometimes be seen in the mucosa adjacent to the main tumor (Fig. 4.15). It seems that the changes found in the adjacent epithelium represent stages of developement from simple hyperplasia through atypical hyperplasia to carcinoma in situ.

3.1.3 The Stroma

In the stroma beneath early esophageal carcinomas are found varying degrees of chronic inflammation. These consist mainly of lymphocytic and plasma cell infiltration, with a

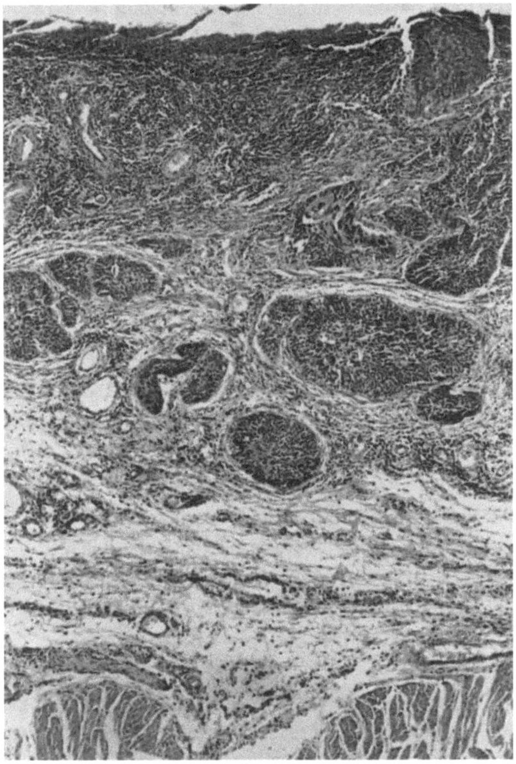

Fig. 4.14. Submucosal carcinoma of the esophagus. Cancer cells are infiltrating the submucosa, but the muscular layer remains intact

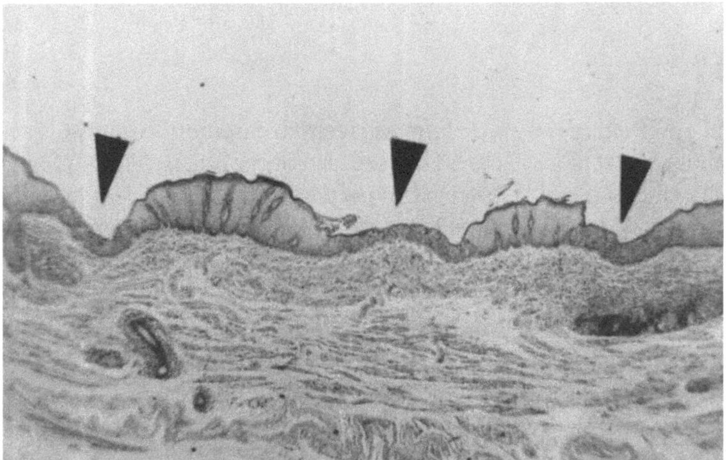

Fig. 4.15. Multicentric carcinomas in situ *(arrows)* in the mucosa adjacent to an advanced invasive squamous cell carcinoma of the esophagus

few cases showing neutrophilic and eosinophilic infiltration. The capillaries are congested and the endothelial cells are markedly hypertrophied. Similar inflammatory reaction, but of different proportions, can often be observed in the lamina propria beneath the epithelium adjecent to carcinoma.

3.2 *More Advanced Stages*

3.2.1. Squamous Cell Carcinoma

The morphology of esophageal squamous cell carcinoma varies depending on differentiation. Well-differentiated carcinoma (Fig. 4.16) may present epidermoid characteristics, including keratinization, pearl formation, and intercellular bridges. Broders's method [24] of classifying carcinomas into four grades according to the degree of differentiation has been employed for many years; however, difficulties exist in its application, and the data thus obtained, as reported in the literature, vary considerably.

A three-grade classification has recently been widely adopted in China. Its basic criteria are as follows.

Grade I. The cancer cells are well differentiated, rather large, polygonal or round, with evident keratinization and intercellular bridges. Mitoses are not frequent.

Grade II. The cancer cells are rather large, of moderate differentiation, round, oval, or polygonal, with a certain amount of pleomorphism. There may be moderate keratinization or a few epithelial pearls. Mitoses are often seen. Intercellular bridges can not usually be found.

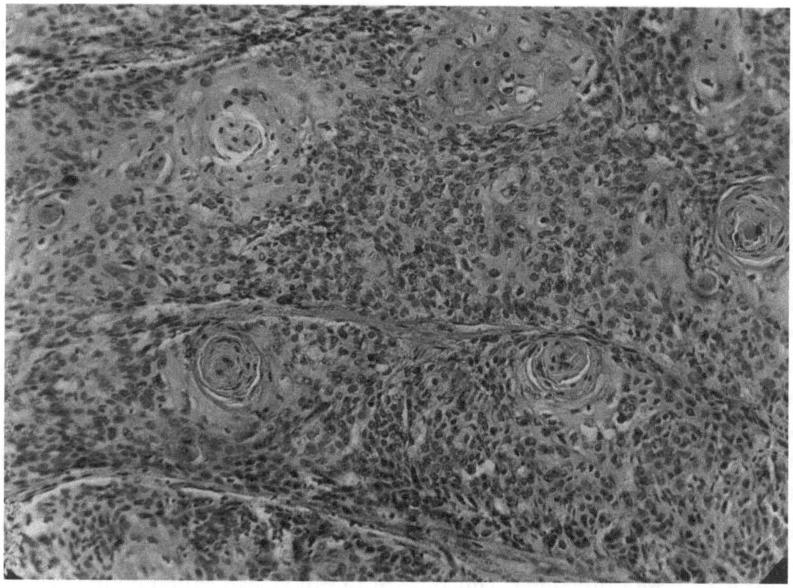

Fig. 4.16. Well-differentiated squamous cell carcinoma of the esophagus. Well-differentiated tumor cells with numerous pearl formations can be seen

Grade III. Most of the tumor cells are spindleshaped, ovoid, or irregular, smaller in size, and with scanty cytoplasm. Mitoses are frequent. No keratinization or intercellular bridges are present. However, the lesion can still be recognized as squamous cell carcinoma and can be distinguished from undifferentiated carcinoma.

This three-grade classification is easy to apply. Liu [8] analyzed 417 resected specimens of squamous cell carcinoma of the esophagus and found the proportions of grade I, II, and III to be 26.1%, 65.3%, and 8.6% respectively. Chen and Lin [25] studied 500 cases from Fujian province and found the proportions to be 24.4%, 64.8%, and 10.8%. The two reports revealed similar findings.

3.2.2 Adenocarcinoma

Adenocarcinoma of the esophagus is not often seen, but its incidence as reported in the literature varies greatly. Verious reports give figures of 0.8% (5/603) [26], 0.8% (10/1312) [27], 0.9% (6/633) [28], 2.4% (45/1859) [29], 3.5% (144/4145) [1, p 415], 3.7% (13/350) [30], 4.7% (21/451) [31], 5.1% (5/98) [32], 6.1% (32/524) [8], 7.3% (23/314) [33], and 8.0% (7/87) [34]. In the data collected by Bosch et al. [30] from various cancer registries in the USA and the USA Third National Cancer Survey, the incidence of esophageal adenocarcinoma is 7.7% (400/5218) and 8.2% (146/1791) respectively.

Some authors incorrectly count adenocarcinoma of the gastric cardia involving the lower portion of the esophagus as adenocarcinoma of the esophagus, and some others confuse adenoacanthoma of the esophagus with squamous cell carcinoma. We suggest that for a diagnosis of adenocarcinoma of the esophagus, the tumor must be (a) clearly seen to arise not from the gastric cardia, but from the esophageal mucosa; (b) definitely located at a certain distance above the squamous-columnar epithelial junction; and (c) unequivocally identified, including confirmation by special staining if it is poorly differentiated.

Adenocarcinomas of the esophagus may be subdivided into simple adenocarcinoma, adenosquamous carcinoma, adenoid cystic carcinoma, and mucoepidermoid carcinoma.

Simple Adenocarcinoma. The tumor cells are cuboidal or columnar, with round, ovoid, or rod-shaped nuclei and coarse chromatin (Fig. 4.17). The degree of glandular structure formation varies greatly. The lesions are usually divided into three grades according to the degree of cell differentiation and glandular structure formation.

Adenosquamous Carcinoma. This type of tumor has also been called adenoacanthoma, acanthoadenoma, or adenocarcinoma with squamous cell metaplasia. Recently, however, most authors have distinguished it from adenoacanthoma – adenocarcinoma with squamous cell metaplasia. In adenoacanthoma, distinctly malignant adenocarcinomatous elements are mixed with clearly benign squamous epithelial cells, while in adenosquamous carcinoma, squamous cell carcinoma and adenocarcinoma elements are present and intimately intermingled. This type of carcinoma is not as rare as is usually thought. Kusalina and Kolycheva [28] reported 20 cases (3.16%) among 633 malignant tumors of the esophagus. Liu found 22 cases (4.2%) in 524 surgical specimens [8], a similar incidence rate.

Adenoid Cystic Carcinoma. This type of tumor is also called cylindroma, adenoid basal cell carcinoma, or cribriform carcinoma. It occurs quite often in the salivary gland, but only rarely in the esophagus. Jacobsohn et al. [35] reported one case and collected 20 more

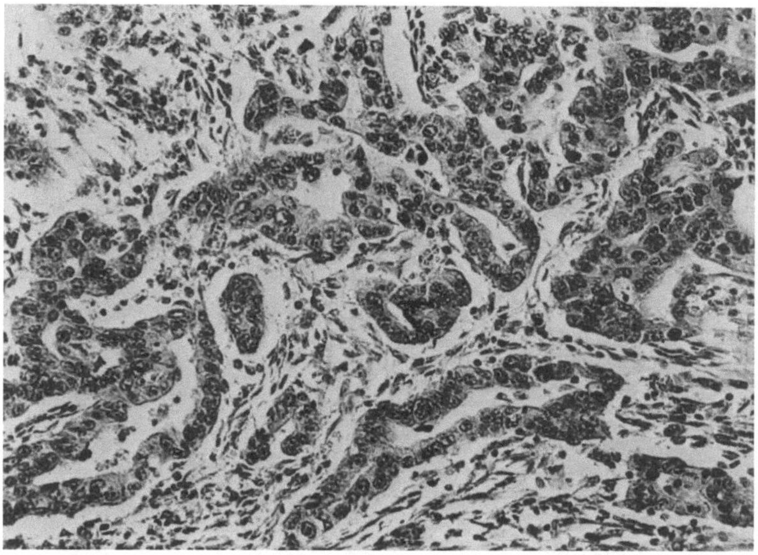

Fig. 4.17. Simple adenocarcinoma of the esophagus. Glandular structures are formed by cuboidal tumor cells

from the literature. The most common location is the middle third of the esophagus (15/21, 71.4%). *Microscopically,* cystic structures of various sizes can be found, lined by flattened cells, and mucoid substance is contained in the cystic spaces.

Mucoepidermoid Carcinoma. This tumor is very rare in the esophagus. Postlethwait and Sealy [1, p. 418] reported one case and collected 13 others from the literature. The most common site is the lower third (10/14, 71.4%). We have seen only one case in over 1000 esophageal cancers. The tumor may originate from the multipotential excretory cells of the submucosal mucous glands. Two elements are mixed in varying proportions: epidermoid cells, sometimes resembling basal cells, and mucin-secreting columnar cells. Irregular adenoid spaces of different sizes containing mucoid material can be observed in the tumor.

3.2.3 Undifferentiated Carcinoma

This type of tumor (Fig. 4.18) is rare in the esophagus. Subdivision into large cell, small cell, and oat cell carcinomas may be made.

In *large cell* undifferentiated carcinoma, the tumor cells are rather large, with abundant cytoplasm and darkly stained nuclei. Bizarre tumor cells are often present. Numerous mitoses may be noted.

In *small cell* undifferentiated carcinoma, the tumor cells are small and have only scanty cytoplasm. The tumor shows a marked infiltrating growth pattern.

Oat cell carcinoma may occur in the esophagus [36]. Tateishi et al. [37] reported six cases, detecting ACTH activity in three of four tumors, and finding neurosecretory type granules in three tumors examined by electron microscopy. However, as described in their material, the three tumors with neurosecretory granules were not the same tumors that

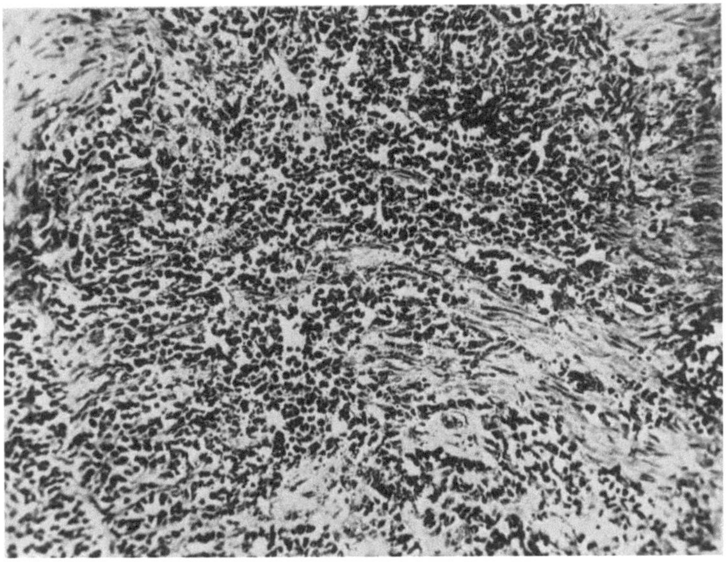

Fig. 4.18. Undifferentiated carcinoma of the esophagus. The tumor consists of diffusely infiltrating undifferentiated tumor cells

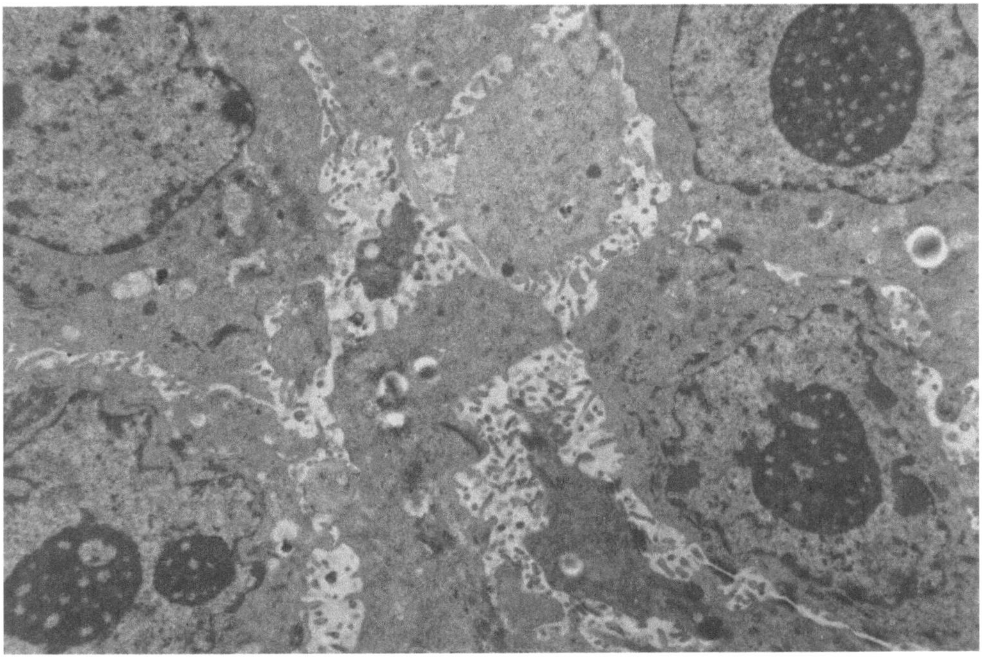

Fig. 4.19. Squamous cell carcinoma of the esophagus. The irregularly arranged tumor cells contain enlarged and irregular nuclei with prominent nucleoli. The dilated intercellular spaces are filled with long, slender cytoplasmic extensions. × 3700

had ACTH activity. Up to 1980, about 20 cases of this tumor had been reported in the literature [38–40], most of them from Japan. A small number of cases have also been observed in China, but few of the patients had evident endocrine activity.

4 Ultrastructure

In recent years several reports [41–47] have been published in China on the ultrastructure of esophageal carcinoma. The material in this section is derived basically from an investigation of 22 cases, including 18 reported previously [43]. The histopathologic diagnosis was carcinoma in situ in four cases, early invasive carcinoma in five cases, and advanced carcinoma in 13 cases. None of the 22 patients received either radiotherapy or chemotherapy.

4.1 The Cancer Cells

The cells of squamous cell carcinoma of the esophagus show certain features which distinguish them from normal esophageal squamous epithelial cells. They are often markedly enlarged, varied in shape, and irregularly arranged. The nuclei may be greatly increased in size, irregular, and hyperchromatic, and frequently show one or more prominent nucleoli (Fig. 4.19). Sometimes a number of nuclear bodies can be seen within a nucleus. The nucleus/cytoplasm ratio is inverted. In some poorly differentiated carcinomas, nuclear pleomorphism is prominent [47], but in a few poorly differentiated tumor cells, the nuclei may be rather round with more evenly distributed chromatin. The changes in the nuclear structure of tumor cells apparently indicate their increased metabolic and proliferative activities and are consistent with their need for intensive nucleus/cytoplasm exchanges of various substances.

The cytoplasm of cancer cells is sometimes richer in mitochondria, but of various sizes and shapes, often swollen, with few cristae. Some cells contain an increased amount of rough endoplasmic reticulum (Fig. 4.20). In most of the cancer cells the amount of free ribosomes is considerably increased. There is little glycogen in the cells. The number of tonofilaments is frequently increased, some of them forming thick bundles of tonofibrils (Figs. 4.20, 21). However, in poorly differentiated cancer cells, tonofilaments are scanty or even absent. This confirms the findings of Fang and Sun [41] and the Henan Medical College team [42]. The above-described changes indicate that in spite of their being less differentiated than normal esophageal epithelial cells, the cancer cells can still continue some of the intensive metabolic and synthesizing functions characteristic of these cells.

In the majority of cases, the intercellular spaces are considerably dilated and filled with innumerable long, slender cytoplasmic extensions (Fig. 4.19). Clearly, such changes may increase the cell surface considerably. In a few cancer cells the intercellular spaces are narrow and the cell surface is rather smooth with few cytoplasmic extensions, which may indicate poor differentiation. The number of desmosomes between cancer cells is often decreased, which may facilitate detachment of the cancer cells from each other and development of invasion and metastasis.

In carcinoma in situ, the basal lamina is generally intact except for occasional small interruptions forming narrow gaps through which a slender cytoplasmic projection of the cancer cell penetrates into the stroma, the so-called microinvasion, not discernible on light

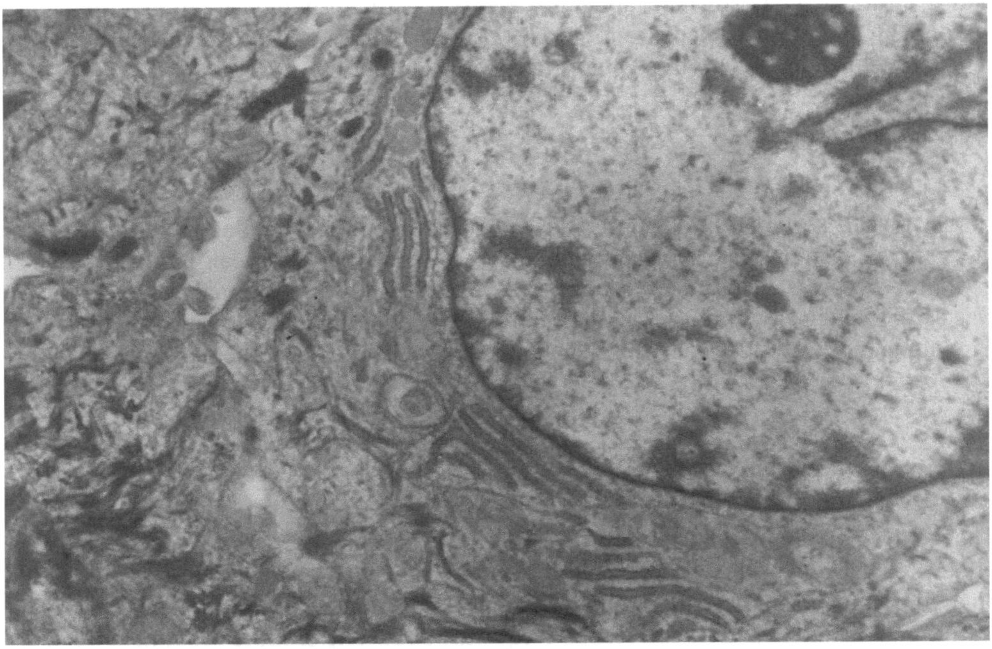

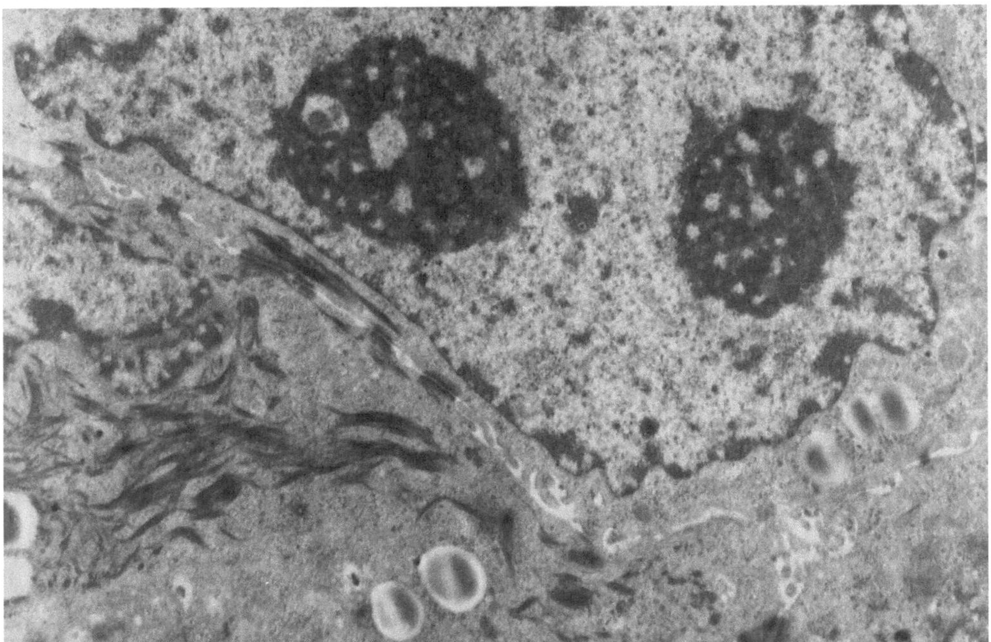

Fig. 4.20 (above). Squamous cell carcinoma of the esophagus. The tumor cells contain increased amount of rough endoplasmic reticulum and bundles of tonofibrils in the cytoplasm. × 15500

Fig. 4.21 (below). Squamous cell carcinoma of the esophagus. Two prominent nucleoli in the nucleus and thick bundles of tonofibrils in the cytoplasm are shown. × 8900

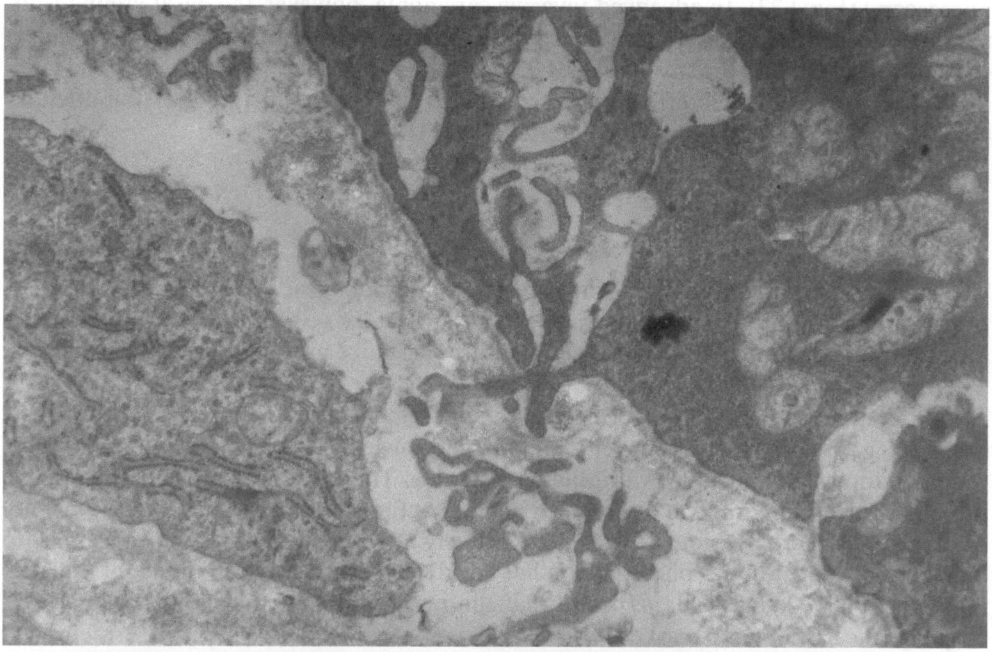

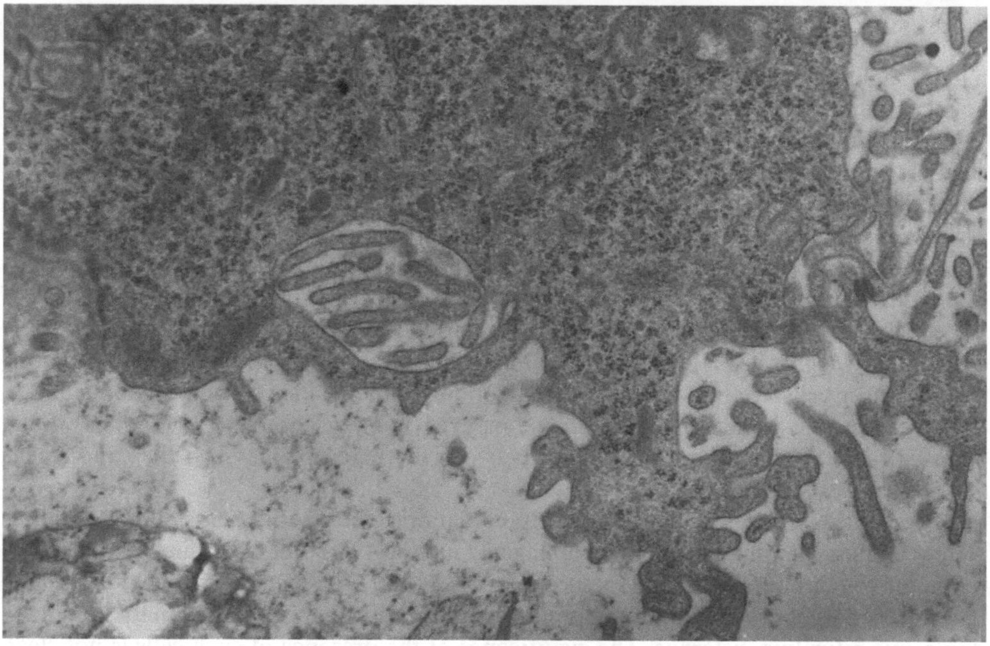

Fig. 4.22 (above). Squamous cell carcinoma of the esophagus. Thin cytoplasmic extensions of the tumor cell are protruding into the stroma through a small gap in the broken basal lamina, so-called microinvasion. A fibroblast is present in the vicinity of the microinvasion site. × 14800

Fig. 4.23 (below). Squamous cell carcinoma of the esophagus. Numerous broad pseudopodia of the tumor cell are protruding into the stroma. No basal lamina can be seen around this cell. × 14500 microscopy (Fig. 4.22). In advanced invasive carcinoma, however, the basal lamina is often incomplete or even absent over a large area, and the broad pseudopodia of the cancer cell protrude deep into the stroma (Fig. 4.23). Zhang et al. [48] reported that the basal lamina is often present in well-differentiated squamous cell carcinoma (grade I), but often incomplete or absent in carcinomas of grades II and III.

4.2 Stromal Reaction

The main manifestations of the stromal reaction in esophageal carcinoma are fibroblast proliferation, an increase in collagen fibers, inflammatory cell infiltration, and capillary alterations. To some extent they reflect the host resistance and defense function against the tumor growth.

Proliferation of fibroblasts is very often seen in the tumoral stroma. The fibroblasts show enlarged and irregular nuclei with enlarged nucleoli and an increased amount of rough endoplasmic reticulum with dilated cisternae. These changes indicate their active protein-synthesizing function. It has been noted that fibroblasts often occur in the vicinity of cancer cell microinvasion, as if they are actively moving up towards the cancer cell to halt its expansion. Similar phenomenon has also been observed in carcinoma of the uterine cervix [48]. Zhang et al. [47] state that the proliferation of fibroblasts in grade III esophageal carcinomas is marked.

In the stroma, the type, amount, and morphology of the inflammatory cells vary. Among the 22 cases examined by Zhou et al. [43] lymphocytes and plasma cells predominate in eight cases each and in the other six cases the two types of cell occur in nearly equal amounts. Of the eight cases in which lymphocytes predominate, in four the lymphocytes have quite smooth cell surface (T-cells?), in three the lymphocytes have numerous slender cytoplasmic (B-cells?), and in one the two types are present in approximately equal numbers. Of the eight cases where plasma cells predominate, in five the rough endoplasmic reticulum cisternae of the plasma cells are narrow and densely arranged, in two cisternae are markedly dilated, and in one both types are present. Zhang et al. [47] reported that there is an increased number of lymphocytes in grade I carcinoma, an increase of plasma cells in grade II carcinoma, and a decreased number of lymphocytes in grade III carcinoma. Macrophages can be seen among the inflammatory cells. In some places, where cancer cells are in contact with macrophages, the cell surfaces are often smooth, their cytoplasmic projections very sparse or even missing completely (Fig. 4.24). Such changes seem to result from interaction between the macrophages and the cancer cells [43].

In one of the 22 cases, some plasma cells containing characteristic crystalline structures were seen in the lamina propria of esophageal mucosa [49], situated within the dilated cisternae of rough endoplasmic reticulum (Figs. 4.25–4.27). It seems reasonable to assume that the crystals consist of immunoglobulin synthesized and accumulated in the rough endoplasmic reticulum cisternae. The significance of the presence of such cells is not clear.

The capillaries in the cancer stroma are considerably congested. Some of the endothelial cells are hypertrophied and occupy a large portion of the lumen. In some capillaries the number of cytoplasmic projections from endothelial cells is increased. Fenestrations (Fig. 4.28) and interruptions of endothelial cells, not observed in the capillaries of normal esophageal mucosa, were noted in 12 and eight cases respectively. Zhang et al. [47] found more fenestrations in grade II carcinoma. In some areas, the basal lamina of capillary en-

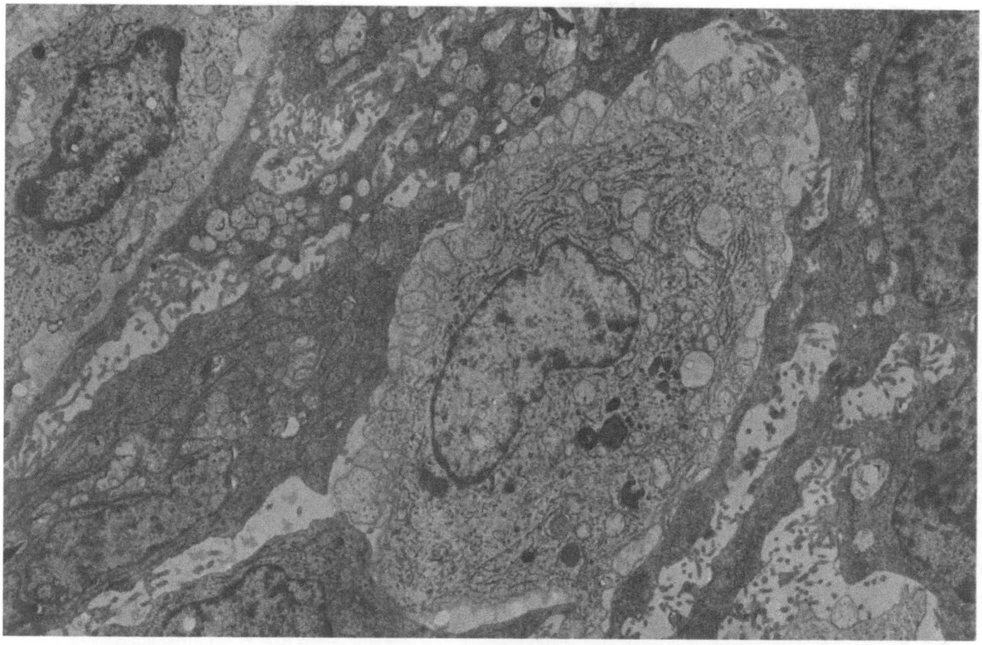

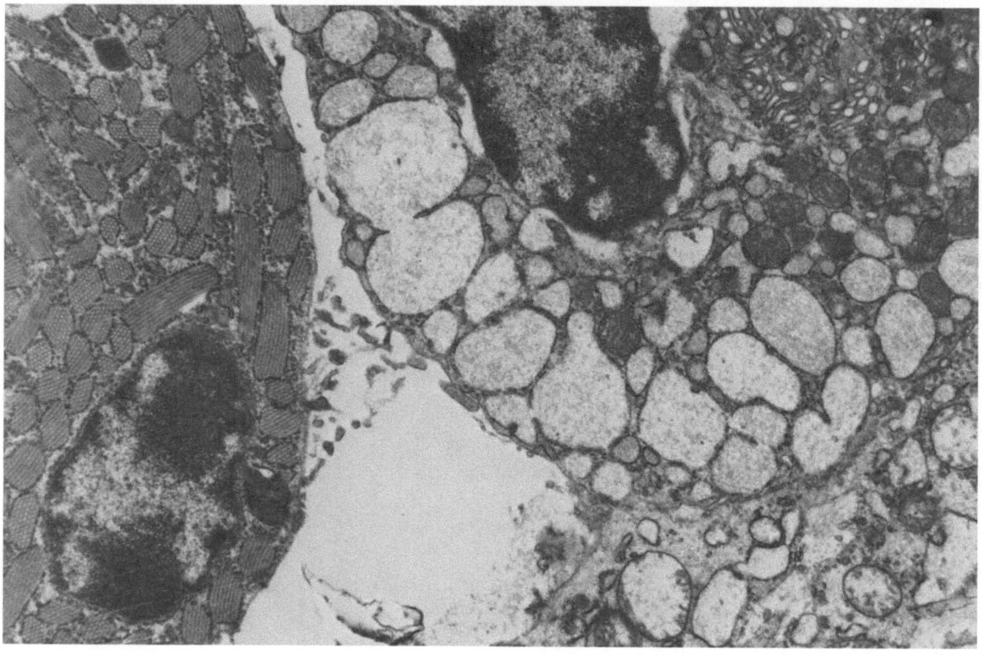

Fig. 4.24 (above). Squamous cell carcinoma of the esophagus. A macrophage is present among several tumor cells. Note that the tumor cell surface adjacent to macrophage is smooth and almost completely deprived of cytoplasmic extensions. × 3100

Fig. 4.25 (below). A plasma cell containing characteristic crystalline structures in the lamina propria of mucosa near the end of a surgical specimen of esophageal squamous cell carcinoma. × 10600

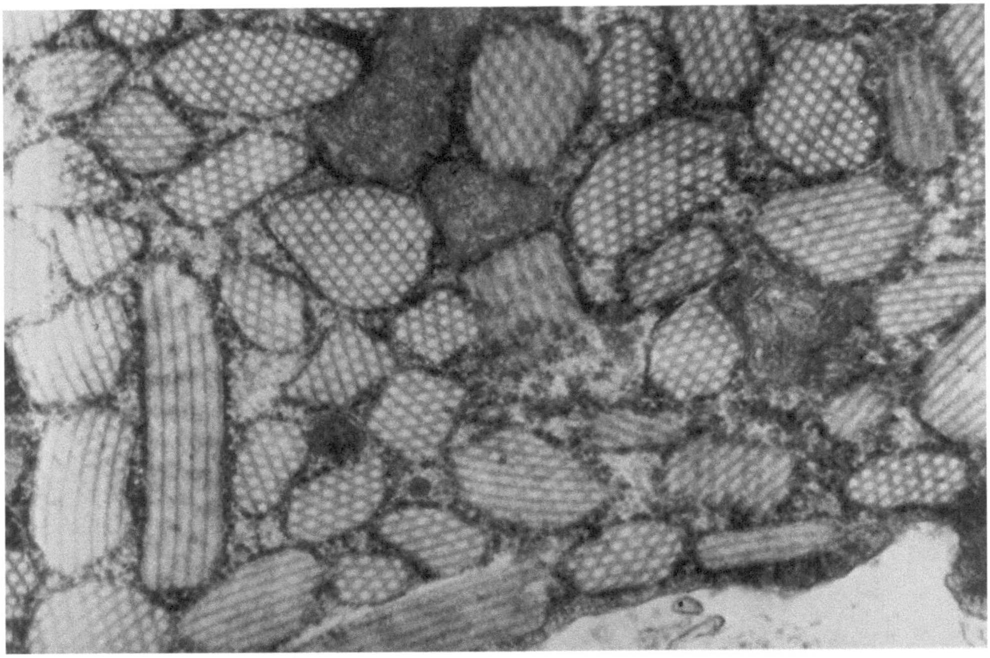

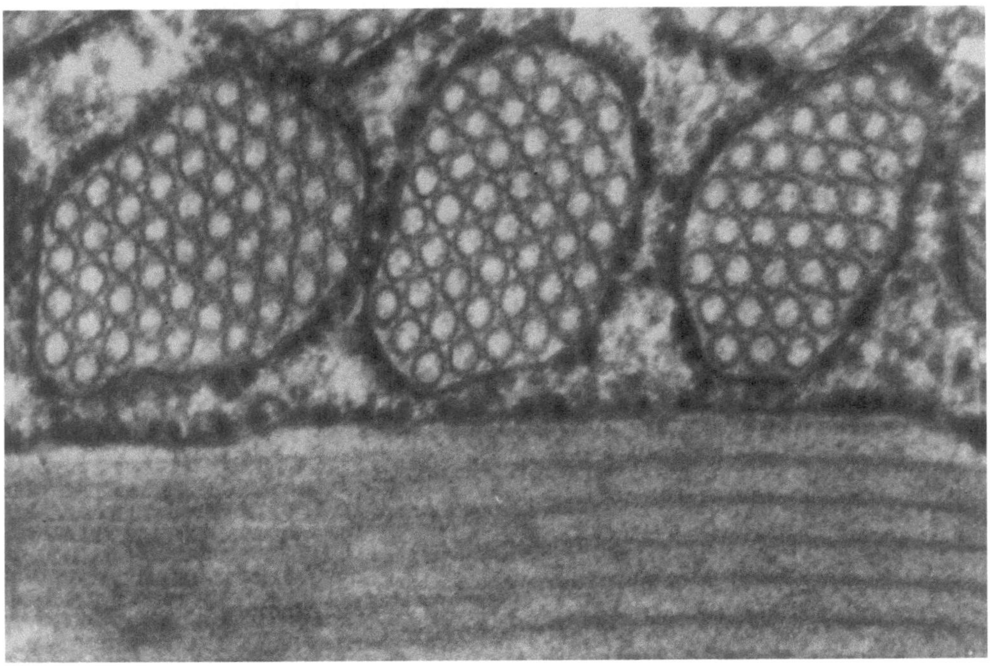

Fig. 4.26 (above). Characteristic crystals in the dilated rough endoplasmic reticulum cisternae of a plasma cell. × 47000

Fig. 4.27 (below). High magnification of the crystals contained in the rough endoplasmic reticulum cisternae of the plasma cell. × 118000 dothelial cells is increased to several layers. Neither the mechanism of formation of these capillary changes nor the relationship between them and the tumor growth and invasion is clear.

No virus particles have been detected in this material, but numerous fungi and bacteria have been observed, within some superficial cancer cells in one case and intercellularly in two other cases (Fig. 4.29).

5 Spread and Metastasis

Esophageal carcinomas spread and metastasize basically in the following ways.

5.1 Intramural Spread

Esophageal carcinoma may spread by infiltration into the esophageal wall or to the surrounding areas, or may permeate the lymphatic vessels in the submucosa or in the plane of the muscular layer to form separate nodules imitating other primary tumors. Such secondaries may be 5–6 cm from the parent tumor. Some authors have stated that carcinoma in situ and carcinomatous changes of basal cells of the epithelium adjacent to the principal tumor are also methods of spreading.

5.2 Direct Involvement of Neighboring Organs

Esophageal cancers very often invade neighboring organs directly. Depending on the location of the tumor, various organs may be involved with different frequency. Thus, carcinoma in the upper segment of the esophagus may invade the larynx, the trachea, and the soft tissues of the neck. Tumors of the middle part may invade the bronchi, invade and perforate the aorta, causing fatal hemorrhage, or involve the thoracic duct, the azygos vein, or the hili of the lungs. Tumors of the lower segment may involve the mediastinum, diaphragm, and gastric cardia. The frequency of involved organs is apparently related to the location of the tumor in the esophagus.

5.3 Lymphatic Spread

Spread via the lymphatics occurs frequently and early in esophageal carcinoma, although in a small number of patients no metastases can be found even in the late stage of disease. The frequency of involved lymph nodes reported in the literature varies depending on the source. Most metastatic lesions are limited to the intrathoracic lymph nodes, but it should be pointed out that in some cases, "jumping" metastasis to the neck or abdominal lymph nodes without intrathoracic involvement can be observed. Liu [8] analyzed 858 cases involving surgical resection and found 361 cases of lymph node metastasis (42.1%). Postlethwait and Sealy [1, p. 357], summarizing nine series totalling 2440 autopsy cases, found that 1876 cases had metastasis or invasion. Among the 1648 sites of lymph node metastasis, the groups of nodes most frequently involved were the mediastinal (484), the abdominal (236), the paratracheal and paraesophageal (220), and the cervical and supraclavicular

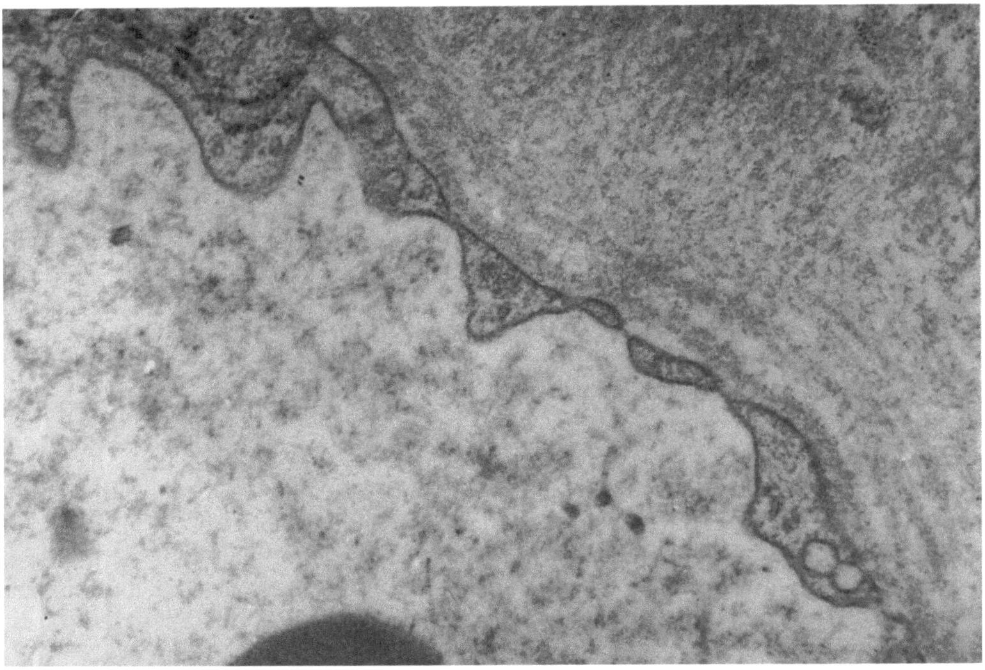

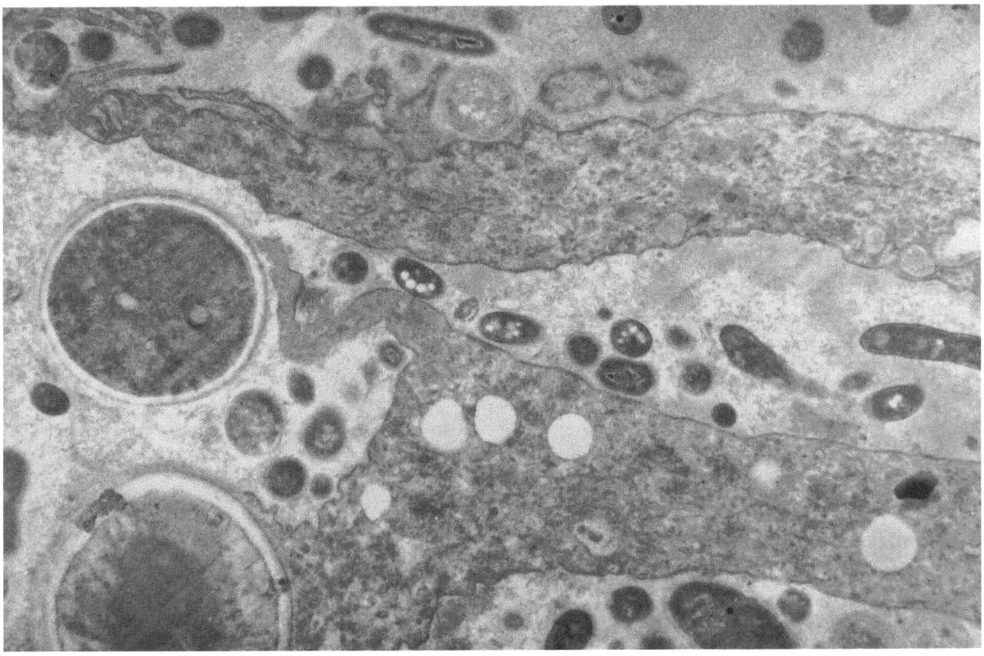

Fig. 4.28 (above). In the stroma of esophageal carcinoma, the capillary endothelial cell shows fenestrations consisting of a thin diaphragm separating the capillary lumen from the surrounding tissue. × 32400

Fig. 4.29 (below). Fungi and bacteria in the intercellular spaces of an esophageal squamous cell carcinoma. × 10700

(136). Yamashita [50] analyzed the dissemination of esophageal cancer from 1132 autopsy records and found metastases in neck and axillary nodes in 213 cases (18.8%), in thoracic nodes in 526 cases (46.5%), and in abdominal nodes in 296 cases (26.1%). Sannohe et al. [51], performing curettage of lymph nodes in esophageal surgery, revealed that of 36 patients with esophageal carcinoma, ten (27.8%) had jumping metastases of the cervical or abdominal lymph nodes without intrathoracic involvement. Hiroko et al. [52] examined 124 esophageal carcinoma patients treated by surgery and found lymph node metastases in 87 (70%), of whom 12 had metastasis in regional nodes, 42 had both regional and distant involvement, and 33 only had jumping metastasis in distant lymph nodes.

5.4 Blood-Borne Metastasis

Metastasis via the blood vessels is common in patients with advanced esophageal carcinoma. In an autopsy series of 824 cases, Dormanns [53] found that the most common distant metastases were in the liver (264), lungs and pleura (176), bone (68), kidneys (59), omentum and peritoneum (44), and adrenals (35). In another group of 41 autopsy cases [54], blood-borne metastases to distant organs were found in the lungs (ten), liver (eight), kidneys (four), skin (three), thyroid, intestine, and pancreas (two each), and trachea, thoracic vertebrae, adrenal, stomach, diaphragm, brain, pituitary, spleen, heart, and peritoneum (one each) in 15 patients. There were no distant metastases in the remaining 26 cases. In Yamashita's statistical analysis of 1132 autopsy cases of esophageal carcinoma, the most frequent blood-borne metastases were found in the lungs (459; 40.5%), liver (328; 29.0%), trachea (137; 12.1%), stomach (122; 10.8%), and adrenals (115; 10.2%). There were 224 cases (19.8%) with metastases in both of the lungs and the liver.

6 Morphologic Factors Affecting Prognosis

6.1 Size of Lesion

Some data indicate that the smaller the cancer, the better the prognosis. Miller [14] analyzed a series of 144 cases treated with surgical resection and found that 5-year survival for patients with tumors of <5 cm, 5–7.5 cm, and >7.5 cm was 20.9% (9/43), 20.4% (11/54), and 4.3% (2/47) respectively. He suggested that tumor size does indeed affect the prognosis in esophageal carcinoma. Endo et al. [55], reporting the results in 469 patients treated with surgical resection, showed that the 5-year survival rate was 27% for patients with cancer smaller than 6 cm on the X-ray film, 20% for 6–7.9 cm, 17% for 8–9.9 cm, and 17% again for 10 cm or more. Huang et al. [56] investigated factors influencing the long-term results of surgical treatment of esophageal carcinoma and found that in 75 patients in whom the tumor measured 3 cm or less in length the 5-year survival rate was 48.0%, while among 901 with tumors over 3 cm it was 28.9%.

6.2 Depth of Invasion

A number of authors [6, 8, 56–59] have pointed out that the depth of invasion of the esophageal wall has a significant influence on the prognosis. In an analysis of 522 cases treated with resection [8] the 3- and 5-year survival rates in the group of patients with cancer infiltrating only a portion of muscular layer of the esophagus were 45.5% and 40.4% respectively, while in the group with cancer penetrating beyond the esophageal wall they were 38.1% and 24.4%. Huang et al. [56] reported the results of surgical treatment in esophageal carcinoma; the 5-year survivals of p-TNM stage I, II, III, and IV cases were 83.3% (5/6), 46.3% (101/218), 26.4% (187/707), and 6.7% (3/45) respectively. The 5-year survival rates of patients with early esophageal carcinoma were reported by several authors as much better than those of patients with advanced invasive carcinoma: Endo et al. [55] reported 64% (18/28), Linxian County Hospital [60] 90.3% (28/31), Huang et al. [17] 85.9% (110/128), and Liu et al [18] 85.5% (59/69).

6.3 Growth Pattern

The results of several histopathologic investigations suggest that the growth pattern of the tumor may affect the prognosis. Xian et al [61] studied 100 cases involving surgical treatment of esophageal carcinoma and found that the 3- to 4-year survival rates among patients with carcinoma displaying sheet, thin strand, network-like and diffuse growth patterns were 3/32, 1/36, 1/27, and 0/5 respectively. Sun and Wu [62] studied 50 patients surviving for less than 2 years and another 50 surviving for over 5 years and found that of those with sheet growth pattern, 35 survived longer than 5 years and only 21 died within 2 years after surgery, while of those with thin strand growth pattern, 29 died within 2 years and only 15 survived for 5 years. Both analyses show that the prognosis for patients with tumors of sheet growth pattern is considerably better than that for those with thin strand growth pattern.

6.4 Stromal Reaction

Some authors have investigated the influence of stromal reaction on prognosis in esophageal carcinoma. Men et al. [63] examined 36 specimens and found that in the areas where the tumor cells were less differentiated and numerous mitoses were present, the amount of argentophil fibers was considerably decreased, while in the areas where the cells were well differentiated with only few mitotic figures, there were many more argentophil fibers surrounding the nests of cancer cells. Yang et al. [64] studied 50 surgical specimens of esophageal carcinoma and found that the number of collagen fibers was inversely proportional to the length of the tumor and that more mature fibrocytes were present in the center of cancer cell nests, while many immature, irregular fibroblasts were present at the periphery of the nests. Sun and Wu [62] found that in patients surviving less than 2 years, the periphery of the carcinoma was often widely infiltrating, while in those surviving more than 5 years, marked degeneration was frequently noticed at the periphery of the tumor tissue. Younghusband and Aluwihare [59] studied the host immune reaction against the tumor, i.e., sinus histiocytosis and follicular hyperplasia in the lymph nodes and lymphocyte infiltration of the tumor, and stated that there was some evidence for the existence of such a reaction. However, more detailed studies are required to see whether it significantly affects the prognosis in esophageal carcinoma.

6.5 *Histologic Grading*

Opinions on the relationship between histologic grading and prognosis vary widely among authors. Wu et al. [57] found that the 5-year survival rates in grades I, II, and III were 40.0% (6/15), 20.5% (8/39), and 20.% (3/15) respectively, and claimed that a definite relationship exists. Liu [8] reported that in a series of 417 cases the corresponding rates were 38.2% (34/89), 23.7% (54/228), and 33.3% (9/27). These results suggest that one may expect a better prognosis in well-differentiated tumors, but there was no parallel relationship between the degrees of differentiation and the prognosis. In studies by Nick et al. [65] and Younghusband and Aluwihare [59], no significant influence of grading of tumors on survival time was shown. Giuli and Gignoux [6] found that undifferentiated or poorly differentiated squamous cell carcinoma appeared paradoxically to have a somewhat better long-term prognosis than well-differentiated forms.

6.6 *Lymphatic Metastasis*

A number of authors [8, 56–59] have noted that the presence or absence of lymph node metastases claerly affects the course and prognosis of the disease. Huang et al. [56] studied a series of 1647 patients treated with resection and found that the 5-year survival rate of 413 patients with lymph node metastases was 12.6%, while of 563 patients without lymph node metastases was 43.3%. Endo et al. [55] reported that among 469 patients with esophageal carcinoma treated by surgery, the 5-year survival rates of those with lymph node metastases were 4%–22%, while that of those without lymph node metastases was 49%.

7 Major Complications and Causes of Death

7.1 *Complications*

Serious complications often occur in patients with esophageal carcinoma. In an autopsy analysis of 41 cases [54], there was pneumonia in 25, chronic pleuritis in 21, hydrothorax in 14, hydropericardium in seven, mediastinitis in six, empyema in six, ascites in four, pulmonary abscess in three, splenic abscess in two, pulmonary thrombosis in one, and subacute endocarditis in one. A number of fistulas were also found: 11 aortic, five esophagotracheal, three anastomotic leak, three esophagotracheomediastinal, two esophagopleural, two esophagoaortotracheal, and one tracheopericardiomediastinal. Palmer [66] summarized six reports totalling 631 cases of esophageal carcinoma and found perforations in 152 cases: 112 into the tracheobronchial tree, 23 into the mediastinum, eight into the pleural cavity, six into the lungs, and one each into the pericardium, the aorta, and the left jugular artery.

7.2 *Causes of Death*

Most patients with untreated esophageal carcinoma die eventually from serious complications, some from cachexia. Taquino and Joseph [67] analyzed 70 cases of esophageal cancer treated nonsurgically and found that the main cause of death was cachexia in 37 cases,

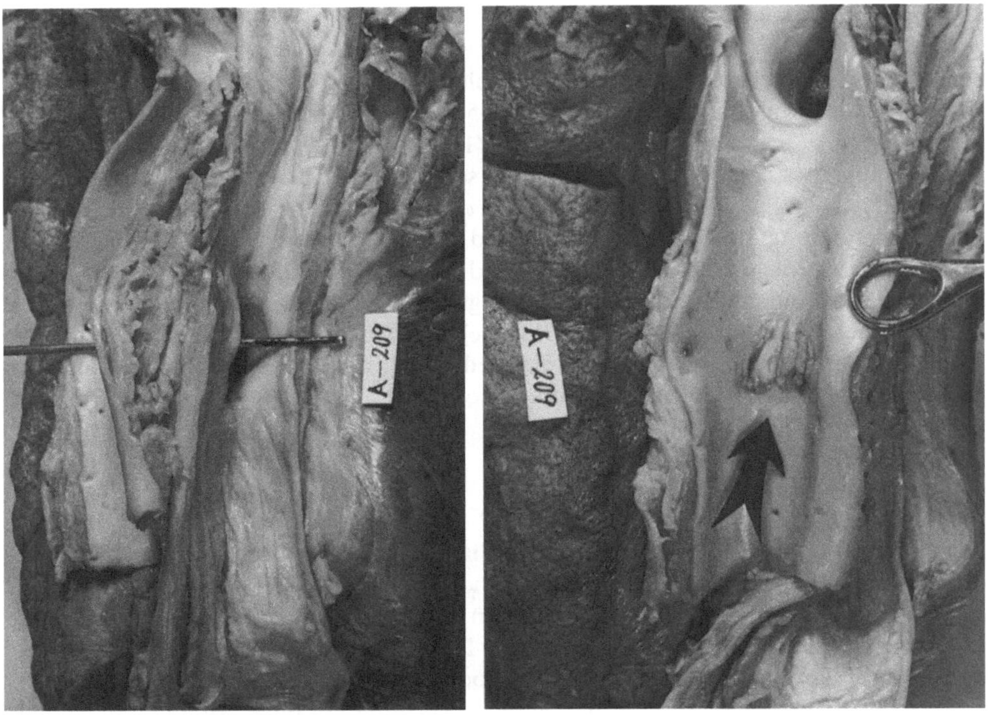

Fig. 4.30. Perforation of aorta caused by esophageal carcinoma. *Left:* Seen from the esophagus; *right:* seen from the aorta. The patient was a 47-year-old woman, Cancer Institute Hospital No. 40229. Squamous cell carcinoma in the middle-lower segment of the esophagus. Four months after radiotherapy (total dose 8000 rads over 10 weeks), the patient died suddenly from hematemesis. At autopsy, a perforation of the esophagus and aorta was revealed. Most of the cancerous tissue in the esophageal wall was replaced by fibrosis, and no obvious radiation damage was seen in the aortic wall

mediastinitis in ten, and pulmonary abscess in seven. Kato et al. [68] reported that of 63 patients treated with radiotherapy, 50% died from cachexia (most of them having dysphagia, indicating recurrence of the tumor); 12.7% from rupture of the aorta; 6.3% from tumor recurrence; and 6.3% from widespread metastasis.

Several reports have been published on fatal hemorrhage caused by esophageal cancer. Alrenga [69] reported four cases and reviewed 99 others from the literature. Aortoesophageal fistula was the cause of fatal hemorrhage in 78 of these 103 cases. Liu [54] analyzed 42 autopsies and found the main cause of death was esophagoaortic fistula (including two esophagotracheoaortic fistulas) in 13 cases (31.7%; Fig. 4.30), esophagotracheal or esophagobronchial fistula in ten cases (24.4%), mediastinitis and abscess caused by various fistulas in ten cases (24.4%), and metastasis or cachexia in nine cases (22.0%).

Several authors have investigated the reasons for aortic rupture in patients with esophageal carcinoma. Marcial-Rojas and Castro [70] and Thomas and Forbus [71] suggested that radiation injury leading to necrosis in the aorta is one of the important causes. Some authors believe that thrombosis may also cause aortic perforation. Soreide et al. [72] reported a case in which the aortic rupture was due to necrosis with infection following irradiation and bleomycin treatment, and suggested that the effects on normal aortic tissue of radiation in combination with cytostatic therapy need further investigation. Postoloff and

Cannon [73] stated that the aortic damage was mainly due to thrombosis of the vasa vasorum leading to ischemia of the aortic wall. Poon et al. [74] demonstrated both histologically and ultrastructurally the changes in a human aorta that ruptured subsequent to radiation during treatment of esophageal carcinoma, and postulated that infection combined with radiation necrosis might have triggered the rupture. All authors have noted that tumor cells infiltrate only the aortic adventitia, never invading the media and intima. Liu [54] compared histologically the irradiated aortic tissue at the site of rupture, the irradiated aortic tissue at a certain distance from the perforation, and the nonirradiated abdominal aortic tissue. There were severe lesions in the intima, media, and adventitia at the perforation site, but in the remote irradiated area he found only occasional mild rupture of elastic fibers in the media, which could not be the cause of perforation. It is probable that the cancerous adhesion of esophagus to aortic adventitia, the inflammatory reaction, and the endo- and perivasculitis of vasa vasorum in the adventitia lead to severe ischemia of the aortic wall, which can no longer withstand the high pressure of blood from inside and eventually ruptures. It follows, therefore, that rupture of the aorta may not be caused directly by radiation damage to the aortic wall.

8 Postirradiation Morphologic Alterations

8.1 Factors Affecting Morphology

The postirradiation morphology of esophageal carcinoma may be influenced by a number of factors. For example, external and intracavitary irradiation may have disparate effects, and different dose levels may cause different morphologic changes. Undifferentiated carcinomas are markedly radiosensitive, squamous cell carcinomas moderately so, and adenocarcinomas relatively resistant. As a rule, the less differentiated the tumor cells, the more sensitive is the tumor to irradiation. Tumor tissue with a rich blood supply reacts more sensitively to irradiation. The morphologic changes are also more pronounced in specimens taken some time subsequent to irradiation than in those taken shortly afterwards. The main tumor of invasive carcinoma of the esophagus is more sensitive to external irradiation than are carcinoma in situ and early carcinoma in the adjacent mucosa.

8.2 Basic Changes

Irradiated esophageal carcinomas show mainly stromal reaction and degeneration and necrosis of cancer cells.

8.2.1 Alterations of Cancer Cells

Postirradiation changes may occur in both nuclei and cytoplasm. Acute irradiation at high dosage often causes acute necrotic lesions of tumor cells. However, chronic irradiation may cause a series of changes of different degrees. Early in a course of irradiation the structure of the nucleus becomes indistinct and the chromatin becomes unevenly distributed. There may then be swelling of the nucleus and aggregation of chromatin near the nuclear envelope, and the nucleoplasm may become transparent, the nucleus coming to resemble a bullseye. In some cells the chromatin is aggregated into coarse clusters and the nuclei become irregular. Multinucleate tumor cells may appear. Sometimes the nucleoli disappear. These changes are usually thought to be reversible.

After heavier irradiation, in some markedly changed tumor cells the nuclei are ruptured and cell debris are scattered in the tumor bed matrix. Cells may be swollen to a certain degree and irregular in shape. Cytoplasm is stained red and scattered acidophilic bodies may be noted. Small or large cytoplasmic vacuoles are often present in which may be found Sudan-III-positive or mucicarmine-positive material, and sometimes PAS-positive but diastase-resistant material. In more severely radiation-damaged tumor tissue, the cells may be pyknotic, swollen, or balloon-like. Large clusters of keratinized material may be present in irradiated squamous cell carcinoma. Mono- and multinucleate bizarre tumor cells can frequently be observed.

8.2.2. Stromal Reaction

Shortly after irradiation, lymphocytes appear around the cancer cells or even inside their cytoplasm. In cases involving greater degeneration of the tumor, lymphocytic infiltration often increases accompanied by proliferation of capillaries in the tumor bed, with the result that granulations are formed. In areas of greater degeneration and marked necrosis, the inflammatory infiltration decreases, pink proteinous substances and cell debris can be seen in the tumor bed matrix, and the number of capillaries declines. Necrotic keratinized material, mono- and multinucleate foreign body giant cells, cholesterol crystals, and even scattered calcification may be observed in the tumor stroma. Endo- or perivasculitis of small or medium-sized arteries with stenosis or obliteration of their lumina may be noticed in the tumor bed.

In tissues markedly changed after irradiation, tumor cells may disappear completely, leaving only mild inflammatory infiltration and sparse capillaries. Fibrous tissue proliferation or scar formation occurs, and finally the radiation damage is repaired.

To summarize, the reaction of esophageal carcinoma to irradiation consists of three consecutive but overlapping stages. The major features of the tissue injury stage are degeneration and necrosis of tumor cells. The stage of elimination of necrotic tissue is characterized mainly by capillary proliferation, inflammatory infiltration, and the presence of foreign body giant cells. The tissue repair stage is marked mainly by granulation, fibroblast proliferation, and scar formation.

8.3 Intracavitary Irradiation

In recent years many cases of early esophageal cancer have been discovered in high-incidence areas in China. Since the results of external irradiation in early lesions were often unsatisfactory, and since sophisticated radiotherapeutic equipment is often lacking in rural areas, intracavitary radiotherapy with ^{60}Co has been undertaken. A number of patients have been operated upon after intracavitary irradiation, with resection of the tumor-bearing part of the esophagus. The present study was based on the pathological examination of 29 such specimens.

Examination of the gross specimens revealed that characteristic annular ulceration was often formed after irradiation (Fig. 4.31). The surface was grayish-white to grayish-yellow

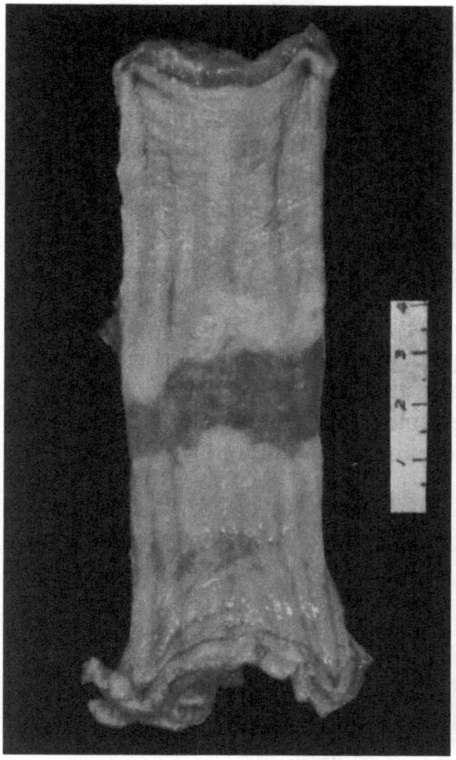

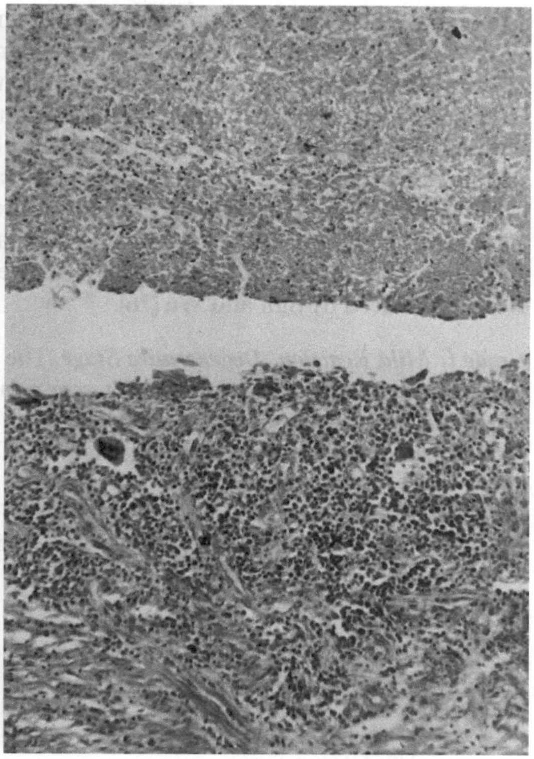

Fig. 4.31 (left). Annular ulceration after intracavitary irradiation. Surgical specimen of early esophageal carcinoma

Fig. 4.32 (right). Early esophageal carcinoma after intracavitary irradiation. The tumor bed is replaced by granulation tissue covered with a pseudomembrane. No tumor cells can be detected in this case

in color, frequently covered with a pseudomembrane (Fig. 4.32), and the border was distinct, hyperemic, and edematous. In seven cases, however, the tumor was rather large without annular ulceration.

Microscopically, all 29 cases showed degeneration and necrosis of tumor cells and a certain stromal reaction. The degree of degenerative changes varied in different layers of the esophageal wall. The most remarkable changes of tumor cells were seen in the mucosa and submucosa. In five of the 29 cases, cytosmear examination showed the presence of tumor cells but the lesions were covered with granulations and histologically no carcinoma could be detected. Of these five, four were early esophageal carcinoma, indicating that intracavitary irradiation is effective in the treatment of this lesion.

8.4 Changes After Preoperative Irradiation

Methods of grading and typing the morphologic changes in irradiated esophageal carcinomas vary among authors. Nakayama [75] used Takazawa's classification to assess the preoperative radiotherapeutic effects, based on the degree of morphologic changes in cancer cells (X_1, X_2, X_3), stromal reaction (S_1, S_2, S_3), carcinoma infiltration (L_1, L_2, L_3), and differentiation of the carcinomatous parenchyma (D_1, D_2, D_3,). Sun and Wu [76] studied 80 resected specimens of esophageal carcinoma treated with preoperative irradiation, grading the effects of radiation as mild, moderate, or marked according to the changes in gross and microscopic features of the tumors and the presence or absence of tumor cells. They concluded that the grading of postirradiation morphologic changes seemed to be related to radiation dose, with doses of over 3000 rads having particularly marked effects.

Liu [8] analyzed 251 resected specimens of preoperative irradiated esophageal carcinoma. Based on changes in tumor cells and stromal reactions, he also classified postirradiation changes of esophageal carcinoma into three grades, using categories very similar to those introduced by Sun and Wu [76].

Grade I: Mild Reaction, Degenerative Stage. The prominent feature in this stage is degeneration of tumor cells. *Grossly,* tumor size remains the same or decreases only slightly (Fig. 4.33). *Microscopically,* only a portion of the tumor cells are degenerated (Fig. 4.34), many others remaining intact. Inflammatory infiltration is pronounced.

Grade II: Moderate Reaction, Granulation Stage. The prominent feature in this stage is granulation formation. *Grossly,* tumor size is greatly reduced and tumor contours are

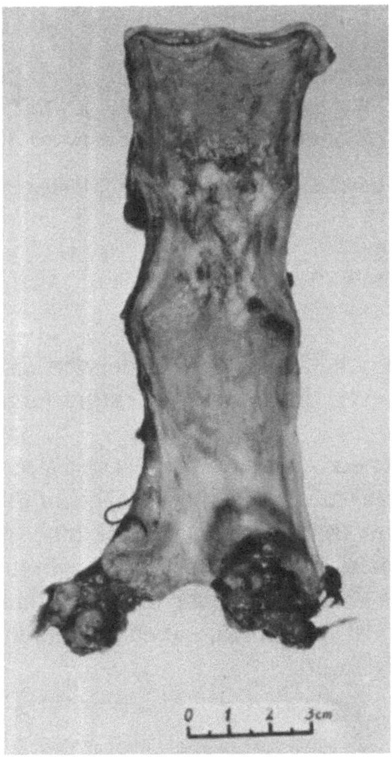

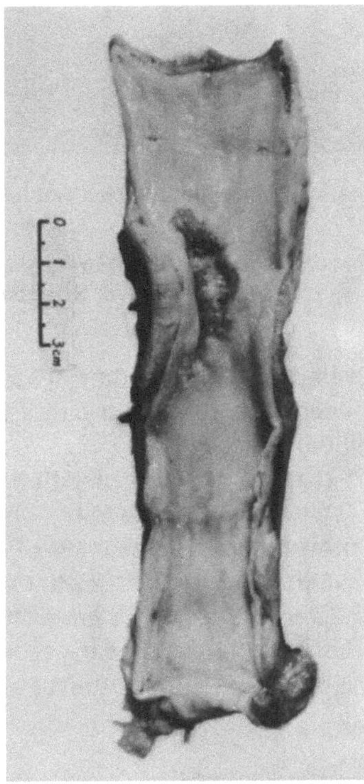

Fig. 4.33 (left). Squamous cell carcinoma of the esophagus, radiation reaction grade I. The gross appearance of the tumor is little changed

Fig. 4.34 see p. 111

Fig. 4.35 (right). Squamous cell carcinoma of the esophagus, radiation reaction grade II. The tumor size is considerably reduced

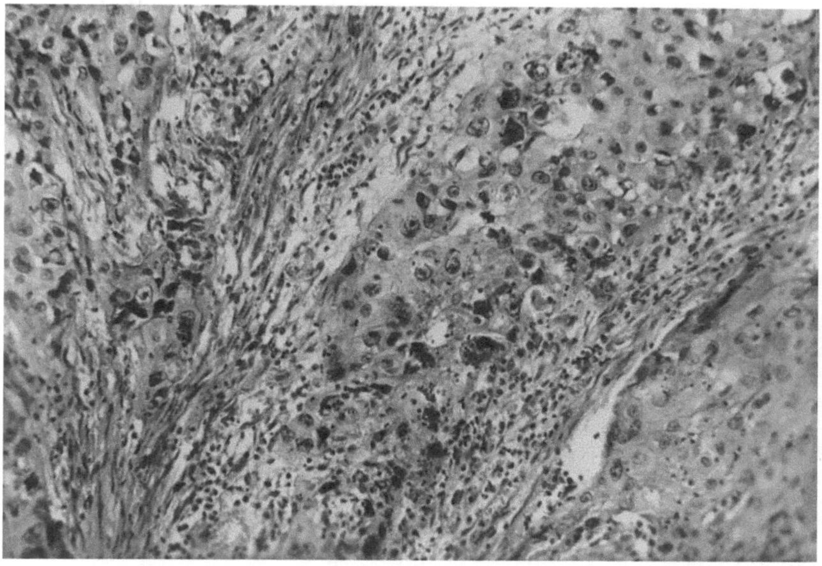

Fig. 4.34. Squamous cell carcinoma of the esophagus, radiation reaction grade I. Some of the tumor cells are markedly degenerated

blurred (Fig. 4.35). The ulceration becomes shallow, possibly even disappearing. On the cut surface the tumor tissue is grayish-red or brownish-red and the border is obscured. *Microscopically,* the majority of tumor cells have disappeared and the remaining degenerated tumor cells are surrounded by fibrous tissue. Keratinized substances (Fig. 4.36), cholesterol crystals, calcification (Fig. 4.37), foreign body giant cells, and neutrophils can be observed in the tumor bed matrix, and capillaries are abundant. Late in this stage inflammatory infiltration may be reduced, while fibrous tissue proliferates.

Grade III: Marked Reaction, Fibrotic Stage. The prominent feature of this stage is proliferation of fibroblasts and scar formation. *Grossly,* no obvious tumor is seen (Fig. 4.38), but occasionally a small, shallow ulceration may be left. On the cut surface, the esophageal wall is thin and its structure is obscured. *Microscopically,* no tumor cells can be found. There is fibrosis or scar formation in the tumor bed, which is lined by a thin layer of squamous epithelium (Fig. 4.39).

Among Liu's 251 cases mentioned above [8], all 22 tumors irradiated with less than 1500 rads showed grade I changes. Of the 41 lesions receiving over 5000 rads, 20 showed grade III alterations and 15 had grade II changes. This illustrated the relationship between radiation dose and postirradiation reaction.

The prognosis of patients with esophageal carcinoma treated by irradiation is influenced by various factors, including morphologic alterations caused by radiation. Liu [8] analyzed 218 cases involving preoperative irradiation; there was no significant difference in 1-year survival rate (67.2%–70.8%) between different postirradiation grades, but a slight difference was found in the 2-year survival rates, and a significant difference in 5-year survival rates (grade I 22.4%, grade II 32.4%, grade III 37.8%). The findings seem to indicate that the long-term survival of patients with esophageal cancer may be improved by preoperative radiotherapy.

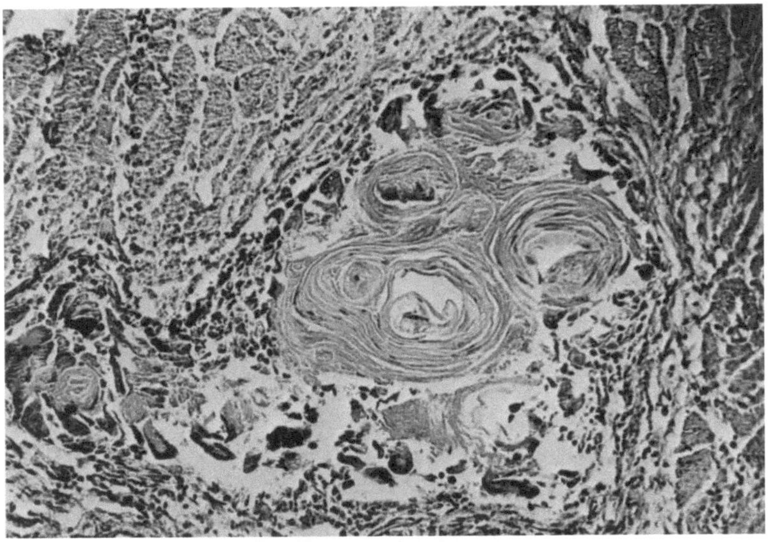

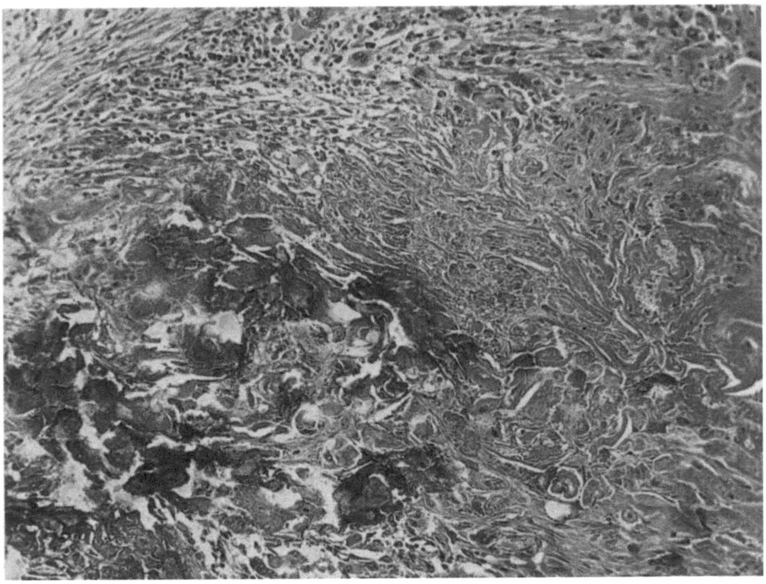

Fig. 4.36 (above). Squamous cell carcinoma of the esophagus after irradiation. The number of tumor cells is considerably decreased. Some keratinized material, granulation tissue, and foreign body giant cells are present

Fig. 4.37 (below). Squamous cell carcinoma of the esophagus after irradiation. Calcification can be seen in the midst of keratinized material

Huang et al. [77] presented the clinical data and evaluation of 408 selected patients with esophageal carcinoma treated by combined preoperative irradiation and surgery. They concluded that adjuvant preoperative irradiation enhanced surgical results in their series.

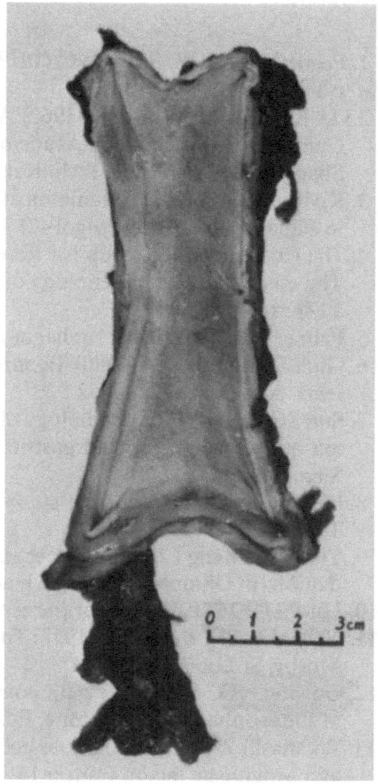

Fig. 4.38. Squamous cell carcinoma of the esophagus, radiation reaction grade III. Grossly, no obvious tumor or ulceration is seen

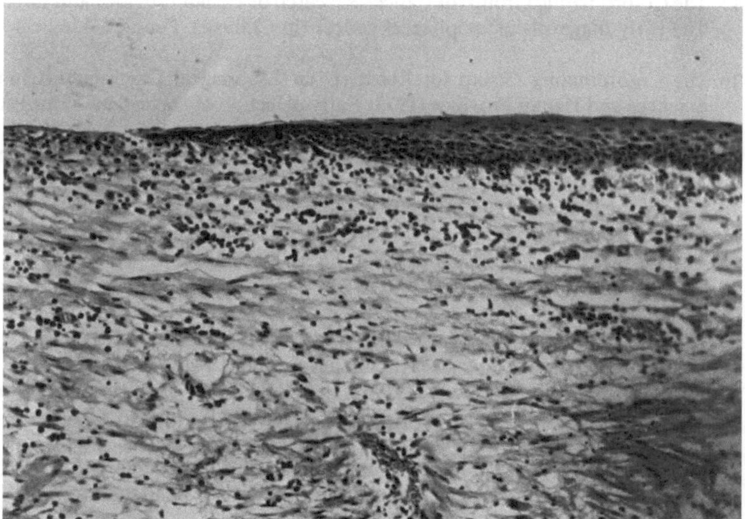

Fig. 4.39. Squamous cell carcinoma of the esophagus, radiation reaction grade III. Marked fibrosis in the tumor bed is covered with newly formed thin epithelium. No tumor cells can be found in this case

References

1. Postlethwait RW, Sealy WC (1979) Surgery of the esophagus. Appleton-Century-Crofts, New York, p 348
2. Li KH, Kao JC, Wu YK (1962) A survey of the prevalence of carcinoma of the esophagus in North China. In: The Chinese Academy of Medical Sciences (ed) Selected papers on cancer research. Shanghai Scientific and Technical Publishers, Shanghai, pp 215–221
3. Kiviranta UK (1952) Carcinoma of the esophagus. Its incidence, age and sex distribution and prognosis in Finland. Acta Otolaryngol 42: 73–88
4. The Co-ordinating Group for Research on the Etiology of Esophageal Cancer in North China (1975) The epidemiology and etiology of esophageal cacer in North China. A preliminary report. Chin Med J 1/3: 167–183
5. Palmer ED (1952) The esophagus and its diseases. Cassell, London, p 375
6. Giuli R, Gignoux M (1980) Treatment of carcinoma of the esophagus: retrospective study of 2400 patients. Ann Surg 192: 44–52
7. Sun SQ, Wu X (1965) Pathology of carcinoma of the esophagus. In: Wu YK, Huang GJ (eds) Carcinoma of the esophagus and gastric cardia (in Chinese). Shanghai Scientific and Technical Publishers, Shanghai, p 27
8. Liu FS (1977) Pathological study of 858 cases of esophageal cancer (in Chinese). Cancer Res Prev Treat 4: 273–277
9. Yin WB, Zhang LJ, Yang ZY, et al. (1980) An analysis of 3798 cases of esophageal cancer treated by radiation (in Chinese with English abstract). Chin J Oncol 2: 216–221
10. Liu FS (1976) Pathology of the esophageal cancer (in Chinese). Cancer Res Prev Treat 3: 74–83
11. Schenken JR, Burns EL (1957) The gastrointestinal tract. In: Anderson WAD (ed) Pathology, 3rd edn. Mosby, St Louis pp 746–747
12. Gowing NFC (1961) The pathology of oesophageal tumors. In: Tanner NL, Smithers DW (eds) Tumors of the esophagus. Livingstone, Edinburgh London, p 94
13. Takahashi K (1961) Squamous cell carcinoma of the esophagus. Stromal inflammatory cell infiltration as a prognostic factor. Cancer 14: 921–933
14. Miller C (1962) Carcinoma of thoracic esophagus and cardia. A review of 405 cases. Br J Surg 49: 507–522
15. The Co-ordinating Group for Cancer Research of Henan Province and Linxian County Hospital (1973) The early diagnosis of esophageal cancer (in Chinese). People's Medical Publishing House, Beijing, p70
16. The Co-ordinating Group for Research on Esophageal Carcinoma, Chinese Academy of Medical Sciences and Henan Province (1973) Early detection of carcinoma of the esophagus (in Chinese). Natl Med J China 53: 451–453
17. Huang GJ, Shao LF, Zhang DW, et al. (1981) Diagnosis and surgical treatment of early esophageal carcinoma. Chin Med J 94: 229–232
18. Liu FS, Li L, Qu SL (1982) Clinical and pathological characteristics of early esophageal cancer. In: Burghardt E, Holzer E (eds) Minimal invasive cancer (microcarcinoma). Saunders, London, pp 539–557 (Clinics in oncology vol. 1, no. 2)
19. Wu YK, Liu Y, Hu MH, et al. (1958) The classification of types of carcinoma of the esophagus (in Chinese). Natl Med J China 76: 213–228
20. Sun SQ, Yu PL, Tang J, et al. (1960) A study on the incidence rate, sex and age distribution and classification of the esophageal cancer (in Chinese). Chin J Pathol 6: 81–87
21. Wu X, Liu YC, Liu YW, Wu YK (1962) Pathologic types of squamous cell carcinoma of the esophagus. In: The Chinese Academy of Medical Sciences (ed) Selected papers on cancer research. Shanghai Scientific and Technical Publishers, Shanghai, pp 163–177
22. Sun SQ, Wu X (1965) Pathology of carcinoma of the esophagus. In: Wu YK, Huang GJ (eds) Carcinoma of the esophagus and gastric cardia (in Chinese). Shanghai Scientific and Technical Publishers, Shanghai, p 35
23. Huang GJ, Gu XZ, Liu FS, Wang ZY, et al. (1981) Further studies on the separate entity of intraluminal type of esophageal carcinoma (in Chinese with English abstract). Chin J Oncol 3: 110–112
24. Broders AC, Vinson PP (1928) The degree of malignancy of carcinoma of the esophagus. Arch Otolaryngol 8: 79–80
25. Chen YY, Lin QX (1964) A clinico-pathological analysis of 500 cases of esophageal cancer from Quanzhou Area, Fujian Province (in Chinese). Tianjin Med J Sect Oncol 2: 118–119

26. Puestow CB, Gillesby WJ, Guynn VL (1955) Cancer of the esophagus. Arch Surg 70: 662–671
27. Raphael H, Ellis FH Jr, Dockerty MB (1966) Primary adenocarcinoma of the esophagus: 18-year review and review of the literature. Ann Surg 164: 785–796
28. Kusalina GK, Kolycheva NI (1974) On adenogenic esophageal cancers (in Russian with English abstract). Vopr Onkol 20/5: 15–20
29. Turnbull ADM, Goodner JT (1968) Primary adenocarcinoma of the esophagus. Cancer 22: 915–918
30. Bosch A, Frias Z, Caldwell WL (1979) Adenocarcinoma of the esophagus. Cancer 43: 1557–1561
31. Ellis FH Jr, Jackson RC, et al. (1959) Carcinoma of the esophagus and cardia. N Engl J Med 260: 351–358
32. Appelqvist P (1975) Carcinoma of the esophagus and gastric cardia at autopsy in Finland. Ann Clin Res 7: 334–340
33. Smithers DW (1956) Adenocarcinoma of the esophagus. Thorax 11: 257–267
34. Dodge OG (1960) Intraesophageal adenocarcinoma. Gut 1: 351–356
35. Jacobsohn WZ, Libson Y, Dollberg L (1980) Adenoid cystic carcinoma of the esophagus. Gastrointest Endosc 26: 102–104
36. McKeown F (1952) Oat cell carcinoma of the esophagus. J Pathol Bacteriol 64: 889–891
37. Tateishi R, Taniguchi K, Horai T, et al. (1976) Argyrophil cell carcinoma (apudoma) of the esophagus; a histopathologic entity. Virchows Arch [Pathol Anat] 371: 283–294
38. Cook MG, Eusebi V, Betts CM (1976) Oat cell carcinoma of the esophagus; a recent recognized entity. J Clin Pathol 29: 1068–1073
39. Imai T, Sannohe Y, Okano H (1978) Oat cell carcinoma (APUDOMA) of the esophagus. A case report. Cancer 41: 358–364
40. Reid HAS, Richardson WW, Corrin B (1980) Oat cell carcinoma of the esophagus. Cancer 45: 2342–2347
41. Fang ZX, Sun SQ (1965) An electron microscopic observation of squamous cell carcinoma of the esophagus (in Chinese). Acta Shandong Med Coll 1: 6–10
42. Henan Medical College (1972) An electron microscopic observation of normal and cancerous esophageal epithelium (in Chinese). In: Proceedings of the Conference on Prevention and Treatment of Esophageal Cancer, Linxian County, Henan Privince, pp 247–252
43. Zhou CN, Li L, Men ZJ (1979) Electron microscopic investigation of human esophageal squamous cell carcinoma (in Chinese). Natl Med J China 59: 7–11
44. Li K, Ma JQ, Wang YY, Liu SD, et al. (1980) The ultrastructure of human esophageal squamous cell carcinoma (abstract in Chinese). Med Inform 7/2: 22
45. Kuo ZQ, Li JH, Li RQ, Zhang JQ, et al. (1980) A preliminary ultrastructural observation of esophageal carcinoma (abstract in Chinese). Med Inform 7/2: 18
46. Ma JQ, Li K, Wang YY, Liu SD, et al. (1980) The ultrastructure of human esophageal epithelium (abstract in Chinese). Med Inform 7/2: 21
47. Zhang J, Li WQ, Wu LNS (1982) A preliminary electron microscopic observation of squamous cell carcinoma of the esophagus (in Chinese). Chin J Pathol 11: 54–57
48. Department of Ultrastructure of an Institute, Chinese Academy of Medical Sciences (1973) Ultrastructure of squamous cell carcinoma of the human uterine cervix (in Chinese). Natl Med J China 53: 286–289
49. Zhou CN (1980) A characteristic crystalline structure in plasma cells in a patient with squamous cell carcinoma of the esophagus (in Chinese). Chin J Cell Biol 2/2: 22–24
50. Yamashita N (1979) A statistical analysis concerning the routes of dissemination of cancer of the esophagus based on the autopsy records (in Japanese with English abstract). J Jpn Soc Cancer Ther 14: 1146–1149
51. Sannohe Y, Hiratsuke R, Doki K (1981) Lymph node metastasis in cancer of thoracic esophagus. Am J Surg 14: 216–218
52. Hiroko IDE, Endo M, Haniw F, et al. (1974) Lymph node metastasis of carcinoma of the thoracic esophagus (in Japanese). Operation 28: 1355–1364
53. Dormanns E (1939) Das Oesophaguscarcinom; Ergebnisse der unter Mitarbeit von 39 Pathologischen Instituten Deutschlands durchgeführten Erhebung über das Oesophaguscarcinom (1925–1933). Z Krebsforsch 49: 86–108
54. Liu FS (1980) Autoptic analysis of 41 cases of esophageal cancer (in Chinese with English abstract). Natl Med J China 60: 218–222
55. Endo M, Kinoshita Y, Yamada, et al. (1980) The present state of surgical treatment of the thoracic esophageal cancer (in Japanese with English abstract). J Jpn Bronchoesophag Soc 31: 199–205

56. Huang GJ, Zhang DW, Wang GQ, et al. (1981) Surgical treatment of carcinoma of the esophagus. Report of 1647 cases. Chin Med J 94: 305–307
57. Wu YK, Huang KC, Chang W (1962) Remote results of resection of squamous cell carcinoma of the esophagus. In: The Chinese Academy of Medical Sciences (ed) Selected papers on cancer research. Shanghai Scientific and Technical Publishers, Shanghai, pp 194–198
58. Appelqvist P, Matilla S, Jyrala A, Tala P (1977) Surgical treatment of carcinoma of the esophagus and cardia. Scand J Thorac Cardiovasc Surg 11: 278–282
59. Younghusband JD, Aluwihare APR (1970) Carcinoma of the esophagus: factors influencing survival. Br J Surg 57: 422–430
60. Co-ordinating Group for Research on Esophageal Cancer, Linxian County, Henan (1975) Early diagnosis and surgical treatment of esophageal cancer under rural conditions (in Chinese). Natl Med J China 55: 845–846
61. Xian MS, Gao GT, Chen XJ, et al. (1964) A pathomorphological study on esophageal cancer. II. Pathological typing, staging and their relationship with prognosis (in Chinese). Tianjin Med J Sect Oncol 2: 317–320
62. Sun SQ, Wu X (1980) Factors influencing the prognosis of patients with squamous cell carcinoma of the esophagus: correlation of the morphology of 100 surgical specimens and the postoperative life span (in Chinese with English abstract). Chin J Oncol 2: 119–124
63. Men W, Chen YR, Shi KL, et al. (1961) The reactive changes of argentophil fibers in esophageal cancer tissue (in Chinese). Acta Shandong Med Coll 6: 32–35
64. Yang MH, Kun SK, Wang BT (1965) Morphological study on stromal reaction of esophageal squamous cell carcinoma (in Chinese). (Unpublished data)
65. Nick R, Green D, McClatchie G (1973) A clinicopathological study of some factors influencing survival in cancer of the esophagus: a survey of ten years' experience. Aust NZ J Surg 43: 3–13
66. Palmer ED (1952) The esophagus and its diseases. Cassell, London, p 409
67. Taquino GJ, Joseph GF (1947) Carcinoma of the esophagus. An analysis of 145 cases with special reference to metastases and extensions. Ann Otol Rhinol Laryngol 56: 1041–1058
68. Kato T, Koike N, Niibe H, Murakami Y (1975) Treatment of cancer of the esophagus by radiation. Part 2. Recurrence and cause of death (in Japanese with English abstract). Nippon Acta Radiol 35: 321–327
69. Airenga DP (1976) Fatal hemorrhage complicating carcinoma of the esophagus. Am J Gastroenterol 65: 422–426
70. Marcial-Rojas RA, Castro JR (1962) Irradiation injury to the elastic arteries in the course of treatment for neoplastic disease. Ann Otol Rhinol Laryngol 71: 945–958
71. Thomas E, Forbus WD (1959) Irradiation injury to the aorta and the lung. Arch Pathol 67: 256–263
72. Soreide O, Janssen CW Jr, Kvam G, Hartveit F (1976) Aorto-oesophageal fistula complicating carcinoma of the esophagus. Review of the literature and report of a case following irradiation and cytostatic therapy. Scand J Thorac Cardiovasc Surg 10: 79–84
73. Postoloff AV, Cannon WM (1946) Genesis of aortic perforation secondary to carcinoma of the esophagus. Report of investigation in two cases. Arch Pathol 41: 533–539
74. Poon TP, Kanshepolsky J, Tchertkoff V (1968) Rupture of the aorta due to radiation injury. JAMA 205: 875–878
75. Nakayama K (1964) Pre-operative irradiation in the treatment of patients with carcinoma of the esophagus and some other sites. Clin Radiol 15: 232–241
76. Sun SQ, Wu X (1965) The pathological alterations of esophageal squamous cell carcinoma treated by ^{60}cobalt irradiation (in Chinese). Chin J Pathol [Suppl] 9: 402–405
77. Huang GJ, Gu XZ, Zhang RG, et al. (1981) Combined preoperative irradiation and surgery in esophageal carcinoma. Report of 408 cases. Chin Med J 94: 73–76

Chapter 5
Pathology of Carcinoma of the Gastric Cardia

Ling Li and Guo Li Pan

---

1 Introduction

Carcinoma of the gastric cardia is one of the malignant tumors with a high incidence in certain regions of China. It has unusual epidemiologic and clinical features, but as a result of its location, experts have failed to agree on whether to assign it to the stomach or the esophagus, and its pathological features, histogenesis, and metastatic properties have seldom been touched upon in the specialized analyses and investigations. In recent years, along with progress in the research into carcinomas of the esophagus and stomach, data and reports on carcinoma of the gastric cardia have gradually accumulated.

2 Classification

There have long been different views about how to classify carcinoma of the gastric cardia. Most investigators call it gastric cancer at the cardia, but interpretations of "cardia" vary. Other authors include it in the category of cancers of the lower segment of the esophagus [1–5]. Still others are in favor of a separate category and define it as a malignant tumor of the stomach, originating often in the stomach but sometimes in the esophagus [6]. The disagreement is due mainly to the fact that most patients with carcinoma of the gastric cardia are seen at an advanced stage, making it difficult to pinpoint the origin of the tumor, and this probably also explains why the incidences reported in the literature vary so greatly. Such discrepancies may also affect further pathological study.

During the past few years, clinicians and pathologists in Japan have conducted certain special investigations and discussions on carcinoma of the gastric cardia. In view of the peculiar histologic features at the esophagogastric junction, carcinoma of the gastric cardia has been proposed as a separate disease entity. However, opinion is by no means unanimous [7–11]. For example, Nishi et al. [7] held that the area up to 2 cm above and below the esophagogastric junction, i. e., 2 cm of the lower segment of the esophagus and 2 cm of the region of the cardiac glands, making a range of 4 cm, has specific anatomic functions, and carcinoma arising in this region should be termed "carcinoma of the esophagogastric junction." Further, those carcinomas located <1 cm, 1–2 cm, and >2 cm below the esophagogastric junction line were respectively given the names of "carcinoma of the junction," "carcinoma of the cardia," and "carcinoma of the stomach related to the cardia."

The Thirtieth Conference on Carcinoma of the Stomach in Japan [8] proposed defining carcinoma of the esophagogastric junction as "a carcinoma having its center within 1 cm of the junction."

Pathologists such as Kato et al. [9] are of the opinion that "carcinomas of the esophagogastric junction" should include those gastric carcinomas with their centers located 2 cm below the junction, i. e., gastric carcinoma at the cardia.

In order to clarify this problem, it is useful to refer again to the peculiar anatomohistologic features of the gastric cardia. Pathological studies on early gastric and esophageal carcinomas adjacent to the junction may also be informative. The gastric cardia is the orifice between the esophagus and stomach and has unique anatomophysiologic characteristics [11–13]. Histologically stratified squamous epithelium of the esophagus and simple columnar epithelium of the stomach are sharply demarcated at the esophagogastric junction. Below this point there is an area which is characterized by irregularly distributed tubular or branched tubular cardiac glands and has been termed "the cardiac portion" or "the region of the cardiac glands" within a range of 0.5–4 cm, mostly about 2 cm, from the junction [11, 14]. Histologic study of the cardiac mucosa in our material shows that the cardiac glands usually extend not more than 2 cm below the junction [15]. In our series, all 18 early carcinomas of the gastric cardia were located within 0–2.5 cm of the junction (centers of lesions within 1.75 cm), which conforms well with the distribution of cardiac glands. There is evidence to show that these early carcinomas, all adenocarcinomas, originate from the columnar epithelium of the cardia [15]. Investigation of early carcinomas of the esophagus also show that early squamous carcinomas adjacent to the junction arise exclusively from the squamous epithelium of the esophagus [16]. It seems reasonable to designate carcinomas of the gastric cardia as those arising from the cardiac region, for which we prefer to set a limit of 2 cm below the junction. Carcinoma of the gastric cardia is a stomach cancer and should be strictly distinguished from cancers in the lower segment of the esophagus, but because of its particular histologic relationship to cardiac epithelium and its dissimilarities in epidemiology, pathology, and clinical manifestations to cancers in other parts of the stomach, it should be singled out as an independent disease entity.

When dealing with advanced carcinomas of the gastric cardia, clinicians may find that many of those which are almost entirely adenocarcinomatous and a few of those which are squamous invade the lower segment of the esophagus, to a distance generally not more than 5 cm; conversely, some squamous carcinomas and a few adenocarcinomas of the lower esophagus invade the cardia. It is extremely difficult to ascertain the exact site of origin of a tumor in such circumstances. For practical purposes, most clinicians would consider adenocarcinomas at the esophagogastric junction area as carcinomas of the gastric cardia and squamous carcinomas at that location as esophageal carcinomas. This classification has proved to be correct in most instances.

3 Gross Types

In the gross typing of carcinomas of the gastrointestinal tract, Borrmann's classification has generally been followed. The basic types are polypoid or fungating, sharply demarcated ulcerating, infiltrating ulcerated, and infiltrating [17]. At the National Collaborative Conference on Gastric Cancer [18] held in China in 1978, eight categories were proposed: plate-like fungating, nodular fungating, localized ulcerative, infiltrating ulcerative, localized infiltrating, diffuse infiltrating, superficial spreading, and unclassifiable or mixed.

Little work has been done on gross classification with special reference to carcinomas of the gastric cardia. In 1963, Sun et al. [19] classified 100 cases of carcinoma of the gastric cardia into three types, cauliflower-like, ulcerating, and infiltrating. Bearing in mind that the gross appearance of carcinomas of the gastric cardia is not so complicated as that of those in other parts of the stomach, it may not be wise to subdivide them into too many types. On the other hand, the ulcerating type in Sun's classification actually includes two distinct forms, one sharply demarcated with raised margins and the other without definite borders, which have different prognoses. We prefer to adopt Borrmann's system and classify carcinomas of the gastric cardia into four types: fungating, localized ulcerating, ulcero-infiltrating, and infiltrating.

Fungating. The tumor forms a nodular, fungating, cauliflower-like, polypoid or bulky mass which protrudes into the lumen, usually with a regular margin and occasionally with shallow ulceration (Fig. 5.1).

Localized Ulcerating. The tumor has a conspicuous deep ulcer with a sharply demarcated and raised margin (Fig. 5.2).

Ulcero-Infiltrating. The tumor appears as an infiltrating and ulcerating lesion without clear demarcation from the surrounding mucosa (Fig. 5.3).

Infiltrating. The cancer cells diffusely infiltrate all layers of the stomach in the cardiac region, resulting in generalized thickening of the diseased gastric wall (Fig. 5.4).

The gross typing is related to histologic classification. The fungating and localized ulcerating types consist mostly of well-differentiated adenocarcinoma and well-differentiated mucinous adenocarcinoma, the fungating type having the highest proportion of well-differentiated carcinoma. In the ulcero-infiltrating type, poorly differentiated adenocarcinoma and poorly differentiated mucinous adenocarcinoma are more frequently seen. The

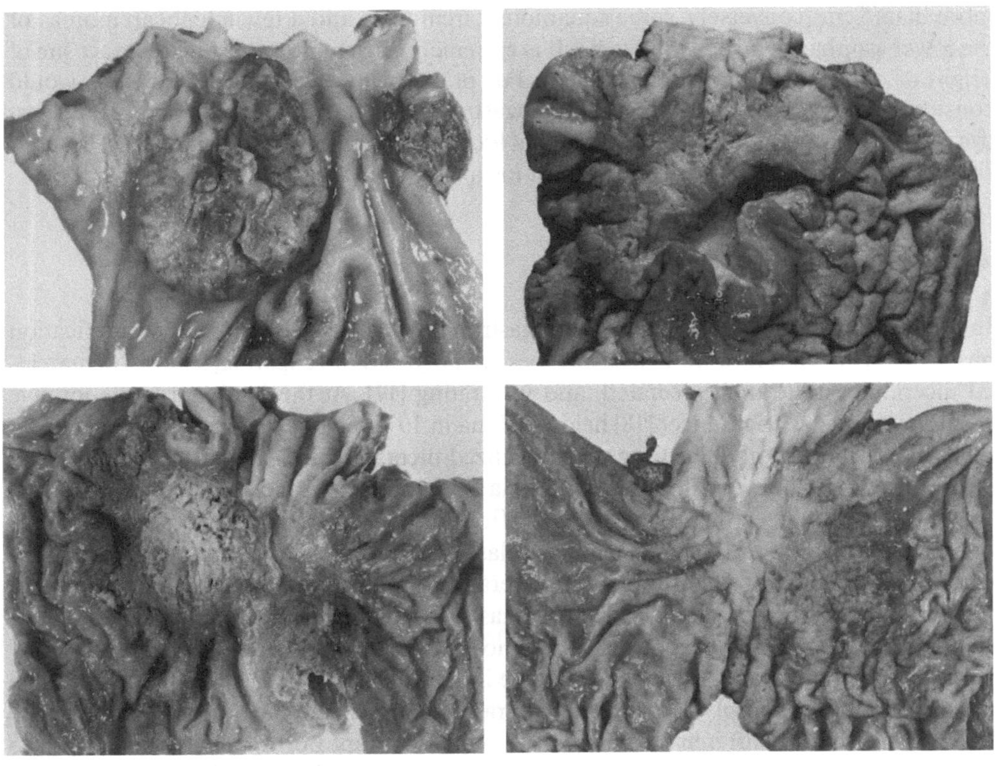

Fig. 5.1 *(upper left).* Fungating carcinoma of the gastric cardia

Fig. 5.2 *(upper right).* Localized ulcerating carcinoma of the gastric cardia

Fig. 5.3 *(lower left).* Ulcero-infiltrating carcinoma of the gastric cardia

Fig. 5.4 *(lower right).* Infiltrating carcinoma of the gastric cardia

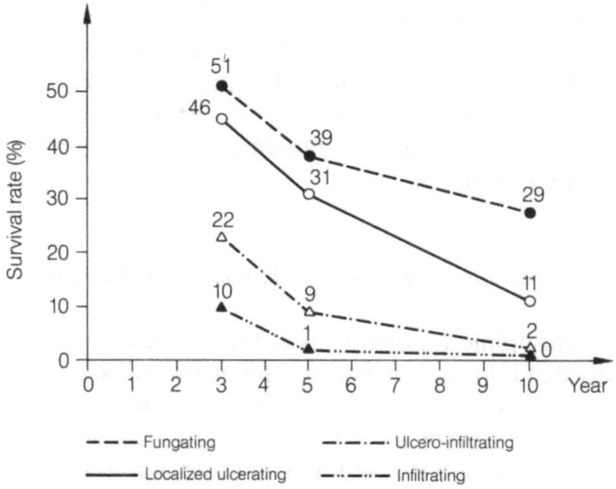

Fig. 5.5. Gross types and prognosis

infiltrating type consists mostly of poorly differentiated or diffuse adenocarcinoma and diffuse mucinous adenocarcinoma.

Among 500 carcinomas of the gastric cardia we have studied, the fungating type was found in 82 cases (16.4%), the localized ulcerating type in 182 cases (36.4%), the ulcero-infiltrating type in 140 cases (28.0%), and the infiltrating type in 96 cases (19.2%). Different types have different prognoses, from the poorest in the infiltrating type to the best in the fungating type (Fig. 5.5) [20].

It has also been observed that there is a limited range of forms of carcinoma of the gastric cardia as compared with the other parts of the stomach, and this is being regarded as one of the distinctive pathological features [7, 20, 21]. Whether or not this observation is valid remains to be clarified by further investigation.

4 Histologic Types

4.1 Classifications from the Literature

As with gross typing, histologic breakdown of carcinoma of the gastric cardia has been done by most investigators in accordance with that of gastric carcinoma. The principal classifications are as follows:

- Lauren [22] classified gastric carcinomas as intestinal or diffuse, according to epidemiology, etiology, clinical manifestations, and prognosis.
- Nakamura [23] also used two broad categories, in his case differentiated and undifferentiated. The principal lesions in the differentiated group were tubular adenocarcinoma, papillary tubular adenocarcinoma, and nodular mucinous adenocarcinoma. Included in the undifferentiated group were mucocellular carcinoma and scirrhous carcinoma. The classification recommended by the National Conference on Gastric Carcinoma in China [18] is broadly similar.
- Nagayo and Yokoyama [17] divided gastric carcinomas into well-differentiated, moderately differentiated, and poorly differentiated.

- Histologic classifications with special reference to carcinoma of the gastric cardia have only been occasionally reported and are generally treated in a simpler way. Sun et al. [19], Ellis [24], and Gunnlaugsson et al. [1] all favored division into adenocarcinoma, adenoacanthoma, and squamous carcinoma. In McPeak's classification [25] there was an additional category of papillary adenocarcinoma. Dodge [26] included undifferentiated and mixed types.

4.2 Adenocarcinoma and Mucinous Adenocarcinoma

In our opinion, carcinomas of the gastric cardia are mostly adenocarcinomas and can be divided into two categories, adenocarcinoma and mucinous adenocarcinoma. Both these categories are wide, ranging from very well differentiated to very poorly differentiated forms. Moreover, a certain proportion of adenocarcinomas have a distinctly diffuse infiltrating appearance, and mucinous adenocarcinomas also have an intermediate type between the well-differentiated and poorly differentiated forms. We therefore subdivide each category into well-differentiated, poorly differentiated, and diffuse.

Well-Differentiated Adenocarcinoma. Highly columnar cancer cells form clearly seen glandular, occasionally papillary or acinar structures (Figs. 5.6, 5.7).

Well-Differentiated Mucinous Adenocarcinoma. The excessive mucin secretion of the cancer cells forms mucous pools, which are usually surrounded by a few layers of fibrous tissue. The cancer cells are well differentiated, some forming glandular structures and others floating in the mucous pools (Fig. 5.8).

Poorly Differentiated Adenocarcinoma. The cancer cells are mostly low columnar, cuboidal, flat, polyhedral, or irregular in shape, and are often small with only scanty cytoplasm. They are arranged in small irregular tubes and threads, and in patterns like "simplex", "medullary", or "cribriform" carcinoma (Figs. 5.9, 5.10).

Poorly Differentiated Mucinous Adenocarcinoma. Histologically this type is between well-differentiated and diffuse mucinous adenocarcinoma, and is sometimes characterized by the conspicuous irregular mucous acini of various sizes (Fig. 5.11).

Diffuse Adenocarcinoma. The cancer cells are mostly small with irregular, deeply stained nuclei and scanty cytoplasm. They tend to infiltrate the tissue individually or in groups of three to five. Some of the cells contain varying amounts of mucus and a few present as typical signet-ring cells (Figs. 5.12, 5.13).

Diffuse Mucinous Adenocarcinoma. The tumor is mainly composed of signet-ring cells which infiltrate the tissue diffusely and are frequently mixed with varying numbers of irregular undifferentiated cells (Fig. 5.14).

Histologic type is apparently linked with prognosis. In 500 carcinomas of the gastric cardia [20], we found well-differentiated adenocarcinoma in 261 cases (52.2%), well-differentiated mucinous adenocarcinoma in 32 cases (6.4%), poorly differentiated adenocarcinoma in 148 cases (29.6%), poorly differentiated mucinous adenocarcinoma in nine cases (1.8%), diffuse adenocarcinoma in 32 cases (6.4%), and diffuse mucinous adenocarcinoma in 15 cases (3.0%).

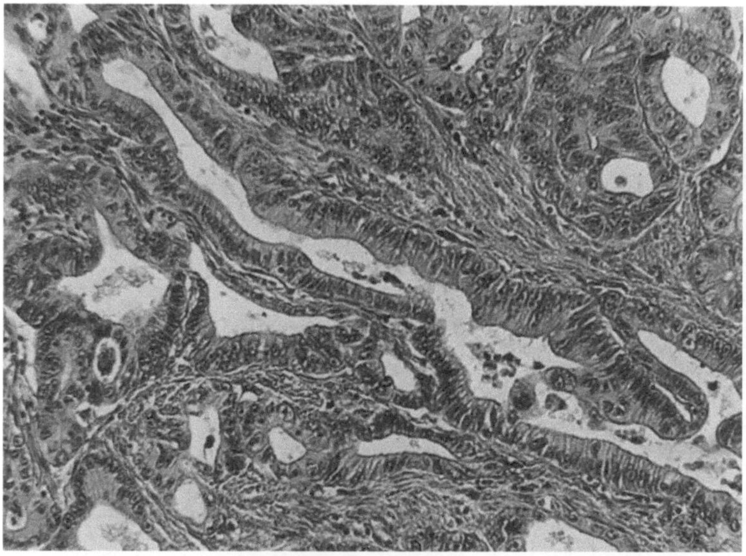

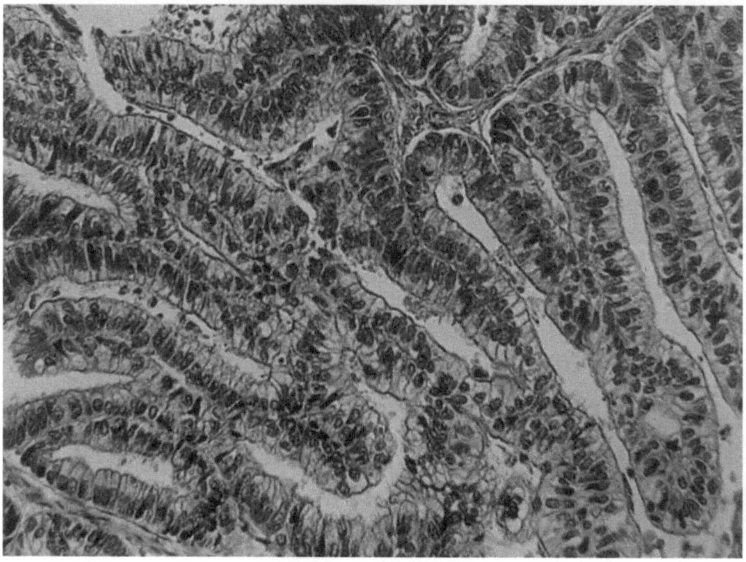

Fig. 5.6 (above). Well-differentiated adenocarcinoma of the gastric cardia. H&E, ×150

Fig. 5.7 (below). Well-differentiated adenocarcinoma of the gastric cardia showing the differentiation of cardiac epithelium. H&E, ×170

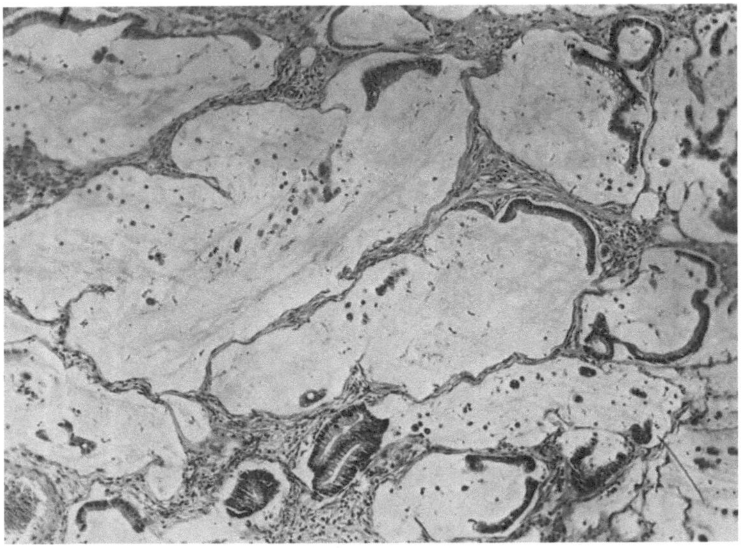

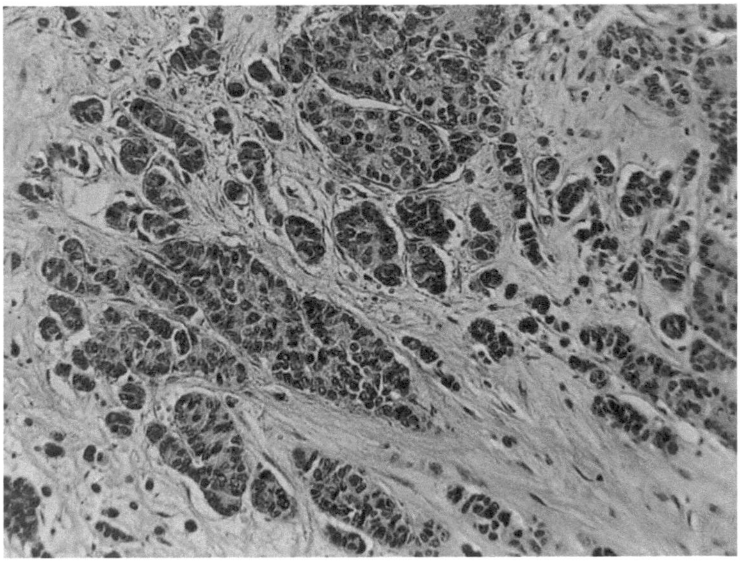

Fig. 5.8 (above). Well-differentiated mucinous adenocarcinoma of the gastric cardia, showing mucus pools. H&E, ×50

Fig. 5.9 (below). Poorly differentiated adenocarcinoma of the gastric cardia. The cancer cells are mainly arranged in the shape of small bands, resembling "simplex" carcinoma. H&E, ×150

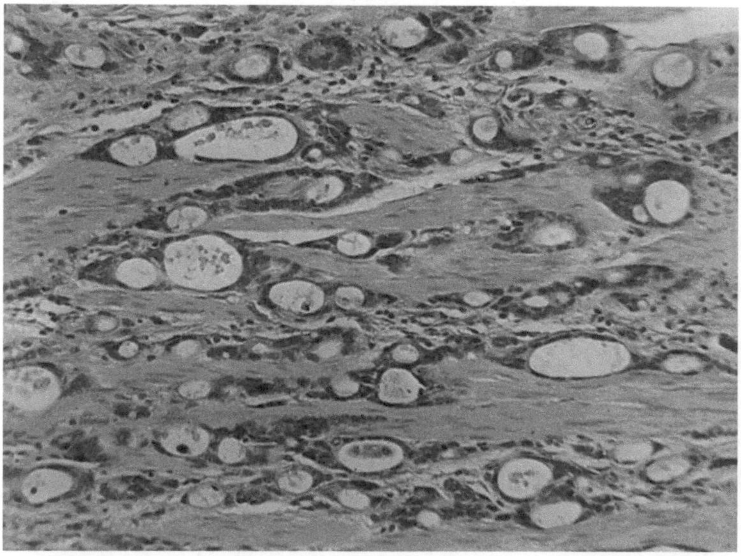

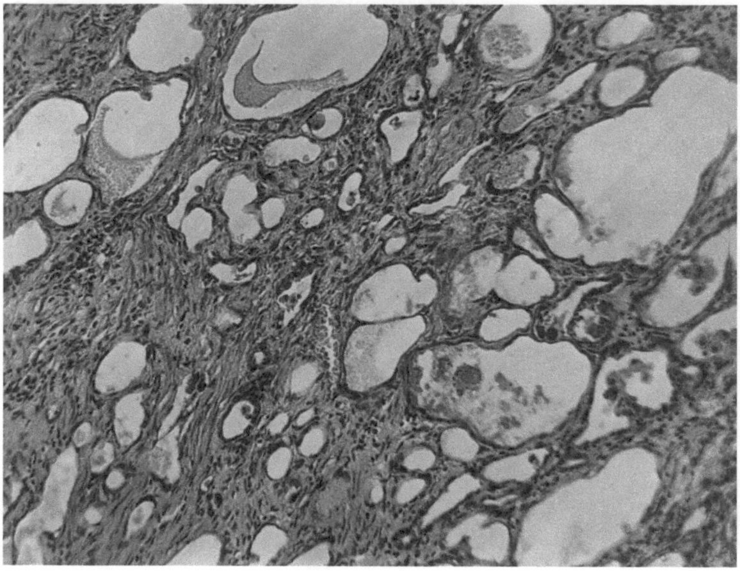

Fig. 5.10 (above). Poorly differentiated adenocarcinoma of the gastric cardia. The cancer cells take the form of small tubes and acini. H&E, 150

Fig. 5.11 (below). Poorly differentiated mucinous adenocarcinoma of the gastric cardia. Various sizes of irregular mucous acini are present. H&E, × 110

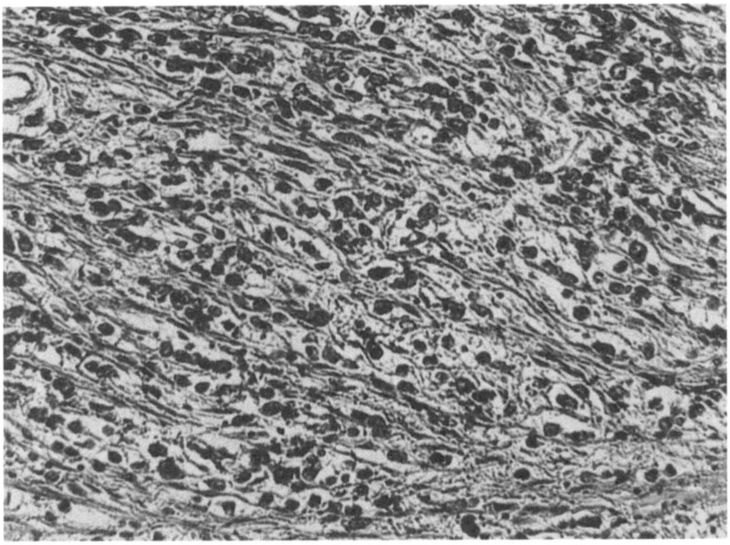

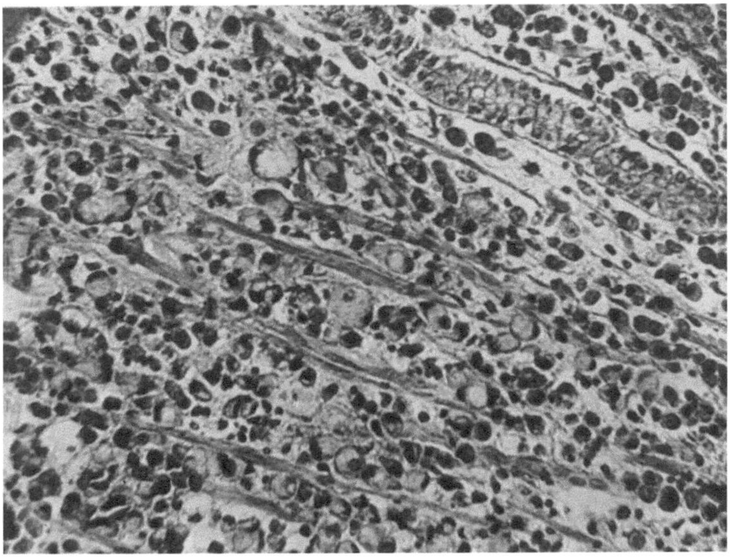

Fig. 5.12 (above). Diffuse adenocarcinoma of the gastric cardia. The cancer cells are anaplastic with deeply stained small nuclei and scanty cytoplasm. H&E, ×200

Fig. 5.13 (below). Another area of the tumor in Fig. 5.12, showing a mixture of anaplastic cells, mucin-producing cells, and signet ring cells. H&E, ×200

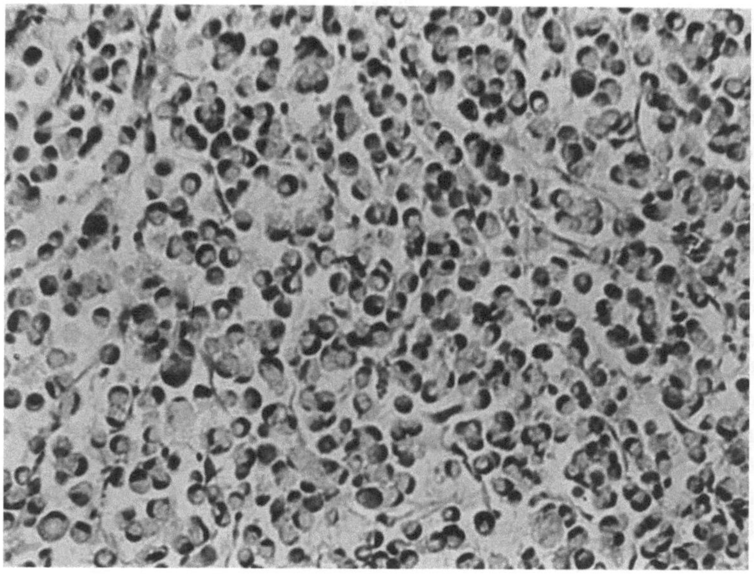

Fig. 5.14. Another area of the tumor in Fig. 5.12. Nearly all the cancer cells are signet-ring cells, revealing a typical pattern of diffuse mucinous adenocarcinoma. H&E, ×200

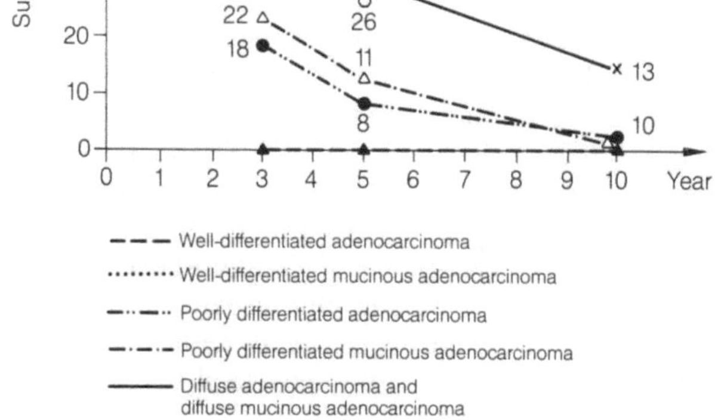

Fig. 5.15. Histologic types and prognosis

There was a clear difference in prognosis between the well-differentiated, poorly differentiated, and diffuse types in each category, but the prognosis was more or less the same in corresponding types, e.g., in well-differentiated adenocarcinoma and well-differentiated mucinous adenocarcinoma (Fig. 5.15).

Some authors [7, 9, 10, 20] have pointed out that one of the pathological characteristics of carcinoma of the gastric cardia is that there is a higher proportion of well-differentiated tumors than in other parts of the stomach. It should be particularly noted that in a small portion of well-differentiated adenocarcinomas, the cancer cells are so well differentiated that they closely resemble the cells of severe or moderate hyperplasia, and in rare cases may hardly be distinguishable from cells of mild atypical hyperplasia. Some of these very well differentiated adenocarcinomas have the features of intestinal epithelium, i. e., highly columnar cells with eosinophilic cytoplasm and occasionally striated borders, and with fusiform, ovoid, or round nuclei close to the basement membrane. Some possess the features of cardiac glandular epithelium, i. e., a single layer of columnar cells with pale (sometimes absolutely clear) cytoplasm, containing abundant mucin and small nuclei located very close to the basement membrane and regularly arranged. These very well differentiated cancer cells take on the shape of regular tubular, acinar, cystic, and occasionally cystic papillary structures, similar in appearance to proliferating cardiac glands (Figs. 5.16–5.18). Some authors deem this to be one of the pathological features of carcinoma of the gastric cardia [20, 27]. Among our 500 cases, 42 (8.4%) have very well differentiated components, including 24 (4.8%) in which such components predominate. We term this type grade I adenocarcinoma. The prognosis is far better than in other well-differentiated adenocarcinomas [20]; the 3-, 5-, and 10-year survival rates after surgery are as high as 67%, 57%, and 40% respectively (Fig. 5.19).

The other well-differentiated adenocarcinomas (grade II adenocarcinoma and papillary adenocarcinoma) also show traces of differentiation toward intestinal or cardiac epithelium. The two patterns of differentiation often coexist in the same lesion. Malignant goblet cells may be found in a number of cases and clusters of clear cells may also be seen.

Papillary adenocarcinoma has been classified by some authors as a separate histologic type [25], but we are of the opinion that it may be included with the well-differentiated adenocarcinomas. Carcinomas with elements resembling papillae or cystic papillae, which are seen in only a few cases, have a prognosis similar to that of well-differentiated adenocarcinoma.

Diffuse adenocarcinoma and diffuse mucinous adenocarcinoma show distinctly diffuse infiltration. Both are composed of varying proportions of undifferentiated cells, signet-ring cells, and forms transitional between the two. Sometimes an extensive desmoplastic reaction can be seen in the stroma.

Depending on the predominant components, which are often not the same at different sites and depths, these carcinomas have frequently been diagnosed as scirrhous carcinoma, signet-ring cell carcinoma, undifferentiated carcinoma, or undifferentiated adenocarcinoma. The prognosis is very poor; among our 500 cases [20], none of the patients in this group survived for more than 3 years. Biologically these types are actually equivalent to undifferentiated carcinoma, but in almost every case the differentiation of gastrointestinal epithelium can be found, exhibiting evidence of a greater or lesser degree of mucin secretion, and we could hardly call them undifferentiated carcinoma. Therefore, it seems that their characteristics are fully described by designation as "diffuse adenocarcinoma" or "diffuse mucinous adenocarcinoma."

The histologic patterns given above are often mixed in the same lesion, though in almost every case one is predominant.

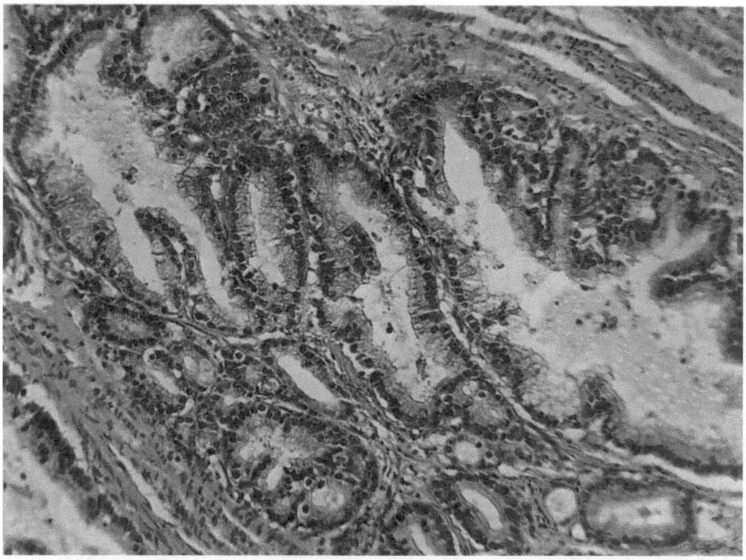

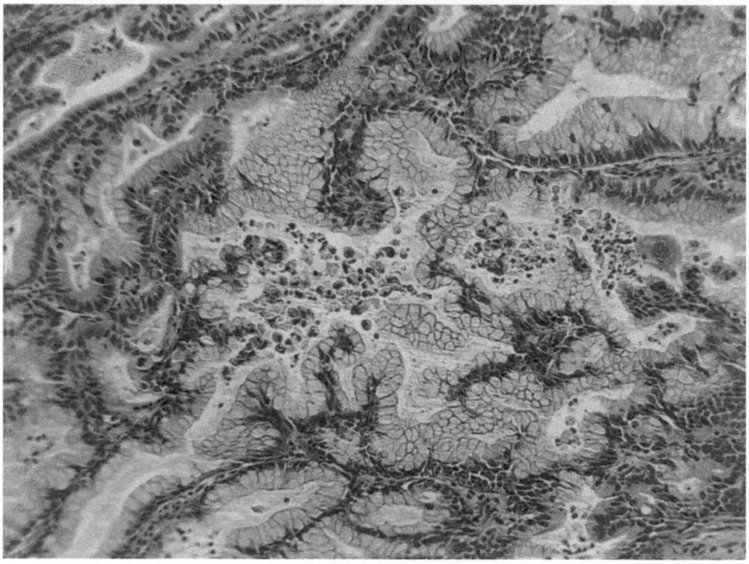

Fig. 5.16 (above). Grade I adenocarcinoma of the gastric cardia. The cancer cells are very well differentiated and resemble the atypical hyperplasia of cardiac glands. H&E, ×110

Fig. 5.17 (below). Grade I adenocarcinoma of the gastric cardia. The very well differentiated cancer cells are rich in mucus and arranged in regular tubular and cystic papillary structures. H&E, ×100

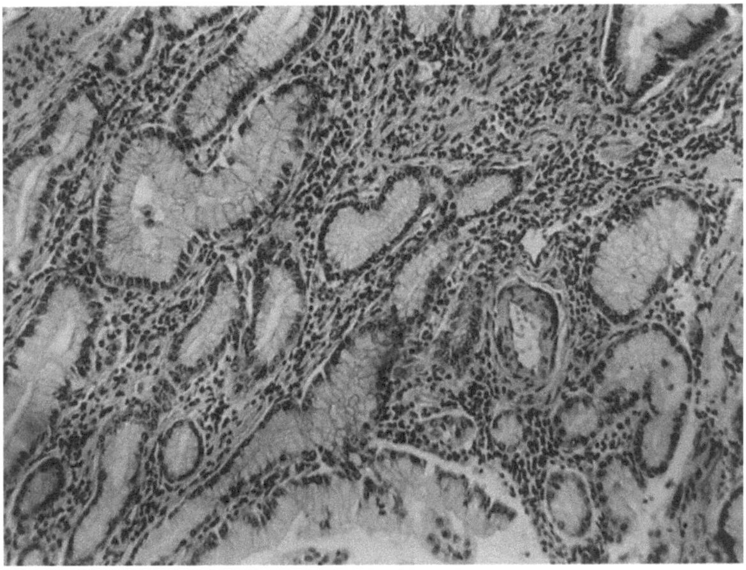

Fig. 5.18. Grade I adenocarcinoma of the gastric cardia. The cancer cells form regular tubes. They are so well differentiated that they closely resemble the simple hyperplasia of cardiac glands. The tumor extends to the serosa with metastasis in local lymph nodes. The patient died 2 years and 6 months after operation. H&E, ×140

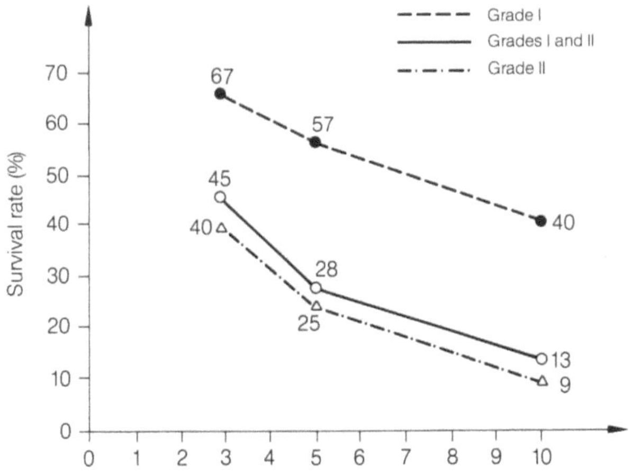

Fig. 5.19. Comparison between prognoses of different grades of well-differentiated adenocarcinoma

4.3 Other Types

Some histologic variants may be encountered at the cardia, accounting together for less than 5% of total carcinomas.

Adenosquamous Carcinoma. Adenocarcinomatous and squamous components are closely intermingled and are sometimes even present in the same nest. Our 500 cases included only three (0.6%) of this type [20].

Squamous Cell Carcinoma. The tumor is characterized by squamous differentiation. Intercellular bridges and keratin can be demonstrated. Because of differences in definition of carcinoma of the gastric cardia, the reported incidence of squamous carcinoma varies greatly. The high figures in some reports are obviously due to the inclusion of some squamous carcinomas of the lower segment of the esophagus [1, 5, 19, 24, 26]. Some authors state that the number of squamous carcinomas with indisputable origin in the cardia should be very small and that the diagnosis of squamous carcinoma can only be made when invasion and metastasis from the esophagus are excluded and origin in the cardiac epithelium is proved. Talerman and Woo-Ming [28] made a detailed study of two cases of squamous carcinoma in the cardia by autopsy and serial sections and found that in each case there was a minute squamous carcinoma in the esophagus which had metastasized lymphatically to the cardia. Of the early carcinomas originating from the cardiac epithelium reported in the recent literature, none were true squamous carcinoma, which reinforces the contention of this lesion's scarcity. Among our 500 cases [20], not one was proved to be squamous carcinoma.

Undifferentiated Carcinoma. The tumor is composed exclusively of undifferentiated cells with deeply stained pleomorphic nuclei and scanty cytoplasm, with no evidence of differentiation toward squamous carcinoma or adenocarcinoma. Pure undifferentiated carcinoma of the gastric cardia is rarely seen.

Carcinoid Tumor (Argentaffinoma). Carcinoid tumors, which originate from Kulchitsky cells, are mostly of low malignancy. They are usually single, small, and circumscribed nodules covered by intact mucosa. Microscopically, they are composed of small columnar or polyhedral cells arranged in trabeculae, islands, acini, and rosettes, usually giving a strong argyrophilic reaction. Carcinoid is seldom seen in the stomach and is even rarer in the cardia. Noncarcinoid adenocarcinoma of the gastric cardia with carcinoid syndrome has been reported [29].

Adenocarcinoma Containing Neoplastic Paneth Cells. Only a few cases of adenocarcinoma containing neoplastic Paneth cells have been reported, almost all from the intestinal tract [30]. Neoplastic Paneth cells in adenocarcinoma of the urinary bladder, nasal cavity, and nasal sinus have also been reported [30, 31]. We have encountered one case of neoplastic Paneth cells in adenocarcinoma of the gastric cardia; the adenocarcinoma was well differentiated and showed features of differentiation toward cardiac epithelium. Cells intermediate in type between neoplastic Paneth cells and mucous cells have also been seen (Fig. 5.20) [32].

Carcinosarcoma. Carcinosarcoma of the gastric cardia has rarely been reported in the literature. Wu and Sun [33] found one case, in which two elements, adenocarcinoma and rhabdomyosarcoma, were closely intermingled.

Acanthosis Nigricans Associated with Adenocarcinoma. Acanthosis nigricans has been classified into three types: benign, pseudomalignant, and malignant [34]. It is generally consid-

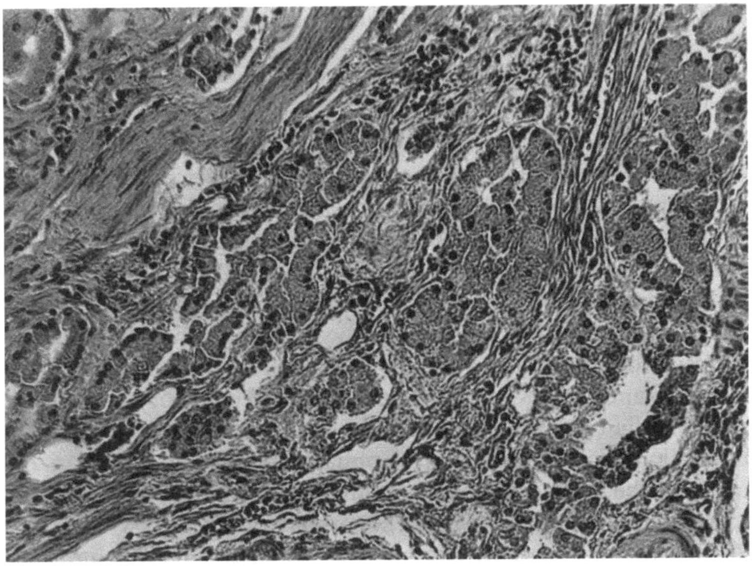

Fig. 5.20. Well-differentiated adenocarcinoma of the gastric cardia containing neoplastic Paneth cells. H&E, ×170

ered that the majority of cutaneous lesions might be related to metastasis of carcinoma in the adrenals and in the sympathetic nervous plexus [35]. Recently, it has been postulated that malignant acanthosis nigricans is caused by the ectopic release of a peptide from the neoplasm [34]. We have seen a case of acanthosis nigricans associated with adenocarcinoma of the gastric cardia. The patient had melanin deposits all over the skin, especially on the face, waist and groin, and died 11 months after operation. Autopsy showed metastases of adenocarcinoma in both adrenal glands [36].

5 Pathology of Early Carcinoma

5.1 Incidence

In recent years, as a result of the extensive use of fiberoptic endoscopy and balloon cytologic techniques, there has been a marked rise in the detection of early carcinomas of the esophagus and the stomach, and much pathological experience has been gained in this field. The study of early carcinoma of the gastric cardia, however, is still at a preliminary stage. Only a few cases of early carcinoma of the gastric cardia have been reported [37–45], and minute carcinomas have been detected even more rarely. Literature reports containing a good number of cases are as follows:

- Suzuki et al., in 1976 [46], found ten cases of early gastric adenocarcinoma less than 2 cm in diameter at the esophagogastric junction, one being a minute carcinoma of 0.5 cm.
- Endo et al., in 1978 [47], reported 18 cases of carcinoma of the gastric cardia with the focal centers located within 2 cm below the esophagogastric junction, seven of the lesions having a diameter of less than 1 cm.

- Matsue et al., in 1978 [10], reported nine early carcinomas of the gastric cardia with the focal centers located within 2 cm below the junction, three of which were less than 1 cm in diameter.

We ourselves have reported 18 cases of early carcinoma of the gastric cardia, mostly found by exfoliative cytologic examination during mass screening in regions with high incidence of esophageal and cardiac cancers. All the focal centers were within 2 cm below the junction, and in 15 cases the lesions were less than 2 cm in diameter, six being minute carcinomas not exceeding 0.5 cm [15].

According to information gathered from the literature, Chinese and worldwide, the number of cases strictly conforming to the criteria of early carcinoma of the gastric cardia has not yet exceeded 100. Due to lack of experience, certain clinicopathological problems still await solution.

5.2 Definition

From the pathological point of view, the term "early carcinoma of the gastric cardia" should be restricted to those lesions in which there is neither invasion of the muscular layer nor metastasis to lymph nodes. This definition includes adenocarcinoma in situ, intramucosal infiltrating adenocarcinoma (or intramucosal carcinoma), and submucosal infiltrating adenocarcinoma (or submucosal carcinoma).

5.3 Macroscopic Features

The macroscopic morphology of early carcinoma of the gastric cardia is quite similar to that of early carcinomas in the esophagus or elsewhere in the stomach. In 1962, the Japanese Gastroenterological Endoscopic Society proposed the following gross classification of early gastric carcinoma [48]:

Type I: Protruded
Type II: Superficial
  IIa: elevated
  IIb: flat
  IIc: depressed
Type III: Excavated

Many combinations of the five basic types can be made. This classification has been accepted by many authors in Japan and in other countries, but there have been some reservations, especially with regard to the combinations, some authors holding that they are superfluous and saying the classification should be simplified [49, 50]. In the cases of early carcinoma of the gastric cardia that we have seen, the macroscopic changes are minimal, usually only slight erosions or slight thickening of the mucosa. About 30% of the cancerous foci show almost no gross abnormality. The carcinomas are usually minute, less than 0.5 cm in diameter. None of this is true of early carcinomas in the other parts of the stomach, over half of which show a markedly excavated or ulcerative appearance. The early cancerous foci with marked ulceration are seldom seen at the cardiac region. Similarly, those early carcinomas with polyp-like features, which may develop in adenomas, rarely occur at the cardia. We propose a division of early carcinoma of the gastric cardia into three simple types: depressed, elevated, and concealed.

Depressed. The cancerous mucosa is slightly depressed and is eroded or occasionally superficially ulcerated, usually with no apparent demarcation from the surrounding mucosa (Fig. 5.21).

Elevated. The cancerous mucosa shows a slightly irregular elevated appearance. It is rough, granular, discolored and feels superficially indurated to the examining finger. Sometimes it forms a distinct patch, occasionally a nodular or polypous lesion (Fig. 5.22).

Concealed. There is almost no gross abnormality except a very slight roughness. On the cut surface, the tumor corresponds in thickness to normal mucosa. The nature and location of this earliest type of early malignancy can only be determined under the microscope (Fig. 5.23).

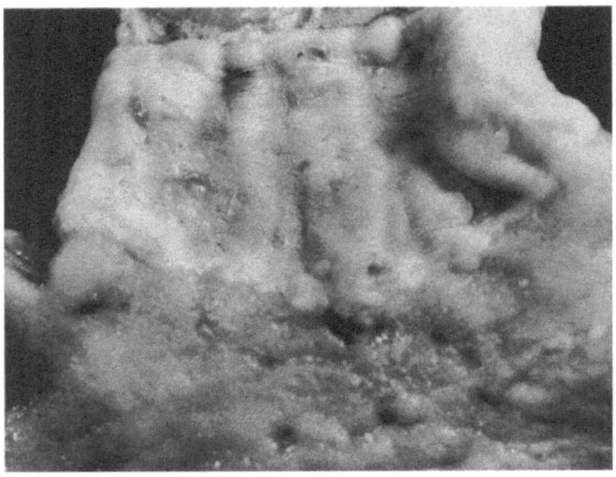

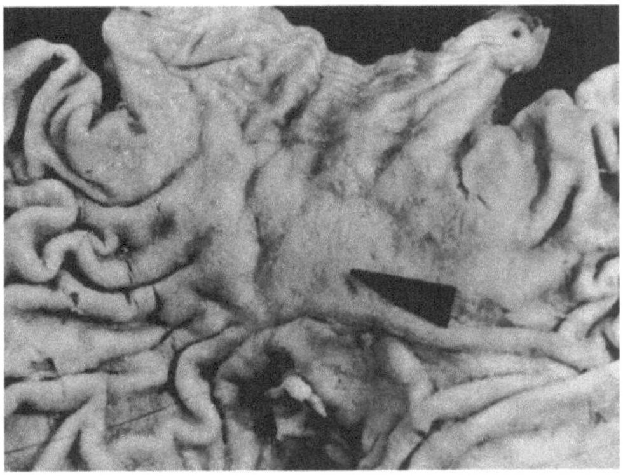

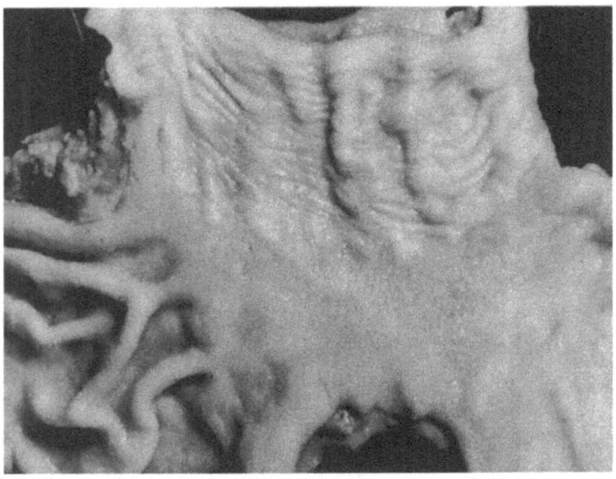

***Fig. 5.21** (upper left).* Depressed early carcinoma of the gastric cardia. The cancerous mucosa is slightly depressed and looks like a superficial ulcer

***Fig. 5.22** (upper right).* Elevated early carcinoma of the gastric cardia. The cancerous mucosa shows slight and irregular elevation

***Fig. 5.23** (lower left).* Concealed early carcinoma of the gastric cardia. No gross abnormality is seen except a very slight roughness

The elevated cases are mainly well-differentiated adenocarcinomas, while the depressed cases are mostly poorly differentiated adenocarcinomas. These two types are the basic forms of early carcinoma of the gastric cardia, from which various types of advanced lesion may develop.

It is not always only the concealed type which presents almost no gross changes; the elevated and depressed types are sometimes hardly distinguishable from hyperplastic lesions. The macroscopic appearance of some evident cancerous foci does not necessarily correspond to the observations under the microscope. Those parts which grossly appear changed may actually be metaplastic or hyperplastic, while other parts which exhibit no gross changes may in fact contain minute cancerous foci. The macroscopic features are much less clear than in early carcinoma of the esophagus.

5.4 Histologic Manifestations

In principle, early carcinomas of the gastric cardia are histologically no different from advanced carcinomas. They can similarly be divided into two categories, adenocarcinoma and mucinous adenocarcinoma, each being further split into several subtypes, depending on the differentiation toward intestinal or cardiac epithelium and the presence or absence of papillary of cystadenopapillary patterns and clear cell nests (the latter occurring only occasionally). However, some authors have noted that the differentiation and histologic typing are somewhat altered as the cancerous foci enlarge and go deeper [15, 23]. Submucosal carcinomas may display far more prominent infiltration and complicated patterns than earlier lesions, and are histologically more similar to advanced carcinoma. With the progression of the tumor, both tubular adenocarcinomas with abundant mucous secretion and signet-ring cell carcinomas may be transformed into well-differentiated mucinous carcinomas. Some signet-ring cells may become undifferentiated in the course of infiltration into the deeper layers. Moreover, poorly differentiated components may sometimes flourish and become the principal constituents of the carcinomatous focus.

However, the histologic appearance of intramucosal carcinomas, especially minute carcinomas, i.e., early adenocarcinomas of less than 0.5 cm [23, 51], seems to be relatively simple. Among neither minute carcinomas nor intramucosal carcinomas is found even a single case of mucinous adenocarcinoma with well-developed mucinous pools or of adenocarcinoma comprising mostly undifferentiated cells and exhibiting diffuse infiltration. This is because the mucus secreted from mucinous cancer cells is freer to go into the gastric cavity and less able to accumulate when the carcinoma is confined to the mucosa. Once the carcinoma invades the submucosa, the passage of mucus may be blocked and mucinous pools formed, resulting in an increase of poorly differentiated types [15, 23].

The various histologic patterns of early carcinoma of the gastric cardia in different stages of infiltration are shown in Figs. 5.24 to 5.32.

Some authors point out that the proportion of grossly elevated and histologically well-differentiated early carcinomas is higher in the gastric cardia than in the other parts of the stomach [7, 10, 15]. Table 5.1 sums up the gross and histologic features of 33 cases of early carcinoma of the gastric cardia with a diameter of less than 2 cm reported in the literature. It demonstrates clearly that the elevated (or I + II a) and concealed (or II b) types are predominant and that the depressed (or II c + III) type is the minor form. This is markedly different from the pattern of early carcinomas in other parts of the stomach.

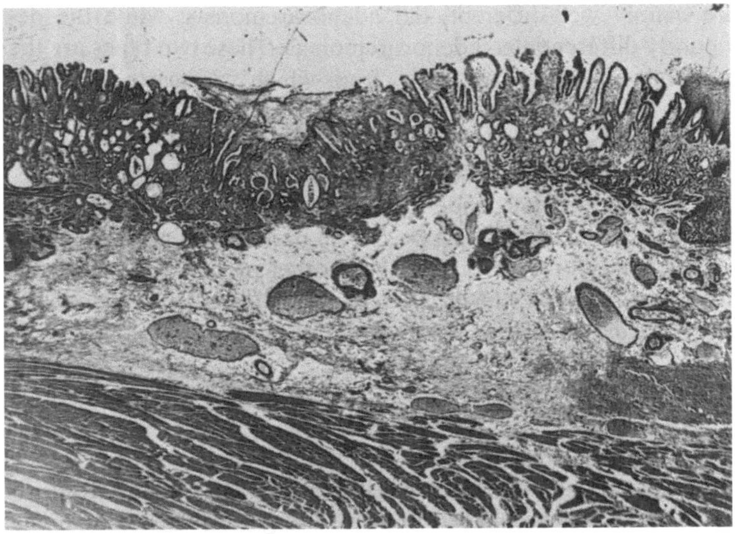

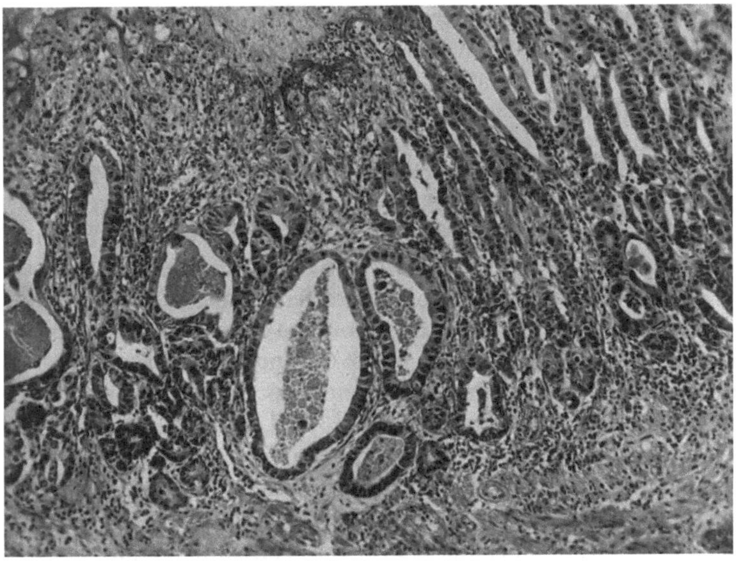

Fig. 5.24 (above). A minute carcinoma of the gastric cardia. The tumor is limited to the mucosa, 0.3 cm from the esophagogastric junction, and 0.2 cm in diameter. H&E, × 15

Fig. 5.25 (below). Higher magnification of the minute carcinoma in Fig. 24. The cancer cells show apparent atypism and form irregular small or large tubes. H&E, × 100

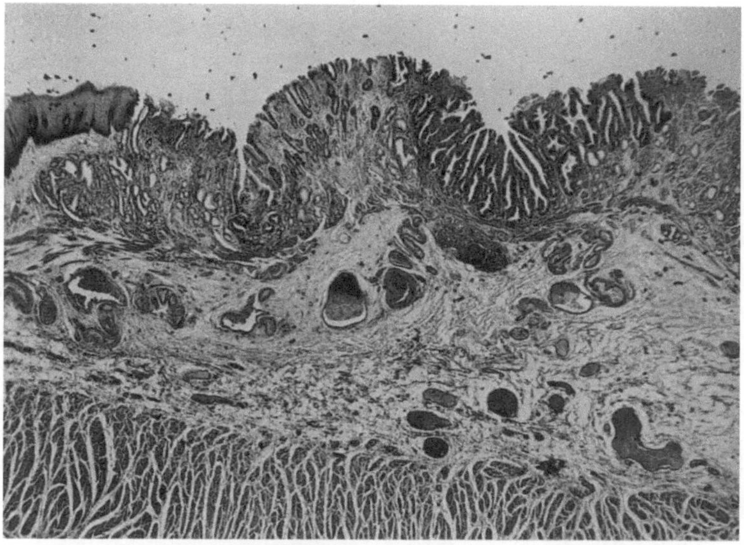

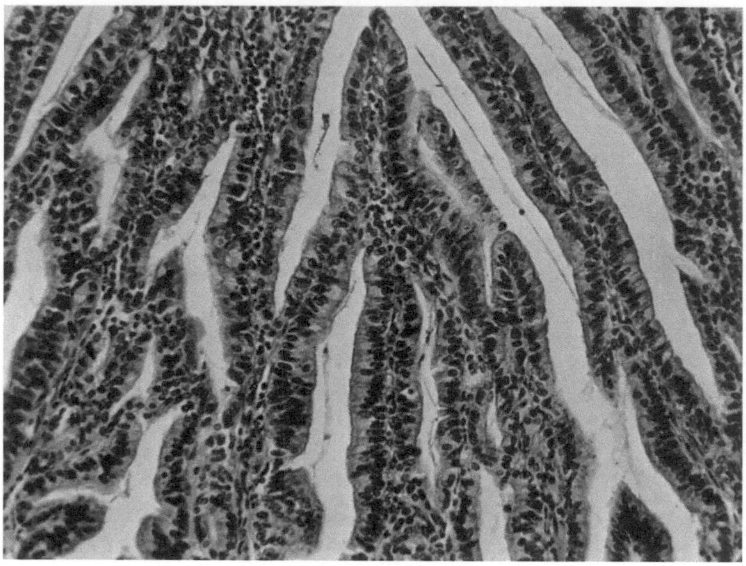

Fig. 5.26 (above). Another minute carcinoma of the gastric cardia. H&E, ×15

Fig. 5.27 (below). Higher magnification of the minute carcinoma in Fig. 26. The cancer cells are well differentiated and arranged in the form of regular glands. H&E, ×130

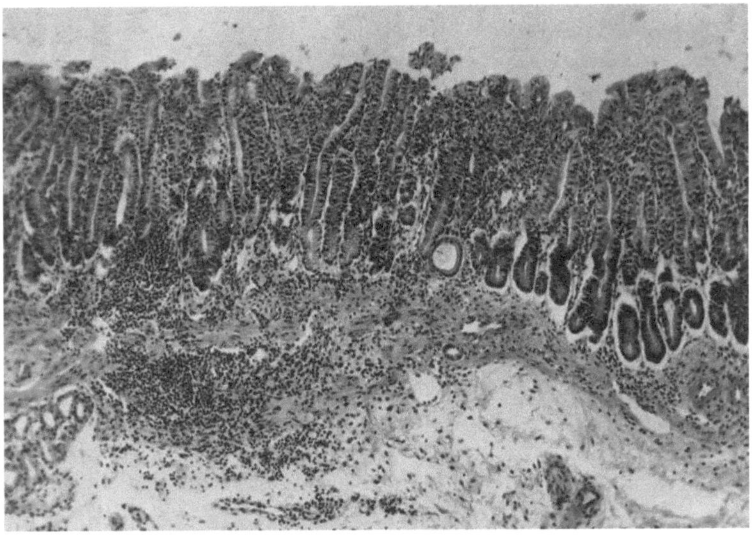

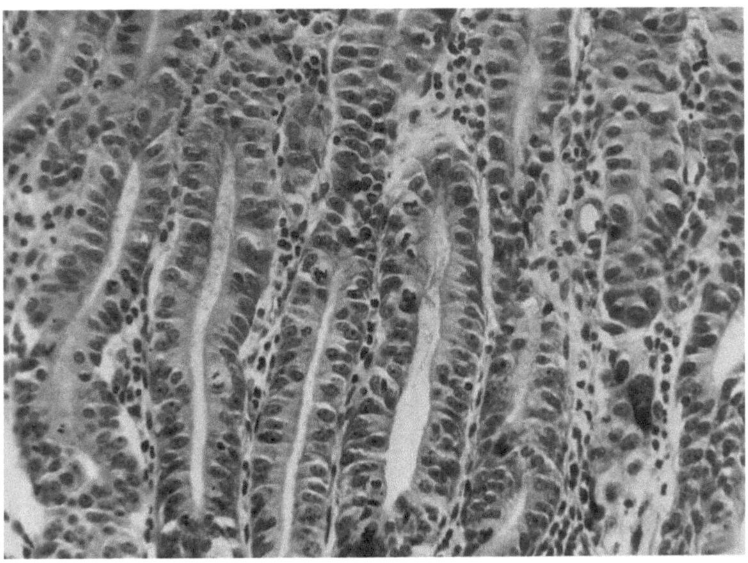

Fig. 5.28 (above). Well-differentiated intramucosal adenocarcinoma of the gastric cardia, with simple and atypical hyperplasia in the lower part of the cardiac glands. H&E, ×50

Fig. 5.29 (below). Higher magnification of Fig. 28, revealing well-differentiated cancer cells, mitoses, atypical mitoses, and bizarre cells. H&E, ×220

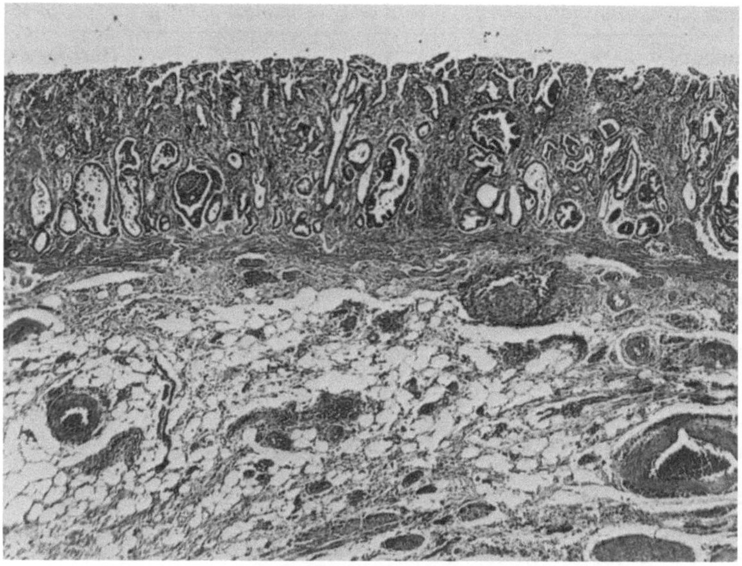

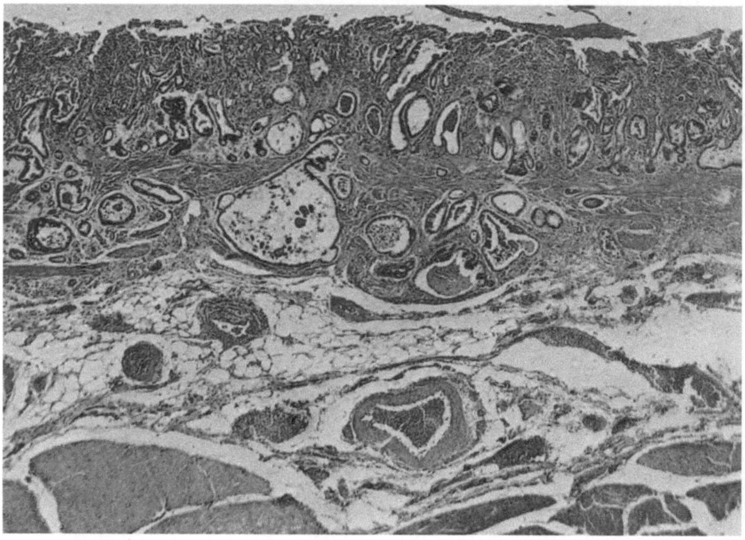

Fig. 5.30 (above). Intramucosal adenocarcinoma of the gastric cardia, showing pleomorphic patterns. H&E, ×25

Fig. 5.31 (below). Another area of the tumor in Fig. 30, showing cancer cells invading the submucosa. H&E, ×25

Table 5.1. Gross and histologic types of early carcinoma of the gastric cardia less than 2 cm in diameter

Authors	Year	No. of cases	Gross types						Histologic types		
			I	IIa	IIa+IIc	IIb	IIc	III	Tubular adeno-carcinoma	Poorly differen-tiated adeno-carcinoma	Mucinous adeno-carcinoma
Sano et al. [37]	1968	1	1						1		
Yoshi Moli [cited in 46]	1969	1	1						1		
Yamauchi et al. [38]	1970	1	1						1		
Nimura et al. [41]	1975	1		1					1		
Murohisa et al. [42]	1975	1				1			1		
Fujita et al. [43]	1976	2		2					1		1
Suzuki et al. [46]	1976	3		3					3		
Endo et al. [47]	1978	4	1			1	1	1			
Matsue et al. [10]	1978	3	2				1				
Liu et al. [44]	1979	1				1			1		
Present authors	1982	15	1	4	1	6	3		13	1	1
Total		33	7	10	1	9	5	1	23	1	2

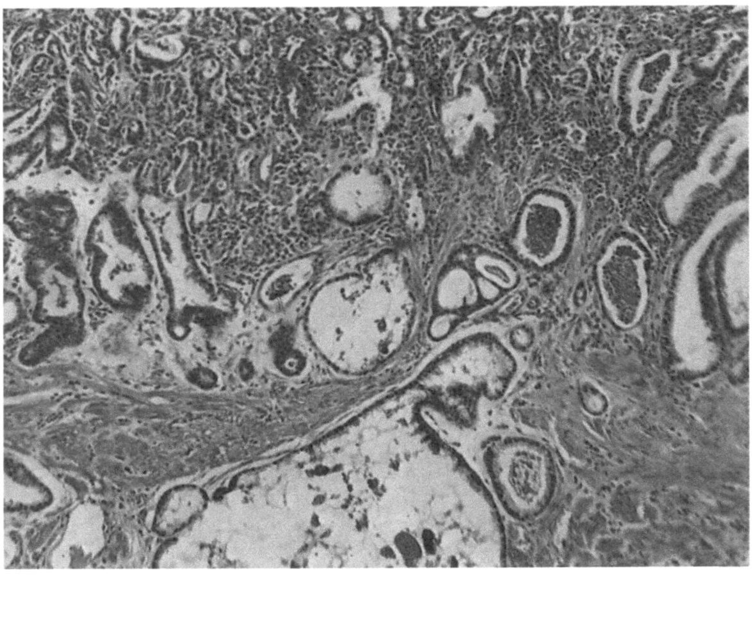

5.5 Adenocarcinoma In Situ

Various authors give different definitions of adenocarcinoma in situ in the gastrointestinal tract. Quite a number hold that, like squamous carcinoma in situ, the term should be used to refer to those very early tumors in which cancer cells are confined to glands and have not penetrated the basal membrane; the term "intratubular carcinoma" has also been used [52–55]. Others, however, doubt the existence of carcinoma in situ in the gastrointestinal tract [56], preferring the term "intramucosal carcinoma" [57, 58]. "Carcinoma in situ" has also been used as a synonym for severe atypical hyperplasia [59]. The borderline lesion (atypical hyperplasia) of the stomach proposed by Japanese pathologists is sometimes described by them in a way which would allow a diagnosis of carcinoma in situ [60]. We believe that the differences of opinion on carcinoma in situ rest on the fact that the mucosa in the gastrointestinal tract has a different histologic structure from that of squamous epithelium and the transition from atypical hyperplasia to the earliest malignancy and on to infiltration is rather rapid. It is thus very difficult in practise to give a diagnosis of adenocarcinoma in situ, but as demonstrated by some workers, such an in situ malignant lesion must exist at some stage in the progression to invasive carcinoma [53]. Understanding of morphology, study of histogenesis, and clarification of the process of cancerous change are aided by theoretical division of gastrointestinal carcinoma into three stages: carcinoma in situ, superficial carcinoma, and infiltrating carcinoma. In our series of early carcinoma of the gastric cardia, three examples of adenocarcinoma in situ and another three similar malignancies adjacent to the main intramucosal carcinomatous foci were revealed by way of serial sectioning [15].

5.6 Differentiation Between Well-Differentiated Early Carcinoma and Atypical Hyperplasia (Dysplasia)

It is sometimes difficult to distinguish the early forms of well-differentiated adenocarcinoma from severe atypical hyperplasia. Many authors who have done a lot of work in this field have stressed the importance of the following morphologic changes in differential diagnosis: In carcinoma the nuclei are mostly round or oval, deeply stained or apparently pale. They are usually arranged irregularly and sometimes project into the lumen. The atypism is prominent. Mitoses and atypical mitoses are often easily seen. The glands are pleomorphic and stiff, closely packed together, and display papillary projections, intraluminal necrosis, bridging, mutual walls, and back-to-back growth patterns. Goblet and Paneth cells are scarce or absent. There is often sharp demarcation between the carcinomatous focus and the surrounding tissue because of the pressure exerted by the carcinoma [61–63]. All these points have proved significant in practise.

However, it is noteworthy that there are morphologic crosses and superimpositions between well-differentiated adenocarcinoma and atypical hyperplasia. Among our 500 cases of advanced carcinoma of the gastric cardia, 4.8% were adenocarcinoma grade I which was morphologically similar to severe, moderate, or even mild atypical hyperplastic epi-

◁ *Fig. 5.32.* Higher magnification of Fig. 30. Some of the cancer cells are well differentiated and arranged in the shape of regular glands, others are poorly differentiated and take the form of small tubes or clusters. H&E, ×60 thelium; in certain individual cases it could be seen that atypical hyperplasia extended directly downward to become just such a very well differentiated adenocarcinoma, and we could hardly tell where the atypical hyperplasia ended and the malignancy began [20]. If this very well differentiated adenocarcinoma were only in the superficial layer, with present techniques it could almost certainly not be distinguished from atypical hyperplasia. Some authors have pointed out that carcinoma and atypical hyperplasia sometimes cannot be distinguished from each other because of this overlap [23, 64]. The difficulty in ascertaining the benign or malignant nature of the lesion is further confirmed by the divergent views of the nature of atypical hyperplasia proposed by Japanese investigators; some authors regard atypical hyperplasia as a proliferative lesion, others assume it to be already malignant, and still others are pondering the possibility of some cases being benign and others malignant [60, 61, 64, 65]. Moreover, though many authors have striven to describe and classify atypical hyperplasia [64, 66], at present only those forms with a transitional relationship to well-differentiated adenocarcinoma are popularly recognized.

To sum up, the nature and the morphology of atypical hyperplasia and its distinction from early adenocarcinoma have not yet been settled.

6 Histogenesis

Chronic peptic ulcer, polyp (adenoma), and atrophic gastritis have long been intensively investigated as to their relationship to gastric carcinoma, and all three were once considered precancerous. However, recent studies throw more light on the subject.

Chronic peptic ulcer is unlikely to undergo malignant change, though this does occasionally happen [58, 67]. Carcinomas alleged to originate from ulcers are in most instances actually carcinomas with superimposed secondary ulcers [23]. The incidence of ulceration in the cardia is far lower than that in the antrum and the body of the stomach. Among the early carcinomas of the gastric cardia clearly described in the literature, there is not one convincing case of origin from a typical chronic peptic ulcer. Even the carcinomas with secondary ulcers are far less common than in the antrum and the body [15]. It seems that ulcers play an insignificant role in pathogenesis at the cardia.

With regard to the frequency of carcinoma developing from a *gastric polyp,* there is wide variation in the statistics [23, 58]. We have observed one case of early carcinoma of the gastric cardia which evidently arose from a polyp (Figs. 5.33, 5.34) [67], confirming that there is some association. Nevertheless, gastric polyps are not at all common, and polyps are seen even less frequently in the cardia. The importance of polyps in carcinoma of the gastric cardia is not great.

The correlation between *atrophic gastritis* and cancer has for many years been one of the vital subjects in research on gastric carcinoma. Remarkable progress has been made but no definite conclusions have yet been reached. Atrophic gastritis and gastric carcinoma have similarities in epidemiology and geographic distribution [68]. Long-term follow-up data show that the incidence of gastric carcinoma in patients with atrophic gastritis is higher than in healthy people [69, 70]. Pathological analyses indicate that concurrent atrophic gastritis is found in most patients with gastric carcinoma. Intestinal metaplasia, one of the main pathological changes of atrophic gastritis, occurs at a rate as high as over 60% [71]. Many authors consider that intestinal metaplasia might be a precancerous lesion [71, 72]. The histogenetic hypothesis proposed by Nakamura, that the differentiated types of adenocarcinoma in the stomach mainly originate from intestinal metaplastic epithelium

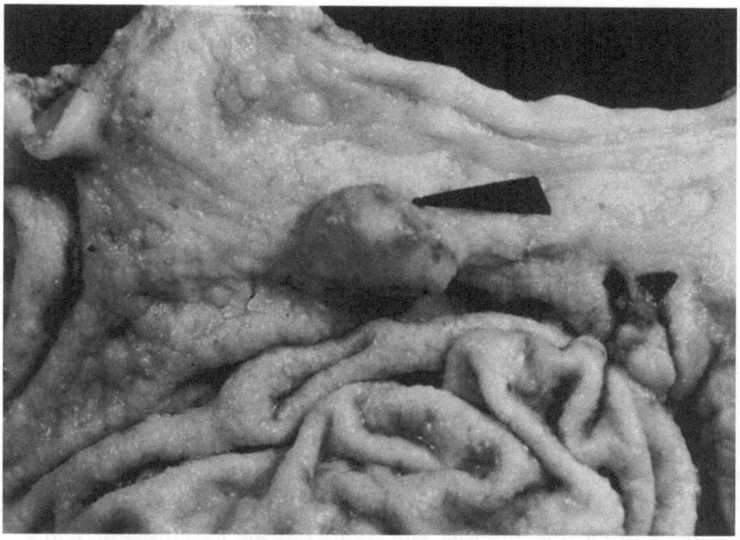

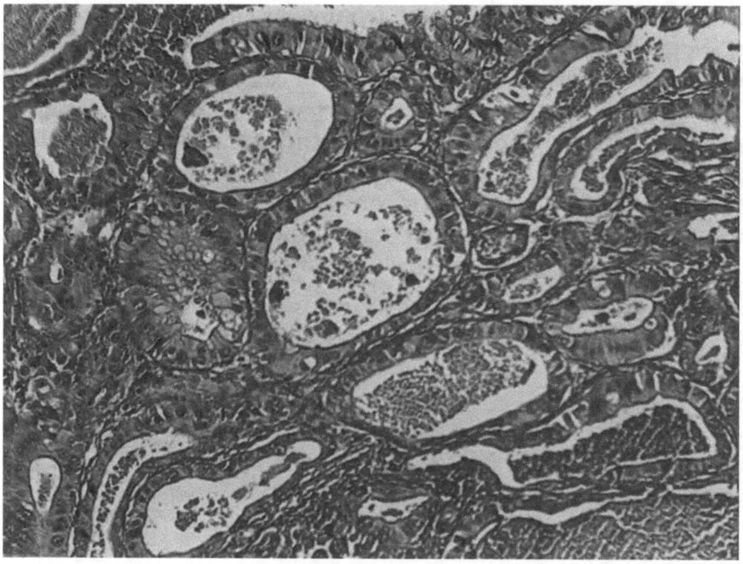

Fig. 5.33 (above). Early carcinoma of the gastric cardia arising from an adenoma at the greater curvature of the cardia of a 50-year-old man. The patient has been alive and well for 8 years since operation

Fig. 5.34 (below). Microscopic view of the tumor in Fig. 33, showing well-differentiated adenocarcinoma. H&E, ×80

while the undifferentiated types develop in the ordinary epithelium [23, 71], has been accepted by many [17, 73]. However, a substantial number of researchers believe that intestinal metaplasia bears no direct relationship to gastric cancer [74, 75]. Recently some authors have proposed that intestinal metaplasia could be divided into two categories, the small intestinal and the colonic, and that only the latter is potentially premalignant [76].

The data obtained through analyses of early and advanced carcinomas of the gastric cardia show that intestinal metaplasia at this site is mild and low in incidence while the proportion of well-differentiated carcinoma is higher than in the gastric antrum and body [7, 9, 15, 20]. These findings cannot be reconciled satisfactorily with Nakamura's histogenetic hypothesis. Our studies on early carcinoma, atypical hyperplasia, and intestinal metaplasia of the gastric cardia indicate the following:

1. The hypothesis that well-differentiated carcinoma of the gastric cardia originates from intestinal metaplastic epithelium, while poorly differentiated or undifferentiated carcinoma comes from cardiac epithelium proper, cannot be satisfactorily proved.
2. It is atypical hyperplasia that is clearly related to carcinoma.
3. Colonic intestinal metaplasia as demonstrated by the culling method is in most instances of atypical hyperplastic nature, being quite different from the small intestinal metaplasia.
4. The site of origin of carcinoma of the gastric cardia is the neck of a cardiac gland (Figs. 5.35, 5.36) [77].

We acknowledge the suggestions of some recent authors that gastric carcinoma originates from the stem cells and that atypical hyperplasia is precancerous [15, 58, 70, 75, 78]. We are of the opinion that carcinoma of the gastric cardia originates from the stem cells of the neck of cardiac glands. The stem cells are carcinogenetically multipotential; the adenocarcinomas formed have the features of either cardiac or intestinal epithelium. Morphologic, ultrastructural, and histochemical studies on early and advanced gastric carcinomas have revealed that the majority of cases present a mixed appearance [15, 20, 70, 75, 79], providing strong support for our view. Atypical hyperplasia is the critical pathological process shared by the supposed "gastric-carcinoma-related diseases" or "precancerous gastric conditions" such as ulcer, polyp, and atrophic gastritis. The incidence of ulcers and polyps is very low in the gastric cardia, and atrophic gastritis and intestinal metaplasia are also less frequent than in other parts of the stomach. These lesions are mostly undergoing

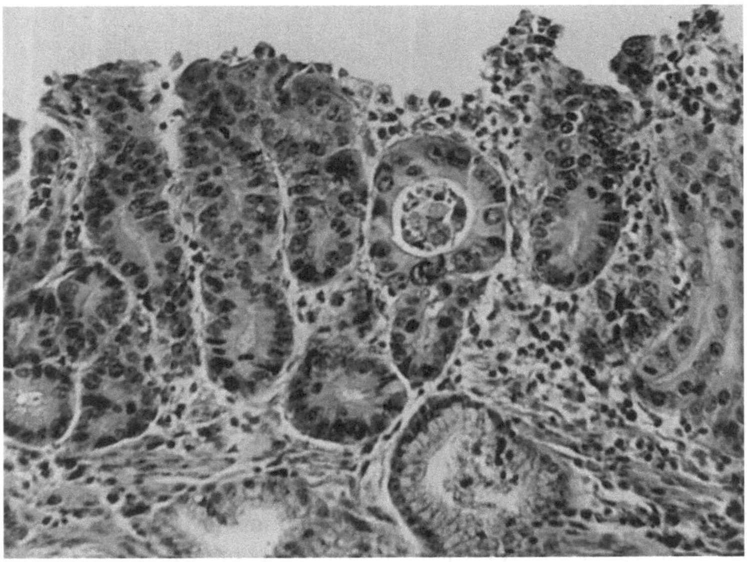

Fig. 5.35. The earliest malignant change in a single gland of the gastric cardia, with surrounding atypical hyperplasia. H&E, ×200

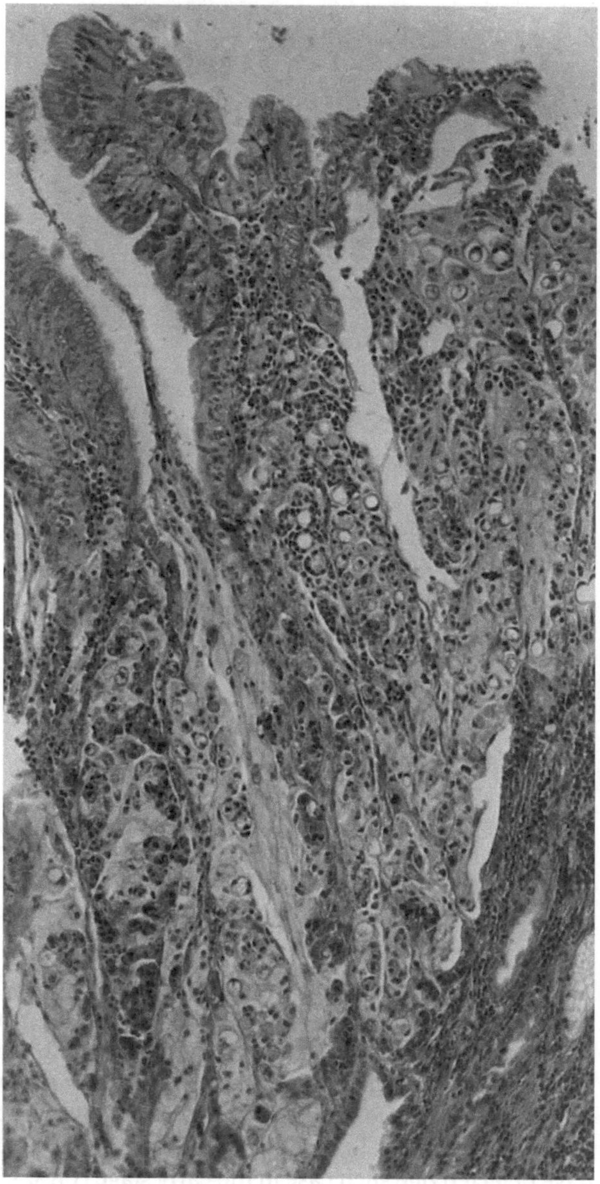

Fig. 5.36. This photomicrograph shows that carcinoma of the gastric cardia arises from the stem cells of the neck of cardiac glands. H&E, ×240

a benign transformation; the transition to carcinoma is only possible when they have the obvious characteristics of atypical hyperplasia. The fact that colonic intestinal metaplasia is mostly atypically hyperplastic in nature merits further investigation.

Some authors claim that reflux esophagitis leading to Barrett's esophagus plays a role in the pathogenesis of adenocarcinoma of the esophagus and the esophagogastric junction. The association between adenocarcinoma of the gastric cardia and Barrett's mucosa may be essentially similar to that between gastric cancer and atrophic gastritis with intestinal metaplasia, and the critical pathologic process is atypical hyperplasia as discussed above.

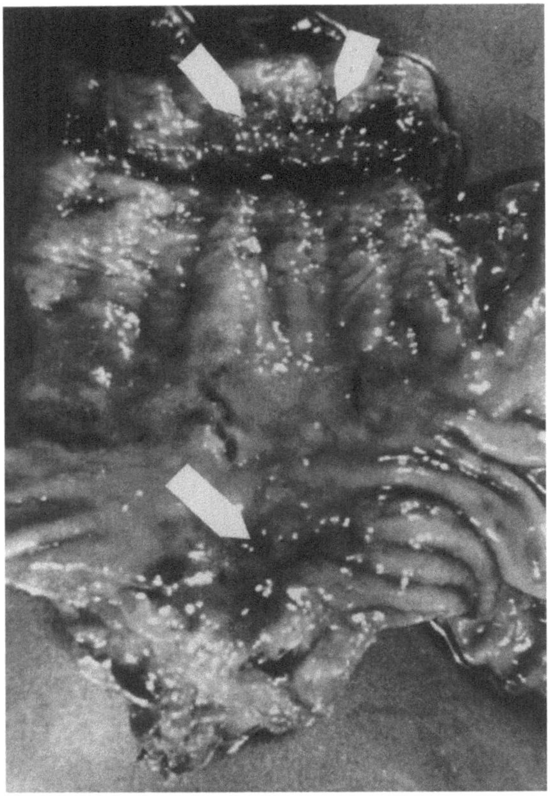

Fig. 5.37. Double primary early carcinomas in the esophagus *(double arrow)* and gastric cardia *(arrow)* from a 55-year-old man. Both lesions are erosion-like in appearance. The patient is still alive 8 years after operation

Under the effect of cancer-inducing factors, stem cell carcinogenesis may present multicentric patterns in a field of cancerization. In a few instances there may be multiple primary carcinomas, with the main tumor situated in the stomach and the others in the stomach, in the esophagus or other digestive organs, or in other systems. These pathological phenomena have been verified by many investigators [51, 55, 81].

Double primaries in esophagus and gastric cardia have often been reported [82–84]. We have detected one such case in the early stage (Figs. 5.37–5.40) [45]. The so-called collision carcinoma of the gastric cardia is actually an unusual variation of this phenomenon; only five cases have been reported so far [85–88]. The primary squamous carcinoma in the lower segment of the esophagus meets the primary adenocarcinoma of the gastric cardia by chance and they fuse to form a collision carcinoma with its unique appearance.

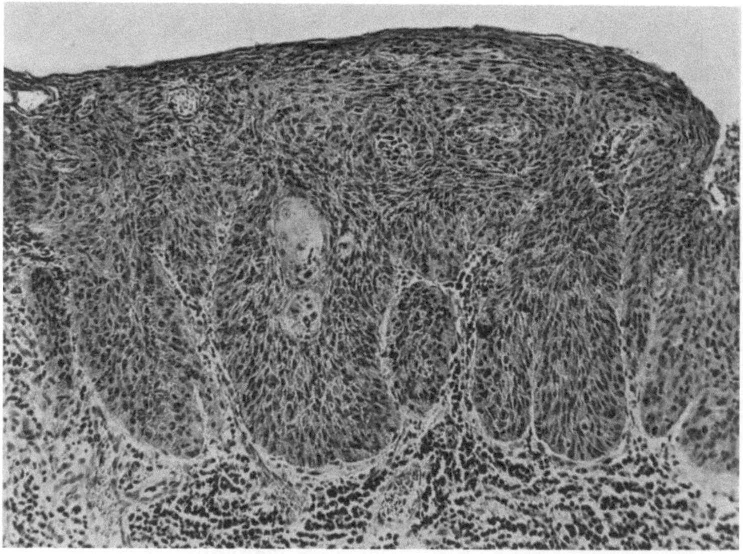

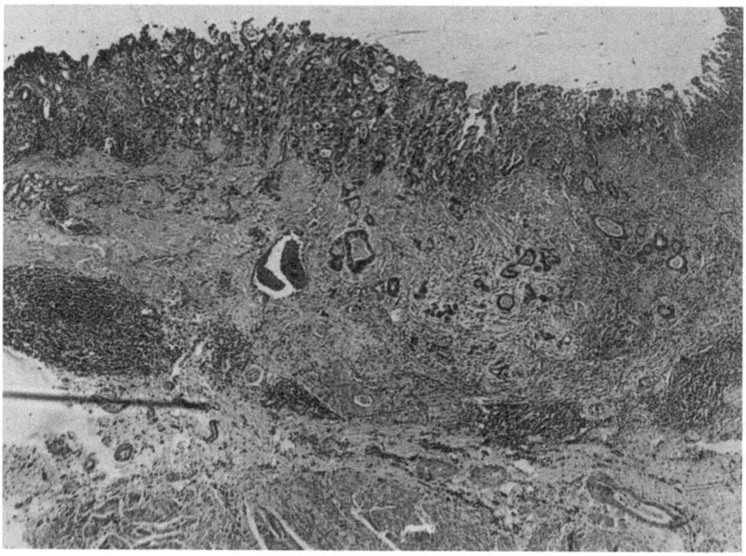

Fig. 5.38 (above). Microscopic view of the early carcinoma of the esophagus in Fig. 37, revealing early infiltrating squamous carcinoma. H&E, ×120

Fig. 5.39 (below). Microscopic view of the early carcinoma of the gastric cardia in Fig. 37, revealing submucosal poorly differentiated adenocarcinoma H&E, ×25

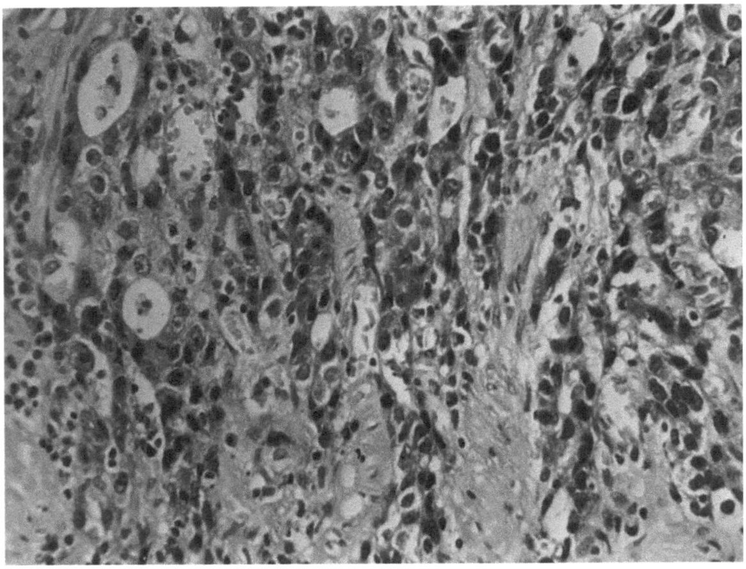

Fig. 5.40. Higher magnification of Fig. 39. Poorly differentiated cancer cells form small bands and small tubes. H&E, × 220

7 Spread and Metastasis

7.1 Direct Extension

It is common for carcinoma of the gastric cardia to directly invade the lower segment of the esophagus, and sometimes this process can hardly be distinguished from esophageal carcinoma invading the cardia. Direct invasion and metastasis are more frequent in the advanced stage. Direct invasion often involves the hiatus of the diaphragm, the left lobe of the liver, the hepatogastric ligament, the tail of the pancreas, the hilus of the spleen, and other retroperitoneal structures, making surgical resection difficult or even impossible.

7.2 Lymphatic Metastasis

There are abundant intramural lymphatic networks in all layers of the gastric cardia, especially in the submucosa and subserosa, which communicate freely with each other and also communicate with the lymphatics of the esophagus. These networks drain into extramural lymphatic trunks which flow down into the celiac axis or up into the mediastinum, both routes leading finally to the thoracic duct. Maruyama et al. [89], using lymphography, determined three lymphatic flow systems arising in the gastric cardia:
1. Ascending flow reaching the mediastinum along the esophageal wall.
2. Right-side flow from the lesser curvature through the cardioesophageal branch and the left gastric artery network to the celiac artery system.
3. Left-side flow from the posterior wall through the greater curvature and the upper border of the pancreas to the retroperitoneum; this is further divided into three channels – greater curvature, posterior gastric, and diaphragmatic.

Along these flow systems are distributed numerous lymph nodes. The first-step nodes in lymphatic metastasis from carcinomas of the gastric cardia are those of the gastric cardia itself, which can be subdivided into left cardia and right cardia, the lower segment of the esophagus, and the lesser curvature. The lymph nodes of the second step are those along the left gastric artery, splenic artery, splenic hilus, and omentum. In the late stage, remote lymph nodes are involved, e.g., celiac artery, aortic artery, hepatic hilus, mediastinal, and supraclavicular nodes.

7.3 *Hematogenous Metastasis*

The most frequent sites of hematogenous metastasis from carcinoma of the gastric cardia are liver, lung, bone, brain, adrenals, and skin. There are two pathways:

1. The normal route is through the portal vein into the liver and then through the vena cava into the systemic circulation.
2. Collateral circulation between organs sometimes exists. Following this route, cancer cells can enter the lung or the systemic circulation directly without using the portal vein [90].

7.4 *Implantation*

Secondary implantation deposits from advanced carcinomas of the gastric cardia are commonly seen in the peritoneum, omentum, and mesentery. In more serious cases there may be serous or bloody ascites.

8 Relationship Between Pathological Factors and Prognosis

Carcinoma of the gastric cardia has a rather poor prognosis, the 5-year survival rate after surgical treatment being 9%–20% (Table 5.2) [1, 18, 91–97].

Size of tumor, depth of invasion, gross type, histologic type, lymph node metastasis, lymphatic and intravascular cancer emboli, and other factors all exert a certain influence on the prognosis, with depth, histology, and lymph node metastasis having particular significance. The depth of invasion directly reflects the progression of the disease; the deeper the invasion, the poorer the prognosis. Advanced carcinoma of the gastric cardia already penetrating muscular layers gives a rather poor 5-year survival rate, while early carcinomas confined to the mucosa or submucosa may have a rate of over 90% [15]. Histologically, well-differentiated lesions have a better prognosis than poorly differentiated ones; this has long been generally acknowledged. The presence or absence of lymphatic metastasis is an important indicator of the stage of development, and its bearing on prognosis has been stressed. Gross type, which reveals the state of differentiation and growth to a certain extent, is also widely used as a prognostic indicator.

In recent years, the possible significance of the pathological changes reflecting the immunologic and other defensive responses of the host has received increasing attention. A lot of data have shown that host immunity to the cancer antigen, indicated by the response of lymphocytes and plasma cells in the cancer margin and the proliferation of T and B

Table 5.2. Postresection survival rates for carcinoma of the gastric cardia

Author(s)	Year	Five-year survival (%)	Ten-year survival (%)
Gunnlaugsson et al. [1]	1970	12.7 (31/238)	
Huang [92]	1975	18.5 (30/162)	
Vantsyan [93]	1978	19.7 (49/249)	
Papachristou and Fortner [94]	1980	8.9 (9/101)	
National Collaborating Group on Gastric Cancer [71]	1981	18.0 (342/1901)	
Zhang et al. [96]	1982	15.4 (104/677)	8.6 (23/266)
Present authors	1982	19.2 (82/426)	8.5 (24/283)

lymphocytes in the regional lymph nodes, is definitely advantageous [18, 98, 99]. Sinus histiocytosis in the regional lymph nodes is not such a definitive indicator of prognosis [99]. There are differing points of view on the significance of the phenomenon of fibrous proliferation surrounding the cancer [18, 100].

We carried out a comparative analysis of histologic host responses and prognosis in 487 cases of advanced carcinoma of the gastric cardia, gaining the following results [97]. It was clear that *immune response* in the regional lymph nodes and *fibrous proliferation* surrounding the cancer were factors favorably affecting prognosis. The prognosis was better in lymphocyte predominance and germinal center predominance in regional lymph nodes than in lymphocyte depletion and unstimulated nodes, and better with lymph cell response at the cancer margin than without. We selected a group of 188 cases of the same histologic type and analyzed the relationship between prognosis and various host responses. The prognosis was poorest in those cases with completely negative host responses, somewhat better with one positive response, and markedly more favorable with two positive responses. In cases where three responses were present, the 3-year survival rate was over 90% (Fig. 5.41).

The *histologic type* reflected the biologic features of the carcinoma, and of all the pathological factors, it exercised the most decisive influence over prognosis. The various pathological changes and morphologic host responses were all closely associated with histologic type. Their influence over the prognosis varies with the degree of cancer differentiation. In the cases of diffuse carcinoma, morphologic changes of host response were seldom seen. Grossly, the majority were infiltrating types with lymphatic metastasis. The postoperative mortality was 100% within 3 years whether there was host response or not. The patients with well-differentiated carcinoma were found to have stronger body immunity, and the gross types were largely fungating or localized ulcerative with less metastasis to lymph nodes; their prognosis was better. The 3-, 5-, and 10-year survival rates for grade I adenocarcinoma were 66.7%, 56.5%, and 40.0% respectively, higher than those of other well-differentiated adenocarcinomas.

These pathological phenomena imply that the tumor and the host are antagonists. The histologic type mainly indicates the invasiveness of the cancer, and the immune active cells at the cancer margin and in the regional lymph nodes reflect the immunologic resistance of the body. These factors are closely interlinked, and their importance in the prognosis depends to some extent on how far the cancer has progressed. In the early stages, when there is better hope of complete eradication, it is obvious that the depth of invasion basically decides the postsurgical prognosis. In the advanced stages, the appearance of

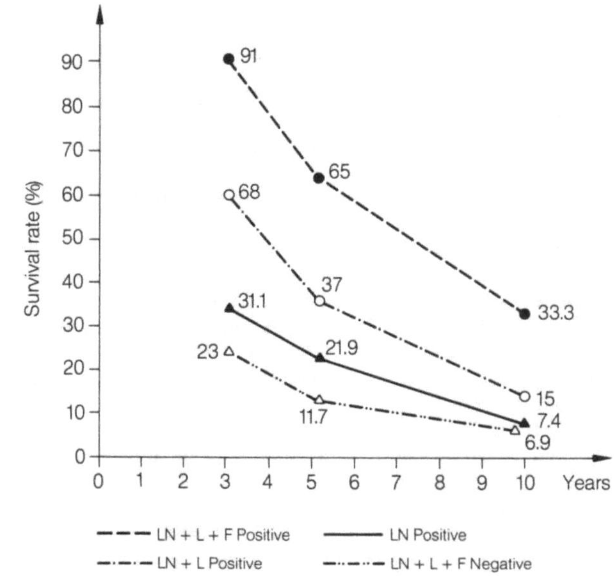

Fig. 5.41. The relationship between different host responses and prognoses in 184 cases of grade II adenocarcinoma. *LN,* immunologic response in regional lymph nodes; *L,* lymphocyte response in cancer margin; *F,* fibrous response in cancer margin

lymphatic metastasis and histologic host responses often has a greater bearing. The biologic behavior of the tumor, reflected in histologic type, is always the most important factor influencing the prognosis.

References

1. Gunnlaugsson GH, Wychulis AR, Roland C, et al. (1970) Analysis of the records of 1657 patients with carcinoma of the esophagus and cardia of the stomach. Surg Gynecol Obstet 130: 997–1005
2. Appelqvist P (1972) Carcinoma of the esophagus and gastric cardia. Acta Chir Scand [Suppl] 430: 1–92
3. Teitler RF, Painter RW, Foster JH (1975) Cancer of the cardia. Am J Surg 129: 89–93
4. Griffith JL, Davis JT (1980) A twenty-year experience with surgical management of carcinoma of the esophagus and gastric cardia. J Thorac Cardiovasc Surg 79: 447–452
5. Welvaart K, Zwaveling A (1980) Carcinoma of the esophagus and gastric cardia. Clin Oncol 6: 203–212
6. Sun SQ, Wu X (1965) Pathology of carcinoma of the gastric cardia (in Chinese). In: Wu YK, Huang GJ (eds) Carcinoma of the esophagus and gastric cardia. Shanghai Scientific and Technical Publishers, Shanghai, p 95
7. Nishi M, Nomura H, Kajisa S, et al. (1978) Surgical problem of carcinoma in the esophagogastric junction (in Japanese). Stomach Intestine 13: 1497–1507
8. Takagi K, Mochizuki T, Okashima K, et al. (1978) Carcinoma of esophagogastric junction (panel discussion) (in Japanese). Stomach Intestine 13: 1517–1528
9. Kata Y, Sugano H, Wada J, et al. (1978) Histogenesis of cardiac carcinoma (adenocarcinoma) in comparison with that of antral carcinoma (in Japanese). Stomach Intestine 13: 1509–1515
10. Matsue H, Hirota T, Itabasi M, et al. (1978) Pathological features and X-ray diagnosis of cancer of the esophagocardiac region (in Japanese). Stomach Intestine 13: 1477–1488
11. Sato H, Isono K (1976) Clinical aspects of carcinoma of the gastric cardia (in Japanese). Kin Kow, Tokyo, pp 7–10
12. Berridge FR, Friedland GW, Tagart REB (1966) Radiological landmarks at the oesophagogastric junction. Thorax 21: 499–511

13. Freeny PC (1979) Double-contrast gastrography of the fundus and cardia: normal landmarks and their pathologic changes. AJR 133: 481–487
14. Weiss L, Greep RO (1977) Histology, 4th edn. McGraw-Hill, New York, p 668
15. Li L, Pan GL, Shen Q (1982) Pathological study of early carcinoma of gastric cardia (in Chinese). Chin J Oncol 4: 93–97
16. Shen Q, Tian DF (to be published) Pathological study of early carcinoma of the esophagus (in Chinese).
17. Nagayo T, Yokoyama H (1978) Recent changes in the morphology of gastric cancer in Japan. Int J Cancer 21: 407–412
18. The National Collaborating Group on Gastric Cancer (1981) The pathological morphology of advanced gastric carcinoma and its prognostic significance in 8523 cases (in Chinese). The National Collaboration Conference on Gastric Cancer.
19. Sun SQ, Wu X, Liu TW (1963) A study of gross classification of carcinoma of the gastric cardia (in Chinese). Chin J Pathol 7: 173–179
20. Li L, Pan GL, Huang GJ (1984) Pathological features of carcinoma of the gastric cardia (in Chinese). Chin J Oncol 6: 37–40
21. Tanai H, Toshimoto Y, Takagi H, et al. (1980) A statistical analysis of dectecting risk factors for stomach cancer patients. In: Lindberg, Kaihara (eds) MEDIFO 80, North-Holland, Amsterdam Oxford New York, pp 974–978
22. Lauren P (1965) The two histological main types of gastric carcinoma: diffuse and so-called intestinal-type carcinoma. Acta Path Microb Scand 64: 31–49
23. Nakamura K (1972) Pathology of gastric carcinoma, histogenesis of minute carcinoma (in Japanese). Ken Hou Do, Tokyo
24. Ellis FH (1964) Surgical aspects of malignant lesions of the esophagogastric junction. In: Cancer of the stomach, 1st edn. Saunders, Philadelphia London, pp 127–140
25. McPeak E, Warren S (1948) Histological features of carcinoma of the cardioesophageal junction and cardia. Am J Pathol 24: 971–991
26. Dodge OG (1961) The surgical pathology of gastro-esophageal carcinoma. Br J Surg 49: 121–125
27. MacDonald WC (1972) Clinical and pathologic features of adenocarcinoma of the gastric cardia. Cancer 29: 723–732
28. Talerman A, Woo-Ming MO (1968) The origin of squamous cell carcinoma of the gastric cardia. Cancer 22: 1226–1232
29. Li HM (to be published) Carcinoid syndrome associated with adenocarcinoma of gastric cardia.
30. Pallesen G (1981) Neoplastic Paneth cells in adenocarcinoma of the urinary bladder. Cancer 47: 1834–1837
31. Schmid KO, Auböck L, Albegger K (1979) Endocrine-amphicrine enteric carcinoma of the nasal mucosa. Virchows Arch A Path Anat and Histol 383: 329–343
32. Li L, Pan GL (to be published) Neoplastic Paneth cells occurrence in an adenocarcinoma of gastric cardia.
33. Wu X, Sun SQ (1979) Adenocarcinoma and rhabdomyosarcoma of the gastric cardia (in Chinese). Chin J Oncol 1: 314
34. Jacobs MI, Rigel DS (1981) Acanthosis nigricans and the sign of Leser-Trelat associated with adenocarcinoma of the gall-bladder. Cancer 48: 325–328
35. Yao BL, Shen DW (1965) Acanthosis nigricans associated with carcinoma of gastric cardia, a case report (in Chinese). Tianjin Med J [Spec Issue Cancer] 3: 153–154
36. Department of Pathology, Cancer Institute, Chinese Academy of Medical Sciences (1975) The atlas of tumor pathology (in Chinese). People's Medical Publishing House, Beijing, p 59
37. Sano K, Kawasaki M, Yanagimoto S, et al. (1968) Early carcinoma originating from esophago-gastric junction: a case report. Nippon Shokakibyo Gakkai Zasshi 65: 295–296
38. Yamamuchi D, Takemoto C, Haneu F, et al. (1970) Type I early carcinoma of the gastric cardia: a case report (in Japanese). Stomach Intestine 5: 671–674
39. Henan Cancer Research Team (1972) Pathological study of early carcinoma of the gastric cardia (in Chinese). Selected papers of National Conference on Prevention and Treatment of Esophageal Cancer by Combination of Chinese Traditional and Western Medicine, pp 223–230
40. Department of Thoracic Surgery, Radiotherapy, and Pathology, Fourth Hospital, Hopei Medical College (1975) Clinical diagnostic experience of early carcinoma of the esophagus and gastric cardia (in Chinese). Hopei Cancer Res 2: 25–29

41. Nimura Y, Takahashi T, Takagi K, et al. (1975) A minute early gastric cancer at the squamocolumnar junction of the cardia (in Japanese). Stomach Intestine 10: 109–113
42. Murohisa B, Yomada T, Waki S, et al. (1975) A case of minute IIb type early carcinoma of the cardia of the stomach diagnosed by exfoliative cytology and aiming biopsy (in Japanese). Stomach Intestine 10: 1305–1308
43. Fujita S, Shimaguchi S, Nagoshi K (1976) Two cases of early gastric cancer at the esophago-cardiac junction of the cardia (in Japanese). Stomach Instestine 11: 203–208
44. Liu ZM, Liu SC, Yang GH (1979) Pathological study of early carcinoma of gastric cardia in four cases (in Chinese). Acta Acad Med Sichuan 10: 46–51
45. Li L (1981) Double primary early carcinomas in the esophagus and gastric cardia (in Chinese). Chin J Oncol 3: 142–143
46. Suzuki S, Nagayo T, Murakami H, et al. (1976) Minute early carcinoma on the esophago-gastric junction (in Japanese). Stomach Intestine 11: 697–704
47. Endo M, Suzuki S, Kawada A, et al. (1978) Endoscopic diagnosis of esophagocardial cancer (in Japanese). Stomach Intestine 13: 1489–1495
48. Murkami T (1972) Pathomorphological diagnosis, definition and gross classification of early gastric cancer. Gan 11: 54
49. Hermanek P, Roesch W (1973) Critical evaluation of Japanese "early gastric cancer" classification. Endoscope 5: 220–224
50. Liu TH, Chen MZ (1981) Early gastric carcinoma: clinicopathologic analysis of 50 cases. Chin Med J 94: 345–354
51. Oohara T (1979) Clinico-pathology of microcarcinoma (in Japanese). Stomach Intestine 14: 1037–1044
52. Machado G, Davies JD, Tudway AJC, et al. (1976) Superficial carcinoma of the stomach. Br Med J 2: 77–79
53. Schade ROK (1974) The borderline between benign and malignant lesions in the stomach. In: Grundmann E, Grune H, Witte S (eds) Early gastric cancer, current status of diagnosis. Springer, Berlin Heidelberg New York, p 46
54. Whitehead R (1979) Mucosal biopsy of the gastrointestinal tract. Saunders, Philadelphia, p 36
55. Ming S (1973) Tumors of the esophagus and stomach. Atlas of tumor pathology, 2nd ser, fasc 7, American Forces Institute of Pathology, Washington, p 162
56. Kraus B, Cain H (1979) Is there a carcinoma in situ of gastric mucosa? Pathol Res Pract 164: 342–355
57. Grundmann E (1975) Histologic types and possible initial stages in early gastric carcinoma. Beitr Pathol 154: 256–280
58. Morson BC, Sobin LH, Grundmann E, et al. (1980) Precancerous conditions and epithelial dysplasia in the stomach. J Clin Pathol 33: 711–721
59. Riddle RH (1976) The precarcinomatous phase of ulcerative colitis. Curr Top Pathol 63: 209
60. Nagayo T (1968) The borderline lesion of the stomach (in Japanese). Jpn J Cancer Clin 14: 465–471
61. Sugano H, Nakamura K, Takagi K (1972) An atypical epithelium of the stomach, a clinico-pathological entity. Gan 11: 258
62. Nagayo T (1975) Borderline lesion of gastric mucosa (in Japanese). Stomach Intestine 10: 1437–1442
63. Zhang YC, Bai YZ, Zhang WF (1979) Histopathologic study of atypical epithelial proliferation of the gastric mucosa and its follow-up study (in Chinese). Chin J Oncol 1: 23–28
64. Yoshii T (1975) Borderline lesion of benign and malignant epithelial cells in stomach (in Japanese). Stomach Intestine 10: 1471–1478
65. Taniguchi H, Tateishi R, Wada A, et al. (1954) Some considerations on a lesion of the stomach which appeared histologically on the borderline between benignancy and malignancy (in Japanese). Stomach Intestine 10: 1449–1454
66. Yoshii T (1972) Gastritis. In: Tzumoka K (ed) All cases of early gastric carcinoma (in Japanese). Nan Ko Do, Tokyo, pp 138–144
67. Pan GL, Li L, Liu FS (to be published) Early carcinoma originated from polyp of gastric cardia
68. Imai T, Kubo T, Watanabe H (1971) Chronic gastritis in Japanese with reference to high incidence of gastric carcinoma. J Natl Cancer Inst 47: 179–195
69. Cheli R, Santi L, Ciancamerla G, et al. (1973) A clinical and statistical follow-up study of atrophic gastritis. Am J Dig Dis 18: 1061–1066
70. Liu TH, Lu ZM, Chen MZ, et al. (1982) Ultrastructure of atrophic gastritis and gastric carcinoma (in Chinese). Chin J Oncol 3: 89–92

71. The National Collaborating Group on Gastric Cancer (1981) The pathological analysis of advanced gastric carcinoma associated with intestinal metaplasia in 4668 cases (in Chinese). The National Collaborating Conference on Gastric Cancer
72. Schade ROK (1977) The pathology of precancerosis of the gastric mucosa. In: Figus AI, Simon L (eds) Gastric precancerosis. Akademiai Kiado', Budapest, p 24
73. Hiroto T, Itahashi M, Suzuki K (1979) Micro- and small early gastric cancer, histogenesis of gastric cancer (in Japanese). Stomach Intestine 14: 1027–1036
74. Johansen AA (1976) Early gastric cancer. Curr Top Path 63: 34
75. Li SH, Tan YC, Chen DY, et al. (1981) Histogenesis of gastric carcinoma (in Chinese). Proceedings of the 3rd National Pathological Conference
76. Teglbjaerg PS, Neilsen HO (1978) "Small intestinal type" and "colonic type" intestinal metaplasia of the human stomach. Acta Pathol Microbiol Scand [A] 86: 351–355
77. Li L, Pan GL (1983) Histogenesis of carcinoma of gastric cardia (in Chinese). Acta Acad Med Sin 5: 169–172
78. Lei DN, Xi YP, Wang YL, et al. (1980) A histogenetic and pathologic classification of gastric carcinoma - 239 cases (in Chinese). Chin J Oncol 2: 55–59
79. Nevalainen TJ, Jarvi OH (1977) Ultrastructure of intestinal and diffuse type gastric carcinoma. J Pathol 122: 129–136
80. Thompson JJ, Zinsser KR, Enterline HT (1983) Barrett's metaplasia and adenocarcinoma of the esophagus and gastroesophageal junction. Hum Pathol 14: 42–61
81. Yamada E, Nakazato H, Koike A, et al. (1974) Surgical results for early gastric cancer. Int Surg 59: 7–14
82. Wang ZH, Gu YZ (1955) Double primary carcinomas of the esophagus and gastric cardia (in Chinese). Chin J Surg 3: 459–460
83. Sun SQ, Liu FS, Wu X, et al. (1964) Five cases of double primary carcinomas of the esophagus and gastric cardia (in Chinese). Tianjin Med J [Spec Issue Cancer] 2: 297–298
84. Liu FS (1979) Double primary carcinomas of the esophagus and stomach, a pathological study of nine cases (in Chinese). Acta Acad Med Sin 1: 67–70
85. Dodge OG (1961) Gastro-esophageal carcinoma of mixed histological type. J Pathol Bacterial 81: 459–471
86. Wanke M (1972) Collision tumor of the cardia. Virchows Arch [Pathol Anat] 357: 81–86
87. Majmudar B, Dillard R, Susann PW (1978) Collision carcinoma of the gastric cardia. Hum Pathol 9: 471–476
88. Spagnolo DV, Heenan PJ (1980) Collision carcinoma at the esophagogastric junction, report of two cases. Cancer 46: 1702–1708
89. Maruyama K, Miwa K, Kawamura J (1978) Lymphatic flow of gastric cardia, a study by endoscopic lymphography (in Japanese). Stomach Intestine 13: 1535–1542
90. Hirayama R, Miyanaga T, Nihei Z, et al. (1978) Clinicoembryological and anatomical study on the metastatic pathways of cancer of esophagocardiac region. Stomach Intestine 13: 1529–1534
91. Gu YZ, Wang ZH, Zhang JQ, et al. (1964) Long-term effects of surgical treatment and radiotherapy of carcinomas of the esophagus and gastric cardia (in Chinese). Chin J Surg 12: 115–120
92. Department of Surgery, Cancer Institute, Chinese Academy of Medical Sciences (1975) Surgical treatment of carcinoma of esophagus and gastric cardia: an analysis of 1432 cases (in Chinese). Chin Med J 1: 60–63
93. Vantsyan EN (1978) Surgical treatment of cancer of the cardia (in Russian). Thorax Surg 3: 87–92
94. Papachristou DN, Fortner JG (1980) Adenocarcinoma of the gastric cardia. Ann Surg 192: 58–64
95. Li C (1980) Surgical treatment of carcinoma of the esophagus and gastric cardia: clinical evaluation of 327 cases (in Chinese). Chin J Oncol 2: 116–118
96. Zhang YD, Du XQ, Zhang W, et al. (1980) Cancer of the esophagus and gastric cardia: experience of surgical treatment in 4310 cases (in Chinese). Chin J Oncol 4: 1–4
97. Pan GL, Li L, Huang GJ, et al. (1983) Prognostic significance of histologic host response in cancer of the gastric cardia. Acta Acad Med Sin 5: 97–101
98. Watanabe H, Enjoli M, Imai T (1976) Gastric carcinoma with lymphoid stroma: its morphologic characteristics and prognostic correlations. Cancer 38: 232–243
99. Phil E, Malahy MA, Khankhanian N (1977) Immunomorphological features of prognostic significance in Dukes class B colorectal carcinoma. Cancer res 37: 4145–4149
100. Tu XR, Chen PH, Zhu SJ (1981) Fibrous stroma response in cancer of the large bowel and its clinical significance (in Chinese). First National Pathological Conference on Cancer of the Large Bowel

Chapter 6
Diagnostic Cytology and Early Detection

Qiong Shen

1 Introduction

Carcinoma of the esophagus is one of the common malignancies in northern China [1, 2]. It is a serious threat to the life and health of the working people, and has been more prevalent in the rural parts of the high-incidence areas. Statistics show that by the time patients begin to suffer from progressive dysphagia and go the city hospitals for treatment, the disease is already in a late stage, with lymph node metastasis already present in more than half of the cases. The results of treatment – surgery, radiology, or any combined regimen – are unsatisfactory.

It has long been the common aim of those working in this field to devise an efficient and practical means of detecting carcinoma of the esophagus and gastric cardia in the early stages, thereby improving the therapeutic success rate. Medical workers in Henan province and of the Chinese Academy of Medical Sciences, Beijing, have since 1959 carried out a joint investigation of esophageal carcinoma in Linxian county, a high-incidence area. They have established a local anticancer organization and have gone directly to the patients' homes, offering medical care and at the same time doing much work on epidemiology and etiology as well as on public anticancer education. They have conducted mass screening for esophageal carcinoma and have been rewarded by the discovery of many early cases. On the basis of extensive surgical treatment in these cases, valuable resources have been created for pathologists, cytologists, epidemiologists, radiologists (both diagnostic and therapeutic), and other workers in the broad field of cancer prevention and research, and many important contributions have been made to the study and control of carcinoma of the esophagus.

After many years of experience, it has been found that balloon cytologic examination is a satisfactory technique for the early detection of carcinoma of the esophagus and gastric cardia. It is simple and effective both in mass surveys and in the daily screening work in clinics, not only for carcinoma, but also for detection and follow-up of esophageal dysplasia, and has been adopted as an important tool in most thoracic and oncologic clinics throughout China [3–6].

The purpose of this chapter is to report our method and results in the early detection of carcinoma of the esophagus and gastric cardia by balloon cytology. The efficacy of this method in the diagnosis of carcinoma and related conditions and in the detection and follow-up of esophageal dysplasia, a subject of growing importance, will also be discussed.

2 Specimen Collection Technique

The apparatus for collecting cytologic specimens is a double-lumen tube (Fig. 6.1 *left*) made of rubber and plastic which is about 65 cm in length and 0.25 cm in diameter and is graduated every 5 cm. At the distal end, it has an inflatable balloon about 5 cm long and 2.5 cm wide covered with a cotton mesh net. At the proximal end it is divided into two tubes, one for air injection and the other for suction. The apparatus is sterilized by soaking in alcohol solution for 1 h after cleansing with soap water. A recently developed alternative is a single plastic tube which may be disposable (Fig. 6.1 *right*).

The examination is usually done in the morning, and the subject is instructed to come with an empty stomach. After intubation through the cardia, the balloon is first inflated with 30 ml air and then slightly deflated so that it can be pulled back past the cardia. When the balloon comes up into the lower segment of the esophagus, it is redistended to obtain

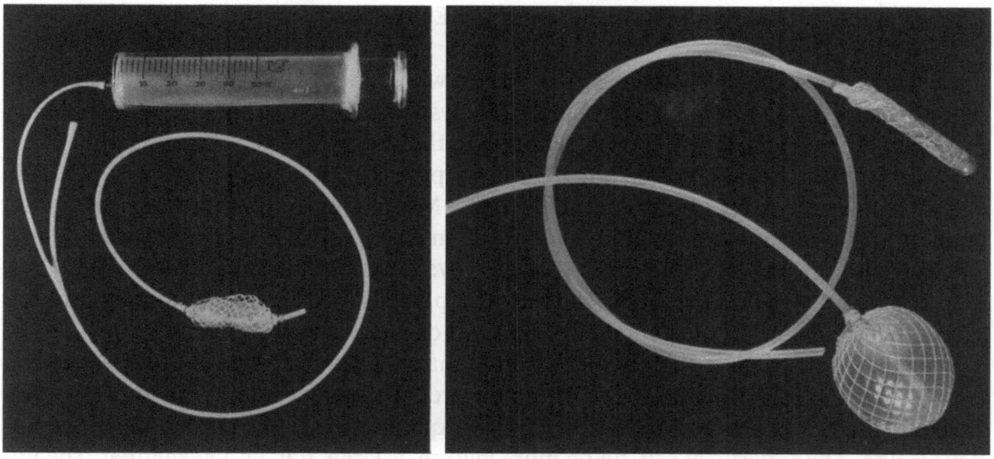

Fig. 6.1. Balloon catheters. *Left:* Double-lumen model with syringe in place. *Right:* Modified single-lumen model with balloon inflated

complete contact with the mucous surface, then slightly deflated. The tube is retracted for 5 cm, and again the balloon is distended and deflated. This process is repeated until the 20-cm mark is reached, when the balloon should be deflated completely and withdrawn.

Direct smears are made onto four slides for each subject, with staining by Papanicolaou's method. Throughout the staining procedure the slides should be kept wet.

Balloon cytology is very safe and easy to perform. To date more than a hundred thousand people have been screened in the outpatient department of Linxian County Hospital and in mass surveys. The single serious complication was a hematemesis which occurred in one early case of esophageal cancer, and this patient was operated on safely.

Contraindications to balloon cytology include recent history of hematemesis, acute pharyngitis, severe liver cirrhosis, heart failure, and late pregnancy.

2.1 Segmental Balloon Cytology of the Esophagus

Sometimes it may be necessary to roughly determine the uppermost limit of a roentgenologically and endoscopically occult early carcinoma of the esophagus by balloon cytology. It may also be desirable to detect the extent or location of a cancerous focus above the main carcinoma by this technique before surgery is performed. The examination consists of successive balloon tests at different levels, starting in the upper part of the esophagus and going down as far as desired. For instance, in the first test the tip of the balloon is inserted to 20 cm from the upper incisors, in the second test to 25 cm, and the third test to 30 cm. X-ray may be helpful in deciding how far down to go, and the height of the subject should also be taken into consideration.

Smears are made separately from the upper and the lower halves of the balloon. By mapping the positive and negative smears at different levels of the esophagus or finding the level where the smear from the lower part of the balloon is positive and that from the upper part is negative, the uppermost limit of the cancerous lesion may be determined.

3 Histology and Cytology of Normal Esophageal Epithelium

In screening the smears, the cytologic picture as a whole should be carefully analyzed. The characteristics of the normal, hyperplastic, and dysplastic cells are all important in the interpretation of pathologic conditions reflected in the smear.

The stratified squamous epithelium may be simply divided into three layers, superficial, intermediate, and deep (parabasal and basal). Morphologically, the basal cell is the smallest in the squamous epithelium. Its cytoplasm is basophilic and its cytoplasmic envelope is round or oval. The nucleus is round or oval and located in the center of the cell. The chromatin granules are deeply stained. The parabasal cell is similar to the basal cell except that the total size of cellular envelope and of nucleus is greater.

The intermediate cell is slightly more mature than the parabasal. In the deeper portion of this layer, the cell tends to be ovoid or elongated in shape, while in the upper portion the cell increases in size and becomes elliptic or quadrilateral. The chromatin of the nucleus is fine. The superficial cell, being more mature, is large, flat, and hexagonal. The nucleus is small, pyknotic, and centrally located. The cytoplasm is red or orange and contains keratohyalin, but it does not undergo true cornification [7].

Biologically, the cells in the different layers of the esophageal epithelium represent different stages of maturation. When the basal cell (germinal cell) divides, one of the daughter cells stays at the basement membrane while the other ascends into the parabasal layer. Thus cells are gradually pushed up further by subsequent mitoses of the germinal cells, and so the epithelium consists of as many clones as there are basal cells. The superficial cells are mature, the basal and parabasal cells immature [8].

Exfoliative Cytology

The exfoliative cells of the esophagus in a normal subject are chiefly of the intermediate type, with 10%–15% superficial cells. Parabasal cells are rarely exfoliated, basal cells usually not (Fig. 6.2).

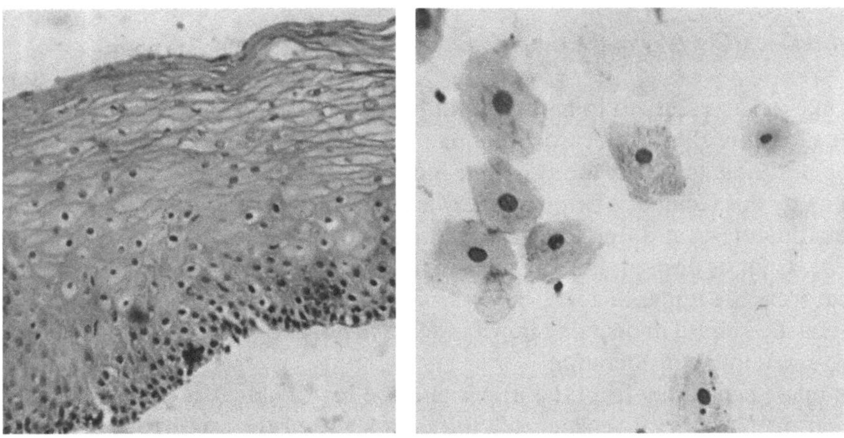

Fig. 6.2. Left: Normal squamous epithelium of the esophagus. × 150. *Right:* Normal exfoliated esophageal epithelial cells of the superficial and intermediate layers. × 150

4 Dysplasia of the Esophagus

4.1 Pathologic Histology

Dysplasia is a disorder of the development and maturation of the epithelium. Histologically, the chief finding of esophageal dysplasia is an increased number of epithelial cells, resulting in increased thickness of the epithelium and vertical arrangement of the epithelial cells. The retardation of maturation is manifested by enlargement of the nucleus and atypism or anaplasia of the cells [9].

Hyperkeratosis is a significant process in association with esophageal dysplasia, preceding it. Acanthosis and parakeratosis are commonly seen in dysplastic esophageal epithelium (Fig. 6.3).

4.2 Cytology

The above-mentioned histologic changes in the upper portion of the epithelium may be reflected in the smear. Hyperkeratosis is demonstrated by the presence of cornified cells in the smear, but cornified epithelium is not frequently found in the section, probably because cornified cells are thin and cannot be seen clearly when they are few in number.

However, cornified cells are a significant finding. For instance, in the brush smears of 30 normal persons in a mass survey by fiberesophagoscopy in an esophageal cancer low-incidence area, no cornified cells was found, whereas in the fiberesophagoscopic brush smears from subjects with various conditions of the epithelium in Linxian, cornified cells were found in nine (30%) of 30 with normal epithelium, 10 (33.3%) of 30 with mild hyperplasia, and 21 (70%) of 30 with marked dysplasia. Wynder and Klein [10] reported that hyperkeratosis of the esophagus in mice with riboflavin deficiency could develop to a very marked degree, so hyperkeratosis in a high-incidence area may be a sign of vitamin deficiency in the community.

Parakeratosis is demonstrated in the smear by the presence of parakeratotic cells, which always appear in sheets in fiberesophagoscopic brush smears (Fig. 6.3).

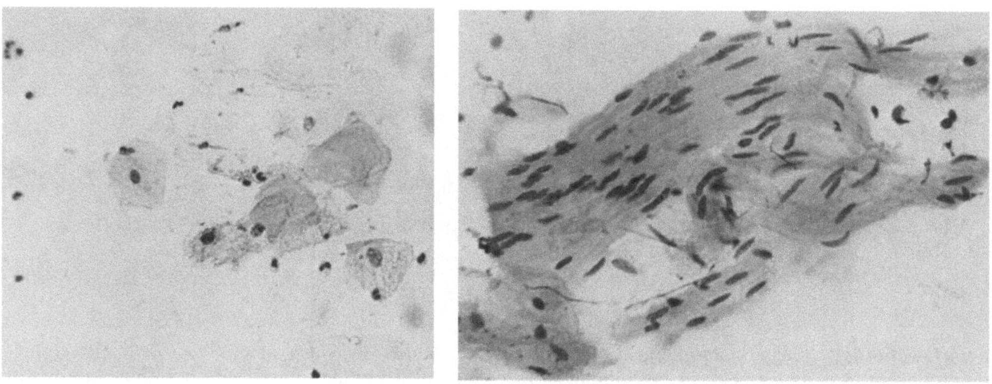

Fig. 6.3. Hyperkeratosis and parakeratosis of the esophagus. *Left:* Anucleated squames in hyperkeratosis. × 150. *Right:* Sheets of superficial parakeratotic cells in a fiberendoscopic brush smear. × 150

Dyskeratosis is not uncommon in dysplastic epithelium of the esophagus, being found in histologic sections as well as in smears. There were 11 cases (13%) with this finding in the section in a series of 84 specimens of early esophageal carcinoma. The dyskeratotic cells show a cornifying property in the cytoplasm of the cells in the intermediate and deep layers of the epithelium when the staining of the smear is optimal.

Anaplasia or atypism denotes that the epithelial cells are not completely differentiated. Their nuclei become enlarged, irregular, and hyperchromatic, although the cytoplasm may appear normal. Nuclear changes in the superficial cells may reflect certain characteristics of the pathologic changes in the intermediate and deep cells.

Such nuclear changes may be used as a diagnostic criterion for dysplasia, in which enlargement of the nucleus is essential. If degree of nuclear change is to be used to denote the diagnostic categories of dysplasia of the esophageal epithelium, all who hear or read the term must know what the entity looks like [11].

4.3 Classification

Dysplastic epithelial cells in the smear are classified into four grades (with early carcinoma as grade V) according to the pathomorphology of the cells, with emphasis on the structural changes of the nuclei [12, 13].

Grade I: Normal. The cytologic picture of normal epithelium in the smear has already been described (Sect. 3).

Grade II: Mild Hyperplasia. There is a mild degree of hyperchromasia of the cells. The chromatin content of the nucleus is increased, and the nucleus in 2 or more but less than 3 times greater than in normal cells in the same layer. The chromatin granules are fine and the nuclear membrane is not thickened (Fig. 6.4).

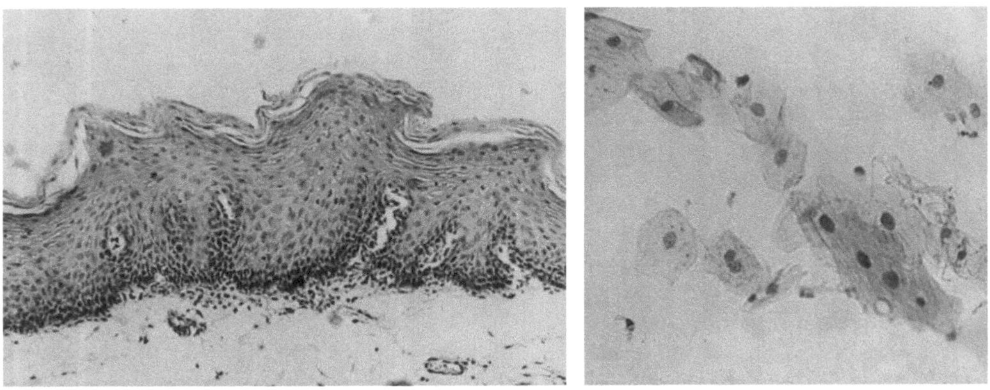

Fig. 6.4. Mild hyperplasia of esophageal epithelium with parakeratosis and acanthosis. *Left:* The epithelium adjacent to early esophageal carcinoma, showing slight thickening in association with acanthosis in the lower portion and parakeratosis in the superficial portion. × 150. *Right:* Mildly hyperplastic cells in smear, presenting nuclei enlarged to double the normal size. × 150

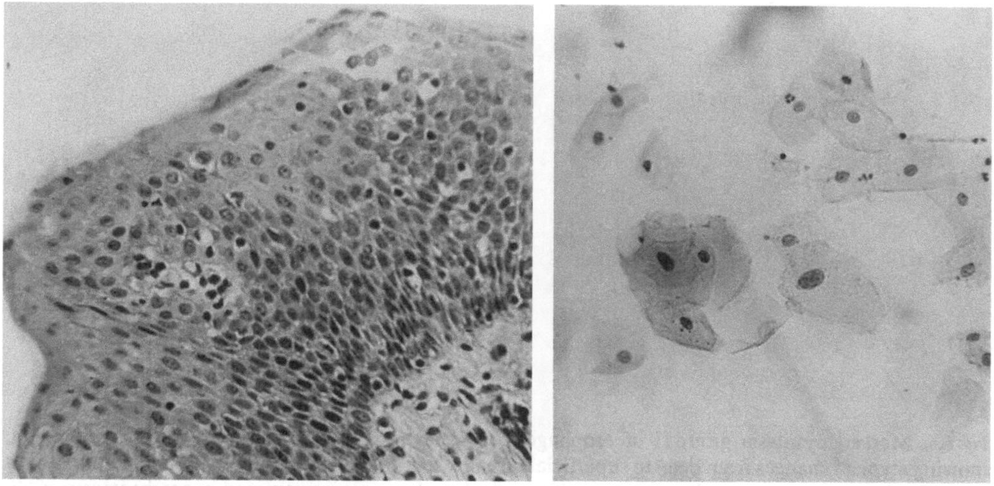

Fig. 6.5. Marked dysplasia group I of esophageal epithelium. *Left:* Atypical changes of epithelium adjacent to early esophageal cancer, showing marked thickening of epithelium and vertical alignment and moderate enlargement of nuclei, fitting the diagnostic criteria of marked dysplasia group I. × 264. *Right:* The single central cell has an enlarged nucleus which fits the same grade in cytology. × 150

Grade III: Marked Dysplasia. The size of the nuclei in dysplastic intermediate cells is 3 times or more that in normal intermediate cells. Hyperchromasia is more marked. The chromatin granules of the nuclei become coarse, but are fairly uniform in size and even in distribution. The nuclear membrane is slightly thickened, but regular. Dysplastic parabasal cells are increased in number. To make a diagnosis, a total of five or more such cells is required. This type of dysplasia may be divided into two groups.

Group I. The nuclear size in dysplastic cells in the intermediate layer is 3 times or more that in normal cells in the same layer (Fig. 6.5).

Group II. The nuclear size in dysplastic cells is 4 times or more that of normal cells in the same layer (Figs. 6.6, 6.7).

Grade IV: Near-carcinoma. The nuclei in the near-carcinoma cells are 5 or more times greater in size than those in the normal cell of the same layer. The chromatin granules of the nuclei are not as coarse as those of typical cancer cells and are evenly distributed in the nuclei. The nuclear membrane is thickened but regular, and the cytoplasm is broader than that in the cancer cells. These are very important points for differentiating near-carcinoma and cancer cells. Near-carcinoma cells always lie in the epithelium adjacent to carcinoma in situ or in the epithelium overlying carcinoma of the basal layers (Fig. 6.8, 6.9).

Grade V: Early Carcinoma. In this category typical cancer cells are present in the smear. The diameter of the nucleus exceeds one-third the total diameter of the cell. The malignant features of the cancer cell nuclei are very distinct. The chromatin granules are coarse, varied in size, and uneven in distribution. All these morphologic characteristics serve to distinguish carcinoma cells from near-carcinoma cells, which is very important in the early diagnosis of cancer by cytology (Fig. 6.10).

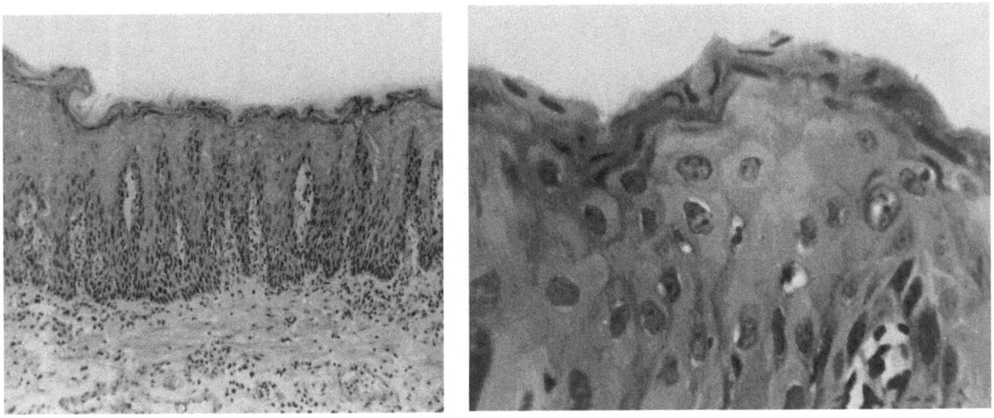

Fig. 6.6. Marked dysplasia group II of esophageal epithelium. *Left:* Epithelium in low magnification, showing atypical changes from deep to superficial layers. × 100. ***Right:*** Upper portion of epithelium in high magnification, presenting cellular changes, with marked nuclear enlargement and hyperchromasia. × 440

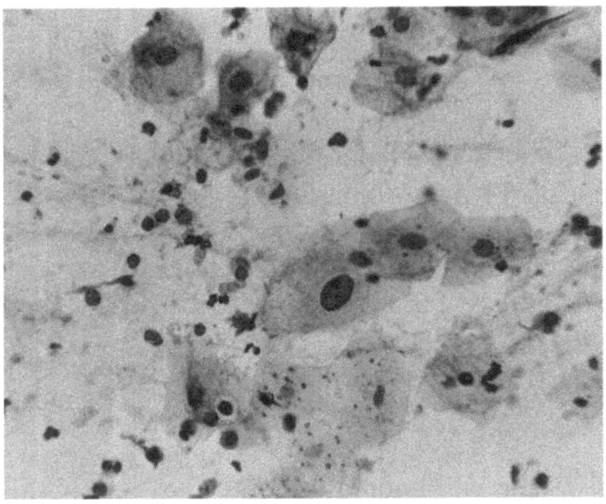

Fig. 6.7. Epithelial cells of marked dysplasia group II. Smear showing a cell in the central portion with hyperchromasia and marked enlargement of the nucleus. × 150

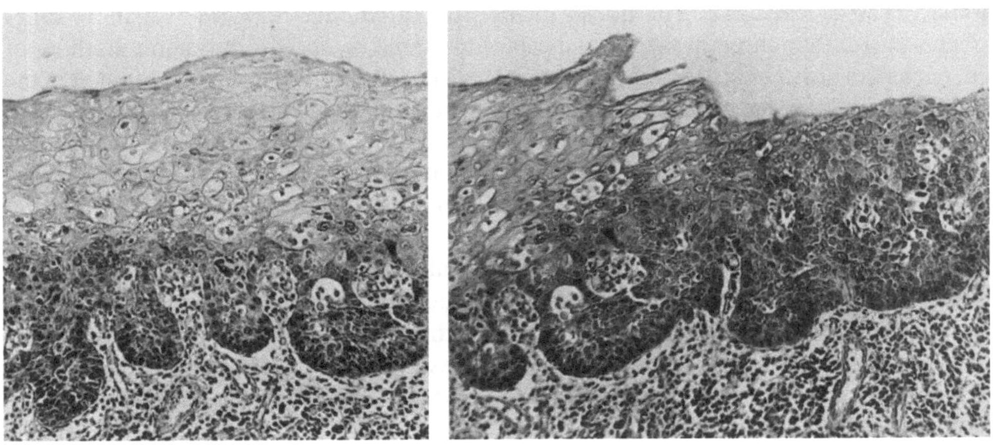

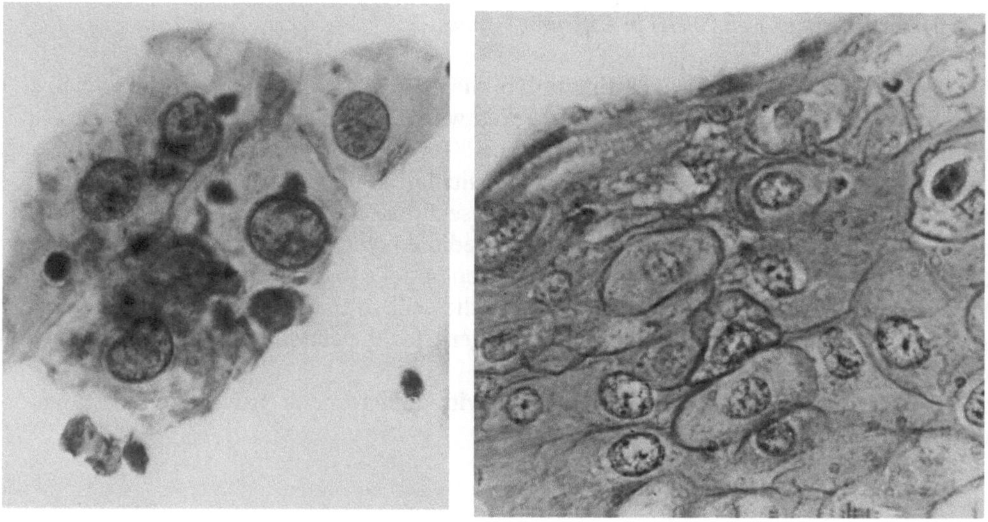

Fig. 6.9. Same case as in Fig. 6.8. Preoperative smear done in November 1962 shows near-carcinoma cells *(left)* closely resembling those in tissue section of the upper portion of the epithelium with carcinoma in basal layer *(right)*. × 570.

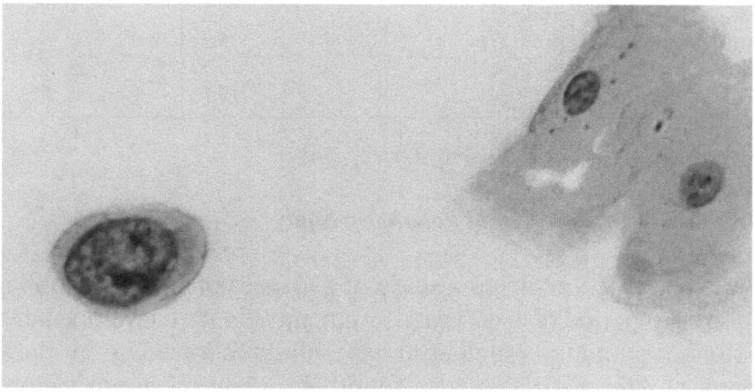

Fig. 6.10. Preoperative balloon cytology of the same case as in Fig. 6.8, from May 1963, shows a cancer cell with full-blown malignant features, its sharp nuclear and cytoplasmic borders suggesting that it is active and fresh. × 570.

◁ *Fig. 6.8.* Tissue section of a small (0.4 × 0.7 cm) esophageal carcinoma in situ, showing carcinoma in the basal layers *(left)* developing into carcinoma in situ *(right)*. The patient was operated upon in July 1963. × 150

4.4 *Measurement of Cell Nuclei in Different Grades*

Grading is established by visual estimation of the degree of enlargement of the nuclei. The reliability of this estimation should be checked with a micrometer, preferably by an experienced cytologist who can select the proper cells for measurement. For each grade 30 cells are measured and the areas of the nuclei are calculated [14].

The same procedure can be applied to tissue sections to measure the cells in the superficial layer and the upper portion of the intermediate layer. From Table 6.1 it can be seen that the ratios of nuclear areas of cells of different grades to those of normal cells are similar in tissue sections and in smears, although the cells in tissue are smaller than those in smears (Figs. 6.2, 6.4, 6.5, 6.7, 6.9). Thus the criteria for the classification of cells in smears can also be applied to those in tissue.

In the cells reported in Table 6.1, checking with a micrometer proved visual estimation of nuclear size to have been reliable.

Table 6.1. Ratio of nuclear areas of various pathologic cells to those of normal cells

Cell type	Ratio in tissue	Ratio in smear
Mild hyperplasia	2.2:1	2.8:1
Marked dysplasia (group I)	3.8:1	3.7:1
Marked dysplasia (group II)	5.2:1	4.7:1
Near-carcinoma	7.3:1	5.9:1
Carcinoma	10.0:1	6.4:1

4.5 *Preliminary Results of Follow-Up Study*

Shu et al. [15] conducted a study of 530 cases of marked esophageal dysplasia. During a follow-up period of 1–12 years, 79 patients (14.9%) developed cancer. In another group of 530 cases with mild esophageal hyperplasia followed up for the same period of time, five cases of cancer (0.94%) were found. In a control group followed up for 1–5 years, no esophageal cancer was found.

Such follow-up studies are very important in the classification of dysplasia of the esophagus. In marked dysplasia, evaluation of group I and group II follow-up results is of importance to determine if one group is reversible and the other not; at present we have no statistically significant data. Individual patients with dysplasia group II have been followed for over 15 years and found to develop cancer of the esophagus eventually (Figs. 6.11–6.14).

In summary, this classification may be considered as a descriptive designation based mainly on morphology. The grading of marked dysplasia of the esophageal epithelium should be correlated with the results of follow-up and checked repeatedly. We have the impression that the cells of marked dysplasia group II slowly but steadily progress to can-

Fig. 6.13. A 1976 follow-up smear of the case in Fig. 6.11 shows an increased number of near-carcinoma cells with huge and multiple nuclei and abundant but faint cytoplasm of superficial origin *(left)*, and enlargement but moderate hyperchromasia of the nuclei of these superficial cells *(right)*. × 440 ▷

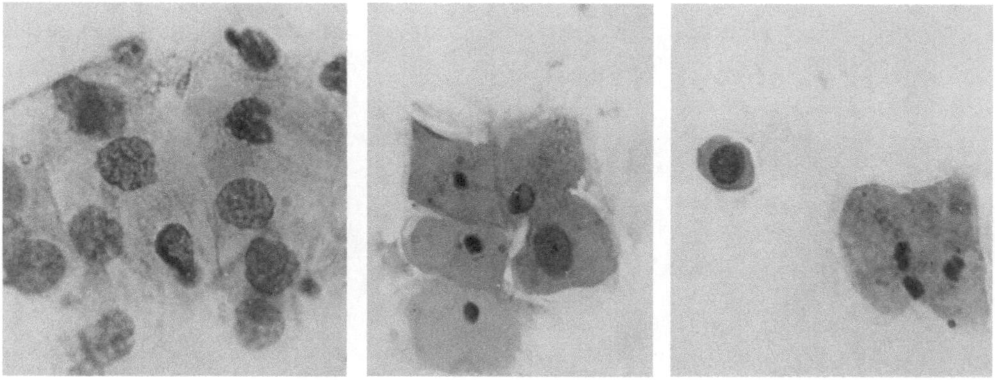

Fig. 6.11. First balloon cytology of this case (May 1965) shows pathologic changes of marked dysplasia group II, with enlarged, degenerated, and swollen nuclei of superficial cells *(left)*, enlarged nucleus with some degree of hyperchromasia of the intermediate cell *(middle)*, and enlarged nucleus and hyperchromasia but indistinct granule of a parabasal cell *(right)*. × 440

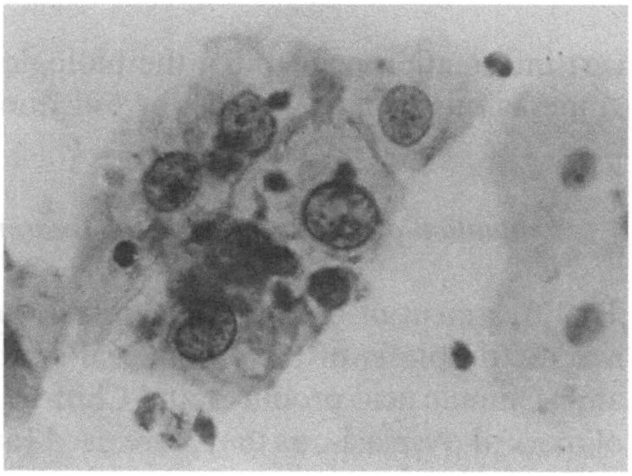

Fig. 6.12. A 1971 follow-up smear of the case in Fig. 6.11 shows a small number of near-carcinoma cells. × 440

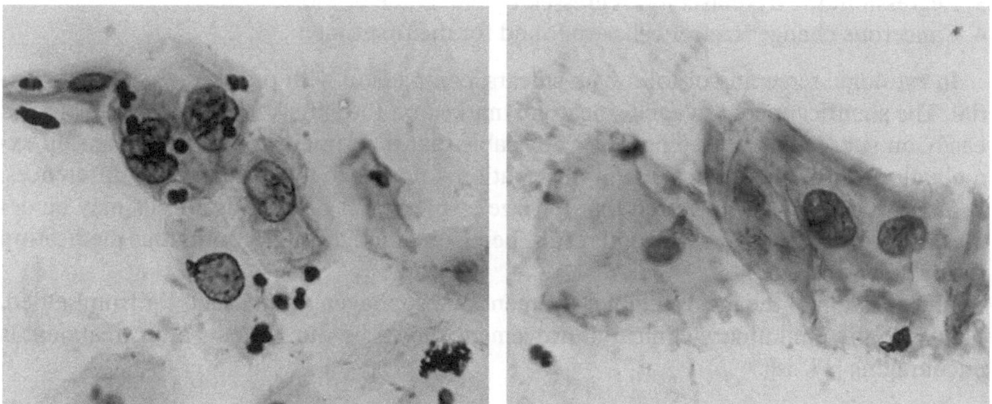

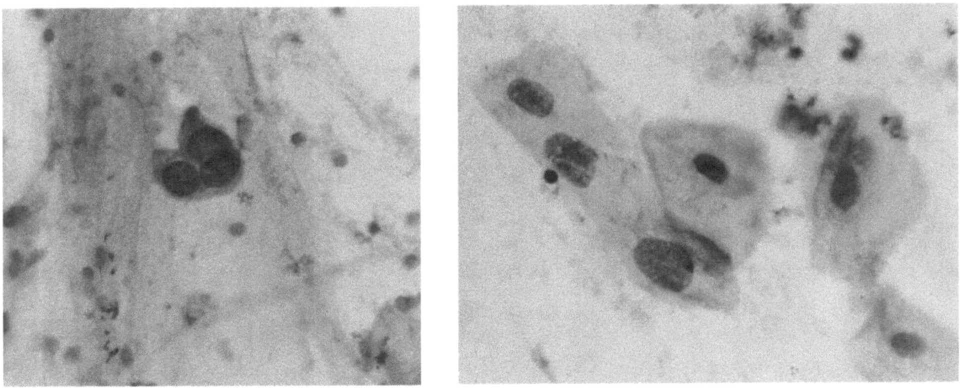

Fig. 6.14. A 1979 follow-up smear of the case in Fig. 6.11 shows near-carcinoma cells and small basal cells *(left)* with moderately enlarged nuclei and hyperchromasia *(right)* × 440. The chromatin distribution here is very similar to the same type of cells in the 1965 smear. It would be proper to interpret this cytologic picture as carcinoma of the basal layer. The patient was well in 1982, with occasional mild dysphagia

cer; information concerning the biologic behavior of cells in the various morphologic grades is fragmentary. Further investigation is necessary.

4.6 *Evaluation of Results of Medical Treatment*

Trial treatment of dysplasia in Linxian has been carried out in groups of subjects with marked dysplasia of the esophageal epithelium for about 10 years. In recent years, vitamins, humic acid products, and Chinese herbal medicines have been used for treatment of marked dysplasia, as they were used for treatment of esophagitis.

Cytologic examination of those who received this treatment was carried out once a year. Evaluation of the results was based on the following criteria [16]:

1. Stabilization: follow-up smears show no significant change since previous examination.
2. Progression: the dysplasia has progressed by one grade or more.
3. Regression: the dysplasia has regressed by one grade or more.
4. Cancerous change: cancer cells are found for the first time.

In cytologic screening of follow-up smears, comparison with previous smears is essential. The significant cells in each smear are marked on the slide so that they can be found easily on subsequent screenings. It is advisable that the same cytologist conducts all examinations throughout the years of observation, in order to avoid subjective differences.

Some authors have suggested that the size of the nuclei of dysplastic cells may be decreased by drug therapy, with good results being obtained through continuous medication for over 5 years.

The question of the most suitable treatment for esophageal dysplasia is far from settled. However, the preliminary clinical improvement shown by our patients after treatment is encouraging [17, 18].

5 Cytology of Carcinoma of the Esophagus

5.1 Early Squamous Carcinoma

The category of early squamous carcinoma includes carcinoma in situ and early invasive carcinoma [19, 20].

Esophageal epidermoid carcinoma in situ is defined as cancerous change of the whole thickness of the esophageal epithelium without invasion of the underlying stromal tissue. Histologically, it may be divided into the following three varieties:

1. Well differentiated. The cancer cells are always polygonal with distinct malignant nuclei. Cornifying cancer cells may be seen in the overlaying layers, and occasionally keratin pearls are formed in the epithelium. This is the commonest variety (Fig. 6.15).
2. Less well differentiated. The majority of cancer cells are ovoid or fusiform with a moderate or scanty amount of cytoplasm (Figs. 6.8, 6.10) [21].
3. Poorly differentiated. The cancer cells are small, the cytoplasm scanty and stained deep blue. The cells are frequently elongated, spindle-shaped, and crowded together without stratification. This variety is rarely seen in resected specimens (Fig. 6.16).

It must be noted that the degree of differentiation of carcinoma in situ is usually not uniform throughout the tumor; for instance, well-differentiated and less well differentiated areas may be mixed in the same section.

When carcinoma in situ becomes an invasive cancer, it may be more differentiated. Keratin pearls are frequently formed in the invasive cancerous tissue developing from a well-differentiated carcinoma in situ, but only rarely in that from a poorly differentiated carcinoma in situ. Evidently, the histologic classification of carcinoma in situ is relative.

As carcinoma in situ progresses and invades beyond the basement membrane underlying the epithelium, it is designated "early invasive cancer" provided there is no lymph

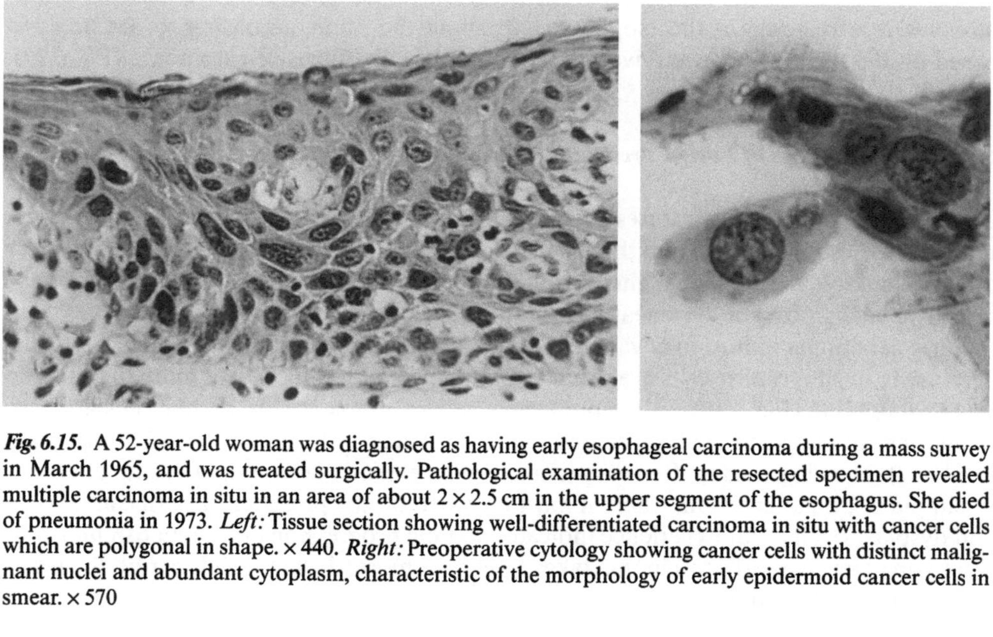

Fig. 6.15. A 52-year-old woman was diagnosed as having early esophageal carcinoma during a mass survey in March 1965, and was treated surgically. Pathological examination of the resected specimen revealed multiple carcinoma in situ in an area of about 2 × 2.5 cm in the upper segment of the esophagus. She died of pneumonia in 1973. *Left:* Tissue section showing well-differentiated carcinoma in situ with cancer cells which are polygonal in shape. × 440. *Right:* Preoperative cytology showing cancer cells with distinct malignant nuclei and abundant cytoplasm, characteristic of the morphology of early epidermoid cancer cells in smear. × 570

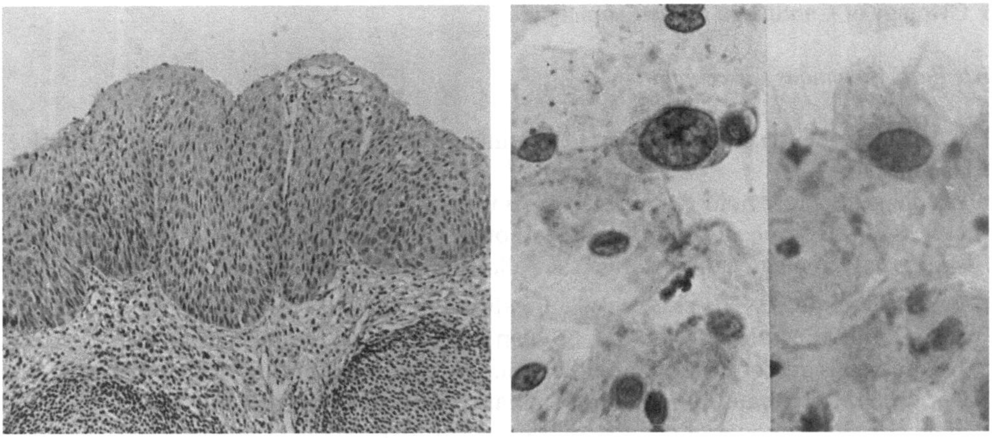

Fig. 6.16. Poorly differentiated carcinoma in situ in a small area (about 0.4 × 0.3 cm). The patient was operated on in 1964 and died of bronchopneumonia in 1972. *Left:* Section showing fusiform and crowded cancer cells. The lymph follicles in the mucosa propria are enlarged. × 150. *Right:* Smear showing fusiform cancer cells. × 570

node metastasis and the invasion is confined to the submucosal layer, not reaching the muscular wall of the esophagus.

We propose calling the cancer "microinvasive" if the invasion does not go beyond the muscularis mucosae. In the case of the uterine cervix, "microinvasive carcinoma" has been defined internationally as a clear invasive epidermoid carcinoma in which the depth of invasion of the stroma does not exceed 5 mm [22]. Invasion to this depth in the esophagus would reach the submucosa. Thus our proposal of defining microinvasive carcinoma as not extending beyond the muscularis mucosae, under which condition the chance of spread is minimal, seems reasonable. The prognosis of carcinoma in situ and that of microinvasive carcinoma of the esophagus are about the same, according to our analysis based on the postoperative survival of patients with microinvasive carcinoma (Fig. 6.17).

5.2 Cytologic Picture of Early Carcinoma

The common microscopic features in smears of carcinoma in situ and early invasive carcinoma of the esophagus are that the dysplastic cells are numerous and the typical cancer cells are variable in number. White cells are not numerous and red cells are scanty or absent. The background of the smear is generally clean (Figs. 6.9, 6.10).

Early carcinoma lesions may vary greatly in the area they cover. In a small (e.g., 1 cm^2) carcinoma in situ, cancer cells are usually found in small numbers, not more than five in one examination (Fig. 6.16). In a more extensive carcinoma in situ, cancer cells are very numerous; in one such case approximately 2700 cancer cells were counted in one slide (Fig. 6.17). The diagnosis is often easy to make in an extensive carcinoma in situ, but is not so simple in a smaller lesion, where it must be based on the presence of both cancer cells and dysplastic cells. Our experience indicates that the progression of a small carcinoma in situ to an extensive early carcinoma takes 5 years or more, during which period the number of cancer cells found in the smears steadily increases.

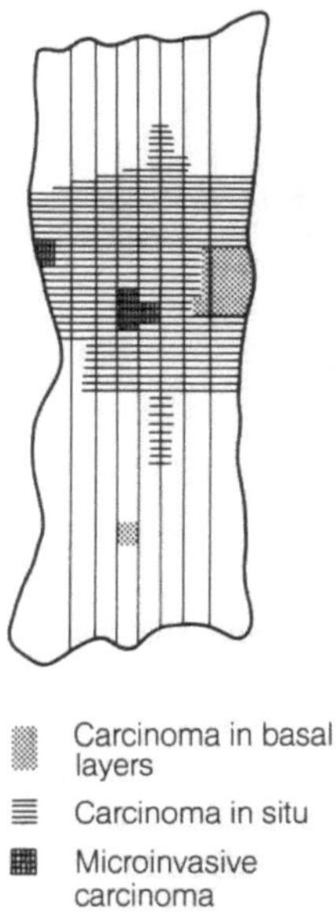

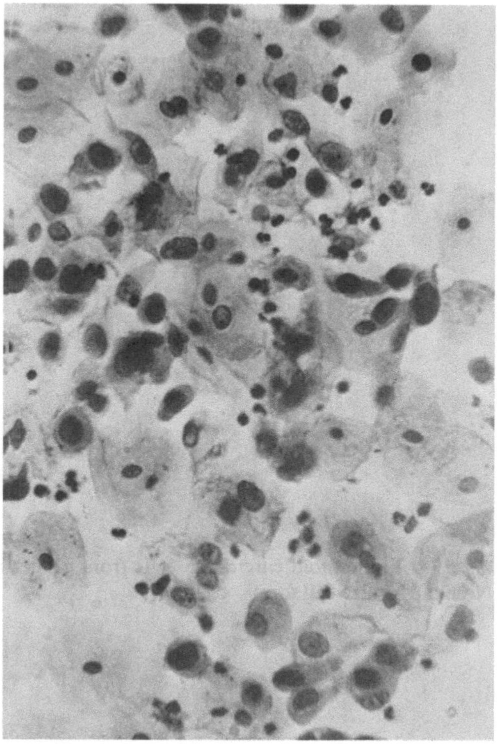

Fig. 6.17. Extensive carcinoma in situ associated with microinvasive carcinoma of the esophagus. The 45-year-old male patient was operated on in December 1966 and remained well on follow-up in 1982. Pathological examination of the resected specimen revealed a carcinoma in situ of about 4.5 × 5 cm with microinvasive lesion in the central portion. *Left:* The distribution of various types of cancer in the specimen. *Right:* Smear showing numerous cancer cells, a few near-carcinoma cells, and a large number of dysplastic cells. × 264

5.3 Cytologic Differences Between Early and Late Carcinoma

In smears from advanced esophageal carcinoma, the striking features are the polymorphism of the cancer cells and the presence of deformed cornified cancer cells, which come from keratin pearls in the deeper tissue. Dysplastic cells are few in number, while inflammatory cells, red cells, and degenerated cells are commonly seen (Fig. 6.18).

In a smear from early esophageal carcinoma, the cancer cells tend to be uniform in shape. Deformed cornified cancer cells are absent and dysplastic cells of all grades are present. These cytologic differences between early and late esophageal carcinoma may be of only relative significance, as the smear of a late case may be similar to that of an early case due to the balloon only having contacted the border zone of the tumor.

5.4 Cytology of Late Squamous Carcinoma

Histologically, late epidermoid carcinoma of the esophagus may be divided into three grades which may have different features in cytologic smears:

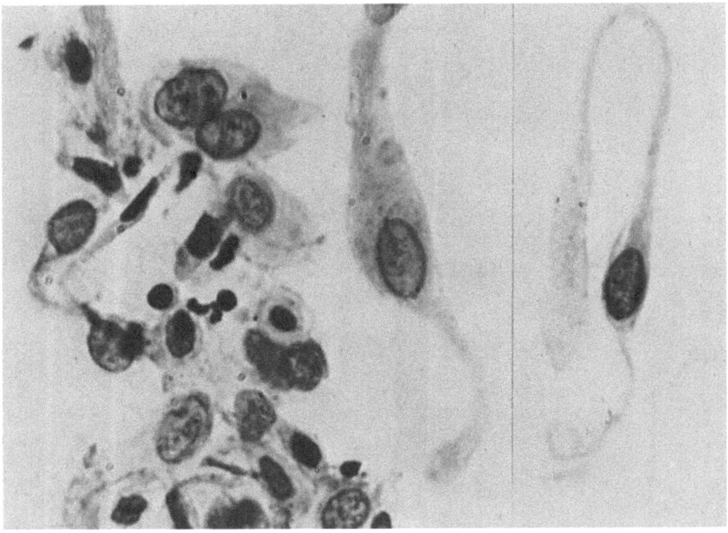

Fig. 6.18. Epidermoid carcinoma cells from a late invasive carcinoma, showing marked polymorphism. Note the bizarre cell forms. × 570

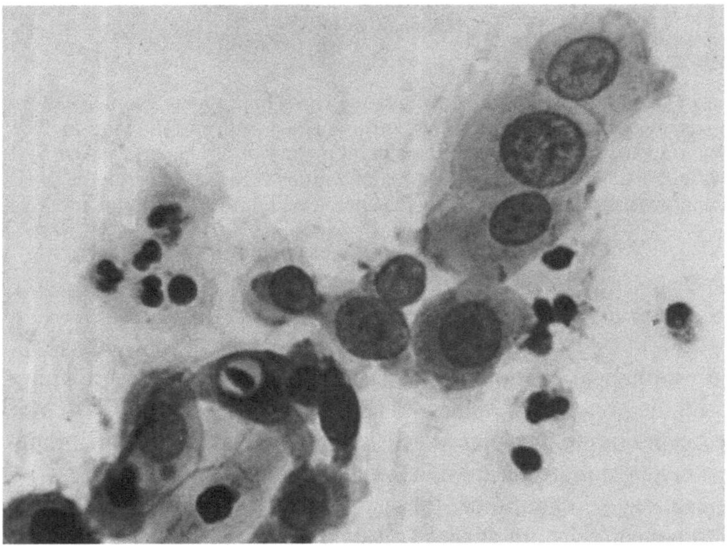

Fig. 6.19. Epidermoid cancer cells of the intermediate differentiated type comparable to parabasal cells with malignant nuclei. × 570

1. The highly differentiated pearl-forming variety comprised about 40% of our specimens. The pearls always lie deep in the invasive cancerous tissue, so deformed cornified cancer cells are rarely seen in the smear.
2. The moderately differentiated variety presents cancerous tissue without pearl formation. The cancer cells in the balloon smear are chiefly of the parabasal type (Fig. 6.19).

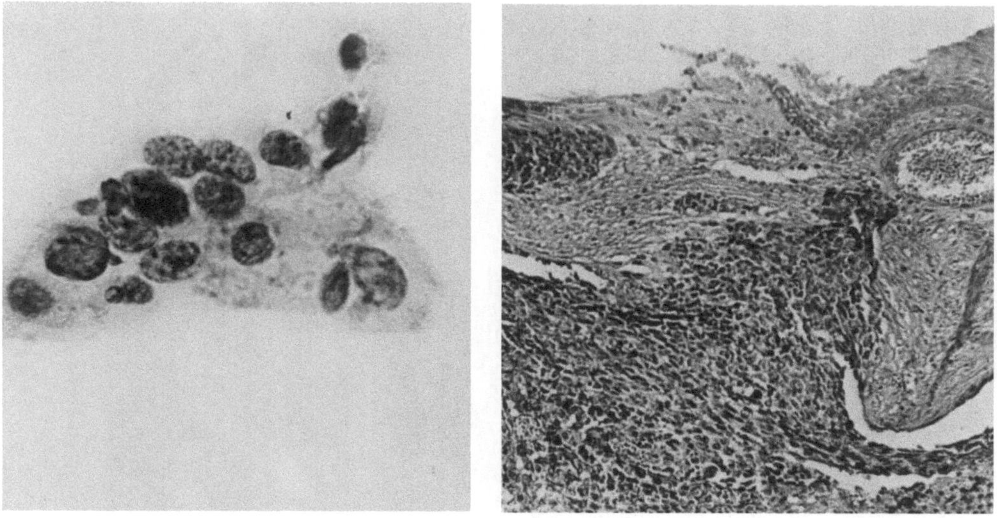

Fig. 6.20. Epidermoid cancer cells of the anaplastic type with scanty cytoplasm or naked nuclei and coarse chromatin granules (*left:* × 570), which are similar to those in tissue section (*right:* × 100)

3. The anaplastic variety was rare in our resected esophageal specimens. The cancer cells are smaller than those of the parabasal type and naked nuclei are frequently found in the smear. The diagnosis is usually made on the basis of the scarcity of parabasal cancer cells (Fig. 6.20); histologic type can be established by smear if anaplastic cells are dominant.

5.5 Adenocarcinoma

There are two types of adenocarcinoma in the esophagus. Adenocarcinoma originating from *ectopic gastric mucosa* has the same histologic and cytologic pictures as gastric carcinoma. It is rarely seen in surgical specimens. We have seen two late cases, one in the middle third and one in the lower third, and one early case was associated with epidermoid carcinoma in situ of the esophagus (Fig. 6.21).

The other type is adenocarcinoma arising from the *esophageal glands proper,* which are small compound glands located in the submucosal layer with richly branched tubuloalveolar secretory portions containing only mucous cells. The branches of the smallest ducts are short and fused into a cyst-like dilated main duct which pierces the muscularis mucosae and opens onto the surface of the esophageal epithelium through a small orifice [23]. The epithelium in the small ducts is low columnar, that in the upper portion of the main duct is stratified squamous, and that in the lower portion of the main duct is commonly transitional.

Adenocarcinoma of the esophageal glands proper commonly develops from tubular epithelium. Its cancer cells as seen in smears are squamous or transitional, medium-sized or small. They may desquamate into the lumen of the tube and be drained to the surface even in the early stage (Figs. 6.22–6.24).

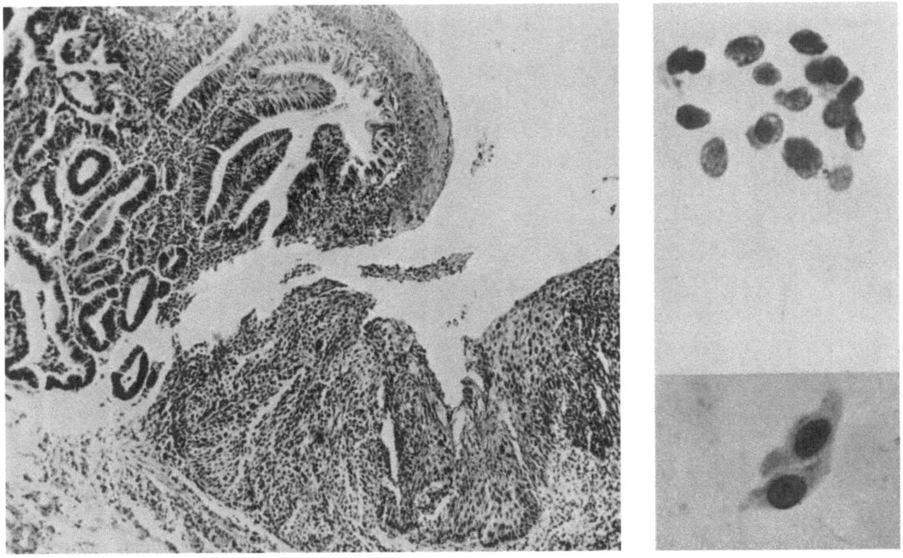

Fig. 6.21. Adenocarcinoma of the esophagus originating from ectopic gastric mucosa with associated epidermoid carcinoma in situ of the esophagus. *Left:* Tissue section showing adenocarcinoma confined to the mucosa propria and bulging up on the surface, about 3 × 2.5 × 2 mm in size; serial sections revealed no connection with the esophageal glands. × 60. *Right:* Smear showing the two types of cancer cells. × 440. The preoperative cytologic diagnosis of squamous carcinoma was revised after histopathologic examination of the specimen

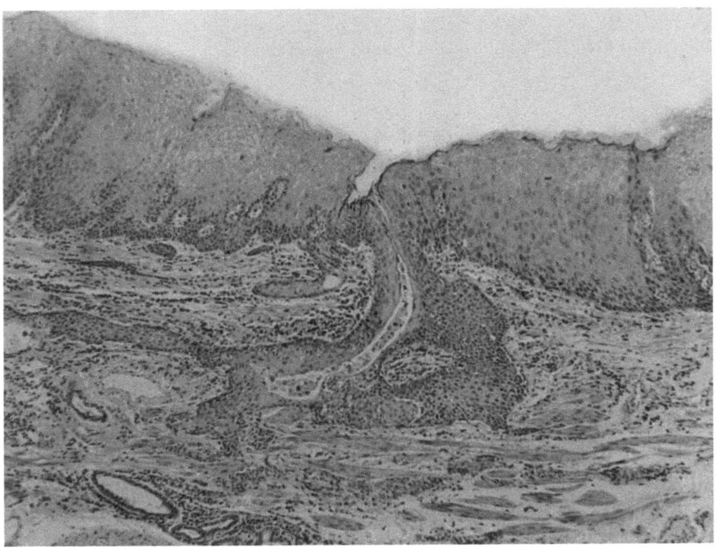

Fig. 6.22. Carcinoma originating from the upper portion of the duct of an esophageal gland. The 48-year-old male patient was treated surgically in April 1965 and died of apoplexy in 1983. The pathological diagnosis was early carcinoma of the gland of the esophagus. × 60

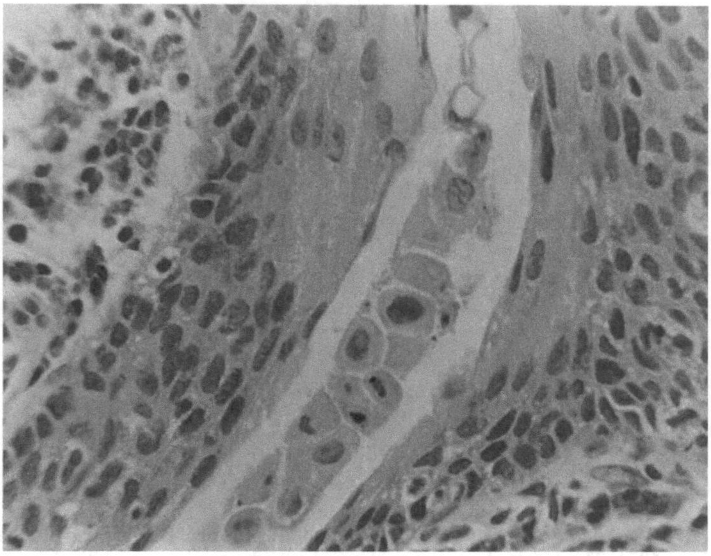

Fig. 6.23. Ductal cancer cells and dysplastic cells desquamated into the lumen of the tube. × 440

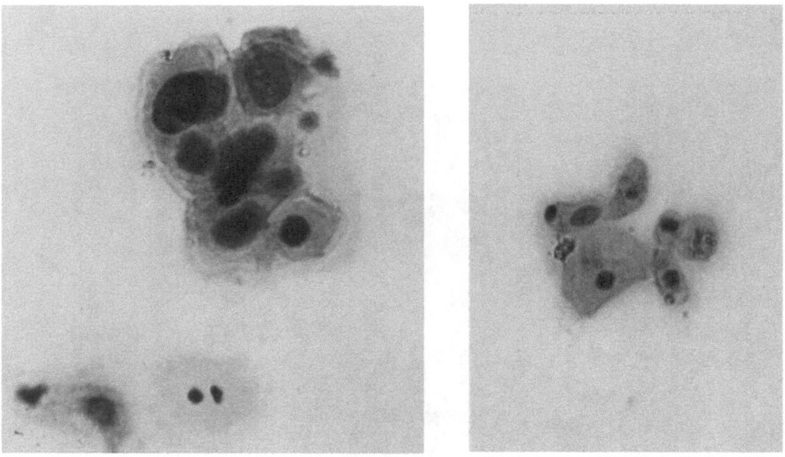

Fig. 6.24. Preoperative balloon cytology of the case in Fig. 6.23, showing cancer cells and dysplastic cells very similar to those in the lumen of the duct. *Left:* Degeneration of cancer cells, possibly due to their long stay in the lumen. × 570. *Right:* The ductal dysplastic cells are smaller than the overlying epithelial cells. × 440

In a late case of adenocarcinoma of the esophageal glands proper, there are cancer cells from the ducts of the glands and from the alveoli. In smears these cancer cells may simulate the shape of those in tissue section (Figs. 6.25–6.27) [24].

Carcinoma of the upper portion of the duct is always associated with carcinoma of the overlying esophageal epithelium. On the other hand, dysplastic cells from the duct are always present in smears of epidermoid carcinoma of the esophagus, so interpretation

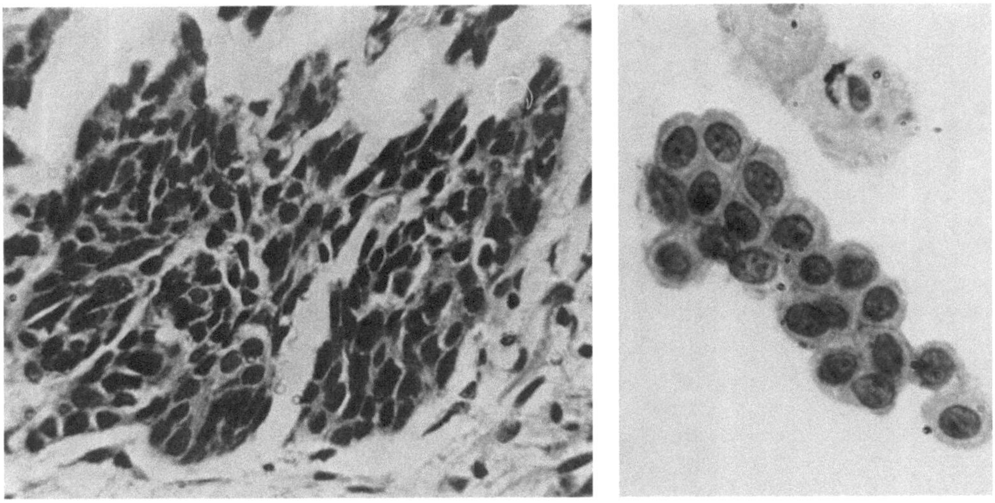

Fig. 6.25. Adenocarcinoma of esophageal glands proper. The 46-year-old male patient was operated on in June 1971. The resected specimen showed an advanced tumor with deep round ulceration in the central portion. Sections showed cancerous tissues developing from the alveoli of the glands. The overlying epithelial tissue was not involved by the cancerous process. A diagnosis of mucoepidermoid carcinoma was made. *Left:* Epidermoid basaloid cancerous tissue derived from ductal epithelium shown in the section. × 440. *Right:* Smear showing ductal cancer cells of basaloid type with prominent nucleoli. × 570

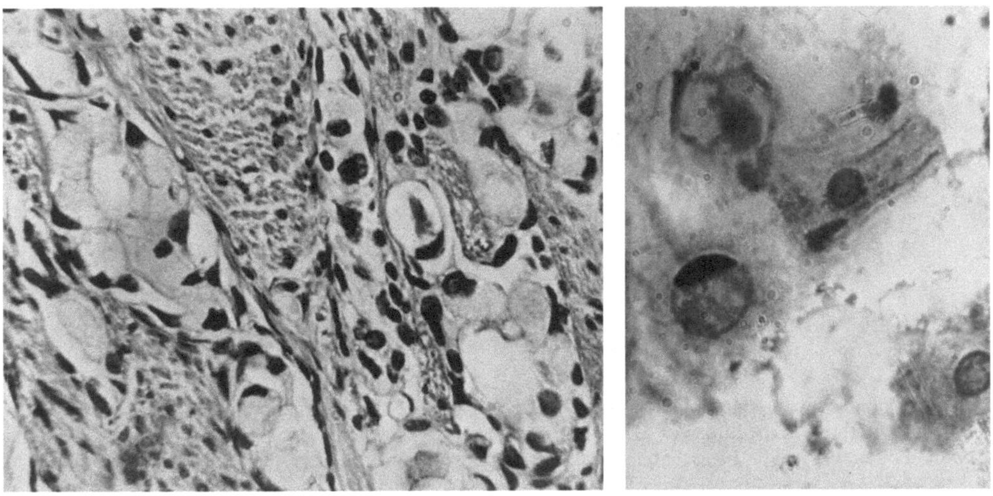

Fig. 6.26. Same case as in Fig. 6.25. *Left:* Mucoid cancerous tissue derived from the alveoli infiltrating into the muscular layer. × 440. *Right:* Mucoid cancer cell in smear similar to those in the tissue. × 570

should be very cautious. The cytologist and the pathologist should bear these pathologic conditions in mind when a smear suggestive of glandular carcinoma of this type is examined.

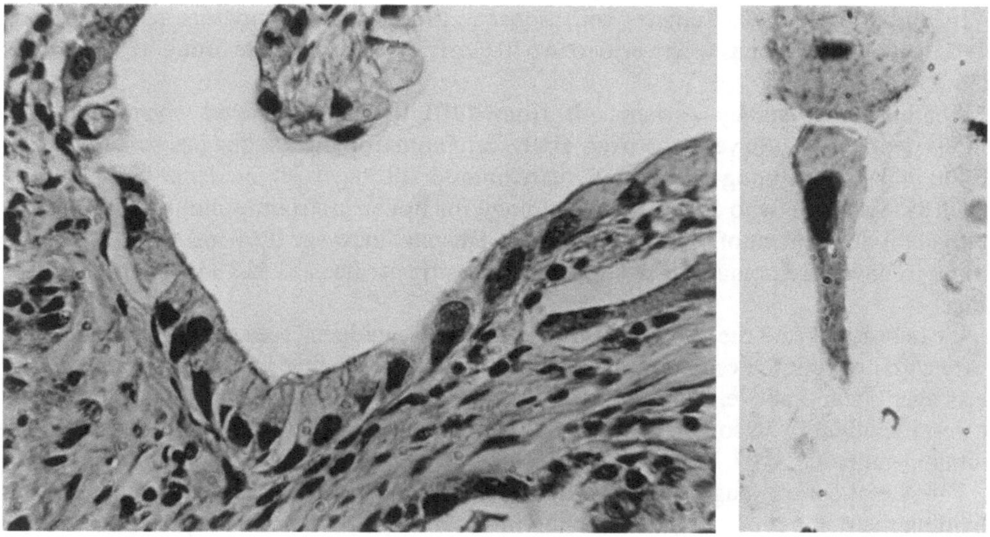

Fig. 6.27. Same case as in Fig. 6.25. *Left:* Alveolar cancer tissue infiltrating the muscular layer. × 440. *Right:* Cylindrical cancer cell found in the smear. × 570

5.6 *Rate of Correct Diagnosis of Carcinoma of the Esophagus and Gastric Cardia by Balloon Cytology*

A total of 256 patients with symptoms suggesting esophageal carcinoma were examined by balloon cytology in the outpatient department of Linxian County Hospital between July 1961 and June 1962. Carcinoma of the esophagus or gastric cardia was eventually verified in 156 of them by means of follow-up studies, pathological examination of the resected specimens, or endoscopic biopsy: 137 (87.8%) had positive cytology. False-negative cases were carefully anlayzed, and subsequent improvements in instrumentation and examination procedures gave higher positive rates in the following years. For example, among 359 patients examined by balloon cytology at the same hospital from June 1968 to May 1969, 124 were eventually verified to have carcinoma; 114 (91.93%) had positive cytology.

The accuracy of balloon cytology in the diagnosis of 110 inpatients of esophageal carcinoma in Linxian County Hospital in 1966 reached 98.1% [5]. In several other hospitals in various provinces, the rates have been about the same or even higher than in Linxian. The most effective way of improving the rate is to repeat the examination when necessary. For instance, in one report of the results of balloon cytology in 52 patients, the rate with a single examination was 65.4%, while that with four examinations was 90.4% [25].

6 Early Detection of Esophageal Carcinoma by Mass Survey

In the 1960s and early 1970s, mass surveys by balloon cytology were carried out in different groups of subjects in Linxian, with varying early detection rates being obtained [24, 26].

In one group of 7686 subjects with upper gastrointestinal symptoms surveyed from 1963 to 1969, carcinomas were verified in 510. Early carcinomas were found in 86, an incidence of 16.9%.

Another mass survey carried out from 1970 to 1972 involved examination of 11,564 people aged 30 years or over. Early carcinoma of the esophagus or cardia was found in 96 cases among a total of 136 carcinoms of all stages, an incidence of 70.6%.

Of 8528 patients who had balloon cytology for upper gastrointestinal illnesses in the outpatient department of the Linxian County Hospital between 1961 and 1971, 3122 were found to have carcinoma of the esophagus or gastric cardia; 212 (6.8%) were in the early stage.

It can be seen from the above data that in this high-incidence area the discovery rate for early carcinoma of the esophagus and gastric cardia was highest in a mass survey of subjects aged 30 and above, lower in a mass survey of subjects with related symptoms, and lowest in patients who sought medical aid. The reverse was true for the discovery of carcinoma in general.

The rate of correct diagnosis by balloon cytology in a mass survey may be calculated by dividing the number of carcinomas found in the survey by that number plus those found in the same group during the next 2 years. For instance, in a 1977 mass survey in the suburban area of the city of Hebi, Henan province, among 5800 people examined, 121 cases of cancer were found at the time of survey and nine more in the following 2 years. The rate of correct diagnosis was therefore 93.1% (121/121 + 9).

7 Cytology of Carcinoma of the Gastric Cardia

7.1 Normal Histology and Cytology

The mucous membrane of all parts of the stomach contains a multitude of glands which open into the bottoms of the gastric pits. The epithelium which lines the gastric pits and covers the mucosa between them is of the same structure.

Each cardiac gland constists of a neck, body, and fundus and is compound and tubular, with the terminal portion opening directly into a gastric pit. The surface and the neck are lined with mucus-producing cells. Parietal cells and chief cells are scanty in the gastric region. The normal gastric glands are situated 5–30 mm below the gastroesophageal junction [23, 27].

The normal cells of the gastric cardia may be fresh and numerous in a balloon cytologic smear if fixation is optimal. The normal glandular cells in a smear are in clusters; the cells in the central portion have a "honeycomb" appearance, and those located peripherally are flattened on the side, quite similar to the gastric lining cells in tissue sections. Singly distributed cells display abundant cytoplasm, a flattened surface, and a tail-like end. The ovoid nucleus is in the central portion of the cell (Fig. 6.28).

7.2 Intestinal Metaplasia

When the normal gastric mucosa is replaced by cells akin to the mucous cells lining the large intestine, the process is referred to as intestinal metaplasia. This may be observed in inflammatory conditions of the stomach, and may occasionally be noted in smears in

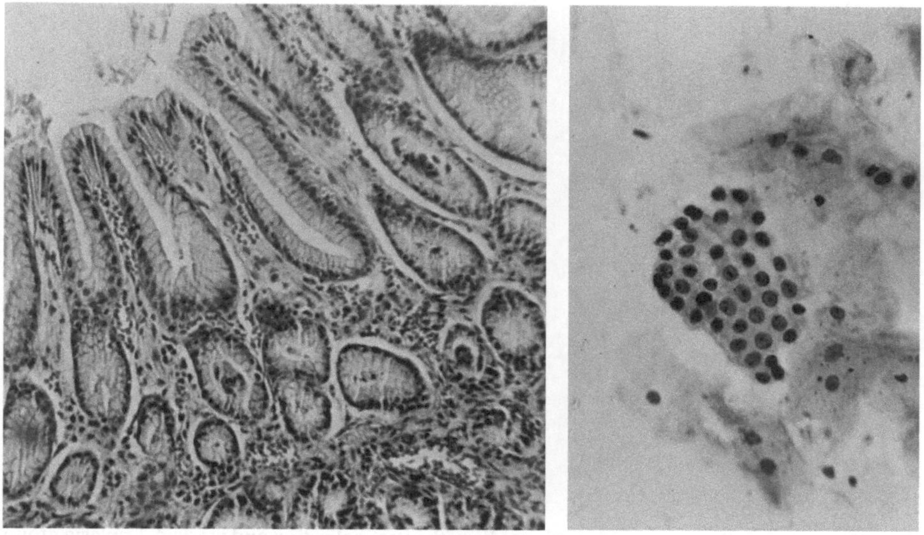

Fig. 6.28. Normal histology and cytology of the gastric cardia. *Left:* Section of biopsied tissue showing normal mucosa of gastric cardia. The epithelial cells of the gastric pits and cardiac glands are normal in arrangement and configuration; lymphoid cells in the propri are scanty. H & E, × 150. *Right:* Cluster of normal superficial epithelial cells showing honeycomb appearance. × 150

which the collumnar cells have the appearance of goblet cells or ring-like cells distended with mucus, but without any sign of malignancy. Many authors believe that chronic gastritis with intestinalization is in a broad sense a precancerous condition [28–30].

In one of our cases, chronic inflammation with intestinal metaplasia and marked dysplasia of gastric cardia was diagnosed by balloon cytology, and cells suggestive of cancer were seen in the smear after 4 years follow-up (Figs. 6.29, 6.30).

7.3 *Dysplastic Changes*

The categories used in classification of dysplastic changes of the epithelium of cardia are similar to those used in the esophagus.

Mild Hyperplasia. *Histologically,* the epithelial cells on the mucosal surface and the lining of the pits are increased in number and irregularly crowded. Their nuclei are slightly enlarged. There may be small papillary growths on the mucosal surface. *Cytologically,* the epithelial cells in a smear show slightly enlarged nuclei and their size may vary a little (Fig. 6.31).

Dysplasia. Our experience of dysplasia is very limited. According to many authors, atypical glandular hyperplasia can be identified cytologically as well as histologically. It may have a biologic significance similar to that of severe dysplasia of the uterine cervix and is helpful in the morphologic identification of high-risk patients [31, 32]. We divide marked dysplasia of the epithelium of the gastric cardia into two groups.

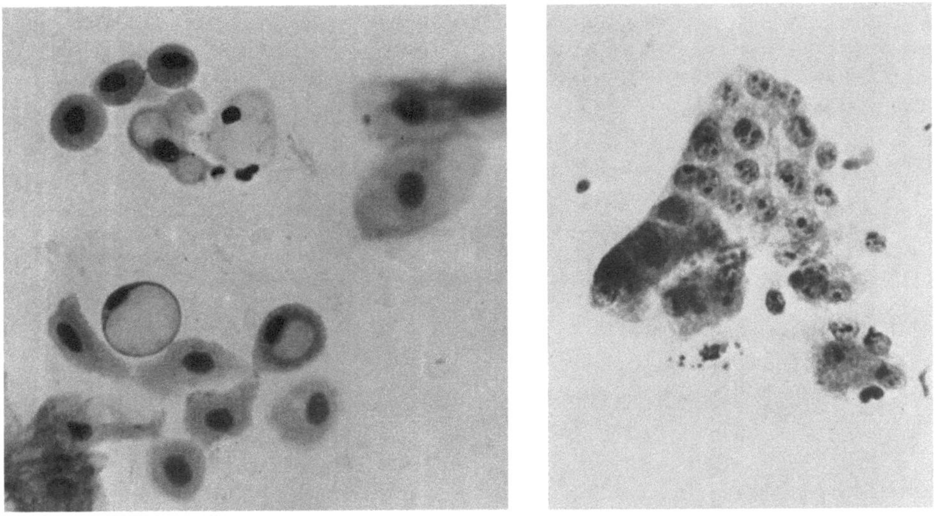

Fig. 6.29. Chronic inflammation of gastric cardia with intestinalization and marked dysplasia group II. The 52-year-old male patient had balloon cytology in 1977 and follow-ups during the next 5 years. The dysplastic changes of the cells seemed to be progressive. *Left:* Smear made in 1977 showing cells with intestinalization. Note the mucous cells in signet-ring form resembling goblet cells. × 440. *Right:* Smear made in 1979 showing marked dysplasia group II or near-carcinoma. × 440

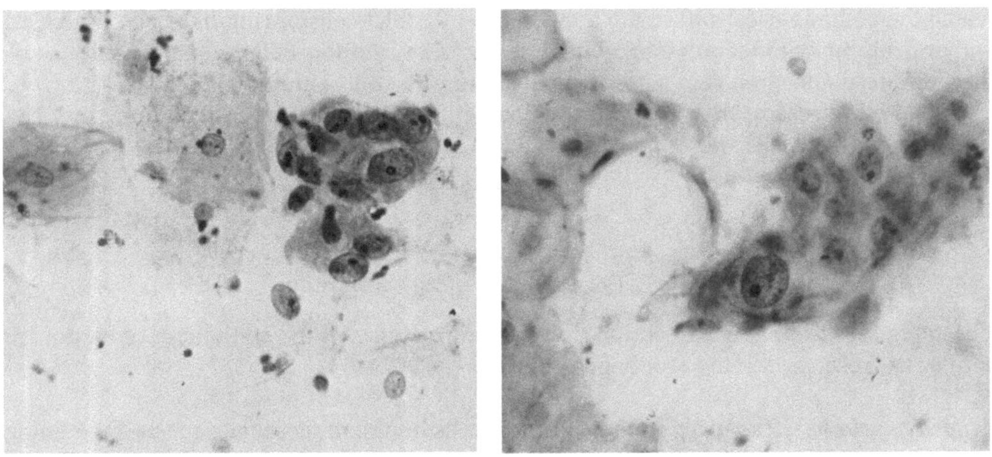

Fig. 6.30. Same case as in Fig. 6.29. *Left:* A follow-up smear in 1981 shows glandular near-carcinoma cells with suspected adenocarcinoma cells arranged in acinar form with prominent nucleoli, but the chromatin granules are not coarse and the nuclear membrane is not thickened. × 440. *Right:* A smear made in 1982 shows glandular cells markedly varied in size with prominent nucleoli. × 440

Group I. Histologically, the glands are increased in number, showing crowding of cells and shifting of nuclei to the upper halves of the cells. Papillary growths are distinct. *Cytologically,* the cells in a smear show enlargement of the nuclei to about twice their normal size or more. The chromatin is increased but not coarse. The nucleolus is conspicuous. In one of our cases, cancer cells turned up in the smear after 15 years follow-up (Fig. 6.32).

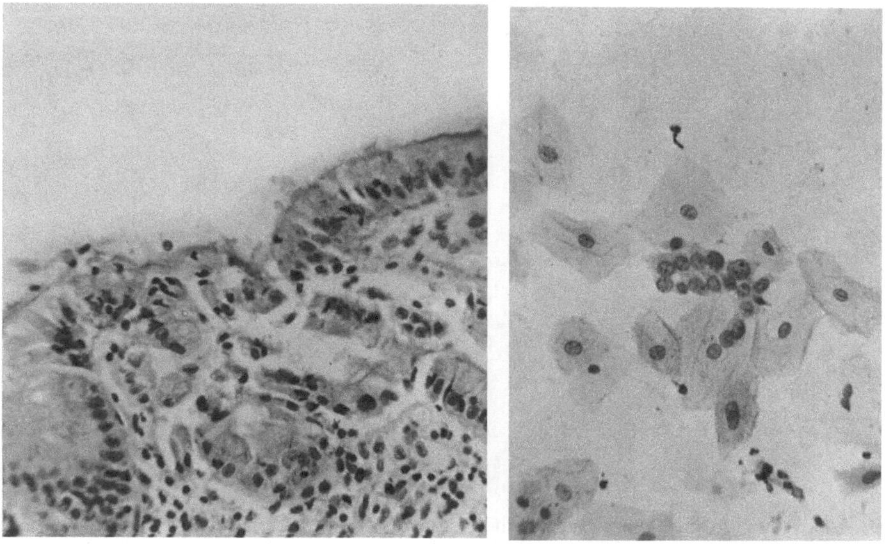

Fig. 6.31. Mild hyperplasia of epithelium of gastric cardia in histology and cytology. *Left:* The superficial epithelial cells are slightly crowded. Their nuclei are somewhat enlarged and are beginning to shift upwards. × 150. *Right:* The nuclei of the glandular cells are slightly enlarged and their size varies a little. × 150

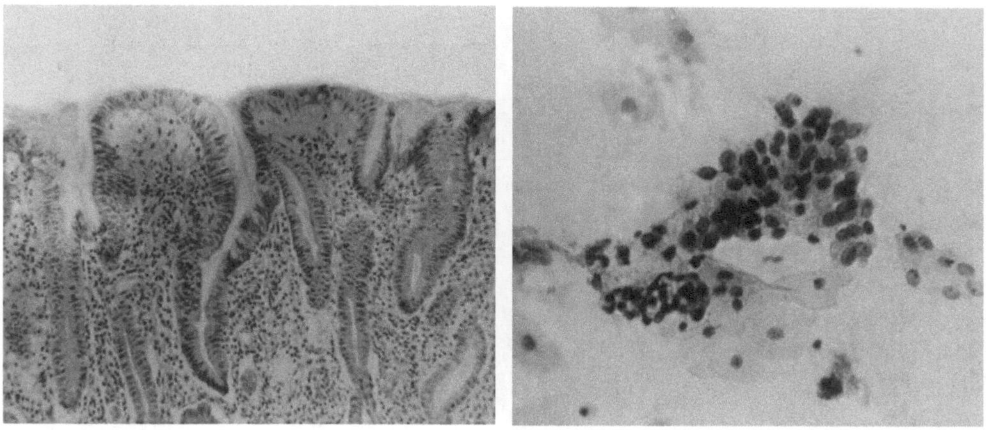

Fig. 6.32. Marked dysplasia group I of the epithelial cells of the cardia. *Left:* Mucosa adjacent to early adenocarcinoma of cardia showing papillary growth of the superficial epithelium and crowding of the glands. The atypism can be discerned without too much difficulty. × 60. *Right:* Smear showing nuclei of glandular cells enlarged and deeply stained, with distinct nucleoli. × 150. The patient was first examined in a 1965 mass survey by balloon cytology; after 15 years follow-up with balloon tests, glandular cancer cells were found in 1980

Group II. Histologically, the glands are further increased in number and the glandular cells are more crowded. Pseudostratification of the epithelium is distinct. The polarity of the cells is preserved (Fig. 6.33). *Cytologically,* the nuclei of the glandular cells are enlarged to three times their normal size or more. The chromatin granules are not coarse. The glandular cells are cohesive.

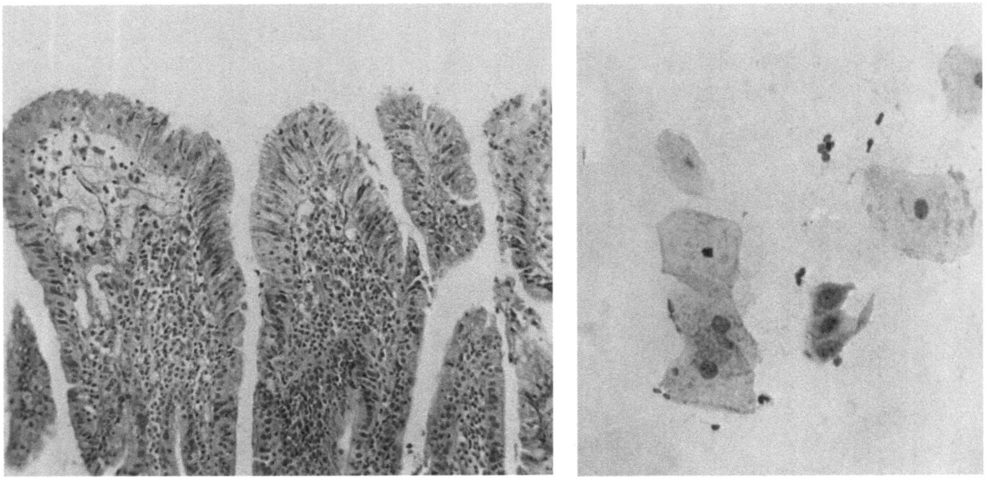

Fig. 6.33. Marked dysplasia group II of the cardiac epithelium. *Left:* Distinct papillary growth of the mucous surface and pseudostratification of the overlying epithelial cells; atypism of the glands is noted. × 150. *Right:* The glandular epithelial cells in the smear show good cohesiveness with markedly enlarged nuclei but regular chromatin distribution. × 150

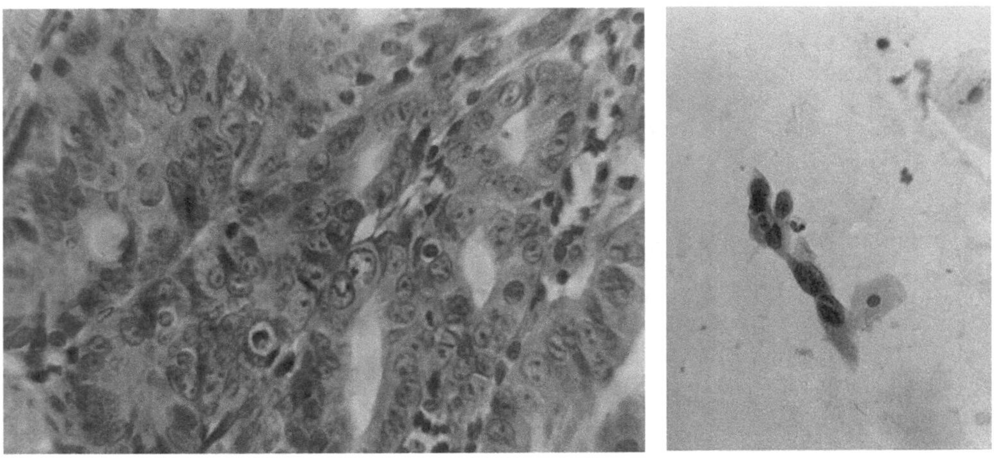

Fig. 6.34. Near-carcinoma of gastric cardia. *Left:* Tissue section showing crowded dysplastic glands in back-to-back formation and benign glandular cells. × 440. *Right:* Smear showing near-carcinoma cells which are apparently benign though the nuclei are large. × 150

Near-Carcinoma. *Histologically,* atypical glands are further increased in number and the back-to-back pattern may be present. The polarity of the glandular epithelium is preserved. *Cytologically,* the nuclei are enlarged to 3–4 times normal size. In clusters the arrangement of the cells is not greatly disrupted. The cohesiveness of the cells is not generally diminished but there seems to be an occasional scattering tendency (Fig. 6.34).

Follow-up observation of the biologic behavior of dysplasia of the gastric cardia is not yet adequate. A case of ours which has been followed cytologically for 17 years may be of interest (Figs. 6.35–6.40).

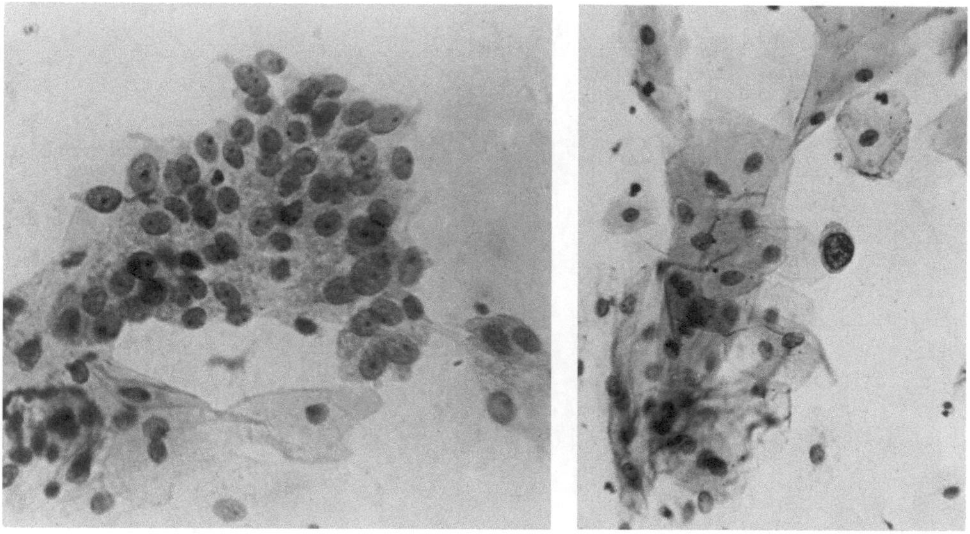

Fig. 6.35. A case of marked dysplasia group II of both the cardia and the esophagus which eventually developed into double primaries in the course of 17 years of follow-up. Smears in May 1965 showed glandular cells of marked dysplasia group I *(left)* and group II *(right)*. × 264

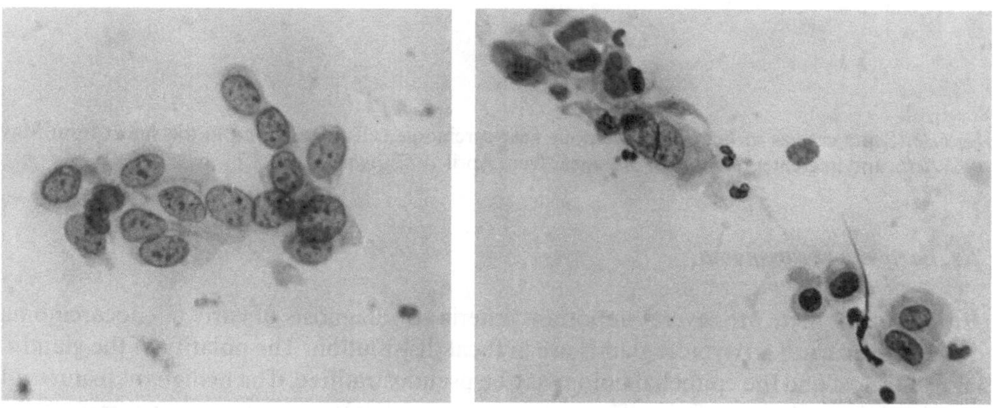

Fig. 6.36. Same case as in Fig. 6.35. *Left:* Smear from April 1972 showing glandular cells of near-carcinoma type. The chromatin granules are not coarse, the nuclear membrane is regular and not thickened, and the nucleoli are not very prominent. × 440. *Right:* Smear from September 1978 showing glandular near-carcinoma cells and cells probably from intestinal metaplasia of gastric cardia. × 440

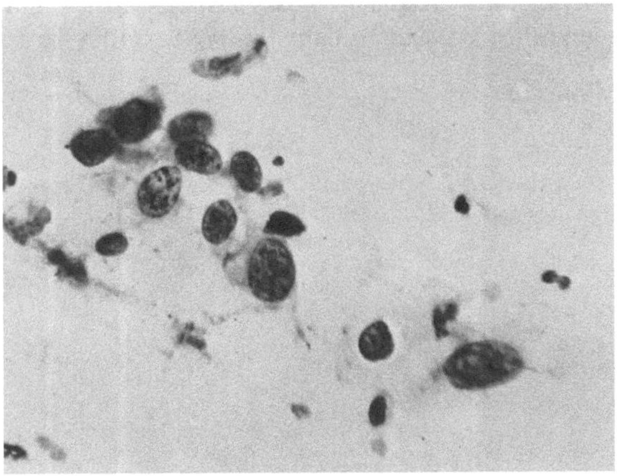

Fig. 6.37. Same case as in Fig. 6.35. Smear from August 1982 showing adenocarcinoma cells in groups. Roentgenography revealed lesion in the cardia. × 440

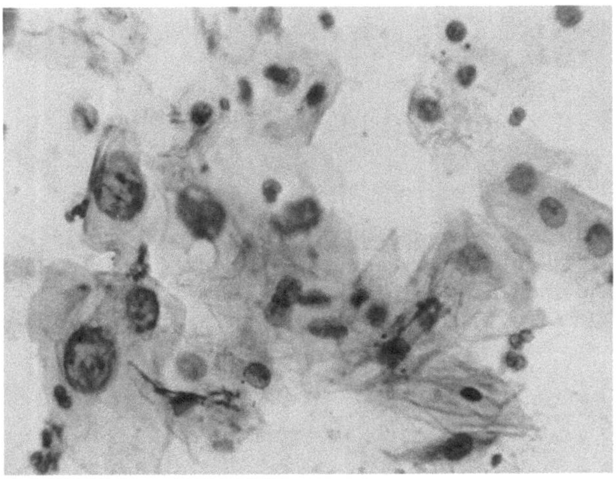

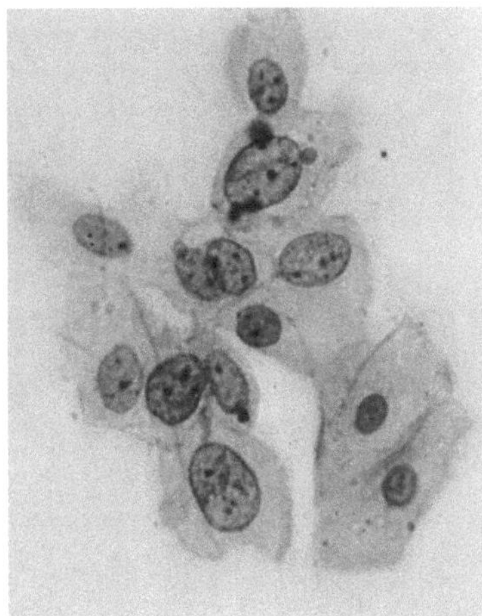

Fig. 6.38. Same case as in Fig. 6.35. Squamous near-carcinoma cells were found in the smear from May 1965 *(left)*, and in greater quantity in the smear from April 1972 *(right)*. × 440

7.4 Early Adenocarcinoma

Histologically, there are several important criteria for diagnosis of early adenocarcinoma of the gastric cardia. Atypical glands are in focal distribution. The polarity of the glandular cells is lost and the epithelial lining may be pseudostratified. The malignant features of the glandular cells are definite. The cancerous focus displays a tendency to compress the surrounding tissue or invade the mucosa propria.

Cytologically, cancer cells of early adenocarcinoma are characterized by a nucleolar diameter of about 5 μm or more. Nuclear chromatin granules are coarse and unevenly distributed, and the edge of the nucleus is jagged. The cancer cells in clusters display scattering, and their size varies. Dysplastic glandular cells are always present in the background of the smear, in distinct contrast to late adenocarcinoma, in which the dysplastic glandular cells are scenty or lacking altogether (Figs. 6.41–6.43).

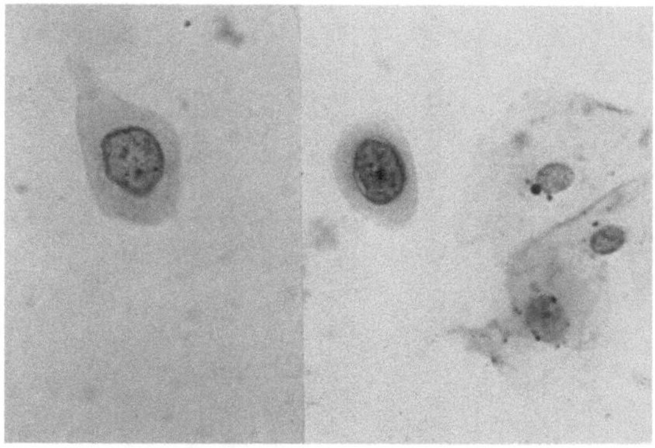

Fig. 6.39. Same case as in Fig. 6.35. Smear from September 1978 showing increased chromatin content of the near-carcinoma cells. × 440

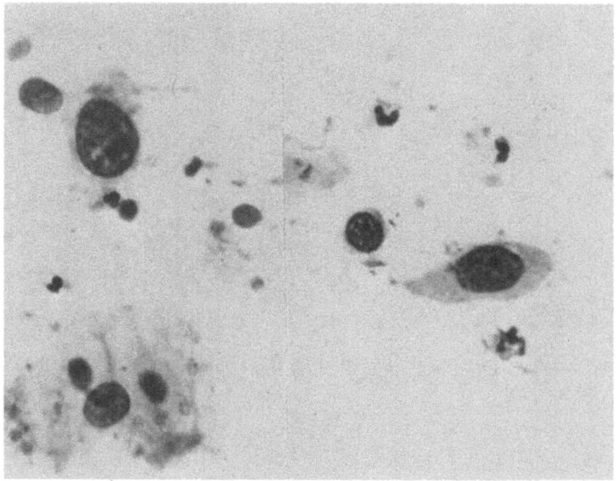

Fig. 6.40. Same case as in Fig. 6.35. Brush smear taken at the 32-cm level under endoscopy in June 1982, showing a small number of squamous cancer cells with distinct malignant features. No tumor was found on endoscopy or roentgenography

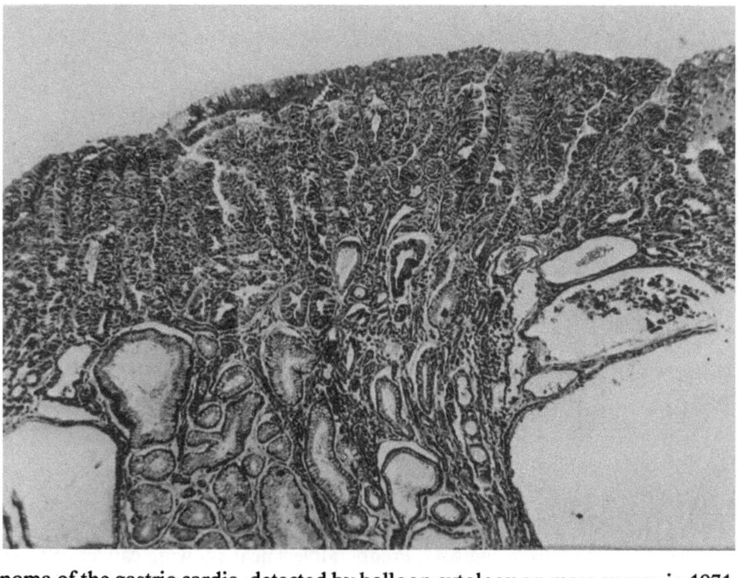

Fig. 6.41. Early adenocarcinoma of the gastric cardia, detected by balloon cytology on mass survey in 1971. The patient was treated surgically and was still alive and well in November 1982. This section of the resected specimen shows cancerous changes chiefly in the upper portion of the mucosa. × 36

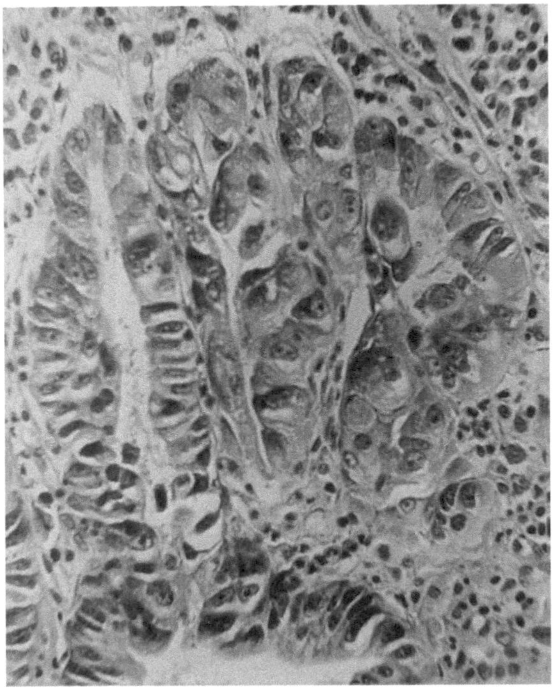

Fig. 6.42. Same case as in Fig. 6.41. Malignant features of the acinus are evident on high magnification. × 570

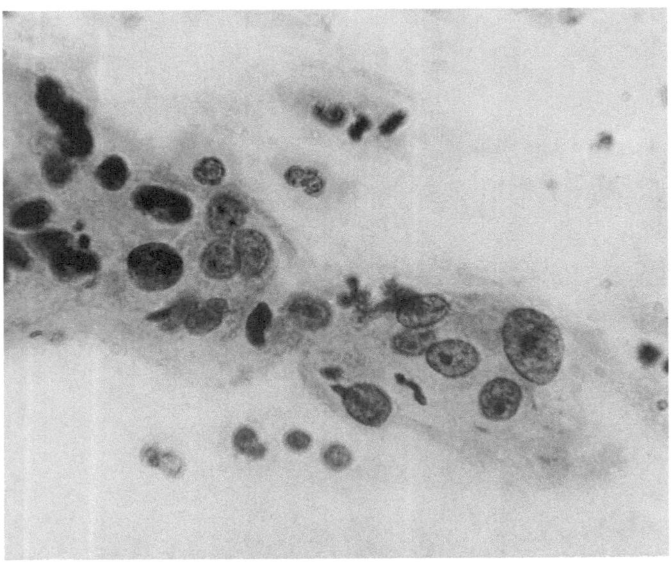

Fig. 6.43. Same case as in Fig. 6.41. Preoperative smear showing cancer cells which were not diagnosed as early adenocarcinoma until after careful re-examination of the slides, when marked dysplastic cells and near-carcinoma cells were found, necrotic cells and fibrinous exudate were not seen, and inflammatory cells and red cells were very scanty or absent. × 570

7.5 *Advanced Carcinoma*

Histologically, most carcinomas of the gastric cardia are one of several types of adenocarcinoma. The well-differentiated type is the most commonly encountered, and is composed of cancer cells with good glandular formation. In the less well differentiated type, the cancer cells are diffusely distributed. The mucoid type is composed of mucoid cancer cells in signet-ring form. The secretion of the tumor cells is usually an acid mucosubstance, easily detected with alcian blue or colloidal iron stains, whereas in normal stomach neutral mucosubstances predominate [33]. The rare anaplastic type is composed of small cancer cells with diffuse infiltration into the deep portion of the gastric wall.

Cytologically, cancer cells of the well-differentiated type may be arranged in acinar patterns. Their nuclei are three-dimensional in appearance with prominent nucleoli, diffuse hyperchromasia, and coarse chromatin granules in the enlarged nuclei. The appearance of the cancer cells is rather uniform (Figs. 6.44, 6.45).

In a smear, cancer cells of the diffuse type show nuclear malignant features similar to those in the well-differentiated type, except that they are more deeply stained. Variation in the size of cancer cells is more marked (Figs. 6.46, 6.47).

Adenocarcinoma of the mucoid type presents signet-ring cancer cells in the smear. The histologic type may be ascertained by cytology if the signet-ring cancer cells predominate (Figs. 6.48, 6.49).

In the case of double early primaries, one in the esophagus and the other in the gastric cardia, both carcinoma pearls and signet-ring cancer cells may be present in the smear. Fiberendoscopy or segmental balloon cytology may help to determine the distance between the two primaries before surgery (Fig. 6.50).

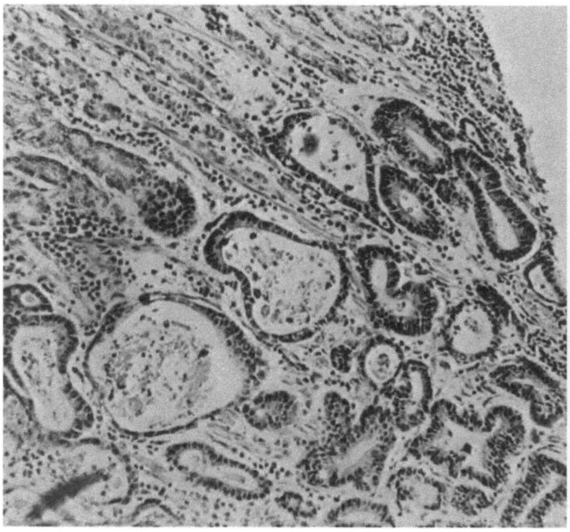

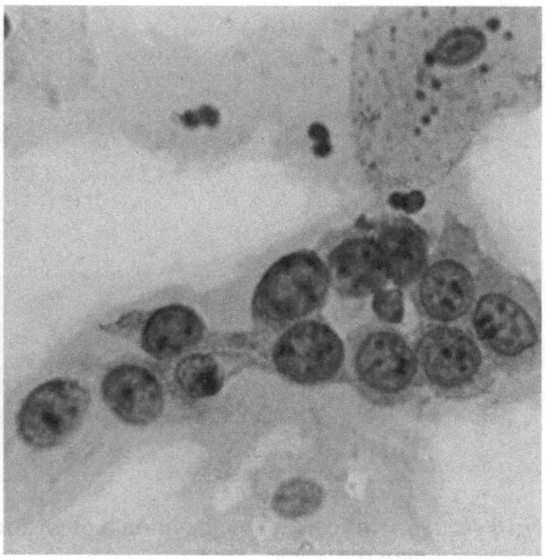

Fig. 6.44 (left). Tissue section showing alveolar structures of well-differentiated adenocarcinoma. × 150

Fig. 6.45 (right). Balloon cytology showing well-differentiated adenocarcinoma cells arranged in alveolar pattern with uniform nuclei of three-dimensional appearance. × 570

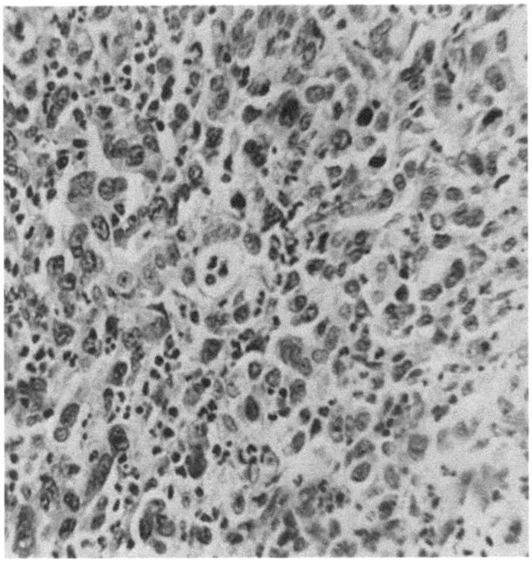

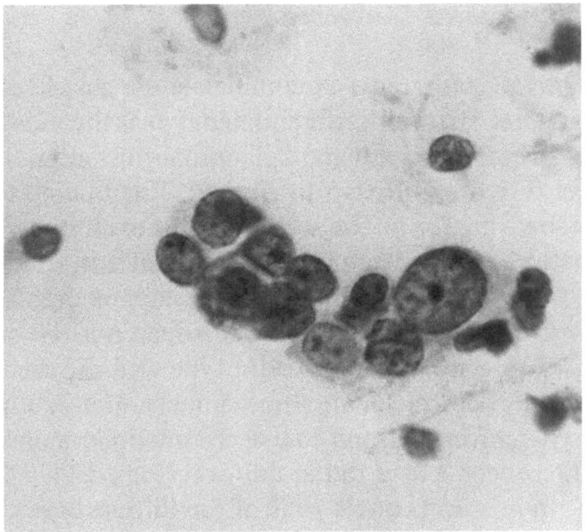

Fig. 6.46 (left). Tissue section of less well differentiated adenocarcinoma (carcinoma simplex) of the gastric cardia, showing diffusely infiltrating cancer cells without acini formation. × 150

Fig. 6.47 (right). Smear of the case in Fig. 6.46, showing cancer cells irregularly grouped and varied in size. × 570

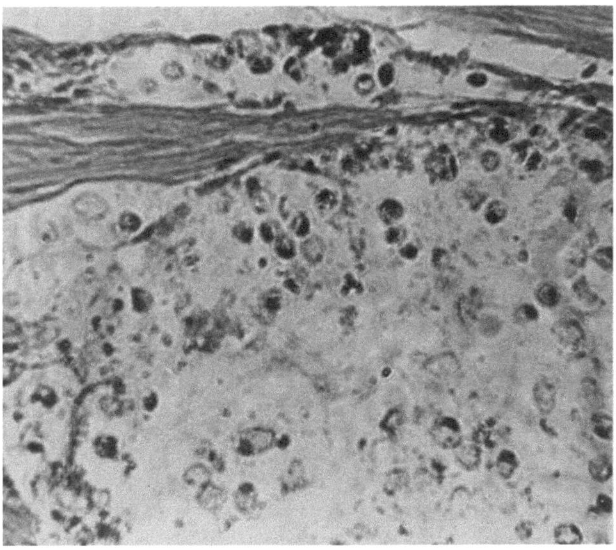

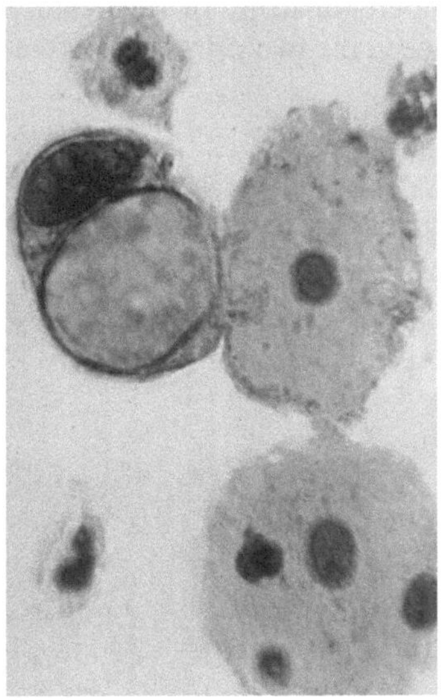

Fig. 6.48. (left). Mucoid adenocarcinoma of gastric cardia with diffuse spread of cancer cells and presence of mucoid material. × 150

Fig. 6.49. (right). The characteristic feature of the mucoid cancer cell is the signet-ring form; the malignant nucleus is pushed to one side. × 570

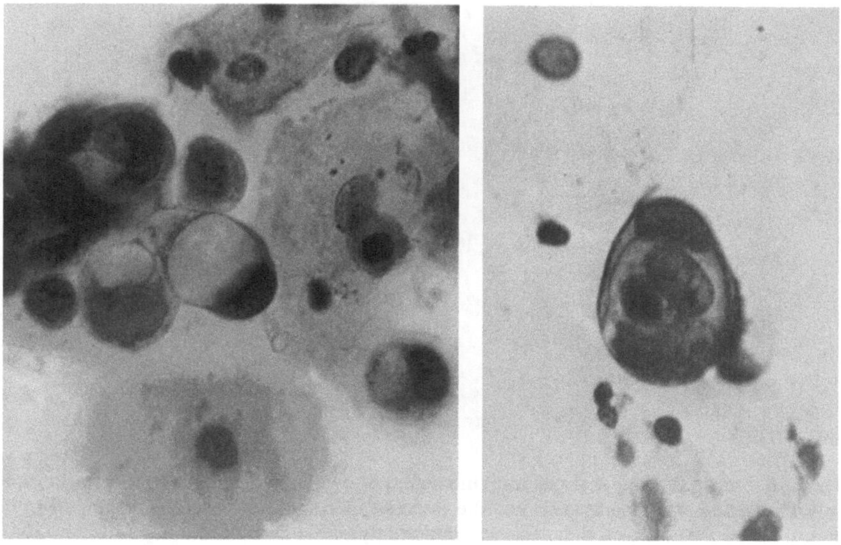

Fig. 6.50. Double primaries: carcinoma of the gastric cardia *(left)* and esophagus *(right)*

7.6 Early Detection of Adenocarcinoma and Its Preliminary Results

Adenocarcinoma of the gastric cardia is a common malignancy, the incidence of which seems to be closely associated with that of esophageal carcinoma. In balloon cytology mass surveys in Linxian in 1974 and 1975, adenocarcinoma cells were found in about a quarter of all cases with positive smears, but early adenocarcinoma of the gastric cardia was rarely operated upon due to lack of symptoms. Unlike early carcinoma of the esophagus, X-ray examination is not very effective for diagnosis.

The inability of balloon cytology to reveal early carcinoma of the gastric cardia in mass surveys is a basic problem, and further investigations have been carried out in an attempt to improve the situation. To increase the understanding of the histogenesis of early carcinoma, the epithelium adjacent to the adenocarcinoma in resected specimens was studied microscopically. After examination of 20 cases, using partial serial sections, it was apparent that the early cancerous changes frequently took place in the neck of the glands and that the surface epithelial cells were often involved. It was concluded that the balloon technique could still be effective in collecting these superficial cancer cells if certain modifications were made.

To modify the balloon, it was necessary to ascertain the dimensions of the field of cancerization at the cardia, and to this end 110 resected specimens of late adenocarcinoma were investigated. The center of the cancerous lesion was taken empirically as the starting point of the whole cancerous process, and the distance between it and the esophagogastric junction was measured. From the data obtained, it was speculated that early adenocarcinoma of the gastric cardia frequently develops in the region 5 cm below the junction, chiefly in the vicinity of the lesser curvature, and that the balloon should be enlarged to obtain wider contact and collect more cells.

The modified balloon with an enlarged, fine cotton mesh net was easily swallowed when wetted and folded. Having passed into the stomach it was inflated with 70–80 ml air

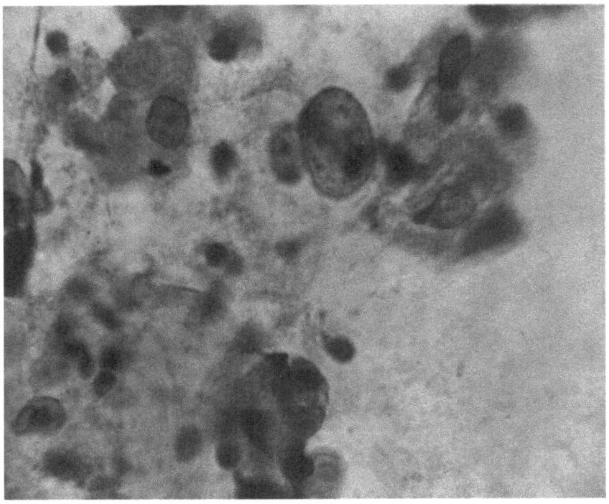

Fig. 6.51. Smear showing a single multinucleated or overlapped cell which was misinterpreted as a cancer cell. The patient was operated on and the resected specimen was carefully examined without finding cancerous tissue. Pathological diagnosis was marked dysplasia group I of the gastric cardia. A cell as inconspicuous as this should be disregarded in making the diagnosis. × 570

and moved up and down several times in the region of the cardia. It was then partially deflated and withdrawn. Gastric cells were found in the smear in about 95% of cases, as compared to 50%–60% with the previous technique. The efficiency of cytologic examination has been greatly improved, as the number of glandular cells in the smear has increased.

Our first mass-survey case of early adenocarcinoma of the gastric cardia was found in 1971. The patient was operated on in good time and was still well when last followed up in November 1982. Pathological diagnosis of the resected specimen was intramucosal adenocarcinoma. However, the lesion was not recognized as early cancer before operation (Figs. 6.41–6.43).

In 1975, 110 people with marked dysplasia of the gastric cardia were found on mass survey. The modified balloon was used for re-examination in 89 of these subjects, and 15 were found to have suspected glandular cancer cells. Three of these patients diagnosed as having early adenocarcinoma were operated upon, and pathological examination of the resected specimens revealed intramucosal adenocarcinoma in two and glandular dysplasia in one. In the smear of the latter case no typical cancer cells were in fact found; the misinterpretation arose from the presence of a few multinucleate dysplastic glandular cells (Fig. 6.51).

In 1977 and 1978, mass surveys were carried out in some other esophageal cancer high-incidence areas. Among 8200 people examined with the modified balloon technique, 144 had cancer cells in the smears, including 32 with glandular cancer cells. Seven patients with adenocarcinoma of the gastric cardia were operated upon, and pathological examination of the resected specimens revealed intramucosal adenocarcinoma in four and early infiltrative adenocarcinoma in three. Lymph node metastasis was not found in any of these cases. They were all still well when last seen in 1982. To date, 25 early cases have been operated on and the results of pathological study of 18 cases have been reported [34].

To sum up, it may be said that the modified balloon technique has led to improvement in the cytologic detection of early carcinoma of the gastric cardia in recent years, but the results are still far from satisfactory. Further investigations are under way.

References

1. Li B, Li JY (1980) National survey of cancer mortality in China (in Chinese) Chin J Oncol 2: 1–10
2. Li GH, Kao RC, Wu YK (1962) A survey of the prevalence of carcinoma of the esophagus in North China. Chin Med J 81: 489–494
3. The Co-ordinating Group for the Research of Esophageal Carcinoma, Chinese Academy of Medical Sciences and Henan Province (1973) Early detection of carcinoma of the esophagus (in Chinese). Sci Sin 14: 457–463
4. Shen C, Qu SL, Chao HT (1963) Cytologic diagnosis of carcinoma of the esophagus: a preliminary report (in Chinese) Chin J Pathol 7: 19–22
5. Department of Pathology, Henan Medical College (1967) The use of exfoliative cytology in clinical diagnosis and mass surveys for cancer of the esophagus. Chin Med J 6: 479–489
6. Huang GJ (KC) (1981) Early detection and surgical treatment of esophageal carcinoma. Jpn J Surg 11: 399–405
7. Ayre JE (1951) Cancer cytology of the uterus. Churchill, London, pp 40–41
8. Mehregen AH, Pinkus H (1964) Intradermal epithelioma: a critical study. Cancer 17: 609–636
9. Cherkassky LA (1962) On larynx cancer morphogenesis (carcinoma in situ) (in Russian) Oncol Quest 8: 29–34
10. Wynder EL, Klein UE (1965) The possible role of riboflavin deficiency in epithelial neoplasia: 1. Epithelial changes of mice in simple deficiency. Cancer 7: 164–180
11. Friedell GH (1976) Carcinoma and carcinoma in situ and "early lesions" of the uterine cervix and the urinary blader: introduction and definition. Cancer Res 36: 2482–2484
12. Shabad LF (1973) Precancerous morphologic lesions. J Natl Cancer Inst 50: 1421–1428
13. Larionov LF (1959) Precancerous condition as a pathological process (in Russian) Arch Pathol 3: 3–9
14. Young WH, Shen Q (to be published) The measurement of dysplastic esophageal epithelial cells in different pathologic changes (in Chinese)
15. Shu YJ, Yuan XQ, Jin SP (1981) Further investigation of the relationship between dysplasia and cancer of the esophagus (in Chinese) Chin Med J 1: 39–41
16. Sporn MB (1976) Approaches of prevention of epithelial cancer during the preneoplastic period. Cancer Res 36: 2699–2702
17. Cai HY, Shu YJ, Wang GQ, Wu AR, Lin PZ, Li SF, Li MX (1980) Therapy of severe epithelial dysplasia of esophagus: I. The therapeutic effects of "antitumor B 3", "antitumor B" and tilorone (in Chinese) Chin J Oncol 2: 92–95
18. Lin PZ, Cai HY, Gan DQ, Bao KJ (1981) Treatment of marked epithelial dysplasia of esophagus: II. Microspectrophotometric studies on DNA content in epithelial cells of esophagus treated with "antitumor B 3" or tilorone (in Chinese) Chin J Oncol 3: 245–248
19. Sun SC, Wu H (1962) Sqmous carcinoma of the esophagus: carcinomatous changes of the epithelium adjacent to the principal lesion (in Chinese) Chin Med J 81: 557–567
20. Department of Pathology, Henan Medical College and Beijing Medical College, and Department of Pathology, Cancer Institute of Chinese Academy of Medical Sciences, Beijing (1968) Study on the morphologic characteristics of early squamous cell carcinoma of the esophagus. Chin Med J 5: 279–304
21. Shen C, Qu SL, Liu FY (1964) Carcinoma in situ of the esophagus: report of one case (in Chinese) Chin J Pathol [Suppl] 8: 405
22. Leham MH, Benson WL, Kurman RJ, Park RC (1976) Microinvasive carcinoma of the cervix. Surg. Obstet Gynecol 48: 571–578
23. Bloom W, Fawcett DW (1964) A textbook of histology, 8th edn. Saunders, Philadelphia London, pp 427–441
24. Medical Team of Henan Province for Preventive and Therapeutic Studies of Esophageal Carcinoma and Linxian County Hospital (1973) Early diagnosis of carcinoma of the esophagus (in Chinese). People's Medical Publishing House, Beijing, pp 46–48
25. Departments of Pathology and Surgery, Yubei Medical School, Chi County, Henan (1966) A cytological study of esophageal carcinoma with the aid of improved balloon method. Chin Med J 1: 76–80

26. Shao LF, Li ZC, Liu SX, Wang MF (1981) Surgical treatment of 210 cases of early carcinoma of the esophagus and gastric cardia (in Chinese) Chin J Surg 19: 259–261
27. Koss LG (1979) Diagnostic cytology and its histologic bases, 3rd edn. Lippincott, Philadelphia Toronto, vol 11/24, pp 832–854
28. Li YQ, Wang ZX, Wu ZM (1980) "Intestinal" gastric carcinoma: analysis of its incidence, pathological typing, and prognosis based on 211 cases (in Chinese) Chin J Oncol 2: 101–106
29. Munoz N, Asvall J (1971) Time trends of intestinal and diffuse types of gastric cancer in Norway. Int J Cancer 8: 144–157
30. Kyoichi Nakamura, Haruo Sugano, Kunio Takagi, Ariya Fuchigami (1966) Histopathological study on early carcinoma of the stomach: criteria for diagnosis of atypical epithelium. Gann 57: 613–620
31. Pilotti S, Rilke F (1977) Atypical epithelium of the protuberant lesions in the stomach. Acta Cytol 21: 1–2
32. Crespi M, Casale V, Grassi A, Maggio C (1978) Results and prospective of a mass screening for gastric cancer and precancerous conditions of the stomach. Acta Endosc 8: 73–85
33. Juan Rosai (1981) Ackerman's Surgical Pathology, vol 2, 6th edn. Mosby, St Louis, p 437
34. Li L, Pan GL, Shen Q (1982) A pathologic study of early carcinoma of gastric cardia (in Chinese) Chin J Oncol 4: 93–97

Chapter 7
Radiologic Diagnosis

Zheng Yan Wang and Ji Hao Su

1 Examination Technique

1.1 Roentgen Examination of the Esophagus

Esophagography with barium meal is a simple and sensitive method of diagnosing tumors of the esophagus [1]. It can determine the anatomic location, nature, and extent of the tumor and its relation to the neighboring organs. The technique is also helpful in clinical staging and in selection of the most suitable therapy. Roentgen examination combined with cytology and esophagoscopy can improve diagnostic accuracy [2].

The subject is instructed to abstain from food and drink for 3–4 h prior to the examination, in order to avoid retention of food particles, decrease secretion by the esophageal mucosa, and render the barium more adherent to the mucosa. Before the barium meal, fluoroscopy of the chest is required to ascertain whether the lungs, heart, blood vessels, and mediastinum are in good condition, as any pathologic change in these organs may affect the contour of the esophagus. Special attention must be paid to the size and shape of the air bubble in the stomach, which may be deformed by the new growth at the gastric cardia. A thicker mixture of barium is needed for esophagography, while with patients suffering from obstruction a thin barium suspension is used. When esophageal perforation is suspected, iodized oil or sterile barium suspension should be used.

Barium esophagography is done with the patient upright and views are taken from various angles in order to obtain images of the entire circumference of the esophagus. The cervical portion of the esophagus is viewed in the AP and lateral positions in roentgen examination. In order to isolate the thoracic portion of the esophagus and bring it into clear relief, the patient is turned to the RAO and LAO positions [3]. As the barium is swallowed, careful attention must be paid to the filling, passing, and emptying states of the esophagus, particularly to the changes in the mucosal folds. Spot films are taken if necessary. The supine and Trendelenberg positions may be used to slow down the barium flow in the esophagus, and are usually helpful in the detection of lesions in the upper esophagus and in the observation of esophageal distensibility and flexibility.

For double-contrast esophagography, the patient can be asked to swallow air or to suck the barium meal through a drilled tube so that air is ingested along with the barium mixture. Another simple technique involves successive swallows of an excellently coating barium mixture and of water to create the double-contrast effect. The esophagus distends to its maximum, while the fine layer of barium coating the mucosa outlines its contours as a fine edging. Double-contrast esophagography has proved helpful in (a) detection of small tumors, (b) delineation of the morphologic features of neoplastic and inflammatory diseases, and (c) assessment of the total vertical extension of the disease [4–8].

During barium esophagography, special attention must be paid to the following points [9]:

Caliber: most malignant tumors of the esophagus produce some degree of narrowing at the site of the lesion, while benign polypoid tumors may cause local dilatation of the lumen.

Intraluminal filling defect: malignant tumors cause irregular filling defects, while in benign tumors the defects are smooth and regular.

Marginal contour: ragged or nodular marginal outlines are most typically produced by primary malignant tumors. Localized protrusions of barium from the main lumen of the esophagus may be due to peptic or neoplastic ulcerations or fistulas. Advanced or extensive carcinoma may cause fistulas into the mediastinum or the tracheobronchial tree.

Distensibility of the wall: spasm and stiffness in the affected segment are frequently observed in esophageal carcinoma.

Mucosal pattern: the normal parallel linear mucosal folds of the esophagus may be distorted or replaced by neoplastic involvement, since primary malignancies are most often of mucosal origin. Benign tumors which are intramural may press on the overlying mucosa, producing varying degrees of diminished prominence of the rugal pattern or complete effacement of it.

1.2 Roentgen Examination of the Gastric Cardia

The complex anatomy of the esophagogastric junction, with its many individual variations, its peculiar topography in relation to the diaphragm, vertebral column, and left lobe of the liver, and its retrocostal position (making it inaccessible to palpation), turn this section of the digestive tract into one of the most formidable for radiologists [4]. Abnormalities of the gastric fundus or cardia are frequently difficult to demonstrate using conventional single-contrast barium study. The double-contrast method is ideal for the examination of the cardia because adequate distension can be achieved without increasing opacity. With good mucosal coating and correct positioning, very fine anatomic and pathologic details can be identified [10, 11].

On examining the cardia, attention must be paid to the shape and size of the gastric bubble. The patient is given an effervescent agent to produce gas in order to distend the gastric fundus, and is then turned to the RAO position and asked to take one mouthful of barium. During the swallow, the lower end of the esophagus, including the distention, the dilatation, and the outline of the cardia, is studied. The mucosal folds are best observed after the barium has passed. Spot films are taken if necessary. The bed is then put in the horizontal position and another 30–50 ml barium meal is given to the patient, who is then turned from side to side 2–3 times in order to get the mucosal surface of the stomach coated. The patient is rotated into the prone position for examination of the fundus and cardia. The pattern of the mucosal folds and the outline, distensibility, and flexibility of the fundus are noted. The patient is then turned to the LAO position with the table tilted head up to about 60°, permitting flow of barium down the lesser curvature into the antrum. The gas is now up in the fundus and cardia, demonstrating *en face* and in double contrast the cardia and the lesser curvature together with the adjacent anterior and posterior wall surfaces [12]. In case of carcinoma, the entire silhouette of the tumor mass, especially that of the ulcer, may be demonstrated. Finally, in the erect position, the barium-coated tumor and the outline of the fundus are easily shown. For the cascade or high horizontal stomach, additional positions such as lateral anterior flexion are necessary to view the cardia [13].

1.3 Computed Tomography

Computed tomography (CT) demonstrates the relation of the esophagus to the neighboring mediastinal structures. The dividing soft tissue planes are normally distinct [14], and blurring or distortion of the interfaces is reliable evidence of tumor involvement. Moss [15] reported that CT is an accurate way of staging esophageal carcinoma preoperatively, providing information previously only made available by surgical exploration. It can also demonstrate the size of the tumor, the extent of mediastinal invasion, local lymph node enlargement, and intra-abdominal metastasis. In carcinoma of the gastric cardia, the size of the tumor, the extent of gastric involvement and extragastric spread, involvement of the neighboring organs and intra-abdominal metastasis can be shown. In addition, the assistance of a CT scan in treatment planning is of great help to surgeons and radiotherapists.

2 Diagnosis of Carcinoma of the Esophagus

2.1 *Early Carcinoma*

Radiologic examination has a significant part to play in the early diagnosis of esophageal carcinoma. As the radiographic abnormalities in the early stage are inconspicuous, they are easily overlooked or misinterpreted. According to the report of the Cooperative Group for Prevention and Treatment of Esophageal Carcinoma in Linxian county, Henan

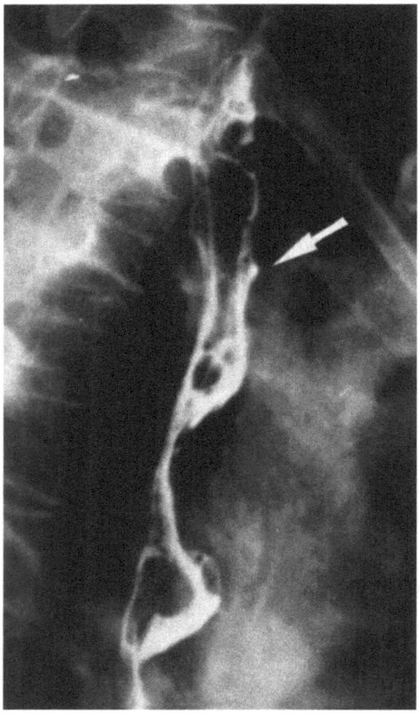

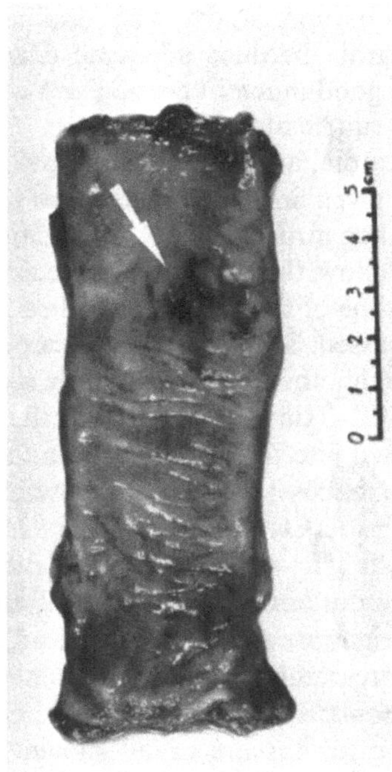

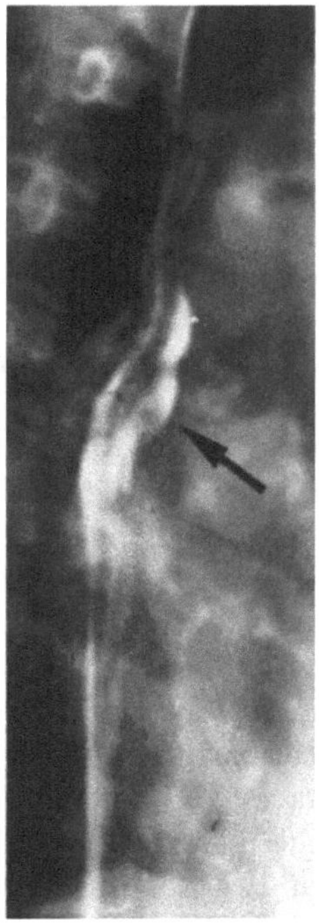

***Fig. 7.1** (left, middle).* Early esophageal carcinoma. A 53-year-old woman (CI Hosp. No. 319399) had dysphagia for 3 months. *Left:* Esophagogram showing irregular superficial filling defect with a small niche *(arrow)* on the anterior wall of the upper esophagus. *Middle:* Surgical specimen showing a 2-cm lesion *(arrow)* with coarse and granular mucosa and superficial erosions. Pathological diagnosis: early erosive squamous carcinoma

***Fig. 7.2** (right).* Early esophageal carcinoma. A 52-year-old symptom-free woman was found to have squamous cancer cells on cytologic screening. Esophagography revealed thickened mucosal folds, stiff wall, and stagnation of barium in the midesophagus *(arrow)*. Pathology of resected specimen: carcinoma in situ province [16], the 5-year survival rate after operation is 90.3% which clearly shows the importance of early diagnosis, the prerequisite for early treatment. In 130 cases of operated early esophageal carcinoma [17, 18], the main radiologic findings were as follows.

Localized Superficial Filling Defect. This is a relatively common finding. The lesion appears as an irregular and superficial defect with rough margins or as a smooth small depression. Macroscopically, it is caused by a plaque-like growth. Sometimes a localized defect is caused by erosion with elevated margins. A polyp-like filling defect may be caused by a papillary or mushroom-like growth protruding into the esophageal lumen (Fig. 7.1).

Changes in the Mucosal Folds. Such changes are the most common finding, appearing as thickening, tortuosity, interruption, destruction, and convergence, thickening and tortuosity being the most frequently observed. Tortuous mucosal folds take the form of lines of dots on X-ray films. Endoscopically, these changes are found in plaque-like and erosive lesions (Figs. 7.2–7.4).

Minute Ulceration. This condition is uncommon. Barium meal esophagography may show single or multiple small niches at the site of the lesion. The mucosal rugae at the margins of these niches are coarse and interrupted (Fig. 7.5).

Spasm and stiffness are often observed in the affected segment.

The following characteristic X-ray features may be observed in the four pathological types of early esophageal carcinoma [16, 19].

Erosive. The mucosal folds at the diseased segment are thickened, interrupted, and tortuous with rough and irregular margins sometimes resembling the early changes of esophageal varicosity. Single or multiple niches, 2–5 mm in diameter, may be observed among the interrupted mucosal folds. *Pathologically,* the esophageal mucosa in the diseased area is slightly depressed or mildly eroded. The lesions are map-like and vary greatly in size. They are clearly demarcated from the surrounding normal mucosa, which is slightly elevated. This type is the most common of the four.

Plaque-Like. Small filling defects are detected in the interrupted mucosal folds, ranging in size from about 0.4×0.4 cm to about 2.0×0.5 cm. Occasionally, minute niches are seen (Fig. 7.6). *Pathologically,* plaque-like elevations are observed on top of swollen mucosa in the diseased areas. The surface is coarse, granular, and clearly delineated from the normal mucosa. Small superficial erosions are seen.

Papillary. The appearance is that of a small, clearly defined filling defect protruding out of the interrupted mucosa into the esophageal lumen. The esophageal wall is distensible (Fig. 7.7). *Pathologically,* the carcinoma presents itself as a papillary or mushroom-like growth protruding into the esophageal lumen. It is clearly demarcated from the surrounding normal mucosa.

Flat. Barium meal esophagography usually displays no obvious filling defect or niche, but the esophageal wall is less distensible and appears rigid. *Pathologically,* there is elevation or depression in the mucosa, but the diseased area is darkly tinged. There is capillary dilatation and congestion with inflammatory infiltrations.

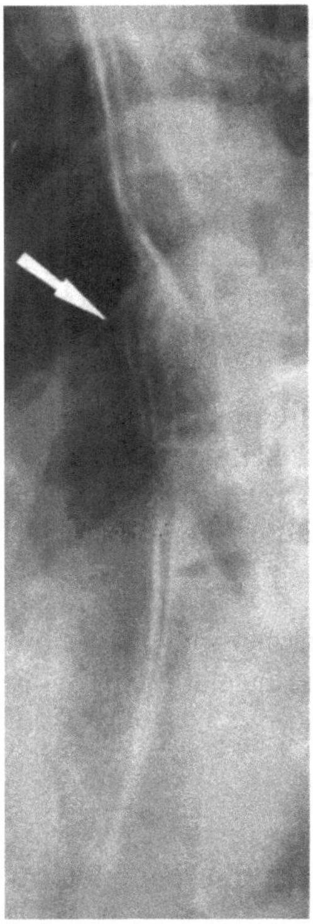

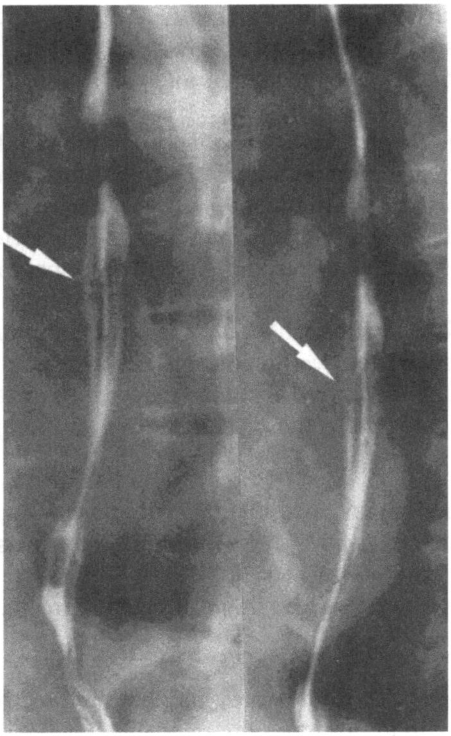

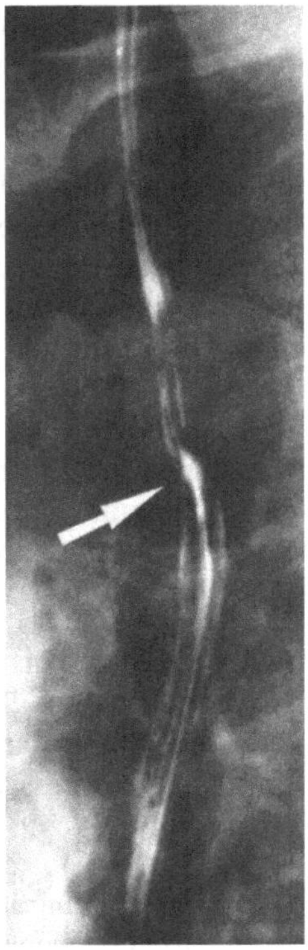

Fig. 7.3 (left). Early esophageal carcinoma. A 48-year-old symptom-free man was found to have squamous cancer cells on cytologic screening. Esophagography revealed thickened and interrupted mucosal folds *(arrow)* in the midesophagus. Pathology of resected specimen: carcinoma in situ

Fig. 7.4 (middle). Early esophageal carcinoma. A 46-year-old man (CI Hosp. No. 218885) had mild dysphagia for 40 days. Esophagography revealed thickened and tortuous mucosal folds as interrupted dots *(arrows)* on the anterior wall of the midesophagus. Pathology of resected specimen: early invasive carcinoma

Fig. 7.5 (right). Early esophageal carcinoma. A 52-year-old man (CI Hosp. No. 280442) had retrosternal pain on swallowing for 2 months. Esophagography revealed slight irregularity in the wall, interruption of the mucosal folds, and a niche at the midesophagus *(arrow)*. Pathology of resected specimen: early invasive carcinoma with superficial erosion

Diagnosis of early esophageal cancer based on roentgenograms should also be correlated to clinical symptoms. It had been thought that patients with early esophageal cancers were symptom-free, but in fact this is not true. Work in high-incidence areas in Henan province has shown that there are mild but definite symptoms [2]. In studies of 70 patients, symptoms such as something sticking during swallowing, retrosternal pain, dry and spastic feeling in the throat, and foreign body sensation in the esophagus were found to occur in the early stage [17]. Cytology and X-ray examinations should be carried out in patients suspected to have esophageal carcinoma, especially those in or from the high-incidence areas [20]. As early lesions are usually superficial and inconspicuous, meticulous attention must be paid to the mucosal pattern and distensibility of the esophageal wall during X-ray examination, and the patient should be viewed in various positions so that the entire circumference of the esophagus is visualized. At least two oblique views should be taken, and double-contrast esophagography is very useful for demonstrating the size and extent

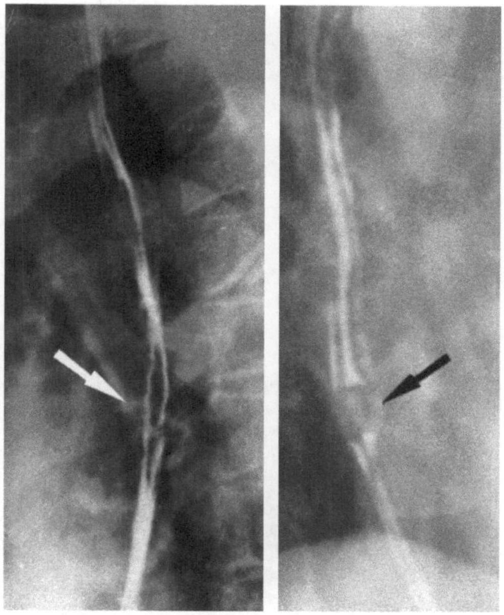

Fig. 7.6 (left). Early esophageal carcinoma. A 50-year-old man (CI Hosp. No. 235573) had mild retrosternal pain on swallowing for 5 years. Esophagography revealed an irregular superficial filling defect with thickened mucosal folds *(arrow)* of the midthoracic esophagus. Pathology of resected specimen revealed early plaque-like esophageal carcinoma

Fig. 7.7 (right). Early esophageal carcinoma. A 47-year-old symptom-free man was found to have squamous cell carcinoma on cytologic examination. Esophagography revealed a 2-cm polypoid filling defect in the lower thoracic esophagus. Pathology of resected specimen: early papillary esophageal carcinoma

of the lesion [21]. Sometimes the lesion is clearly demonstrated on a tangential view. Benign diseases of the esophagus such as esophagitis and tuberculosis may also give rise to mucosal thickening, irregularity, or even ulceration, which it is difficult to differentiate from carcinoma by radiologic examination alone [22]. The final diagnosis may have to be established by cytology, endoscopy, or pathology.

2.2 *Clinicopathological Types*

A classification of esophageal carcinoma into four clinicopathologic types – medullary, fungating, ulcerative, and scirrhous – according to pathological characteristics, X-ray findings, and clinical manifestations has been in wide use in China since 1958 [1]. Further study at the Cancer Institute of the Chinese Academy of Medical Sciences [23, 24] revealed a fifth type, intraluminal. The five types are characterized as follows.

Medullary. *Roentgenologically,* the lesion appears as irregular filling defects. The margin between the upper and lower borders of the lesion and the normal esophagus is sloping and the esophageal lumen is narrowed. There is destruction of the mucosal folds in the diseased areas, usually with niches of various sizes. A soft tissue mass is usually noted. There is usually marked obstruction of the barium meal (Fig. 7.8). *Grossly,* all the layers of

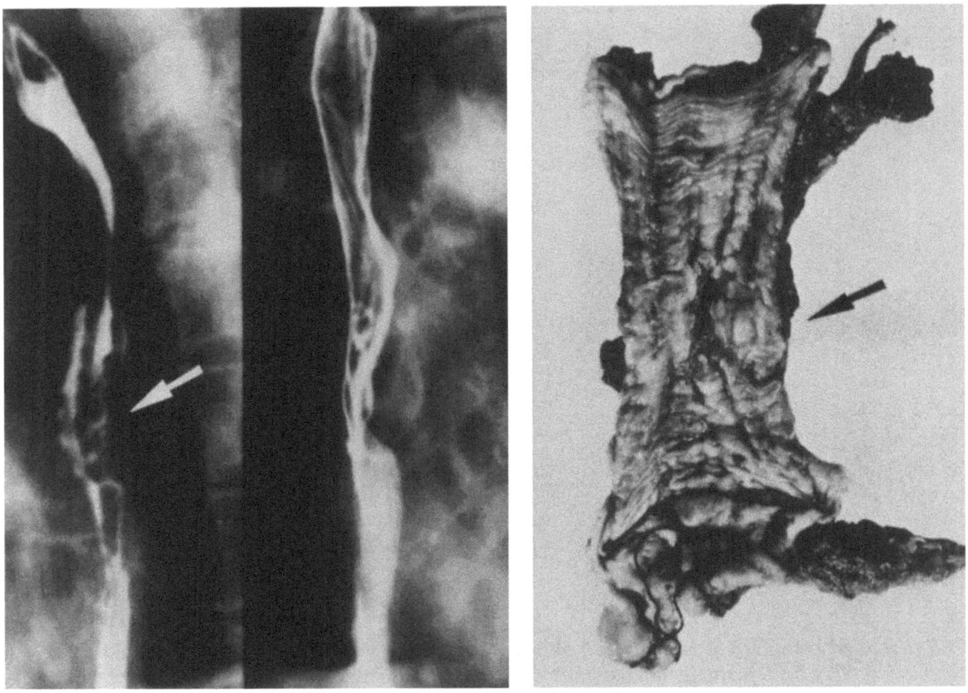

Fig. 7.8. Medullary esophageal carcinoma. A 62-year-old man (CI Hosp. No. 190965) had progressive dysphagia for 1 year. *Left:* Esophagograms showing irregular filling defect and mucosal destruction of about 5 cm in the midthoracic esophagus. *Right:* Surgical specimen showing a tumor mass of about 3.1 × 2.1 × 1.2 cm with central ulceration. Pathology: squamous cell carcinoma

the esophagus are infiltrated by the tumor. The involved wall of the esophagus is markedly thickened. The lesion may involve all or part of the circumference of the esophagus. The lesion protrudes into the lumen or outside it. Ulcers are usually found in the middle of the lesion.

Fungating. *Roentgenologically,* there is a conspicuous filling defect with sharply defined, curved upper and lower borders. The demarcation between the diseased and normal portions is abrupt and clear. There may be linear superficial niches. The mucosal folds, of the diseased portion are interrupted and the esophageal lumen is as a rule only mildly obstructed (Fig. 7.9). *Grossly,* the tumor appears ovoid and flat in shape, protruding into the lumen like a mushroom. Its edge is elevated and prominent. There is superficial ulceration on the surface of the lesion, which usually involves only a part of the esophageal circumference.

Ulcerating. *Roentgenologically,* the lesion appears as a large, punched-out niche which goes deep into the wall and may even protrude out of the esophagus on tangential view.

Fig. 7.10. Ulcerating esophageal carcinoma. A 55-year-old man (CI Hosp. No. 173354) had retrosternal pain on swallowing for 4 months. *Left:* Esophagogram showing an irregular filling defect about 6 cm in length with a deep longitudinal niche in the midthoracic esophagus. *Right:* Surgical specimen showing a tumor with a deep, punched-out ulcer in its center. Pathology: squamous cell carcinoma ▷

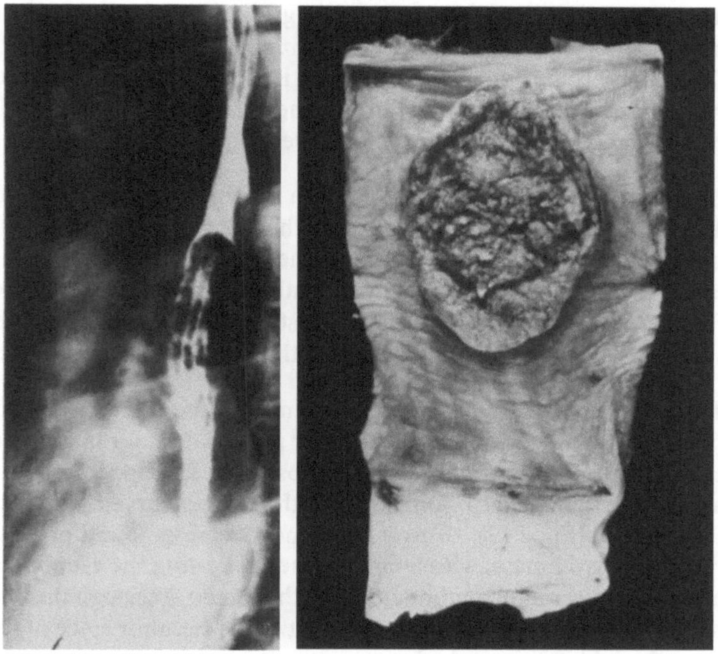

Fig. 7.9. Fungating esophageal carcinoma. A 40-year-old man (CI Hosp. No. 269371) had retrosternal pain and dysphagia for 1 year. *Left:* Esophagogram showing a filling defect about 7 cm in length with a curved, sharp upper border in the midthoracic esophagus. *Right:* Surgical specimen showing a fungating mass about 5.3 × 4.0 × 0.7 cm with superficial ulceration. Pathology: Squamous cell carcinoma

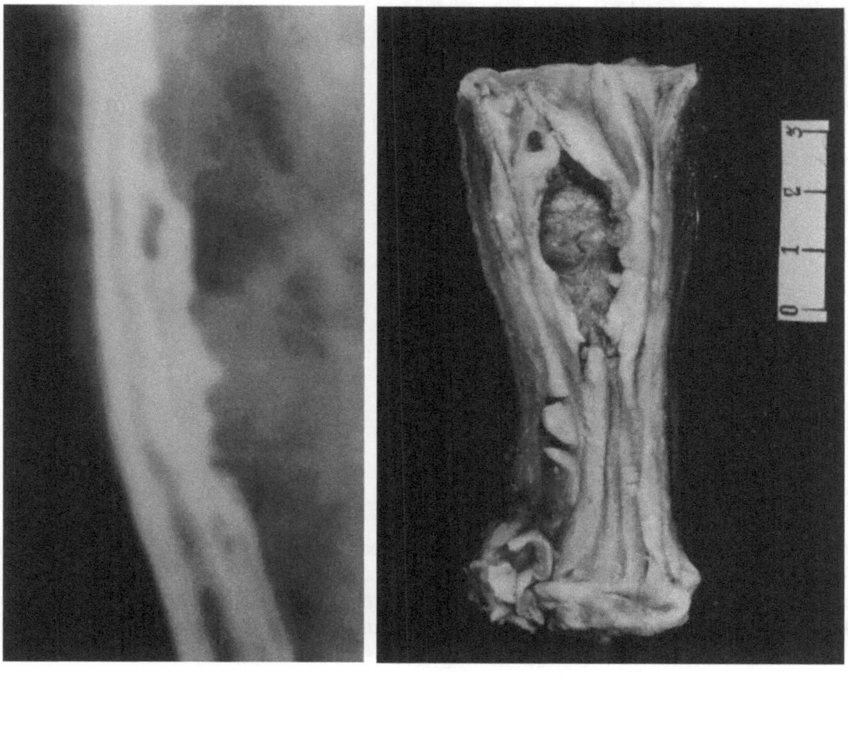

The edge of the ulcer is elevated and gives a positive meniscus sign. Obstruction of the barium meal is only mild (Fig. 7.10). *Grossly,* a deep punched-out ulcer is found on the surface of the tumor, the edge of which is slightly elevated or undermined, with its floor reaching or even penetrating through the muscular layer. In most lesions, only a portion of the esophageal circumference is involved.

Scirrhous. *Roentgenologically,* there is a fusiform or annular stenosis with a smooth wall. The lesion is rather short, usually less than 3 cm from upper to lower border. Obstruction of barium flow is usually severe, with the proximal segment of the esophagus markedly dilated (Fig. 7.11). *Grossly,* the lesion is rather narrow but usually involves the entire circumference of the esophagus, forming a distinct annular stenosis. The mucosal folds are convergent. There is marked dilatation of the proximal portion of the esophagus.

Intraluminal. *Roentgenologically,* the lumen of the diseased portion is dilated and usually fusiform and filled with an irregular or polypoid tumor mass. The surface of the tumor is spotted with barium. Niches may be observed. The upper and lower borders of the lesion are clear-cut and sharp, sometimes with obvious curved margins. Obstruction of barium flow is mild (Fig. 7.12). *Grossly,* the tumor is chiefly found protruding into the lumen as a round or ovoid mass, with a broad base infiltrating the esophageal wall. There is usually erosion or ulceration on the surface of the tumor. Although the tumor is bulky, obstruction to barium flow is not severe as only part of the circumference of the wall is involved. There is marked dilatation of the lumen in the diseased segment.

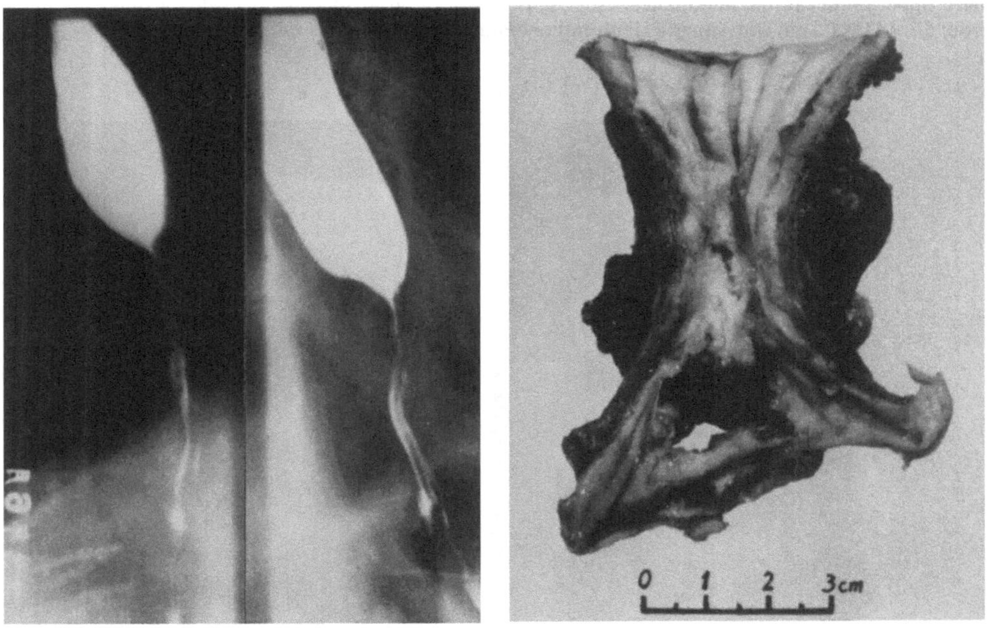

Fig. 7.11. Scirrhous esophageal carcinoma. A 64-year-old woman (CI Hosp. No. 198221) had dysphagia for a year. *Left:* Esophagogram showing linear narrowing about 4 cm in length in the lower thoracic esophagus and marked dilatation of the proximal portion. *Right:* Surgical specimen showing a $4.0 \times 2.5 \times 1.3$ cm tumor mass encircling the lumen and causing annular stricture. Pathology: squamous cell carcinoma

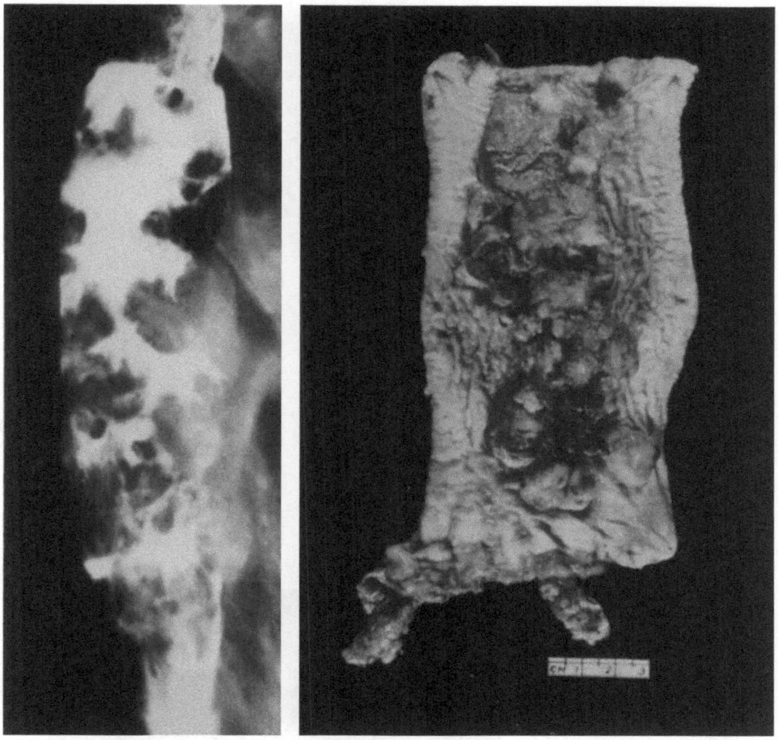

Fig. 7.12. Intraluminal esophageal carcinoma. A 58-year-old man (CI Hosp. No. 84151) had retrosternal pain and dysphagia for 2 months. *Left:* Esophagogram showing a large filling defect in the middle and lower segments of the esophagus with marked dilatation of the lumen. *Right:* Surgical specimen showing a large intraluminal nodular tumor mass. Pathology: squamous cell carcinoma

2.3 CT Findings

The normal esophagus is easily demonstrated by thoracic CT. The soft tissue planes separating the esophagus from its adjacent mediastinal structures are distinct. Blurring or distortion of these tissue interfaces is a reliable indication of disease. In general, the thoracic esophagus, the descending aorta, and the azygos vein should be clearly delineated as separate and distinct structures in a normal case (Fig. 7.13) [14]. Air in the esophagus is considered normal; the diameter of the esophagus depends on the amount of air within. The thickness of the esophageal wall is usually less than 5 mm on CT scan [15].

Based on CT findings, esophageal carcinoma can be classified into four stages as proposed by Moss [15]:

Stage I: Intraluminal mass without esophageal wall thickening
Stage II: Esophageal wall thickening
Stage III: Esophageal wall thickening and contiguous spread of tumor into adjacent mediastinal structures such as trachea, bronchi, aorta, or atrium
Stage IV: Evidence of distant metastases

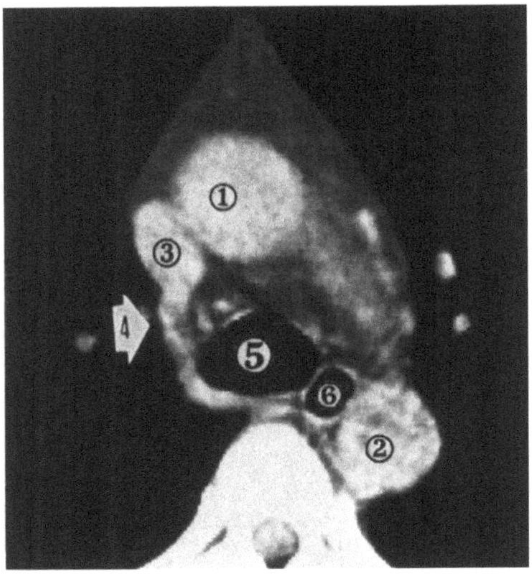

Fig. 7.13. CT scan of the thorax showing normal esophagus. *1* Ascending aorta; *2* descending aorta, *3* superior vena cava; *4* arch of azygos vein, *5* bifurcation of trachea; *6* esophagus

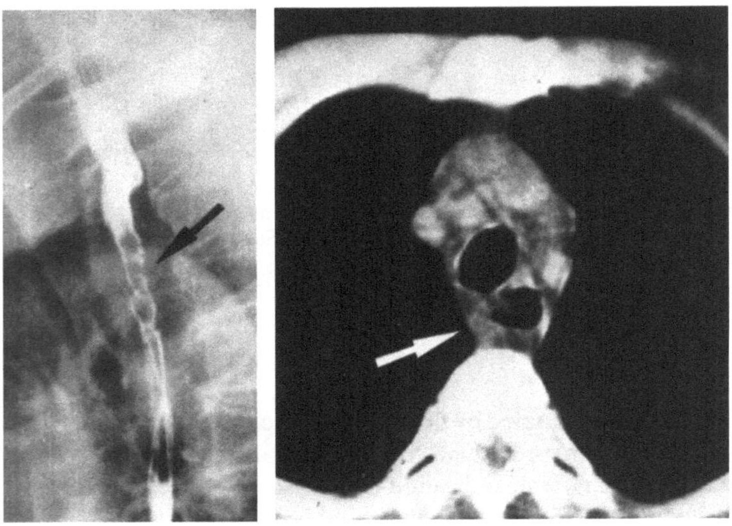

Fig. 7.14. Esophageal carcinoma. A 49-year-old man (CI Hosp. No. 355148) had dysphagia for 6 months. *Left:* Esophagogram showing an irregular filling defect *(arrow)* about 5.5 cm in length in the upper and middle segments of the esophagus. *Right:* CT scan showing thickening of the esophageal wall with nodular tumor mass protruding into the lumen *(arrow)*. Pathology: squamous cell carcinoma

Paraesophageal extension of tumor is usually manifested on CT by the loss of normal fat planes between the esophagus and the adjacent mediastinal structures. Intra-abdominal spread is diagnosed by enlarged retrocrural, celiac, and mesenteric lymph nodes or by evidence of hepatic metastases [25].

CT staging of esophageal carcinoma correlates well with surgical findings, and local extension, regional adenopathy, and tumor size are evaluated better than by other methods. CT offers a noninvasive means of detecting extraesophageal extension of disease and thus

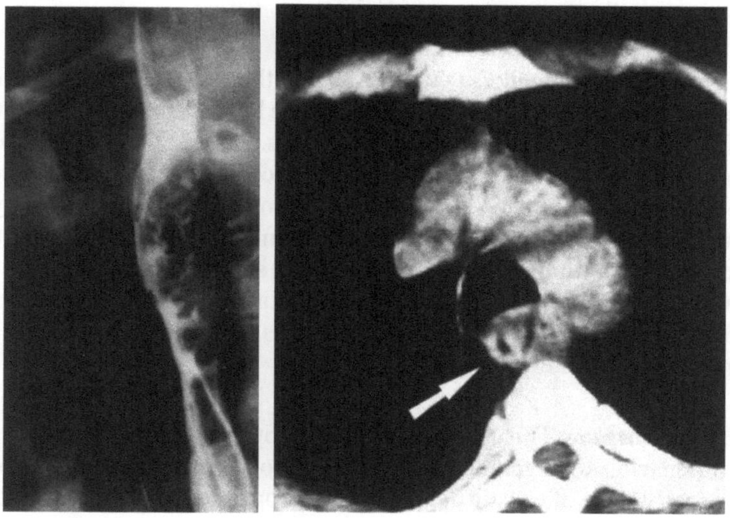

Fig. 7.15. Intraluminal esophageal carcinoma. A 55-year-old man (CI Hosp. No. 355350) had dysphagia for a month. *Left:* Esophagogram showing polypoid filling defect in the upper thoracic esophagus with dilated lumen. *Right:* CT scan showing thickening of the esophageal wall and an intraluminal mass, compressing the membranous part of the trachea *(arrow)*. Pathology: squamous cell carcinoma

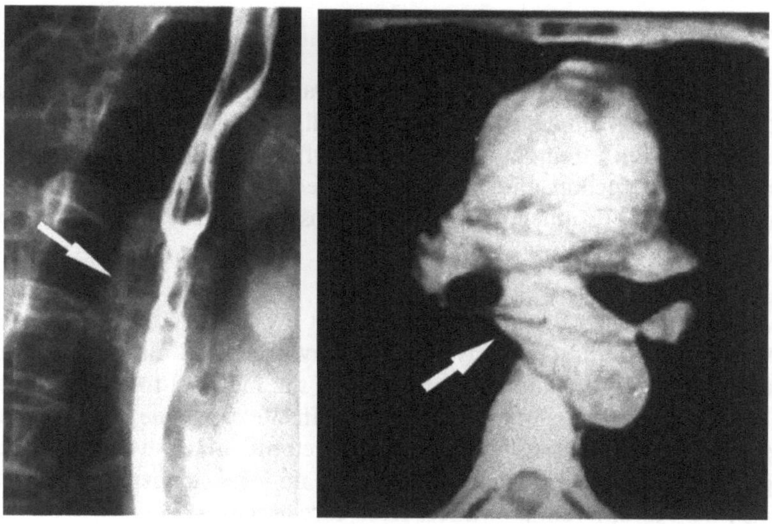

Fig. 7.16. Esophageal carcinoma. A 61-year-old man (CI Hosp. No. 354683) had dysphagia for 4 months. *Left:* Esophagogram showing an irregular filling defect of about 4.5 cm in the midthoracic esophagus with adjacent soft tissue shadow *(arrow)*. *Right:* CT scan showing loss of tissue planes between esophagus, bronchus, and aorta *(arrow)*. Surgery confirmed periaortic invasion. Biopsy of the paraesophageal lymph node revealed squamous cell carcinoma

identifying the patient with unresectable tumor without resorting to surgery. The ability of CT to accurately delineate the extent of disease and thereby help surgeons and radiotherapists in treatment planning should never be underestimated (Figs. 7.14–7.16).

2.4 *Differential Diagnosis*

Peptic Esophagitis and Esophageal Ulcer. In the early stage, the radiologic findings in peptic esophagitis usually consist of spasm of the lower esophagus, narrowing of the lumen, and thickening or blurring of the mucosal folds. Pathological findings are congestion and edema. When erosion and slight superficial ulceration appear, the mucosal folds are irregular, even with small niches. As the disease progresses, stenosis of varying severity develops, with smooth or serrated borders. The lumen may dilate during the passage of a large amount of barium, while in carcinoma the stenosis is constant. Mucosal folds can be seen in the narrowed portion. There is no distinct margin between the diseased and normal parts of the esophagus. Peptic esophagitis is usually accompanied by hiatal hernia and gastroesophageal reflux [26].

Benign Stricture. This is generally caused by the intake of caustic materials such as lye or strong acid. Roentgen diagnosis must be correlated with clinical history. X-ray findings in the early stage of caustic damage to the esophagus usually consist of thickening and tortuosity of the mucosal folds and narrowing of the esophagus due to spasm. In the late stages the lumen is narrowed, with serrated borders, disappearance of normal mucosal folds, and stiffness of the wall due to scar tissue formation. The strictures are characterized by tapering edges, and can distend slightly during filling and contract in a segmental fashion during emptying, whereas in carcinoma, the margins between the narrowed segment and the normal portions are distinct and the diseased segment is associated with irregular filling defects [27].

Tuberculosis. Esophageal tuberculosis is rare. Radiologically, there may be narrowing of the esophageal lumen, stiffness of the wall, and ulceration with filling defects, and differentiation from carcinoma may be very difficult. In tuberculosis, however, filling defects, mucosal destruction, and narrowing of the lumen are usually not as conspicuous as in carcinoma [28]. Esophagoscopy and biopsy are necessary to establish the diagnosis (Fig. 7.17).

Varices. Esophageal varices mostly affect the lower portion of the esophagus, with the midthoracic portion possibly becoming involved if the disease is extensive. The radiologic findings are thickening and tortuosity of the mucosal folds with nodular filling defects. The contour of the esophagus is uneven. In late cases, the lumen is dilated with decreased peristalsis and the passage of barium is retarded. However, the esophageal wall remains pliable with fair contractility, and there is no local stenosis or obstruction. These findings may help to differentiate varices from carcinoma.

Leiomyoma. Radiologic examination shows a round or ovoid smooth filling defect protruding into the lumen. The sharp angle at the proximal and distal margins, where the tumor meets the normal esophageal wall, and the stretched mucosa over the tumor with the "smear effect" usually suffice to differentiate leiomyoma from carcinoma (Fig. 7.18). Multiple adjacent leiomyomas may cause multiple filling defects and a tortuous lumen, but the filling defects have smooth and regular outlines and can thus be differentiated from those in esophageal carcinoma [29]. In case of doubt, however, esophagoscopy and biopsy must be resorted to.

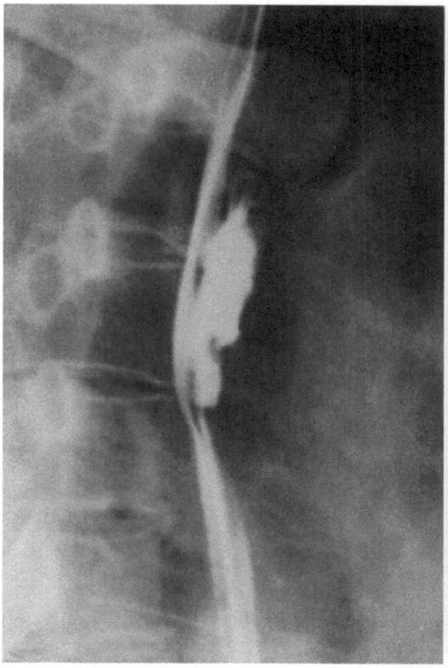

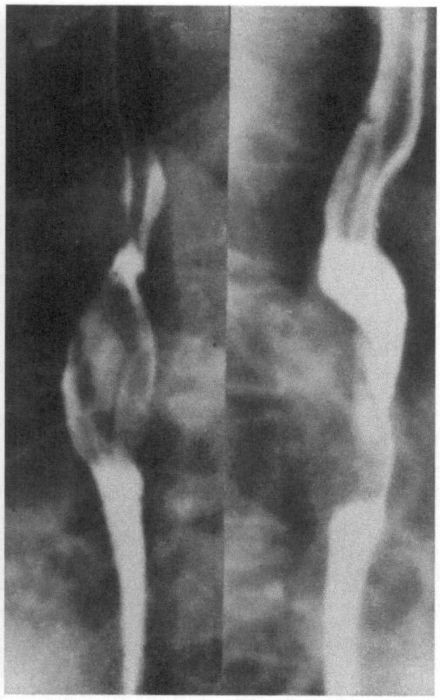

Fig. 7.17 (left). Tuberculosis of the esophagus. A 50-year-old woman (CI Hosp. No. 181796) had dysphagia for 3 weeks. Esophagography revealed a large irregular niche with mucosal destruction in the midthoracic esophagus. Esophagoscopic biopsy proved tuberculosis. The lesion disappeared after antitubercular treatment

Fig. 7.18 (right). Esophageal leiomyoma. A 45-year-old man (CI Hosp. No. 204477) had mild dysphagia for a year. Esophagography revealed an ovoid filling defect in the midthoracic esophagus with smear effect of the mucosa. The tumor was enucleated and pathology showed leiomyoma of the esophagus

Carcinosarcoma. Esophageal carcinosarcoma is rather rare. The tumor is polypoid in shape, usually pedunculated, and protrudes into the lumen. The surface of the tumor is usually smooth and covered with intact mucosa. Occasionally, scattered superficial ulcerations or erosions may be seen. Radiologic examination shows a bulky polypoid filling defect with expansion of the esophageal lumen. Carcinosarcoma of the esophagus may be distinguished from intraluminal esophageal carcinoma by its more marked dilatation of the lumen and its typical fusiform tumor mass, which is usually smooth with occasional superficial niches. There is no marked destruction of the esophageal wall as seen in cases of intraluminal esophageal carcinoma. There is only mild obstruction in most cases of carcinosarcoma, and the smear effect is often observed in the mucosa of the diseased portion of the esophagus (Fig. 7.19) [24].

Changes Due to Extrinsic Factors. Esophageal compression due to enlargement of the mediastinal lymph nodes is common. An enlarged carinal lymph node may displace the esophagus, and is best demonstrated in oblique positions. There is a crescent impression, usually with smooth contour on the esophageal wall but without mucosal destruction (Fig. 7.20). The esophageal lumen is narrowed due to compression, but the passage of barium is not interrupted. If the enlarged lymph node is adherent to the esophagus, or even infiltrates into the esophageal wall, differentiation from intrinsic disease of the esophagus may be very difficult.

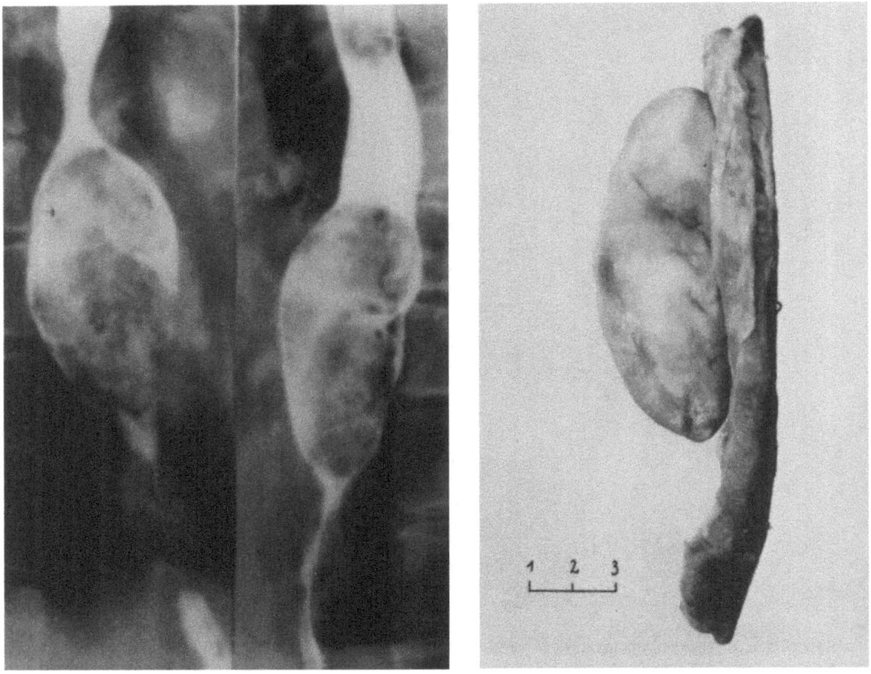

Fig. 7.19. Esophageal carcinosarcoma. *Left:* Esophagograms showing a large polypoid filling defect with smooth, clear-cut outline and dilatation of the lumen in the midthoracic esophagus. *Right:* Surgical specimen showing an oval elevated tumor mass with smooth contour. Pathology: carcinosarcoma of the esophagus

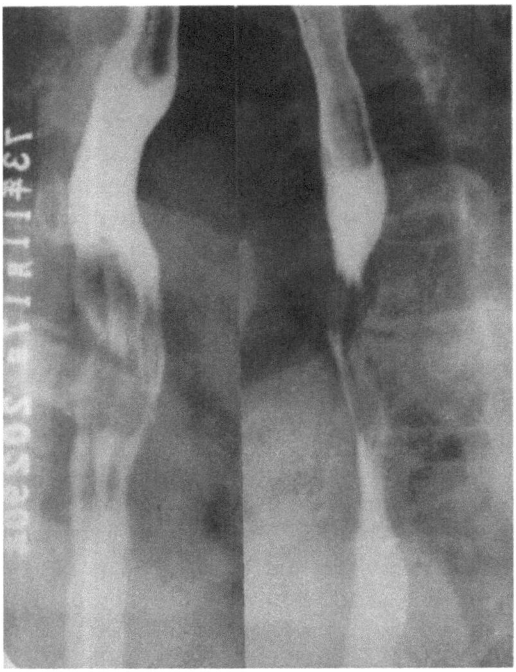

Fig. 7.20. Extrinsic compression of the esophagus by enlarged mediastinal lymph nodes (CI Hosp. No. 202904). Esophagography revealed slight displacement of the midthroacic esophagus with filling defect, but the unbroken mucosal folds indicated extrinsic compression. Surgical exploration revealed enlargement of the subcarinal lymph nodes

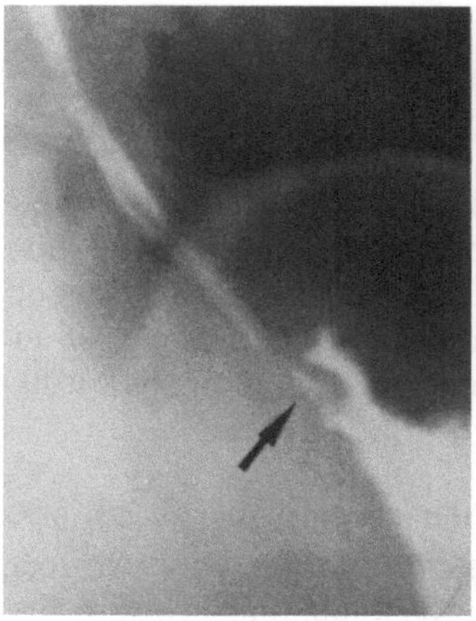
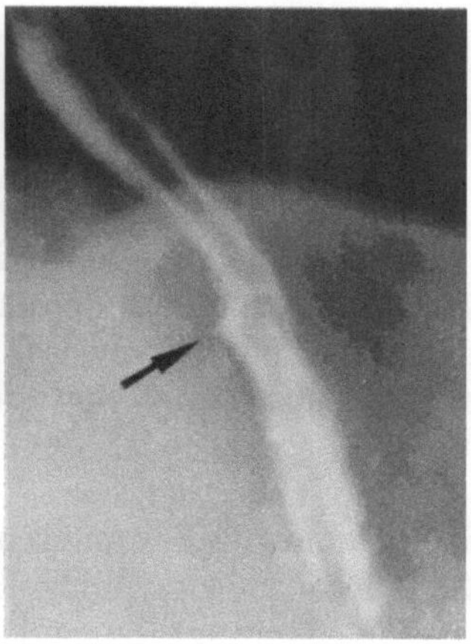
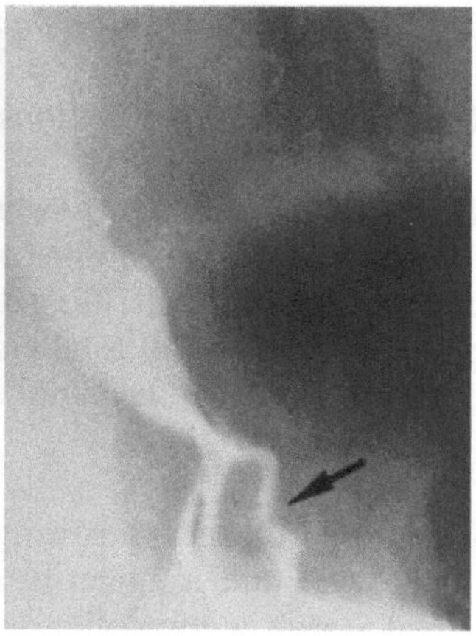

Fig. 7.21 (left). Early carcinoma of the gastric cardia. A 59-year-old woman was discovered to have adenocarcinoma cells on cytologic screening. Esophagography revealed irregularity of mucosal folds at the cardia with localized filling defect. Resection was carried out and pathology showed early adenocarcinoma of the gastric cardia with erosion of the mucosa

Fig. 7.22 (middle). Early carcinoma of the gastric cardia. A 54-year-old symptom-free man was found to have adenocarcinoma cells on esophageal cytological screening. Esophagography revealed a spicule-like small niche *(arrow)* at the cardiac region. Pathology of resected specimen: adenocarcinoma of the gastric cardia with erosion of the mucosa

Fig. 7.23 (right). Early carcinoma of the gastric cardia. A 65-year-old symptom-free woman was found to have adenocarcinoma cells on cytologic screening. Barium swallow revealed slight narrowing of the cardia with a small filling defect below *(arrow)*. Pathology of resected specimen: early adenocarcinoma of the gastric cardia

3 Diagnosis of Carcinoma of the Gastric Cardia

Carcinoma of the gastric cardia is also common in esophageal carcinoma high-incidence areas, with frequency about half that of the eosphageal cancer [30]. As most cases are in the advanced stage when first seen, further work on early diagnosis is of great importance.

3.1 Early Carcinoma

The *mucosal folds* in the cardia are thickened, irregular, interrupted, or even absent. Such changes appear very early in the course of the disease and may be taken as early X-ray manifestations of carcinoma (Fig. 7.21). A *minute niche* or *barium retention* in thickened mucosal folds may appear as a spike, spicule, or plaque (Fig. 7.22). The protruding tumor tissue on interrupted mucosal folds may present as *filling defects* on barium examination (Fig. 7.23).

Various degrees of *narrowing* of the cardia may be found, mainly due to spasm. The cardia can still be distended on the passage of a large amount of barium. Barium flows freely and there is no soft tissue mass in the fundus [30].

The *jet sign* is seen only rarely. It occurred in two of our 21 early cases.

3.2 *More Advanced Carcinoma*

The radiologic manifestations of more advanced cardiac carcinoma are many [31–33].

Destruction of Normal Mucosal Pattern. This damage presents as (a) thickening, blurring, flattening, or disappearance of mucosal folds; (b) interruption and disappearance of mucosal folds with small filling defects; (c) tortuosity, abnormal pattern, and displacement of mucosal folds; or (d) total eradication of normal mucosal folds, with the presence of an irregular filling defect and complete absence of the normal markings of the cardia (Fig. 7.24).

Narrowing. Cardiac narrowing is a common finding and is often accompanied by stiffness of the wall and irregularity of the local mucosal folds. Barium passage is obstructed. When a large amount of barium is forced through the rigid cardia under high pressure, the jet sign may be observed (Fig. 7.25).

Dilatation with Polypoid Tumor Mass. Sometimes the lower end of the esophagus and the cardia are dilated with polypoid filling defects and destruction of the mucosal folds but without obvious obstruction to barium flow.

Soft Tissue Mass in the Cardiac Region. The mass may appear nodular, lobulated, band-like, or unevenly wave-like, with indistinct borders. Sometimes double-contrast gastrogra-

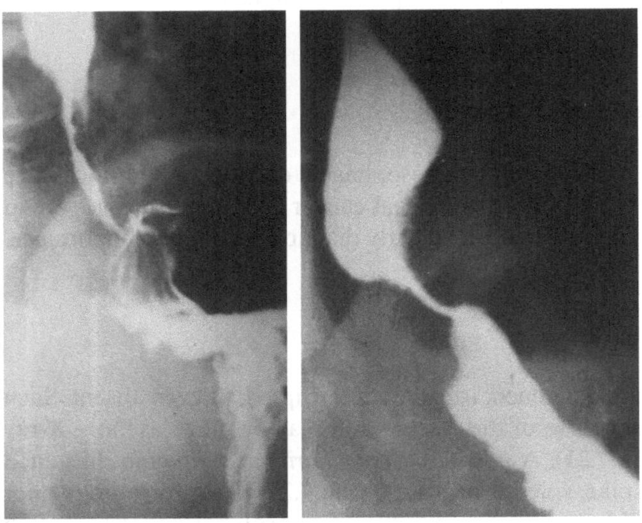

Fig. 7.24 (left). Carcinoma of the gastric cardia invading the lower portion of the esophagus. A 55-year-old man (CI Hosp. No. 332705) had dysphagia for 8 months. Barium swallow shows narrowing and irregular filling defect in the lower portion of the esophagus. The mucosal folds in the cardia are blurred and irregular; some have disappeared. Pathology of resected specimen: adenocarcinoma of the cardia

Fig. 7.25 (right). Carcinoma of the gastric cardia involving the lower end of the esophagus. A 43-year-old man (CI Hosp. No. 261491) had progressive dysphagia for a year. Esophagography revealed narrowing of the distal part of the esophagus and the cardiac orifice, with stiffness of the wall. The lower portion of the esophagus was dilated. Pathology of resected specimen: adenocarcinoma of the gastric cardia phy shows localized thickening of the inner wall of the gastric fundus. The surface of the tumor, being coated with barium, is silhouetted against the translucency of the gastric air pocket. The outline of the tumor mass is clear (Fig. 7.26, 7.27).

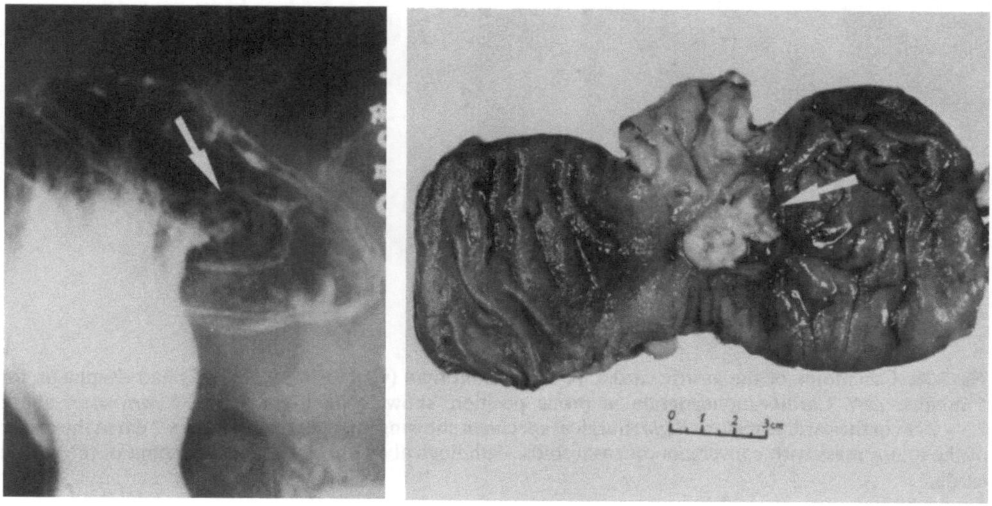

Fig. 7.26. Carcinoma of the gastric cardia. A 59-year-old man (CI Hosp. No. 332112) had dysphagia for 3 months. *Left:* Cardioesophagogram in prone position, showing a tumor mass *(arrow)* with clear outline, measuring about 3 × 2 cm, in the cardiac region. *Right:* Surgical specimen showing a lobular mass *(arrow)* about 3 × 2 cm in size just below the esophagogastric junction. Pathological diagnosis: adenocarcinoma of the gastric cardia

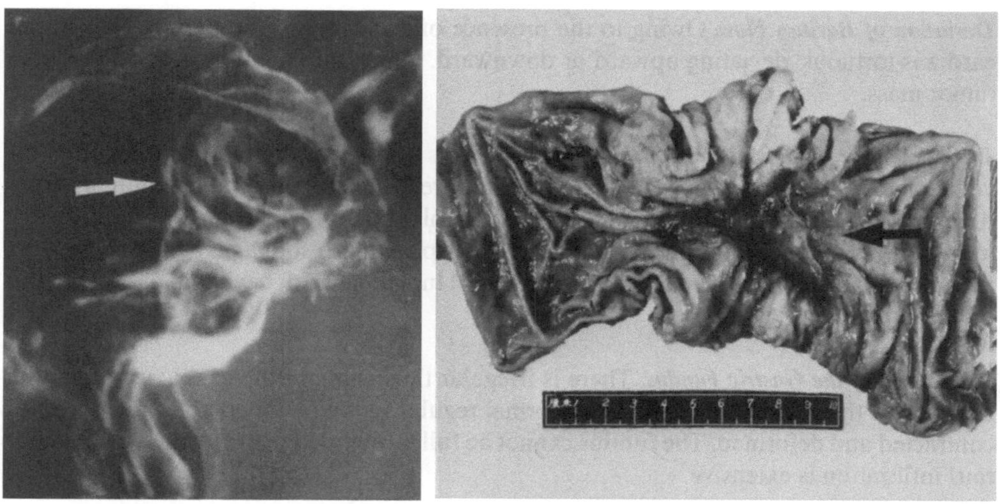

Fig. 7.27. Carcinoma of the gastric cardia. A 43-year-old man (CI Hosp. No. 281890) had progressive dysphagia for 4 months. *Left:* Cardioesophagogram in prone position, showing a large lobulated soft tissue mass at the cardia and lesser curvature of the stomach, with mucosal destruction and niche *(arrow)*. An irregular filling defect is also noted at the lower and of the esophagus. *Right:* Surgical specimen showing a tumor mass with a large ulcer in the center *(arrow)*. Pathological diagnosis: adenocarcinoma of the gastric cardia

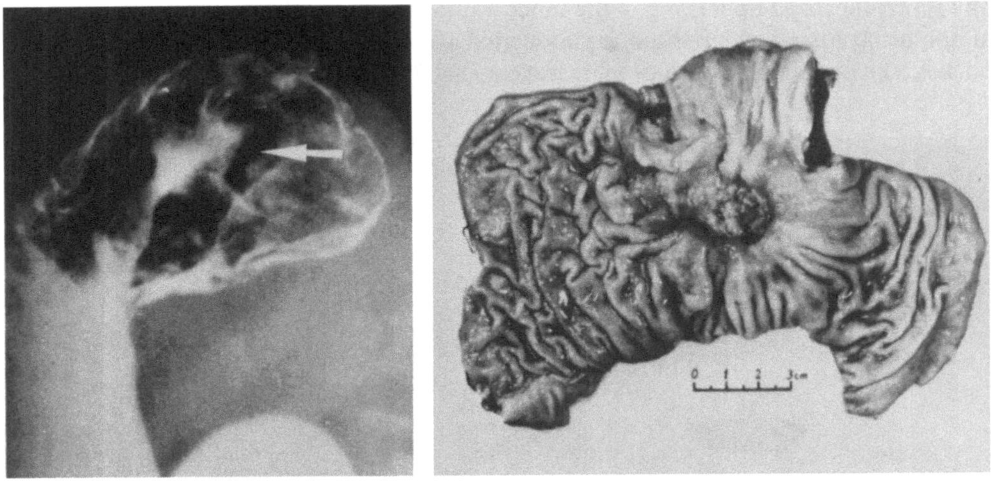

Fig. 7.28. Carcinoma of the gastric cardia. A 48-year-old man (CI Hosp. No. 337982) had dysphagia for 5 months. *Left:* Cardioesophagogram in prone position, showing an irregular niche *(arrow)* of about 2.5 × 2 cm in the cardiac region. *Right:* Surgical specimen showing an ulcer of about 2.5 × 2 cm in the center of the tumor mass with convergent mucosal folds. Pathological diagnosis: adenocarcinoma of the gastric cardia

Niches. A considerable number of cases of cardiac carcinoma display niches of variable size and depth with irregular margins. In some cases, elevated tumor tissue within the niche may lead to a filling defect. Sometimes the niche is inconspicuous, presenting itself as irregular folds (Fig. 7.28).

Deviation of Barium Flow. Owing to the presence of tumor mass, the barium flow at the cardia is tortuous, deviating upward or downward. Sometimes the flow is divided by the tumor mass.

Involvement of the Distal Part of the Esophagus. This portion of the esophagus is often involved in cardiac carcinoma. The main findings are (a) thickening, interruption, destruction, and disappearance of esophageal mucosal folds; (b) irregular narrowing of the lumen, rigidity of the wall, and dilatation of the proximal esophagus; (c) polypoid or irregular filling defects in the involved esophageal lumen; and (d) deviation or obstruction of barium flow.

Infiltration of the Gastric Fundus. There is irregular thickening of the gastric wall near the cardia, and the gastric bubble loses its normal regular semicircular contour and becomes contracted and deformed. The fundus cannot be fully distended with air when carcinomatous infiltration is extensive.

Infiltration of the Lesser Curvature. The lesser curvature of the stomach is often involved in carcinoma of the cardia, and may display irregular margins, stiffness of the wall, filling defects, and niches. There is destruction and disappearance of mucosal folds. The involved portion of the gastric wall is delineated clearly from the normal wall (Fig. 7.29).

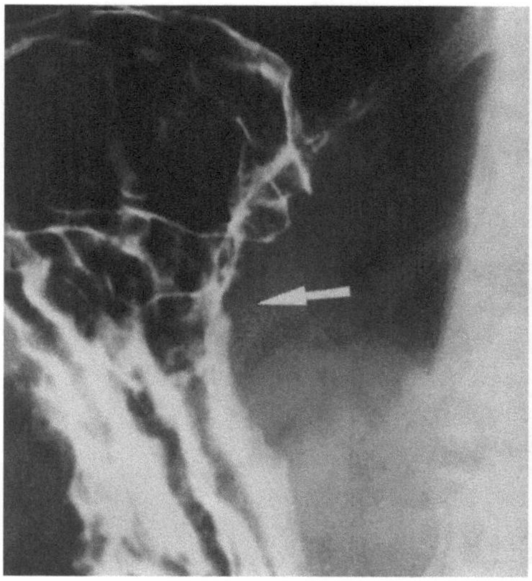

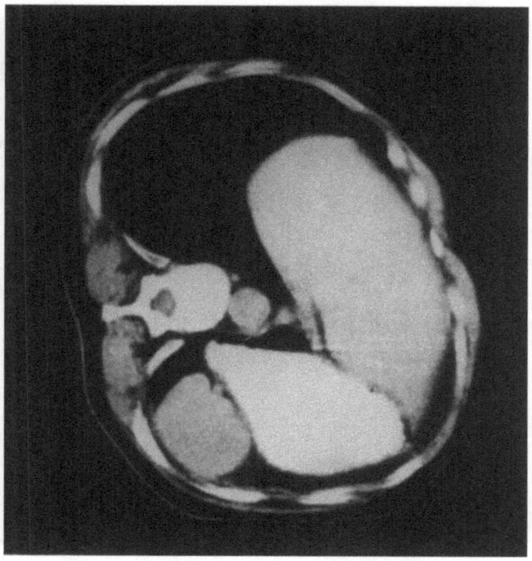

Fig. 7.29 (left). Carcinoma of the gastric cardia involving the lesser curvature of the stomach. A 40-year-old man (CI Hosp. No. 235853) had upper abdominal pain for a year. Barium swallow showed a tumor mass in the cardiac region with an irregular filling defect of the lesser curvature. Pathology of resected specimen: adenocarcinoma of the gastric cardia with invasion of the lesser curvature

Fig. 7.30 (right). CT scan of the upper abdomen in left decubitus position, showing normal gastric cardia with smooth gastric wall

3.3 CT Findings

The outline of the normal gastric fundus and cardia is usually smooth and regular on CT scan. There is neither a filling defect nor a soft tissue mass within the gastric cavity in the left decubitus position (Fig. 7.30). In a small number of cases there is thickening at the esophageal entrance into the stomach, or a focal mass-like shadow in this region. Marks et al. [34] reported that this configuration relates to the transverse anatomic plane of section through the normal esophagogastric junction and cardia, influenced by the degree of distension in the stomach. It is helpful to place the patient in the left posterior oblique position, give some additional contrast material orally, and do a repeat scan. The additional contrast material, change in position, and variation in distension of the stomach, particularly at the esophagogastric junction, can induce disappearance of the soft tissue mass. On CT scan, the cleft separating the caudate lobe of the liver from the lateral segment of the left lobe will be pointing directly toward the region of the esophagogastric junction.

CT scanning is used for preoperative staging in carcinoma of the gastric cardia. The outline of the fundus and cardia is irregular with filling defects on the scan. In the left decubitus position, there is a soft tissue mass in the gastric cavity clearly coated with contrast medium. CT can demonstrate the size of the tumor; its local extension and relation to the adjacent structures, e.g., invasion of the liver, spleen, and diaphragm; and metastases in the intra-abdominal lymph nodes, retrocrural lymph nodes, and liver metastases.

Freeny and Marks [35] reported that CT correctly identified 16 of 21 patients as having unresectable adenocarcinoma of the esophagogastric junction. The most reliable criteria of unresectability were metastases, regional lymph node enlargement, and local extension

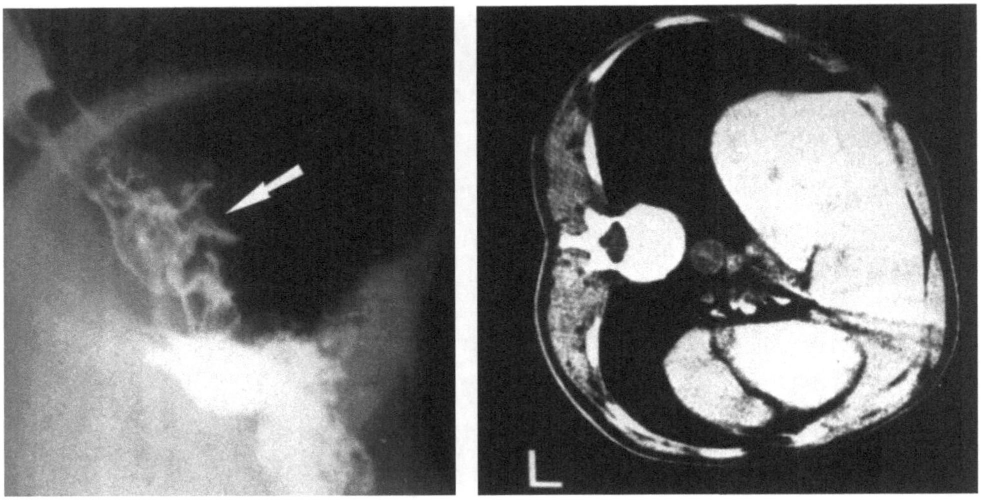

Fig. 7.31. Carcinoma of the gastric cardia involving the lower end of the esophagus. A 48-year-old man (CI Hosp. No. 340278) had dysphagia for 7 months. *Left:* Barium swallow showing a cauliflower-like mass in the cardia and a filling defect of the lower esophagus. *Right:* CT scan of the upper abdomen in left decubitus position, showing a nodular mass in the gastric lumen at the cardiac region. Pathology of resected specimen: adenocarcinoma of the gastric cardia

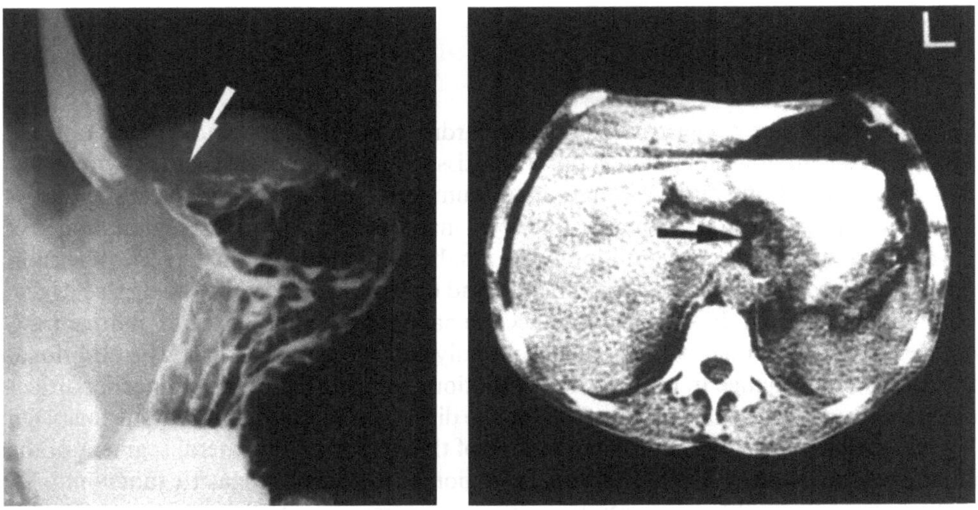

Fig. 7.32. Carcinoma of the gastric cardia involving the lower end of the esophagus. A 58-year-old man (CI Hosp. No. 355554) had dysphagia for 4 months. *Left:* Barium swallow showing irregular filling defects involving the lower end of the esophagus, the cardia, the fundus, and the lesser curvature *(arrow). Right:* CT scan of the upper abdomen, showing barium filling defects in the cardia, fundus, and lesser curvature *arrow)* and blurring of the hilar structures of the spleen. Surgical exploration revealed a tumor mass in the cardiac region involving the fundus and lesser curvature, the liver, the diaphragm, and the spleen, with intra-abdominal lymph node metastases. Biopsy diagnosis: adenocarcinoma

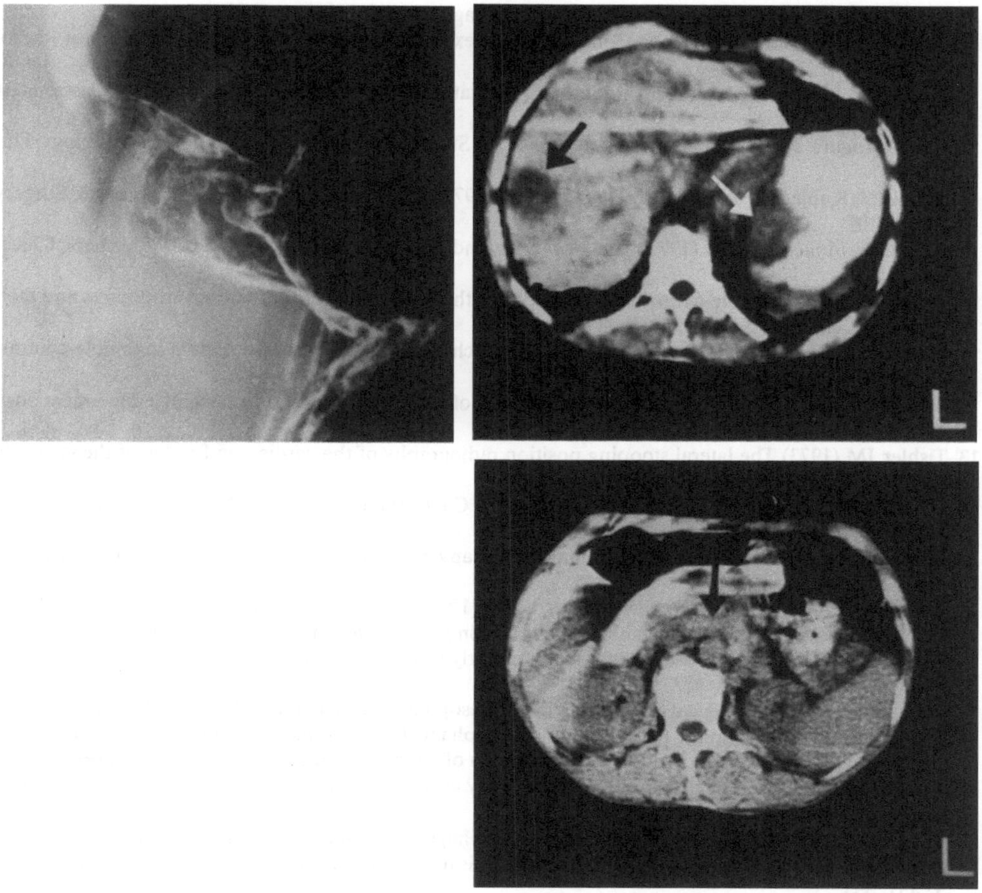

Fig. 7.33. Carcinoma of the gastric cardia involving the lower portion of the esophagus. A 56-year-old man (CI Hosp. No. 355778) had dysphagia for 5 months. *Left:* Barium swallow showing a cauliflower-like mass in the cardia and fundus and filling defects of the distal esophagus. *Right, below:* CT scans of the upper abdomen, showing barium filling defects of the gastric cardia and fundus and metastases to the liver, spleen, and intra-abdominal lymph nodes *(arrows)*

of tumor. The ability of CT to diagnose and stage adenocarcinoma of the esophagogastric junction may avoid an unnecessary operation and can also be important in helping clinicians plan the optimal treatment (Figs. 7.31–7.33).

References

1. Wu YK, Huang GJ (1965) Carcinoma of the esophagus and gastric cardia (in Chinese) Shanghai Scientific and Technical Publishers, Shanghai, pp 29–32, 107
2. The Coordinating Group for the Research on Esophageal Carcinoma of Henan Province, Linxian County Hospital (1973) Early diagnosis of esophageal carcinoma (in Chinese) People's Medical Publishing House, Beijing, p 54
3. Buskstein J (1953) The digestive tract in roentgenology, vol 1. Lippincott, Philadelphia London Montreal, pp 32–34

4. Brombart M (1961) Clinical radiology of the esophagus. Wright, Bristol, pp 3, 311
5. Goldstein HM, Dodd GD (1976) Double-contrast examination of the esophagus. Gastrointest Radiol 1: 3–6
6. Zornoza J, Lindell MM Jr (1980) Radiologic evaluation of small esophageal carcinoma. Gastrointest Radiol 5: 107–111
7. Itai Y, Kogure T, Okuyama Y, Akiyama H (1978) Superficial esophageal carcinoma. Radiology 126: 597–601
8. Suzuki H, Kobayashi S, Endo M, Nakayama K (1972) Diagnosis of early esophageal cancer. Surgery 71: 99–103
9. Stein GN, Finkelstein AK (1973) The esophagus and stomach. Year Book Medical Publishers, Chicago, pp 2–4
10. Freeny PC (1979) Double-contrast gastrography of the fundus and cardia: normal landmarks and their pathologic changes. AJR 133: 481–487
11. Herlinger H, Grossman R, Laufer I, Kressel HY, Ochs RH (1980) The gastric cardia in double-contrast study: its dynamic image. AJR 135: 21–29
12. Schatzki R, Gary JE (1958) Face-on demonstration of ulcers in the upper stomach in a dependent position. AJR 79: 772–780
13. Tishler JM (1973) The lateral stooping position radiography of the cardia and fundus of the stomach. Clin Radiol 24: 333–336
14. Halber MD, Daffner RH, Thompson WM (1979) CT of the esophagus: I. Normal appearance. AJR 133: 1047–1050
15. Moss AA (1981) Esophageal carcinoma: pretherapy staging by computed tomography. AJR 136: 1051–1056
16. Editorial Committee for "A Practice in Oncology" (1979) Tumor of the esophagus and gastric cardia (in Chinese) People's Medical Publishing House, Beijing (A practice in oncology, vol III, pp 266–301)
17. Su JH, Tian ZS, Han JF (1975) X-ray study of early esophageal carcinoma: analysis of 100 cases (in Chinese) Chin Med J 55: 573–575
18. Wang ZY (1980) Radiological appearance in early esophageal carcinoma. J R Soc Med 73: 849–852
19. The Coordinating Group for the Research on Esophageal Carcinoma of Henan Province, Coordinating Group for Research on Esophageal Carcinoma of Chinese Academy of Medical Sciences, Linxian County Hospital (1974) Pathological study of early esophageal squamous cell carcinoma (in Chinese) Cancer Res Prev Treat 2: 26–35
20. The Coordinating Group for the Research on Esophageal Carcinoma of Chinese Academy of Medical Sciences and Henan Province (1973) Early diagnosis of esophageal carcinoma (in Chinese) Chin Med J 8: 451–453
21. Koehler RE, Moss AA, Margulis AR (1976) Early radiographic manifestations of carcinoma of the esophagus. Radiology 119: 1–5
22. Moss AA, Koehler RE, Margulis AR (1976) Initial accuracy of esophagograms in detection of small esophageal carcinoma. AJR 127: 909–913
23. Departments of Surgery, Pathology, and Diagnostic Radiology, Cancer Hospital, Chinese Academy of Medical Sciences (1973) Study on the separate entity of "intraluminal type" of esophageal carcinoma (in Chinese) Cancer Res Prev Treat 3: 8–12
24. Huang GJ, Gu XZ, Liu FS, Wang ZY, Zhang DW, Zhang RG, Wang GQ, Lin H, Wang LJ, Cheng GY (1981) Further studies on the separate entity of intraluminal type of esophageal carcinoma (in Chinese) Chin J Oncol 3: 110–112
25. Daffner RH, Halber MD, Postlethwait RW, Korobkin M, Thompson WM (1979) CT of the esophagus. II. Carcinoma. AJR 133: 1051–1055
26. Vantrappen G, Hellemans J (1974) Diseases of the esophagus. Springer, Berlin Heidelberg New York, pp 505–513
27. Editorial Committee of "Diagnostic Roentgenology", Shanghai First Medical College (1978) Abdomen (in Chinese) Shanghai Scientific and Technical Publishers, Shanghai (Diagnostic roentgenology, vol III, pp 974–975)
28. Wang ZY, Zhang LD (1980) Tuberculosis of the esophagus (in Chinese) Chin J Tuberc Respir Dis 3: 115–116
29. Wang ZY, Zhong S (1982) Radiological diagnosis of smooth muscle tumors of the esophagus (in Chinese) Chin J Radiol 16: 29–31
30. The Coordinating Group for the Research on Esophageal Carcinoma of Henan Province, Linxian

County Hospital, Chengguan Commune Clinic (1974) Study on the X-ray diagnosis of early cardiac carcinoma (in Chinese) Cancer Res Prev Treat 2: 7–10
31. Stewart WH, Illick HE (1934) Roentgen diagnosis of carcinoma of the cardia. AJR 32: 43–51
32. Yang WZ, Cai C (1965) X-ray diagnosis of cardiac carcinoma and abdominal metastases (in Chinese) Chin J Radiol 10: 208–212
33. Lin G, Zhang ZN, Han XY (1981) X-ray diagnosis of cardiac carcinoma (in Chinese) Chin J Radiol 15: 185–187
34. Marks WM, Gallen PW, Moss AA (1981) Gastroesophageal region: source of confusion on CT. AJR 136: 259–362
35. Freeny PC, Marks WM (1982) Adenocarcinoma of the gastroesophageal junction: barium and CT examination. AJR 138: 1077–1084

Chapter 8
Fiberesophagoscopic Diagnosis

Da Wei Zhang

1 Introduction

Nearly 120 years have passed since 1866, when Semeleder and Stoerk first attempted to view the esophageal lumen directly. At first, simple rigid tubes were used, but later illumination devices were employed and optical systems were added to make the visual field clearer. In 1958 Hirschowitz, taking advantage of the discovery that light could be transmitted around curves through glass fibers, invented the flexible fibergastroscope. Five years later the first fiberesophagoscope became available [1–4], supplied with cold light, fully flexible, and double-channelled to allow for pumping of air or water, introduction of biopsy forceps, and the use of suction. Indeed, the invention of the fiberscope opened a new era in endoscopy.

The merits of the fiberscope as compared with the rigid metal esophagoscope may be summarized as follows:

- The fiberscope is much more slender, having an outside diameter of only 1.2 cm. Together with the flexibility – the single most significant advantage – this allows the patient to assume a comfortable position and renders the examination much safer and less painful. The procedure is therefore more acceptable to the patient.
- By using cold light transmitted through the fibers from an outside source, a bright visual field can be obtained without producing heat. The focusing and magnifying ability of the inbuilt lens system gives so sharp an image that even fine submucosal capillaries can easily be identified.
- The bending mechanism of the tip of the scope greatly increases the field of vision. Not only the esophagus but also the entire esophagogastric junction can be thoroughly examined, leading to a marked increase in the detection rate of carcinoma of the gastric cardia.
- The esophageal lumen is inflated with air instead of being forced open by the tip of the scope. The elasticity and motility of the esophagus can thus be assessed satisfactorily.
- The fiberscope permits examination in patients with severe spinal deformities such as kyphosis or bamboo spine. Many contraindications for the rigid scope, including aortic aneurysms and esophageal varicosis, no longer pose problems.

However, fiberesophagoscopy has some limitations. Therapeutic measures such as removal of foreign bodies or dilatation of strictures cannot be carried out directly. Being finely constructed, the fiberscope is very delicate and is easily damaged if not handled with great care. The pharyngoesophageal junction usually remains constricted and cannot be inflated by the fiberscope, and is therefore the only region that is better investigated by the rigid scope.

2 Equipment

A fiberesophagoscope has five main elements (Fig. 8.1). The *control part* is composed of eyepiece, tip-turning knob, valve for insertion of biopsy forceps or cytology brush, and inflation, rinse-control, and suction buttons. The *body* of the scope is about 1 cm in caliber and contains an air/water channel, a suction/biopsy channel, light-guiding fiber bundles, image-transmitting bundles, and a tip-controlling wire. Communicating with the body through the control part is the *main cord*, which is composed of an air/water channel, light-guiding fiber bundles, a suction channel, and an adapter for the scope socket of the

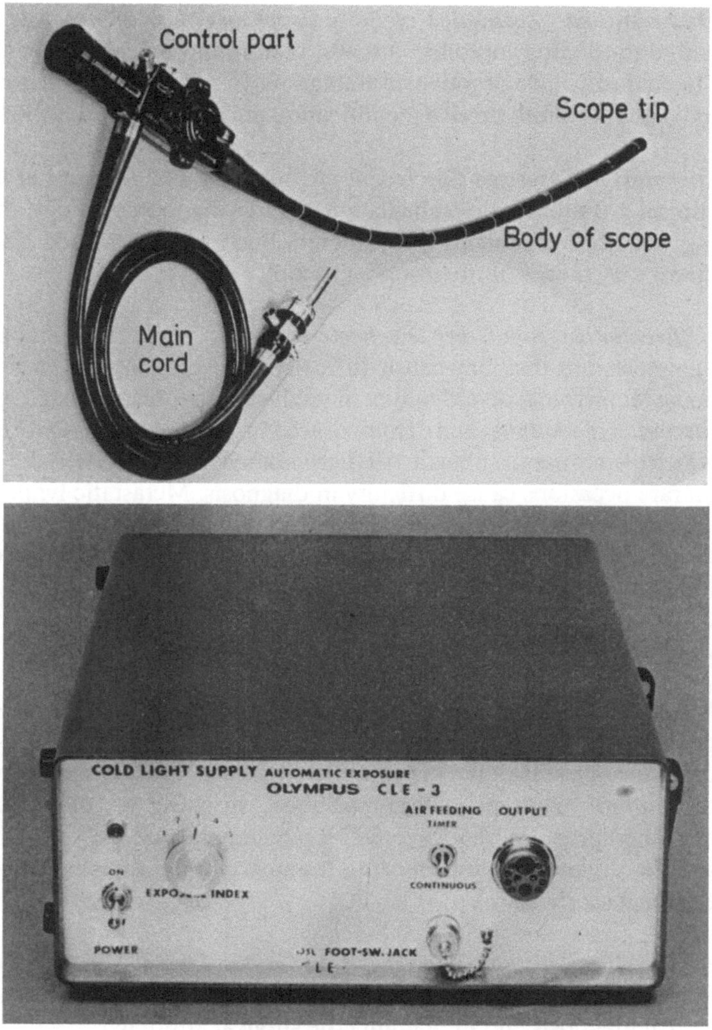

Fig. 8.1. Above: Fiberoptic esophagoscope; *below:* cold light supply

light supply. The *scope tip* is made up of an objective, windows for light-guiding fiber bundles, an air/water outlet, and a protective rubber cuff. Its flexible neck enables it to bend through 180° vertically and 120° horizontally. The *cold light supply* (Fig. 8.1 *below*) is a unit containing halogen lamp, air pump, cooling fan, and automatic exposure system.

Accessories available for further investigation and documentation of any visible mucosal change are biopsy forceps, cytology brush, and medical camera.

3 Indications

As already mentioned, the fiberesophagoscope has much wider indications than the rigid scope. The indications for fiberesophagoscopy in patients with carcinoma of the esophagus and gastric cardia are as follows.

Diagnosis and Localization of Early Esophageal Carcinoma. The patients usually present with only slight symptoms, and are often found on mass screening by balloon cytology. The majority have negative or ambiguous X-ray findings. Fiberesophagoscopy is usually indicated for more precise identification and localization of the lesion.

Diagnosis of Suspected Carcinoma of Esophagus and Gastric Cardia. Patients with definite clinical symptoms of dysphagia but negative balloon cytology and unspecific X-ray findings are not infrequently encountered. Such situations need clarification through direct viewing by means of fiberesophagoscopy.

Differentiation from Other Dysphagic Diseases. There are a number of other benign or malignant lesions that may cause difficulty in swallowing, the most commonly encountered being leiomyoma, diverticulum, hiatal hernia, peptic esophagitis, and achalasia. Carcinosarcoma, melanoma and leiomyosarcoma are relatively rare esophageal malignancies which also cause dysphagia. All these lesions have characteristic X-ray features, but might on rare occasions cause difficulty in diagnosis. Metastatic lymph nodes from a lung cancer may compress the esophagus and should never be missed in differential diagnosis of dysphagia. In some benign esophageal lesions signs of malignant change may appear on follow-up, e.g., the obliteration of a diverticulum by a tumor or the appearance of a filling defect on X-ray in the dilated esophagus of a patient with achalasia. Fiberesophagoscopy will be indicated in these cases.

Follow-Up of Various Treatment Modalities for Esophageal Carcinoma. Recurrence of dysphagia after either surgery or irradiation for esophageal carcinoma demands further endoscopic investigation. Anastomotic cicatricial stenosis should be differentiated from local stump recurrence. Postirradiation stricture or ulcer formation often puzzles radiotherapists, and endoscopic biopsy may be needed to verify the diagnosis. The response of cancer to a given drug therapy may be assessed through biopsy under fiberesophagoscopy.

Advanced Carcinoma of Esophagus or Gastric Cardia. Diagnosis can usually be made "at first sight" on X-ray, but endoscopy may be necessary in ascertaining the precise pathological diagnosis and in planning the surgical approach.

Note: Mental disorders, severe heart and lung diseases, and cachexia are considered contraindications.

4 Preparation and Technique

Although the flexible fiberscope does not, as a rule, give patients as much discomfort as the rigid scope, this does not imply that it carries no operative risks. For instance, fiberesophagoscopy perforation rates of 0.093%–1.6% have been reported in the literature [5, 6]. The success and safety of fiberesophagoscopy, as of rigid endoscopy, depend on the taking of proper measures by the endoscopist and on good preparation of the patient.

4.1 Measures to Be Taken by the Endoscopist

Prerequisites for a safe and fruitful examination are a brief history and a workup of the patient and careful review of the X-rays. The patient must be told the purpose of the endoscopy and be warned of the possible discomfort during the procedure. Patients are often scared simply because they do not know what esophagoscopy is, but once they know what will happen, they cooperate.

A complete check of the instruments should be made before the examination. The endoscopist must be satisfied that all parts are in good working order. Interruption of the examination by mechanical accidents is a sure sign of bad practise.

4.2 Preparation of the Patient

No water or food should be allowed orally for at least 4 h before examination, and oral hygiene measures such as brushing of teeth and gargling should be undertaken if necessary. Any dentures present should be removed.

In adults, 0.5 mg atropine and 0.1 g sodium luminal are injected intramuscularly half an hour before examination. The former is for reduction of upper digestive tract secretion, the latter for sedation and counteraction of any side effects of topical anesthesia.

Spraying of 1% xylocaine over the base of the tongue and the oropharynx affords sufficient topical anesthesia in most cases; it is preferable to perform the examination with the patient conscious [7]. The amount of 1% xylocaine used should not exceed 10 ml. Cocaine and dicain have long been abandoned because of their high toxicity.

The patient is asked to lie relaxed on his left side. In this position any saliva accumulating in the oral cavity can flow freely out of the corner of the mouth, avoiding aspiration into the airway.

4.3 Technique

When everything is ready and the patient is properly positioned with a mouthpiece between his incisors, the endoscopist stands facing the patient and inserts the scope tip into the patient's mouth. Under direct vision he guides the scope tip toward the entrance of the esophagus while an assistant holding the scope body exerts gentle forward pressure. The patient may be asked to swallow, thereby relaxing the cricopharyngeal sphincter and facilitating insertion. The esophageal lumen is inflated by intermittent pumping of air into the esophagus, and the endoscopist starts inspection. In order to avoid overdistension of the upper gastrointestinal tract and the agonizing pain which may result, as little air as possible should be introduced. The endoscopist should at first take a brief bird's-eye view of the entire length of the esophageal lumen. From the upper cervical segment the extrinsic compression by the pulsating aortic arch and next to it the left main bronchus, running obliquely from right to left on the anterior wall, can easily be identified. At midthoracic level the left atrial indentation is also clearly visible. In order to avoid disorientation, the marking notch of the visual field must be kept pointing toward the posterior wall. If the inspection performed from above downward reveals nothing of any importance, the procedure should be repeated in the reverse direction. Such a to-and-fro examination is sometimes necessary because fine changes can easily be missed, particularly when the mucosal folds have not been fully distended. The endoscopy should never be deemed complete until the cardiac region has also been examined thoroughly; carcinoma of the gastric cardia ranks second only to carcinoma of the esophagus as a cause of dysphagia.

In the days of rigid endoscopy, many cases of carcinoma of the gastric cardia were missed because of the "blind zone." In one study [8] endoscopic diagnostic accuracy was only 63% (19/30). There is no blind zone with fiberesophagoscopy; the cardia and the lesser curvature can be seen clearly.

In advanced cases of carcinoma of the esophagus and gastric cardia, positive mucosal changes can usually be seen at the site suggested by X-ray. The appearance, nature, color, and extent of the changes should be defined carefully, and the lesion should be photographed before it is contacted with instruments, as a control for possible subsequent iatrogenic changes.

4.4 Cytology and Biopsy

After careful study by direct observation, the lesion should be histologically identified by means of cytology and biopsy.

Biopsy should generally be performed before cytology. The biopsy forceps is inserted through the biopsy channel and directed toward the lesion by pressure on the forceps itself, adjustment of the scope tip, or a combination of both maneuvers. The opening and closing of the forceps is done by an assistant. In order to raise the rate of positive results, biopsy should be performed at the periphery of the lesion, avoiding the central necrotic portion. The chance of a positive result has been related to the number of specimens taken, and generally at least three should be obtained. After pinching with the biopsy forceps the target areas should be checked for bleeding. Slight oozing is not important, but active bleeding must be stopped by electric cautery or other means. Because the esophagus is a tubular organ with a thin wall and no serosa, any biopsy must be superficial to avoid perforation. No biopsy should be attempted for submucosal lesions, as in these cases no positive result can be obtained.

Brush cytology is usually done after biopsy. Additional benefit from this procedure has been documented, as the two investigations are complementary. A more than 10% increase in correct diagnosis has been reported [9–11]. Brush cytology has been especially helpful in patients with stenotic esophageal cancer [12]. It is our practice to withdraw the scope with the brush in the distal portion of the channel and to obtain smears by pushing the brush out again from the scope tip. If the brush were withdrawn from the scope directly before the smear was made, a certain amount of exfoliated cells would be lost as the nylon brush squeezed through the biopsy channel, with a corresponding reduction in the rate of detection.

Endoscopic cytology can be performed in several other ways, such as saline lavage, suction through a Teflon tube with a beveled metal tip, and imprint smears from biopsy samples [13].

5 Early Esophageal Carcinoma

5.1 Detection

Fiberesophagoscopy has been proved to be of great value in detecting early esophageal carcinoma during the past two decades. Mass surveys using balloon cytology as the main screening measure has been carried out in Linxian county, Henan province, with gratifying results. At the Yaocun Commune Hospital in Linxian, fiberesophagoscopy was performed in some 400 patients with esophageal carcinoma up to the end of 1980. There were 125 early cases, giving a ratio of early to advanced of 1:2.2. During about the same period, 1662 fiberesophagoscopies were performed for various conditions at the Cancer Institute of the Chinese Academy of Medical Sciences, Beijing, where among 329 cases of endoscopically diagnosed esophageal carcinoma, only 38 were proved to be in the early stage, giving a ratio of about 1:7.7.

In a series of 135 cases of early esophageal carcinoma (125 from Yaocun Commune Hospital and 10 from the Cancer Institute), the detection rates of balloon cytology, roentgen examination, and fiberesophagoscopy were 97.7%, 38%, and 85.2% respectively. Early esophageal cancer has been characterized by its minute volume and superficial location. Under these conditions balloon cytology has proved to be the most rewarding diagnostic method, but it cannot identify the site precisely, even if repeated at different segments, as suggested by some workers. Roentgen examination has the advantage of being simple and noninvasive, but the detection rate is low, because its powers of resolution are not sufficient to reveal small lesions. The direct vision offered by fiberesophagoscopy is very helpful in detection, location, and exact definition of extent of early esophageal carcinoma, but in a small proportion of cases the lesion may not be found. It is evident, therefore, that the three diagnostic methods are complementary and should be employed in combination [14, 15].

5.2 Endoscopic Appearance

The recent progress in early detection of esophageal carcinoma as a result of the development and refinement of new diagnostic instruments, together with the performance of mass surveys in high-risk areas, has provided excellent resources for Chinese surgeons, endoscopists, and pathologists in their investigation of the various aspects of early lesions. Based on the fiberesophagoscopic examination of 117 of the above-mentioned 135 cases, the gross endoscopic appearances of early esophageal carcinoma may be summarized as follows.

Mucosal erosion was the most frequent finding, occurring in 62 cases (53%). It is characterized by an area of patches of denuded mucosa interposed with normal pink mucosa, and is often described as map-like. Upon touching, the lesion bleeds easily. The cancer cells infiltrate no deeper than the submucosa, and the contractility of the esophageal wall usually remains unaffected (Figs. 8.2–8.8).

Focal congestion was the second-ranking change, detected in 45 cases (38.5%). It usually presents as an area of hyperemia with indefinite fuzzy demarcation. As with mucosal erosion, there is no derangement of peristalsis (Figs. 8.9–8.11)

Coarseness of mucosa was seen in 32 cases (27.4%). In appearance the mucosa resembles sandpaper, with numerous minute whitish granules (Fig. 8.12).

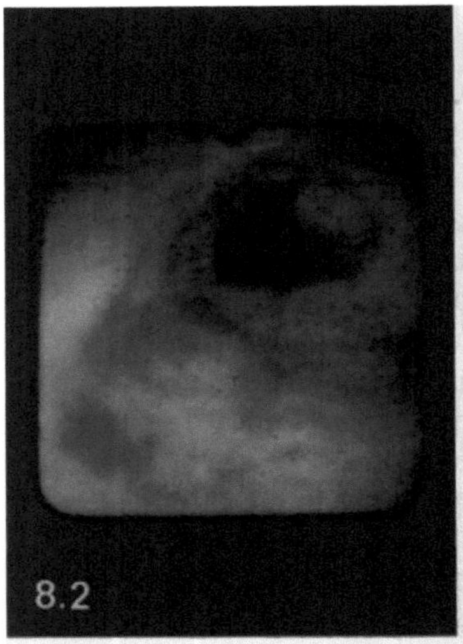
8.2

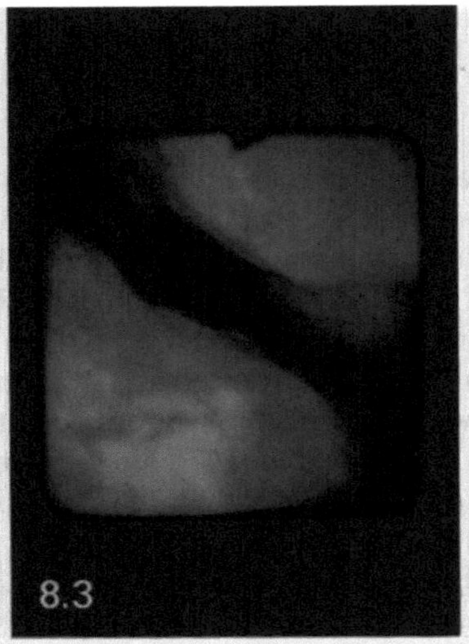
8.3

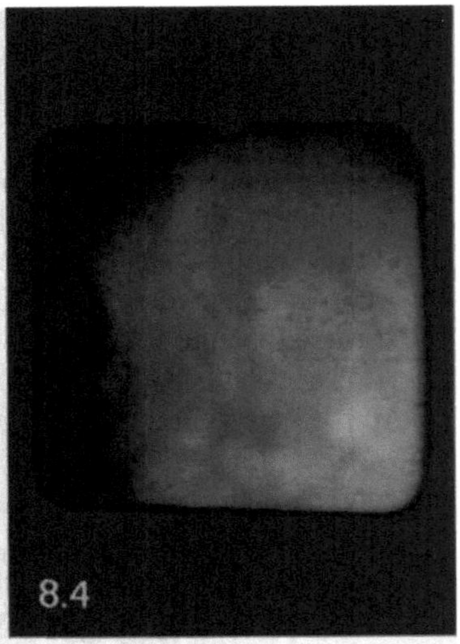
8.4

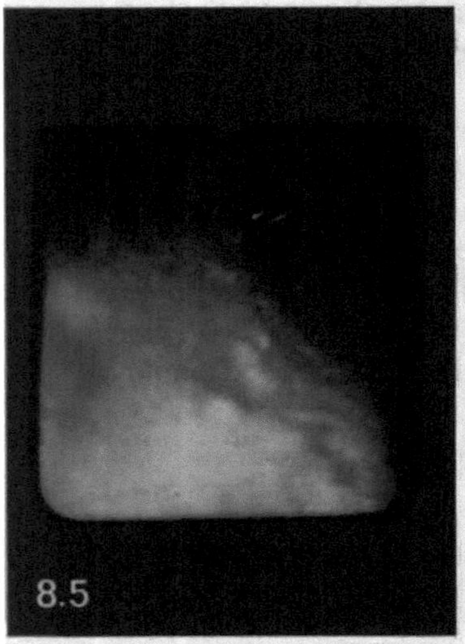
8.5

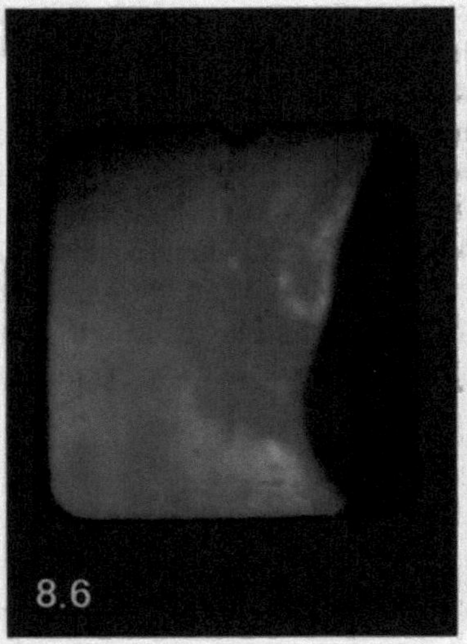
8.6

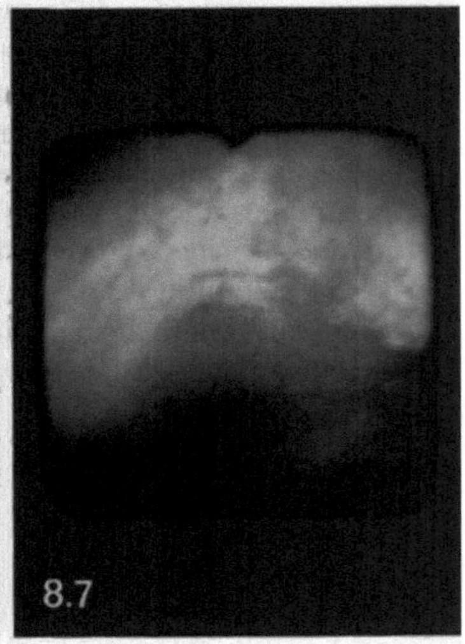
8.7

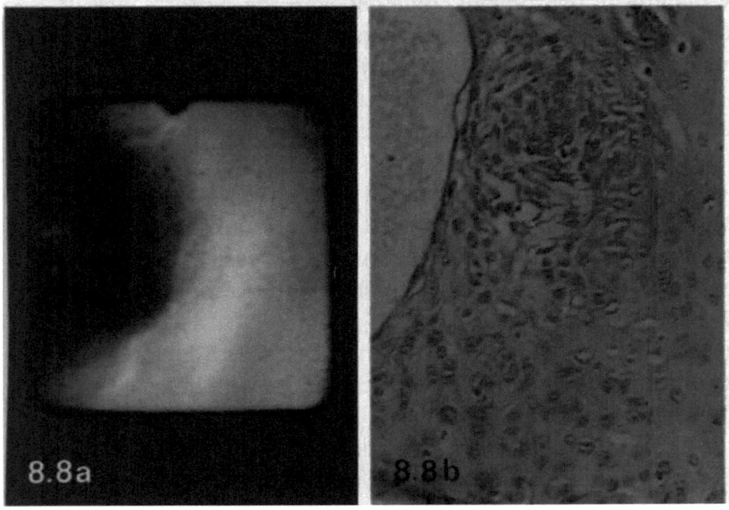
8.8a 8.8b

Other less common changes include small nodules (Figs. 8.13, 8.14), tumor mass, ulcers, and small speckles (Figs. 8.15, 8.16), with incidences of 9.4%, 9.4%, 6.8%, and 6.8% respectively. The cancer occasionally grows in the form of a polyp with a slender stalk.

5.3 Size

The size of lesion was estimated in 92 of our 135 cases. The length varied from less than 1 cm to 13 cm, being under 1 cm in 4.3% (4/92), 1–4.9 cm in 84.8% (78/92), and over 5 cm in 10.9% (10/92). The reliability of these measurements was checked in 37 surgical specimens, and in 26 they were found to be accurate to within 1 cm, for a coincidence rate of 70.3%. In eight of the remaining 11 cases, endoscopic reading was too low, suggesting a tendency toward underestimation.

5.4 Segmental Distribution

The distribution data derived from 116 of our 135 cases conformed quite well with that of more advanced cases. Of these lesions, 10.3% (12/116) were in the upper thoracic segment, 74.1% (86/116) in the midthoracic segment, and 15.5% (18/116) in the lower thoracic segment (Table 8.1).

Table 8.1. Location of lesions in 116 cases of esophageal carcinoma

Location	(*n*)	(%)
Cervical	0	0
Upper thoracic	12	10.3
Midthoracic	86	74.1
Lower thoracic	18	15.5

◁ ***Fig. 8.2.*** Early invasive squamous cell carcinoma of the midthoracic esophagus with erosion of the right anterior wall

Fig. 8.3. Early invasive squamous cell carcinoma of the midthoracic esophagus with erosion of the right wall

Fig. 8.4. Early squamous cell carcinoma of the midthoracic esophagus with erosion of the left posterior wall. The patient died 4 years after irradiation

Fig. 8.5. Early squamous cell carcinoma of the midthoracic esophagus with erosion of the right wall. The patient is alive and well 5 years after irradiation

Fig. 8.6. Carcinoma in situ of the midthoracic esophagus with erosion and congestion of the right wall

Fig. 8.7. Early squamous cell carcinoma of the midthoracic esophagus with erosion of the right wall

Fig. 8.8 a, b. Carcinoma in situ of the midthoracic esophagus. ***a*** Erosion of the left anterior wall. ***b*** Histology showing intact basal membrane

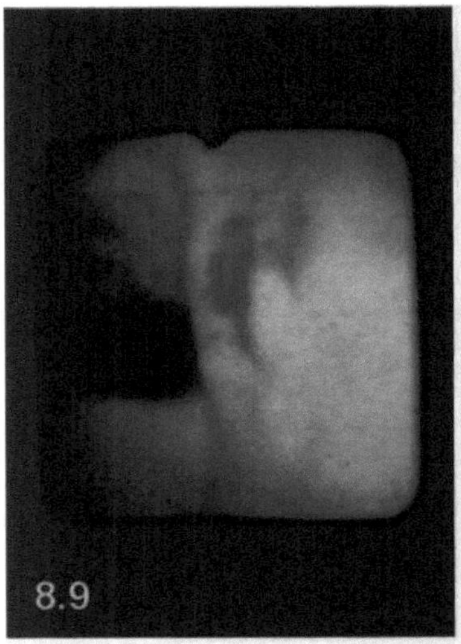
8.9

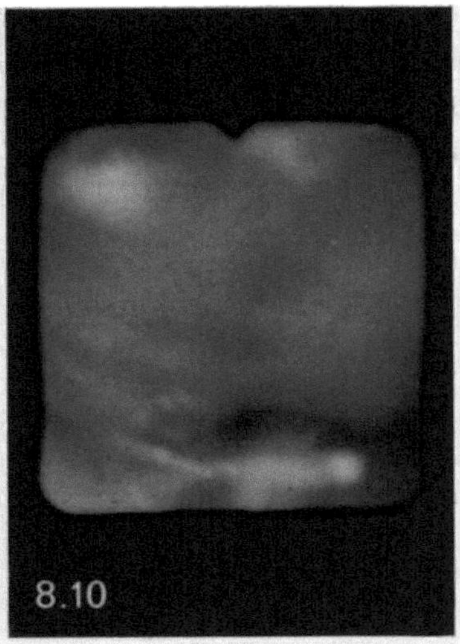
8.10

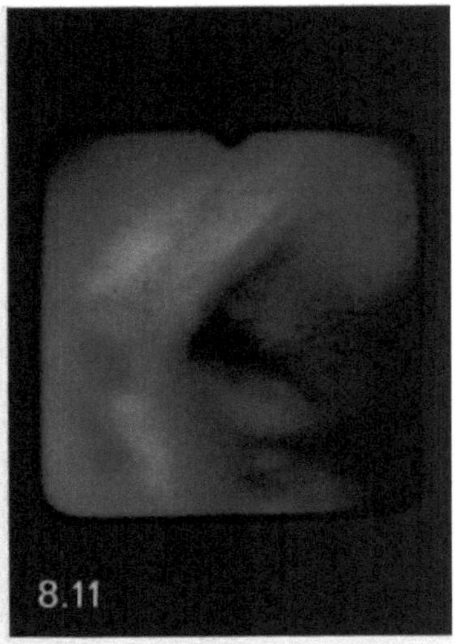
8.11

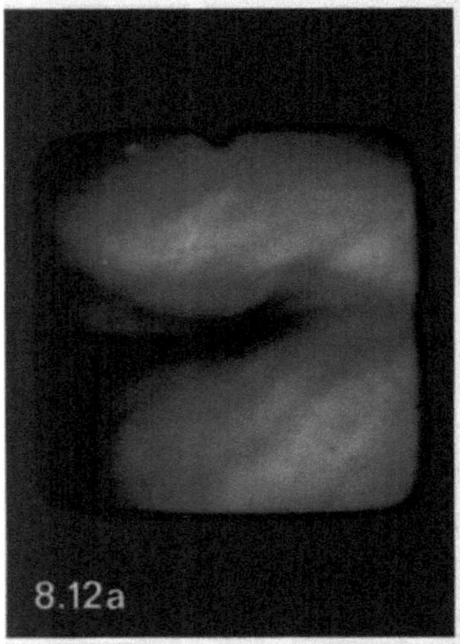
8.12a

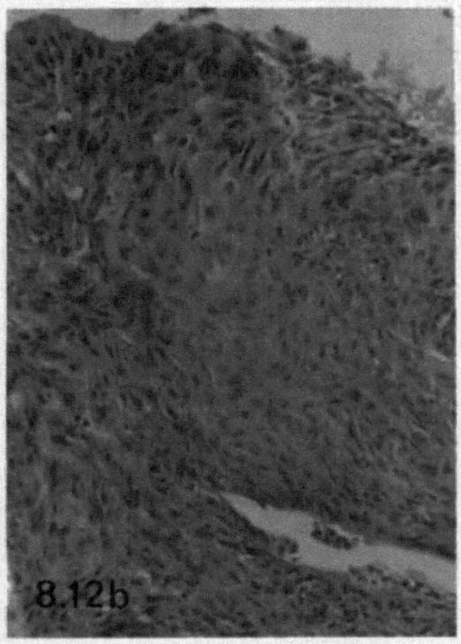
8.12b

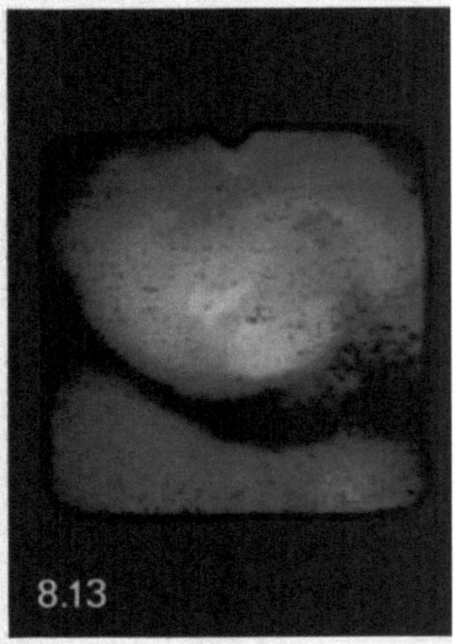
8.13

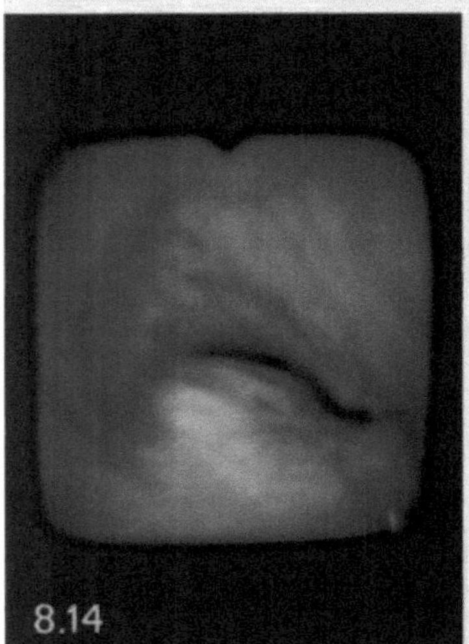
8.14

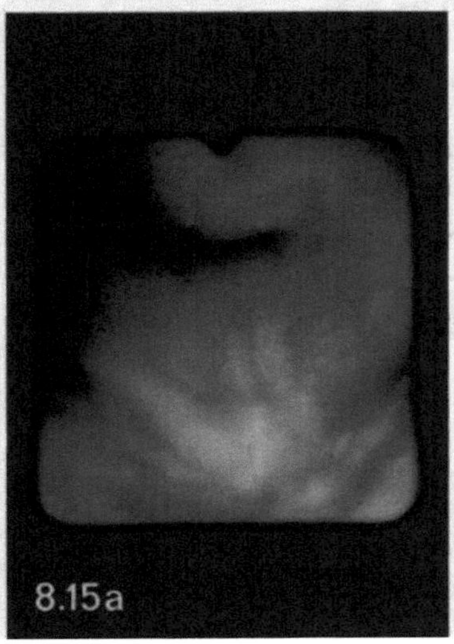
8.15a

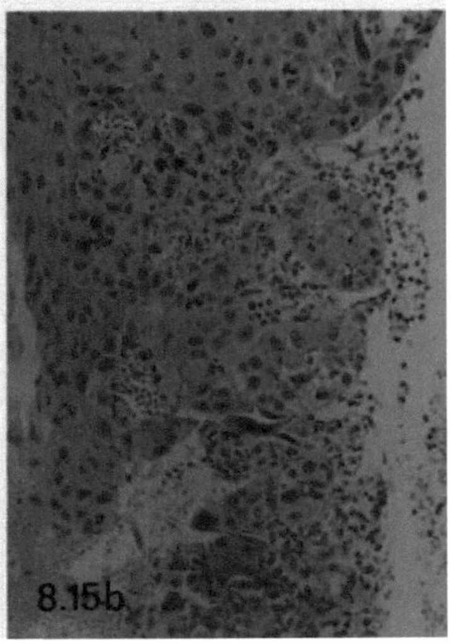
8.15b

5.5 *Circumferential Distribution*

Data enabling the investigation of possible preference of site were available in 110 of our 135 cases. The circumference of the lumen was divided into eight sectors, namely anterior (A), right anterior (RA), right (R), right posterior (RP), posterior (P), left posterior (LP), left (L), and left anterior (LA). Of the 110 lesions, 60.9% (67/110) were confined to one quadrant, 31.8% (35/110) involved two quadrants, and 7.3% (8/110) spread over three or four quadrants. There were 30 lesions on the left (LP+L+LA) and 32 on the right (RA+R+RP), a ratio of 1:1.07. The ratio of anterior (LA+A+RA) to posterior (RP+P+LP), however, was 1:1.42 (31 cases to 44), suggesting that the posterior wall of the esophagus might be more vulnerable to cancer than the anterior wall (Fig. 8.17).

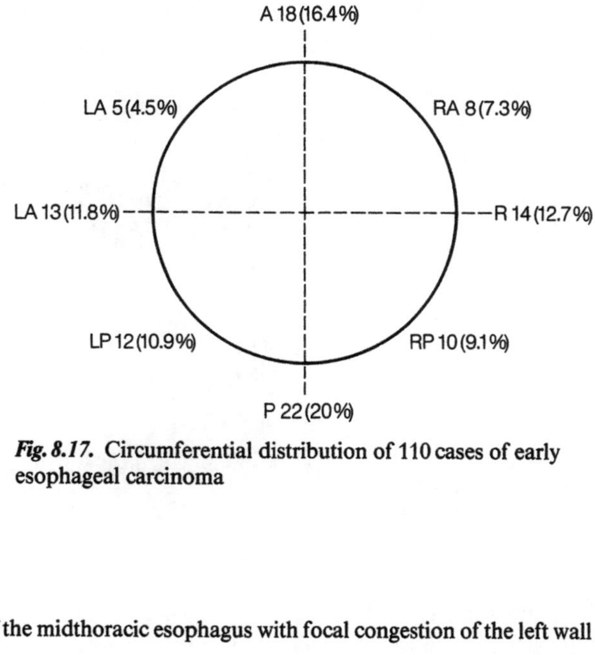

Fig. 8.17. Circumferential distribution of 110 cases of early esophageal carcinoma

◁ ***Fig. 8.9.*** Early squamous cell carcinoma of the midthoracic esophagus with focal congestion of the left wall mucosa

Fig. 8.10. Early squamous cell carcinoma of the midthoracic esophagus with focal congestion of the left posterior wall mucosa

Fig. 8.11. Early squamous cell carcinoma of the midthoracic esophagus with congestion and erosion of the right wall. The patient died over 3 years after irradiation

Fig. 8.12 a, b. Early squamous cell carcinoma of the midthoracic esophagus. ***a*** Sandpaper-like coarseness of the mucosa of the left anterior wall. ***b*** Squamous cell carcinoma

Fig. 8.13. Early invasive squamous cell carcinoma of the lower thoracic esophagus with a polyp-like tumor on the posterior wall

Fig. 8.14. Early squamous cell carcinoma of the midthoracic esophagus with small nodules on the anterior wall

Fig. 8.15 a, b. Early squamous cell carcinoma of the midthoracic esophagus. ***a*** Slightly elevated speckles and congestion of anterior wall. ***b*** Squamous cell carcinoma. The patient survived for 5 years after surgery

Fig. 8.16 see p. 228

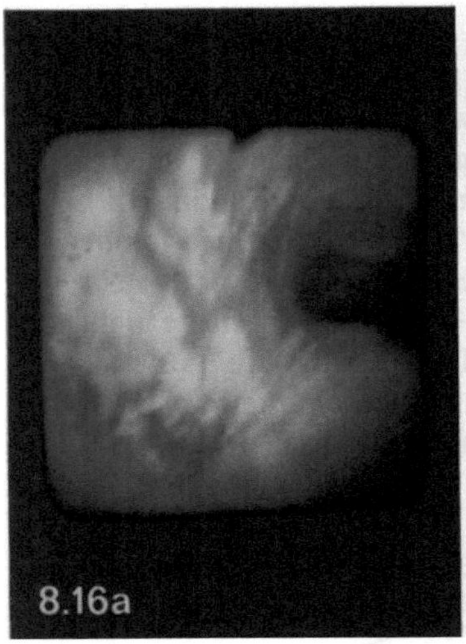

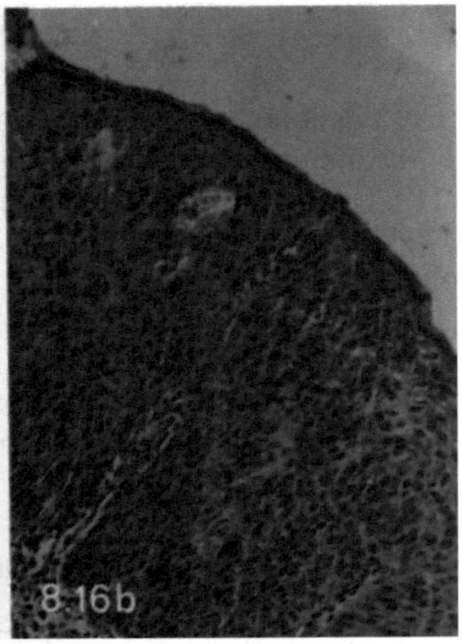

Fig. 8.17 see p. 227

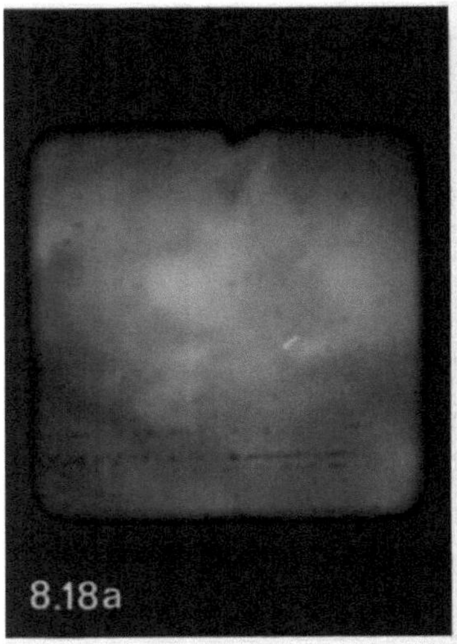

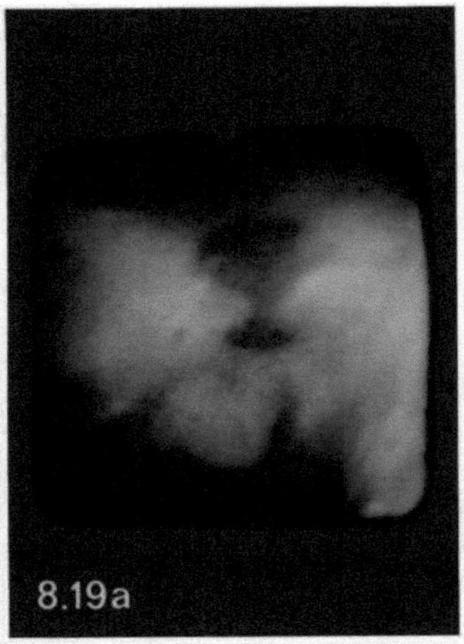

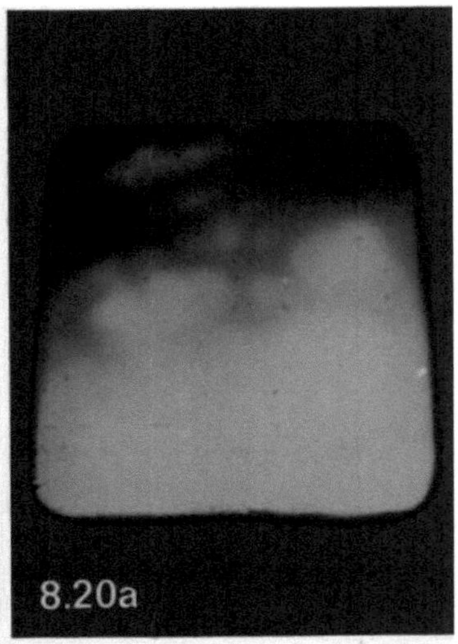

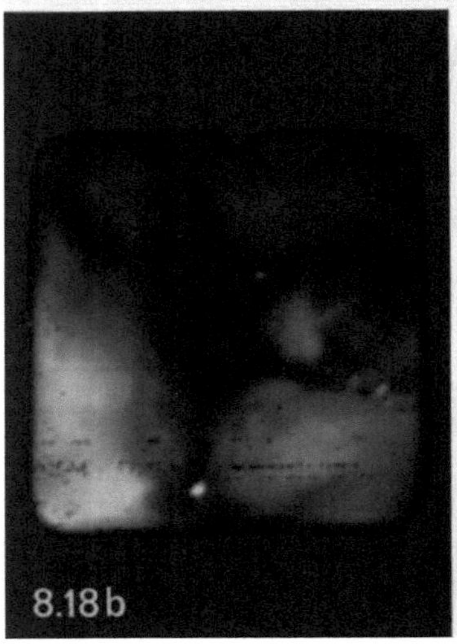

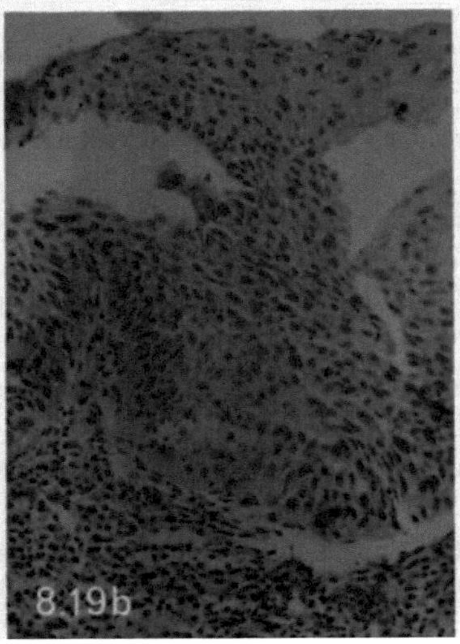

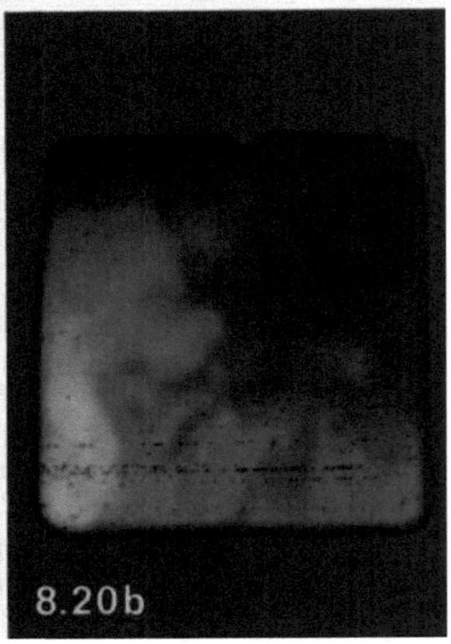

5.6 *Comparison Between Endoscopic Biopsy and Brush Cytology*

Endoscopically gross visible changes needed further confirmation by either biopsy or brush cytology. In our 135-case series the positive rates were 63.3% (31/49) for biopsy and 72.2% (70/97) for brush cytology. The overall detection rate, putting biopsy and brush cytology together, was 70.3% (78/111). In the 40 cases where biopsy and brush cytology were carried out simultaneously, biopsy was positive in 70% and brush cytology in 67.5%. Our data revealed no statistically significant difference between these two diagnostic procedures.

5.7 *Endoscopic In Vivo Staining*

All but one of our 135 patients with esophageal carcinoma had unmistakable positive balloon cytology. To our disappointment, however, 16 cases were missed on endoscopy, demonstrating clearly that endoscopic diagnosis in early esophageal carcinoma may present difficulties even for the experienced endoscopist [16]. In vivo staining with toluidine blue [17–19] or Lugol's solution has been employed in an attempt to improve the diagnostic accuracy of direct vision endoscopy.

5.7.1 *Toluidine Blue*

Toluidine blue acts as a nuclear stain of cancer cells. It infiltrates an esophageal lesion to a depth of five or six cell layers and combines with living cells as well as degenerated tissue, hence making some occult lesions visible to the naked eye. Its main disadvantage lies in the fact that it also stains inflammatory lesions.

Since March 1976, toluidine blue staining has been used in cases of early esophageal carcinoma at Yaocun Commune Hospital. During endoscopy, 10 ml 1% toluidine blue is instilled into the esophageal lumen through a plastic tube inserted via the biopsy channel. After an interval of 3 min the liquid is rinsed off with water and removed by suction. The diseased areas are then stained deep blue while the healthy mucosa retains its normal appearance (Figs. 8.18–8.20). Positive staining of the lesion was obtained in 57 of 62 cases with positive balloon cytology. Among 52 cases with positive biopsy results, 14 (26.9%) which were negative under direct vision turned out to have visible lesions after staining.

◁ ***Fig. 8.16 a, b.*** Early squamous cell carcinoma of the midthoracic esophagus. ***a*** Speckles and congestion of the right wall. ***b*** Differentiated squamous cell carcinoma

Fig. 8.17 see p. 227

Fig. 8.18 a, b. Early squamous cell carcinoma of the esophagus. ***a*** Speckles and erosion of the posterior wall mucosa. ***b*** Same lesion after 1% toluidine blue staining, tumor turning blue

Fig. 8.19 a, b. Early squamous cell carcinoma of the esophagus. ***a*** Staining by 1% toluidine blue. ***b*** Biopsy showing squamous cell carcinoma

Fig. 8.20 a, b. Early squamous cell carcinoma of the esophagus. ***a*** Speckles and erosion of the anterior wall. ***b*** Same lesion stained by 1% toluidine blue

The biopsy positive rate increased from 72.3% without staining to 83.9% with staining ($n = 62$). The staining of inflammatory lesions leads to a false-positive rate of about 20% [20].

5.7.2 Lugol's Solution

We have no personal experience with in vivo Lugol's solution staining, but this method has been widely used in other countries [21–23]. The mechanism is that Lugol's solution turns intraepithelial glycogen particles black in normal squamous epithelium. Usually a 3%–5% solution is used. Normal epithelium is stained brown and pathologic epithelium remains unstained.

Some authors have tried double staining with toluidine blue and Lugol's solution simultaneously, the joint use of the two dyes giving the full benefit of both methods [24]. The two stains have proved useful for the detection, identification, and delineation of carcinoma in situ as well as early invasive carcinoma, and hence greatly facilitate evaluation and treatment planning of both types of lesion.

5.8 Hematoporphyrin Derivative Fluorescence and Photoradiation for Localization and Treatment

The fact that hematoporphyrin derivative (HPD) accumulates and is retained to a higher degree in neoplastic, embryonic, and regenerating tissues and in lymph nodes than in normal tissues has been known for more than 30 years. Illuminated by violet light, the tumor is shown up by the fluorescence of the HPD it contains while the surrounding tissue is dark. Quartz fibers and image intensifiers have been used to produce a clearer image. Early lung cancer only 100 μm thick has been detected by fluorescence bronchoscopy [25]. Usually a dose of 2–2.5 mg/kg HPD is injected intravenously and the fluorescence endoscopy is performed after an interval of 48–96 h. No toxic effects have been observed, but some patients have exhibited sensitivity to sunlight in the form of erythema. This can be controlled by keeping the patients out of direct sunlight for 10–30 days or by covering the skin with clothing or a sunscreen lotion [25].

When activated by red light (> 600 nm), HPD in the tumor tissue can produce the cytotoxic agent singlet oxygen, resulting in rapid necrosis of tumor tissue without damage to the surrounding tissue [26]. In recent years various dye lasers and yttrium aluminum garnet (YAG) lasers have been widely used. Good results have been reported from the use of photoradiation in treating malignant tumors in animal experiments as well as in clinical trials [26–29]. Photoradiation therapy was originally limited to treating easily accessible cutaneous or superficial tumors such as those of the oropharynx and uterine cervix, but the ability of fiberoptics to deliver light directly and effectively to the tumor mass extends the applicability of photoradiation to virtually any anatomic site which can be reached by endoscopes. The fiber can easily be threaded through the biopsy channel of a fiberendoscope and subsequently inserted into the tracheobronchial tree or the esophagus [27]. Our experience with HPD fluorescence fiberesophagoscopy and photoradiation is still limited, but from clinical trials we believe that the prospects for localization and cure of early superficial esophageal carcinomas are promising. This new technique will also be helpful in palliation of advanced stenotic esophageal cancer in elderly patients and in those with severe heart or lung diseases.

6 More Advanced Carcinoma

The majority of carcinomas of the esophagus or gastric cardia are already at an advanced stage when the patient is first seen at a municipal hospital. The usual marked dysphagia and characteristic X-ray findings are sufficient for diagnosis. Unfortunately, about two-thirds of these patients are too late for curative treatment. In a total of 15978 cases of carcinoma of the esophagus and gastric cardia diagnosed at the Cancer Institute of the Chinese Academy of Medical Sciences, Beijing from 1973 to 1981, only about one-third (5150) received some form of definite treatment.

During the same period 1662 patients underwent fiberesophagoscopy, of whom altogether 722 had carcinoma of the esophagus or gastric cardia. In 520 of these cases the endoscopy was for confirmation of diagnosis and in the other 202 it was part of a post-therapeutic workup for one of various reasons, e.g., suspicion of postirradiation recurrence or postresection anastomotic relapse. Miscellaneous esophageal or gastric cardia lesions were found in another 392 cases, and the remaining 548 patients had negative endoscopic findings (Table 8.2). Fortunately, not a single complication was observed in this series.

6.1 Endoscopic Findings

The common endoscopic findings in advanced carcinoma of the esophagus and gastric cardia are as follows:

Tumor mass was the most frequent finding, being observed in 63.9% of our 520 cases. It is either nodular or cauliflower-like, bulges out of the mucosal surface from a broad base, is grayish-white in color, hard but fragile, and bleeds easily when traumatized. In most cases the overlying mucosa is destroyed.

Erosion and *ulceration* had incidences of 48.3% and 29.2% respectively. Carcinomatous ulceration, unlike the inflammatory form, tends to resemble a volcano, rising upward from the periphery with a central depression. Its rugged surface is usually covered by necrotic tissue and exudate. *Edema* and *congestion,* the natural consequences of ulceration, were found in about 50% of the 520 cases.

Narrowing of the lumen and *loss of distensibility* of the affected esophageal wall occurred in 16.5% of the 520 cases. Normal peristaltic activity of the esophageal wall is impaired or abolished by the cancerous infiltration and destruction of the muscular coat, and the space-occupying tumor mass obstructs the esophageal lumen progressively. These mechanisms make swallowing all the more difficult.

Table 8.2. Findings in 1662 fiberesophagoscopies

Findings	(*n*)	(%)
Carcinoma of esophagus	496	29.8
Confirmed after endoscopy	329	
Post-therapeutic follow-up	167	
Carcinoma of gastric cardia	226	13.6
Confirmed after endoscopy	191	
Post-therapeutic follow-up	35	
Miscellaneous	392	23.6
Negative	548	33.0

Esophageal carcinoma occasionally takes the form of a polyp, with a protuberant head and a thin stalk of variable length. The mucosa overlying the mass may appear roughened and adherent. These are also usual findings of an esophageal carcinosarcoma.

Biopsy of the cancerous lesion was performed in 445 of our 520 cases. In 378 cases the results were positive, a detection rate of 84.9%. Brush cytology was done in 109 cases, with 30 positive results, a detection rate of only 27.5%.

6.2 Endoscopic Differential Diagnosis

Esophageal *leiomyoma* has not infrequently been misdiagnosed as cancer clinically, and conversely, now and then cancer is misdiagnosed as leiomyoma. Among 329 cases of esophageal carcinoma confirmed after endoscopy, seven (2.2%) were originally considered to be leiomyoma. In our miscellaneous group of 392 endoscopies there were 270 cases involving one of various esophageal diseases, including 95 cases (35.2%) of leiomyoma. Leiomyoma ranks first among the benign conditions that might cause dysphagia. Endoscopic differentiation is mandatory and not too difficult. A submucosal, intramural, and round, oval or bizarre mass is the characteristic endoscopic finding in leiomyoma. The overlying mucosa is normal in color and texture, and the mass seems to roll under the mucosa when a wave of peristalsis passes. Contrary to the reports in the literature that the tumor is most commonly located in the lower thoracic segment, in 71.6% of the 95 cases in our series it was located in the midthoracic segment (Table 8.3).

Rarely, esophageal carcinoma behaves paradoxically. Instead of fungating and protruding into the lumen, the carcinoma spares the mucosa and infiltrates the submucosal and muscle layers. On X-ray examination the filling defect resembles that of leiomyoma in every detail. Two points might be helpful in endoscopic differentiation; first, there is fixation of the overlying mucosa to the tumor mass in carcinoma, and second, local infiltration of the muscle layer by the carcinoma deranges its distensibility.

No biopsy should be attempted if leiomyoma is suggested endoscopically. Biopsy may cause formation of scar adhesion between the mucosa and the tumor and hence increase the risk of mucosal perforation on subsequent operative enucleation.

Esophageal diverticulum was the second most common lesion in our series of 270 miscellaneous endoscopically diagnosed esophageal lesions, with 59 cases (21.9%). Dysphagia, when occurring, is usually mild and may have been present for a long period of time. Esophagography usually reveals a smooth, round or oval bulging of the esophageal wall. Sometimes the periesophageal inflammation may result in multiple foci of scar traction, giving an X-ray picture of an irregular filling defect. Endoscopically there is a smooth round hole, almost always on the anterior wall. The neck is usually broad and the dimensions of the bulge vary greatly with respiration and peristalsis. The lining epithelium is of the normal pinkish color and soft texture. Because of the possible coexistence of benign diverticulum and malignant tumor in different parts of the esophagus, the endoscopist should never be content with finding a diverticulum but should complete a thorough examination of the entire esophagus and the gastric cardia.

Hiatal hernia and reflux esophagitis is relatively rare in China. It occurred in 30 cases (7.7%) among the group of 392 endoscopically diagnosed miscellaneous diseases. The incidence was 25.0% (30/120) in esophagogastric junction lesions alone. The irregular, coarse mucosal folds seen extending from the stomach into the lower esophagus on X-ray often lead to a diagnosis of cancer of the gastric cardia. Endoscopically, the esophagogas-

Table 8.3. Location of lesions in 95 cases of leiomyoma of the esophagus

Location	(*n*)	(%)
Cervical	0	0
Upper thoracic	9	9.5
Midthoracic	68	71.6
Lower thoracic	18	18.9

tric junction is usually located at a lesser distance from the incisors. Beyond the junction, a ring-like stricture formed by the extrinsic pinching of the crus of the diaphragm can be identified. The spectrum of esophagitis may range from mild congestion and edema to marked scarring and stenosis. Brush cytology and biopsy are necessary to achieve differentiation from cancer of the gastric cardia.

Achalasia or cardiospasm usually affects teenagers and young adults with a protracted history of dysphagia. Despite the dysphagia, most patients are able to maintain a rather satisfactory general condition. In our series of 1662 endoscopies, three of 191 cases (1.6%) of carcinoma of the gastric cardia had been misdiagnosed as achalasia before endoscopy. There were 26 cases of achalasia (21.7%) among the 120 miscellaneous gastric cardia lesions. Under endoscopy the achalasic esophagogastric junction stays in spasm, but the scope tip can be introduced into the stomach with steady gentle pressure. In contrast, in most cases of carcinoma of the gastric cardia the stenosis is so inflexible that the scope tip cannot even be forced through. The lower esophageal lumen is distended tremendously in achalasia as a result of long-standing obstruction. The dilated esophagus should be well prepared by lavage and aspiration before endoscopy to ensure that no small coexistent tumor is missed.

There were 73 cases (18.6%) of *inflammatory changes* among 392 miscellaneous lesions. The conditions could be subdivided into 63 nonspecific and 10 specific (tuberculosis). Roentgenologically, most cases resemble carcinoma, and clinical differentiation is difficult.

The etiology of the *nonspecific inflammatory changes* remains uncertain. Edema, congestion, and/or stenosis were the common endoscopic findings and biopsy usually revealed nothing except chronic inflammation. A correct diagnosis can only be obtained by postoperative pathological examination.

Strictly speaking, *primary tuberculosis* of the esophagus is very rare. Most of the lesions resulted from the extension of tuberculous processes from periesophageal mediastinal lymph nodes. In our series, nine of the ten patients were female and most of them were below 40 years of age. Endoscopically, a fistula with draining pus was the characteristic finding. Sometimes the lesion may appear cancerous, with erosion, ulcer, and tumor mass; in such a case the tuberculous nature can only be confirmed by biopsy. If clinically such a diagnosis is strongly suggested, surgery should not be attempted until specific chemotherapy has proved ineffective.

Changes due to *extrinsic compression* were not infrequently encountered clinically, as they often caused dysphagia. Our 392 miscellaneous cases included 39 (9.9%) of extramural compression of the esophagus. Seven of these cases were diagnosed as vascular compression, the remainder being caused by mediastinal metastatic lymph nodes from primary foci in lung or undefined abdominal viscera, by posterior mediastinal tumors or cysts, or by nonspecific lymphadenitis. Though the etiology varied, endoscopically these lesions were characterized by a normal mucosa. In cases of abberant subclavian artery, innominate artery, or right aortic arch, pulsating compression can be seen on the posterior or anterior wall of the midthoracic esophagus. Compression from metastatic lymph nodes usually causes much more severe stenosis, and not infrequently the esophageal wall is infiltrated by tumor from the muscle layer right through to the mucosa.

Carcinosarcoma, leiomyosarcoma, fibrosarcoma, and *melanoma* are rare esophageal malignancies. Roentgenologically, they present as intraluminal masses, and endoscopically, they appear not much different from esophageal carcinoma of the intraluminal type. Melanotic melanoma has a characteristic grayish-black tinge, but the nonmelanotic variety can only be diagnosed pathologically.

6.2 Gastric Cardia

Adenocarcinoma of the gastric cardia merits special consideration because of the difficulties encountered in its diagnosis. Routine upper GI X-ray examinations, exfoliative cytology and rigid endoscopy have all failed to reveal a proportion of cases of this "occult" carcinoma. Since the invention of the fiberesophagoscope, however, the rate of diagnosis has improved greatly. The blind zone around the esophagogastric junction, which was inaccessible to the rigid scope, can now be viewed. However, the problems in diagnosis of cancer of the gastric cardia have not been wholly solved. In our series of 1 662 cases, 424 fiberesophagoscopies were performed for the identification of esophagogastric junction changes, and 191 carcinomas and 76 benign lesions were diagnosed. In a further 116 cases there were no significant changes, and in the remaining 41 (9.7%) erosion, congestion, and stricture were noted singly or in combination but biopsy and/or brush cytology yielded no positive result.

A low endoscopic discovery rate can be explained by two basic factors. The first is the growth pattern of gastric cardia cancer, which is often characterized by its submucosal invasion of the lower esophagus. In such cases fiberesophagoscopy may only reveal stenosis and stiffness of the esophagogastric junction with nodular bulging or thickening of the mucosa, which may appear pale and edematous but is usually nonulcerated. It is difficult to differentiate these findings from cicatricial stenosis resulting from reflux esophagitis, and biopsy and cytology are rarely positive.

The second factor is that the esophagogastric junction can only be viewed tangentially through the fiberesophagoscope, and on this plane the visual acuity is not so good as it is *en fące*. Fungating carcinoma can easily be recognized, but infiltrating carcinoma, with the mucosa slightly roughened and elevated, may be missed. In highly suspicious cases, multiple fiberendoscopies would be the only way of establishing or ruling out the diagnosis of carcinoma of the gastric cardia.

References

1. Hirschowitz BI, Curtiss LE, Peters CW, Pollard AM (1958) Demonstration of a new gastroscope, the "Fiberscope". Gastroenterology 35: 50
2. Hirschowitz BI (1963) A fiberoptic flexible esophagoscope. Lancet 2/1: 388
3. Hirschowitz BI (1979) A personal history of the fiberscopy. Gastroenterology 76: 864–869
4. Henley KS (1980) History of fiberoptic endoscopy. Gastroenterology 78: 1123–1124
5. Savary M, Miller G (1978) The esophagus: handbook and atlas of endoscopy. Gassmann, Solothurn, p 16
6. Shahmir M, Schuman BM (1980) Complications of fiberoptic endoscopy. Gastrointest Endosc 26/3: 86–91
7. Yamada K, Holyoke ED, Elias EG (1975) Endoscopy in patients with malignant conditions of the gastrointestinal tract. Surg Gynecol Obstet 141: 903–906
8. Block GE, Lancaster JR (1964) Adenocarcinoma of the cardioesophageal junction. Arch Surg 88: 852
9. Prolla JC, Reilly RW, Kirsner JB, Cockerham L (1977) Direct-vision endoscopic cytology and biopsy in the diagnosis of esophageal and gastric tumors: current experience. Acta Cytol (Baltimore) 2/3: 399–402
10. Bruni HC, Nelson RS (1975) Carcinoma of the esophagus and cardia: diagnostic evaluation in 113 cases. J Thorac Cardiovasc Surg 70: 367–370
11. Kasugai T, Kobayashi S, Kuno N (1978) Endoscopic cytology of the esophagus, stomach and pancreas. Acta Cytol (Baltimore) 22: 327–330
12. Winawer SJ, Sherlock P, Hajdu SI (1976) The role of upper gastrointestinal endoscopy in patients with cancer. Cancer 37: 440–448
13. Young JA, Hughes HE, Lee FD (1980) Evaluation of endoscopic brush and biopsy touch smear cytology and biopsy histology of the lower esophagus and cardia. J Clin Pathol 33/9: 811–814
14. Suzuki H, Kobayashi S, Endo M, Nakayama K (1972) Diagnosis of early esophageal cancer. Surgery 71/1: 99–103
15. Little G, Mathews HR (1980) Endoscopic assessment of esophageal disease. Br Med J 281: 1269–1270
16. Maimon HN, Dreskin RB, Cocco AE (1974) Positive esophageal cytology without detectable neoplasm. Gastrointest Endosc 20: 156
17. Shedd DP, Hukill PB, Bahn S (1965) In vivo staining properties of oral cancer. Am J Surg 110: 631–634
18. Yamakawa T, Hofe E, Kagan R, Morgenstern L (1972) The use of tolonium in the diagnosis of malignant gastric lesions. Arch Surg 104: 773–777
19. Kawai K (1978) Endoscopic examination of the digestive tract using dyes. Nippon Rinsho [Suppl.] 36: 2144–2145
20. Wang GQ, Chang FB, Tien ZJ, Tang J (1980) The clinical application of toluidine blue stain in vivo for the diagnosis of early esophageal carcinoma (in Chinese). Chin Med J 60/2: 93–95
21. Schiller W (1933) Early diagnosis of carcinoma of the cervix. Surg Gynecol Obstet 56: 210
22. Mandard AM, Toureux J, Gignoux M, Blanc L, Segal P, Mandard JC (1980) In situ carcinoma of the esophagus, macroscopic study with particular reference to the Lugol test. Endoscopy 12: 51–57
23. Toriie S, Kohli Y, Akasaka Y, Kawai K (1975) New trial for endoscopical observation of esophagus by dye scattering method. Endoscopy 7: 75–79
24. Yoshida M, Hayashi T, Suzuki S, Endo M, Tamemoto T (1976) Endoscopic toluidine blue-iodine method of the esophagus (in Japanese). Stomach Intestine 11: 359–365
25. Doiron DR, Profio E, Vincent RG, Dougherty TJ (1979) Fluorescence bronchoscopy for detection of lung cancer. Chest 76/1: 27–32
26. Dougherty TJ, Kaufman JE, Goldfarb A, Weishaupt KR, Boyle D, Mittleman A (1978) Photoradiation therapy for the treatment of malignant tumor. Cancer 38: 2628–2635
27. Dougherty TJ, Thoma RE, Royle DG, Weishaupt KR (1981) Interstitial photoradiation therapy for primary solid tumors in pet cats and dogs. Cancer Res 41: 401–404
28. Forbes IJ, Cowled PA, Leong ASY, Ward AD, Black AJ, Jacka FT (1980) Phototherapy of human tumors using hematoporphyrin derivatives. Med J Aust 2: 489–493
29. Dougherty TJ (1982) Variability in hematoporphyrin derivatives. Cancer Res 42: 1188

Chapter 9
Clinical Diagnosis

Guo Jun Huang and Wu Ying K'ai

1 Carcinoma of the Esophagus

1.1 Symptomatology

Clinical studies of early esophageal carcinoma in high-incidence areas in China during the past two decades have shown that approximately 90% of patients have mild but definite complaints related to deglutition. The most common are retrosternal discomfort or pain and senses of friction, burning, or slow passage during swallowing of food. These symptoms unsually come and go for months or even years, causing the patient no great concern until they become increasingly consistent and severe. They appear only on deglutition and are more marked when the food is coarse or hastily eaten.

Observation in the high-incidence areas has revealed that these symptoms of early carcinoma of the esophagus are usually of quite long duration; they may have been present for 2–3 years without the lesion having progressed beyond a relatively early stage. In a group of 23 untreated patients with early esophageal carcinoma established by cytologic examination, reported by Pei et al. [1], the average survival period was 43.6 months (range 20–78 months) from the time of cytologic diagnosis.

The symptoms of early esophageal carcinoma should be distinguished from those of chronic pharyngitis and esophagitis, which are also common in esophageal carcinoma high-incidence areas. Patients with chronic pharyngitis or esophagitis usually complain of an obstructive or "foreign body" sensation or of a boring, distending discomfort in the hypopharynx and the upper retrosternal region. These symptoms occur while the patient is not eating or when he merely performs the act of swallowing, but are absent on actual ingestion of food, in sharp contrast to the symptoms of early esophageal carcinoma, which appear only on swallowing food. Final differentiation, however, depends on cytologic and/or endoscopic examination.

The above-mentioned symptoms of early esophageal carcinoma are usually recorded retrospectively after a postive cytologic examination during mass screening in high-incidence areas. As they are usually mild and may appear only for a brief period of time following a long remission, they may often be ignored or forgotten, only to be recalled by the patients when they are questioned during the screening. A small number of patients, however, do seek medical examination, probably due to more marked symptoms or to their heightened awareness, and are thus more promptly diagnosed. It is apparent that public education to increase the level of awareness of both medical workers and the general population to the symptoms of early esophageal carcinoma is of utmost importance if early diagnosis and treatment of this malignancy are to be achieved. This has been carried out in some of the high-incidence areas, with good results.

Perception of sensation in the esophagus is chiefly through the vagi conected with the cerebral cortex. Spasm of the esophagus, excessive distension, cold or heat, inflammatory infiltration, swelling, etc. will give rise to pain or discomfort. The complaints in early esophageal carcinoma are probably related to local spasm, infiltration, or inflammation of the esophagus, and are aggravated during swallowing. The pain/discomfort is often felt behind the sternum, usually at a point higher than the lesion itself, but may be felt in the epigastrium if the lesion is in the lower esophagus.

Gnawing pain deep in the chest or in the back is usually produced by lesions in the mediastinum, such as periesophageal invasion by cancer, perforation of the esophagus, or mediastinitis. Acute inflammation, ulceration, and impending perforation of the esophagus may cause severe pain behind the sternum. "Heartburn," a burning sensation in the pharynx and upper retrosternal region, may occur in patients with cancer of the esophagus, but the mechanism has yet to be explained. Occasionally stimulation of the esophagus by cancer may cause precordial pain simulating angina pectoris, from which it must be differentiated. Our understanding of the symptomatology of early esophageal carcinoma remains incomplete. Further study is needed of the causes of related symptoms such as regurgitation, belching, and indigestion.

Dysphagia, a typical textbook symptom of carcinoma of the esophagus, is the most frequent major complaint of patients seeking medical aid, but is unfortunately a symptom of the late stage. The normal esophageal wall is highly elastic and distensible, and dysphagia appears only when the entire circumference is infiltrated by the cancer.

In about 10% of the patients with rather advanced disease dysphagia does not appear, and their reasons for seeking medical advice are epigastric or substernal pain, belching, or hematemesis. In rare cases the disease may be so late as to involve vocal cord paralysis, distant metastasis, perforation of the esophagus, etc. and yet there is still no obvious dysphagia.

The symptom of dysphagia is usually intermittent at first or appears only when the patient swallows hard or coarse food, but later becomes persistent. In some cases it may progress rapidly, becoming so servere that after a matter of weeks the patient can hardly swallow liquids. In others, difficulty in swallowing may advance only slowly or not at all right up to the time when terminal complications become manifest.

The degree of dysphagia is generally related to clinicopathological type, being most marked in medullary and scirrhous carcinomas, less so in fungating and ulcerative tumors, and least prominent in intraluminal lesions.

Dysphagia in carcinoma of the esophagus may be abruptly aggravated by impaction of food, or much relieved as a result of partial necrosis and sloughing of the obstructing tumor mass. Local inflammation and swelling of the esophageal mucosa and the tumor tissue usually aggravate dysphagia. Dysphagia is often severe when the patient is seen at the outpatient clinic after a long tiring trip but greatly alleviated after admission to the hospital, a good rest, and proper meals. In general, it may be said for carcinoma of the esophagus that once dysphagia has developed it tends to be progressive, but temporary partial relief is common. It follows, therefore, that a change in the severity of dysphagia during the course of the disease must not be taken as an indication of the efficacy of therapeutic measures.

Reports by Wu [2] and Pei [1] showed that the average survival time of patients with carcinoma of the esophagus after the appearance of dysphagia is approximately 9 months. This indicates that dysphagia is usually a late symptom and that the late stage occupies only a fraction of the life history of this malignancy. The appearance of dysphagia clearly does not represent the onset of the disease, nor can its disappearance be taken as indicating regression.

Another common symptom of esophageal carcinoma is the bringing up into the mouth of copious clinging mucus, which increases in volume when esophageal obstruction is severe. The mucus is so thick and tenacious that it can hardly be spat out, which is very annoying for the patient and may disturb his sleep. The mucus is produced by a reflex increase in the secretory activity of the esophageal and salivary glands as a result of inflammation and tumor infiltration of the esophageal mucosa, and esophageal retention due to tumor obstruction. Secretion decreases during sleep, but the mucus collected in the esophagus often causes coughing at night and may be the source of aspiration infections.

Carcinoma of the lower esophagus with marked obstruction often gives rise to regurgi-

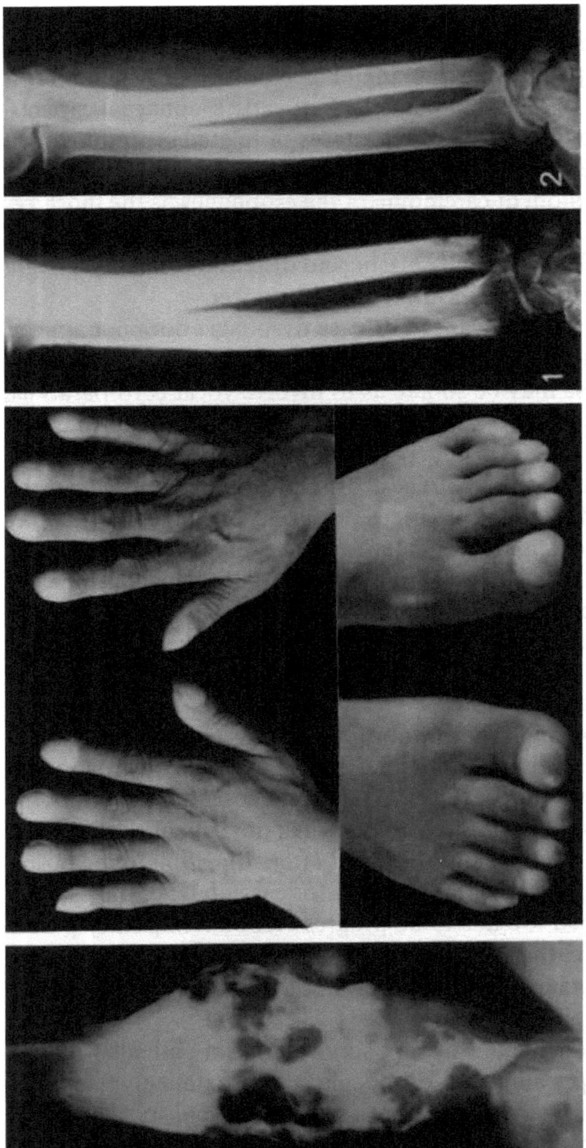

Fig. 9.1. Adenocarcinoma of the esophagus with hypertrophic osteoarthropathy. A 54-year-old man (CI Hosp. No. 292616) had low-grade fever for 9 months and dysphagia for 1 month. Barium swallow showed a 10-cm intraluminal carcinoma of the midesophagus (*left*). The patient had marked clubbing of the fingers and toes (*middle*), which subsided soon after resection of the tumor in 1978, and marked periosteal hyperplasia (*right 1*), which had disappeared by 1 year after operation (*right 2*). Pathological study of the resected specimen showed esophageal adenocarcinoma of low differentiation and adjacent intraepithelial squamous cell carcinoma

tation and belching due to retention and fermentation of ingested food material in the dilated esophagus above the tumor. When the carcinoma is located high in the esophagus, obstruction by the tumor often causes aspiration into the airway and leads to pulmonary infections. Such conditions sometimes need to be differentiated from certain late complications such as esophagotracheal fistula.

Bleeding from the esophagus giving rise to hematemesis or tarry stool is rare (unlike in carcinoma of the gastric cardia), but may be the first symptom of esophageal carcinoma. Very occasionally, particularly with intraluminal type carcinoma, there may be osteoarthropathy, with clubbing of fingers and/or toes and swelling of the ankle and knee joints (Fig. 9.1).

With advancement of the disease and progression of dysphagia and other symptoms there is a gradual deterioration: development of malnutrition, weight loss, emaciation, dehydration, constipation, general weakness, etc. During the terminal stage of the disease, marked cachexia may set in and may often be accompanied by distant metastases or other fatal complications. Common eventual conditions of patients with carcinoma of the esophagus are as follows:

1. Extreme cachexia, dehydration, and generalized debility.
2. Metastases to vital organs such as liver, lung, and brain causing jaundice, ascites, hepatic coma, dyspnea, etc.
3. Metastases to mediastinal and cervical lymph nodes leading to such problems as pain, vocal cord paralysis, tracheal compression, and airway obstruction.
4. Local invasion by the tumor causing perforation and mediastinal abscess, peritonitis, esophagotracheal fistula, pneumonitis, lung abscess, pericarditis, or rupture of large blood vessels.

Occasional patients may present one or more of the above conditions as the earliest occurring or chief symptom when first seen. Such patients may not have marked dysphagia, and this may divert the attention of the attending clinician away from esophageal carcinoma as the underlying cause.

1.2 Physical and Laboratory Examinations

In patients with relatively early carcinoma of the esophagus, physical examination may not reveal any abnormality, whereas those with more advanced disease often appear chronically ill with varying degrees of dehydration and emaciation. Some patients may have bad oral hygiene, with carious teeth and pyorrhea alveolaris. Those with marked dysphagia often have foul breath due to infection of the tumor and putrefaction of food retained in the esophagus. The clinical search for metastasis should be painstaking. The supraclavicular lymph nodes are by far the most common site of metastasis discovered on physical examination. They are often found behind or lateral to the two heads of the sternocleidomastoideus muscle and less often in the paratracheal regions or in front of the scalenus anterior muscle, being more frequently on the left than on the right. The involved lymph nodes are usually enlarged and firm and may be one or several in number, either discrete or matted together. They are often fixed to the underlying structures and hence not freely mobile. When they are small they can only be detected by careful, gentle palpation. Superficial lymph nodes in other regions, such as the axilla, are only rarely involved. Abdominal palpation to ascertain whether there are intra-abdominal or hepatic metastases is another integral part of physical examination in carcinoma of the esophagus.

Malnutrition is a common finding in patients with advanced carcinoma of the esophagus, manifested by decrease in plasma protein, dehydration, electrolyte imbalance, and multivitamin deficiency. These conditions should be carefully assessed and corrected preoperatively.

Laboratory examinations may show anemia and hypoproteinemia. As patients may be suffering from dehydration and hemoconcentration on admission, these tests should be repeated later.

1.3 Special Diagnostic Measures

The general assumption among the members of the medical profession that the diagnosis of esophageal carcinoma is simple is not only incorrect, but also dangerous. It is only true in patients with rather advanced disease where dysphagia is marked and the filling defects are conspicuous on barium swallow, most of whom can unfortunately no longer be effectively treated. In patients with earlier lesions and hence better prognoses, diagnosis is by no means easy.

Techniques for early diagnosis of carcinoma of the esophagus have been investigated extensively during the past 20 years in China [3]. Abrasive cytology by means of a blloon catheter has been developed and used in high-incidence areas, with gratifying results. A great number of cases of early esophageal carcinoma have been detected by this technique in mass screening in combination with roentgenography and fiberesophagoscopy, and the rate of early diagnosis for esophageal carcinoma has been greatly increased during the past two decades. However, a large number of cases are still not diagnosed early, and false-negative results do occur in the cases screened. In a certain number of cytologically positive cases, there still remains the difficulty of determining the site of the lesion, which may not be visualized by either fiberesophagoscopy or roentgenography. It is apparent that diagnosis of esophageal carcinoma at an early stage is still a difficult problem and needs further study.

Balloon cytology is indicated in suspected early esophageal carcinoma in which X-ray has shown nothing definite. If cytology is positive, barium swallow is repeated or esophagoscopy is performed to determine the site of the lesion. Esophagoscopic biopsy and brush cytology are done as indicated. If cytology is negative, esophagoscopy and X-ray examination may also be performed, or follow-up examination performed at intervals of 1–3 months.

Barium swallow is an important diagnostic examination for carcinoma of the esophagus and must be executed meticulously and in close correlation with clinical manifestations. In early cases where the lesion is confined to the mucosa or the submucosa with no gross destruction of the esophageal wall and no obstruction to the barium flow, it is unlikely that X-ray examination will yield definite findings. Experience in high-incidence areas has shown that only about half the cases with positive cytology had definite findings on X-ray, e.g., local thickening, tortuosity, and interruption of mucosal folds; minute ulcerations; superficial filling defects; and localized stiffness of the esophageal wall [3]. These findings cannot always be easily differentiated from irrelevant changes or the artifacts commonly seen in barium swallow films. Due to limitations in clinical facilities and equipment in hospitals in the high-incidence areas, the potential of roentgenography in the diagnosis of early esophageal carcinoma may not be fully realized. It is believed, therefore, that with more sophisticated equipment and further improvements in technique, a higher diagnostic rate of early esophageal carcinoma could certainly be achieved.

Cases involving the simultaneous presence of more than one primary carcinoma in the esophagus or of a squamous cell carcinoma in the esophagus and an adenocarcinoma of the gastric cardia have been reported quite frequently in recent years [4]. It is therefore necessary that the whole length of the esophagus and the gastric cardia be thoroughly examined during roentgenography. One should not be satisfied with the discovery of one tumor, as there is always the possibility of finding a second. A few patients with esophageal carcinoma may complain of epigastric discomfort or pain on their first visit to the clinic, and it is not exceptional for the attending clinician to request a barium examination of the stomach instead of the esophagus. If the roentgenologist then focuses his attention solely on the stomach, he is likely to miss a lesion in the esophagus.

The value of CT in the diagnosis of early esophageal carcinoma is doubtful, as the lesion in the mucosa is only very superficial. A CT scan is not necessary for the diagnosis of more advanced cases of esophageal carcinoma, but may have a place in the assessment of extraesophageal tumor invasion and of lymph node metastases.

Fiberesophagoscopy is a very important procedure in the diagnosis of early esophageal carcinoma. The fiberscope is far superior to the old rigid scope by virtue of its flexibility, smaller caliber, and much clearer and brighter visual field. Its diagnostic accuracy can be much enhanced by combination with balloon cytology, roentgenography, and intraluminal vital staining. In cases with positive balloon cytology, e.g., in mass screening in the high-incidence areas, fiberesophagoscopy is usually resorted to when roentgenography fails to confirm a lesion. Experience has shown [3] that only in 75% of the early cases detected by balloon cytology could the lesion be visualized under esophagoscopy, as local congestion, roughening, maceration, minute papillary growths, or granular appearance of the mucosal surface; in the remaining 25%, esophagoscopy did not reveal any abnormality. Endoscopic biopsy or brush cytology was positive in only 54% of the cases showing mucosal changes. In cases with positive cytology but negative roentgenography and esophagoscopy, repeat examinations should be performed at short intervals.

Intraluminal vital staining of the esophageal mucosa with 1% toluidine blue may assist visualization of early lesions under esophagoscopy. This dye stains the cancer cells but not the normal mucosa, and so can be used as an indicator in localization of the lesion. Its use has increased the rate of positive biopsy to about 80% [5]. However, a small number of false-positive and false-negative staining results occur.

In very early cases of esophageal carcinoma, there may be discrepancies between roentgenologic and endoscopic findings as regards the location and character of the lesions. In such instances it is preferable to perform a repeat roentgenography.

Accurate preoperative determination of the site and extent of an early carcinoma is very important, because such a lesion is hardly palpable during operation and the extent of resection of the esophagus may therefore not be precise. Preoperative balloon cytology repeated at different levels of the esophagus may help the surgeon by giving a rough impression of the upper limit of the lesion, but the accuracy of this technique cannot be absolutely relied on.

1.4 Clinicopathological Staging

Staging of esophageal carcinoma, as at other sites, is of importance in planning therapeutic regimes and in the evaluation of treatment results, and since 1959 has been the subject of clinicopathological studies of a large number of advanced and early cases in China. A practical clinicopathological classification was established after many years of trial and repeated modification, and was eventually agreed upon at the Yangchuan Conference on Esophageal Carcinoma in 1976 (Table 9.1).

From the clinical point of view, stages 0 and I may be designated "early", stages II and III "moderately advanced", and stage IV "late", encompassing severe complications such as esophagotracheobronchial fistula and metastases to vital organs.

In case in which neither operation nor necropsy is performed and hence the extent of pathological involvement is not known, the staging is clinical and is based chiefly on the

Table 9.1. Clinicopathological classification of esophageal carcinoma

Stage	Length of lesion	Depth of invasion	Metastasis
0	Unspecified	Confined to mucosa	None
I	<3 cm	Mucosa and submucosa	None
II	3–5 cm	Part of muscle coat	None
III	>5 cm	Beyond muscle coat with extraesophageal invasion	Regional
IV	>5 cm	Gross invasion of contiguous structures or with severe complications	Distant

roentgenographic findings of the lesion and the state of metastases as assessed on clinical grounds. When pathological findings are available, the staging is clinicopathological and is based chiefly on the extent of tumor invasion and the state of metastasis. When the lesion is confined to the mucosa without metastasis it is classified as stage 0, and is either a carcinoma in situ or an early infiltrative carcinoma. The length of such a lesion is difficult to assess and may exceed 5 cm, and is therefore not taken as a criterion for classification. When the tumor invades the submucosa but not the muscle coat, it is classified as stage I. Stages 0, I, and II include only cases without evidence of lymph node metastasis; when there is lymph node involvement, the carcinoma is classified as stage III or IV, depending on whether the metastasis is regional or distant.

Postsurgical clinicopathological classification is based upon findings from clinical examination, operative exploration, and pathological studies of the resected specimen at the time of surgery, and in general is not to be revised by subsequent findings on follow-up.

Regional lymph node metastasis in carcinoma of the midthoracic esophagus means involvement of the mediastinal nodes. Involvement of nodes outside the mediastinum, such as cervical or intra-abdominal nodes, is considered distant. In carcinoma of the cervical or upper thoracic esophagus, however, involvement of the cervical (including supraclavicular) nodes is still considered regional. Likewise, in carcinoma of the lower thoracic or abdominal esophagus, metastasis to lymph nodes of the lower mediastinim (below the level of tracheal bifurcation) and to the paracardiac lymph nodes is considered regional.

The clinicopathological classification of esophageal carcinoma used in China is essentially the same as the TNM classification published by the UICC in 1978 [6]. One difference is that the former classification is probably a little more convenient because it applies equally well to the cervical, thoracic, and abdominal parts of the esophagus. It is to be noted that stage I in the TNM system encompasses stages 0 and I as classified in China.

1.5 Natural History

On the basis of correlated studies in epidemiology, pathogenesis, pathology, and clinical course, we propose dividing the natural history of esophageal carcinoma into four phases: initial, developing, overt, and terminal.

Initial Phase. The initial phase of esophageal carcinoma covers a long period, possibly 20 years or more. The first changes are mild to moderate hyperplasia of the basal epithelial cells of the esophageal mucosa. As the pathologic process progresses, more marked hyperplasia and dysplasia of the epithelial cells are seen, involving not only the basal layer but also the intermediate layer of the mucosa. Hyperchromatism and dyskaryosis are evident in these cells. The changes may progress or regress depending on subsequent circumstances; they are precancerous in nature but may still be reversible. Preventive measures may be effective in this phase.

Developing Phase. The next step is the development of cancer in situ, which is clinically latent and may remain so for a long time. Eventually the growth breaks through the basal layer and becomes an infiltrative cancer, which may present as a granular plaque, protruding nodule, or depressed shallow ulcer (Figs. 9.2, 9.3). These changes are definitely cancerous and irreversible, but the lesion remains within the limit of the mucosa and submucosa for some time. In the clinicopathological classification this is stage I. In a series of 253 cases of stage I esophageal cancer reported by Shao and Huang, there were 99 carcinomas in situ (39.1%) and 154 early infiltrative carcinomas (60.9%) [7].

Overt Phase. This is the main clinical phase, including all stage II and III esophageal carcinomas, with obvious symptoms and signs, such as progressive dysphagia and characteristic roentgenologic findings of filling defects and obstruction (Fig. 9.4). The cancer may be of the medullary, fungating, ulcerative, scirrhous, or intraluminal type [8, 9]. Once the cancer is in this phase it progresses rather rapidly. In some cases it may gradually enlarge from an originally small localized early lesion and in the process invade the deep layers of the esophageal wall, and in others it may develop from a superficial but large stage I

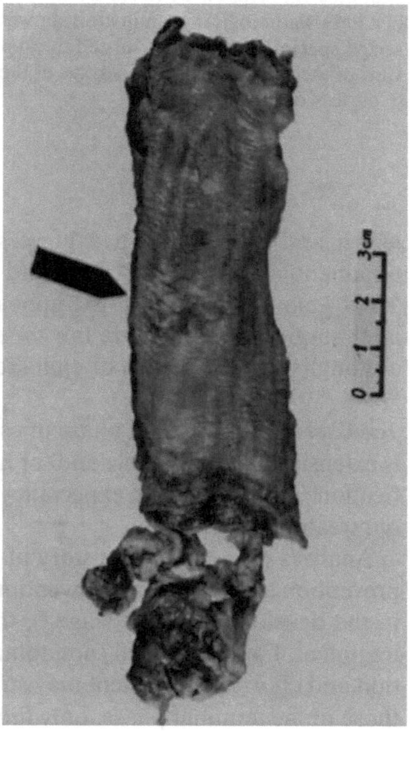

Fig. 9.2. Resected specimen of early infiltrative (stage I) carcinoma of the esophagus showing depressed shallow ulceration. A 52-year-old man had retrosternal discomfort on swallowing for a year. Balloon cytology (during mass screening) was positive and fiberesophagoscopy revealed ulceration of the mucosa at 32 cm, shown on biopsy to be squamous cell carcinoma. Resection with intrathoracic esophagogastrostomy was performed in October 1981, followed by smooth recovery. (Courtesy of Anyang Tumor Hospital)

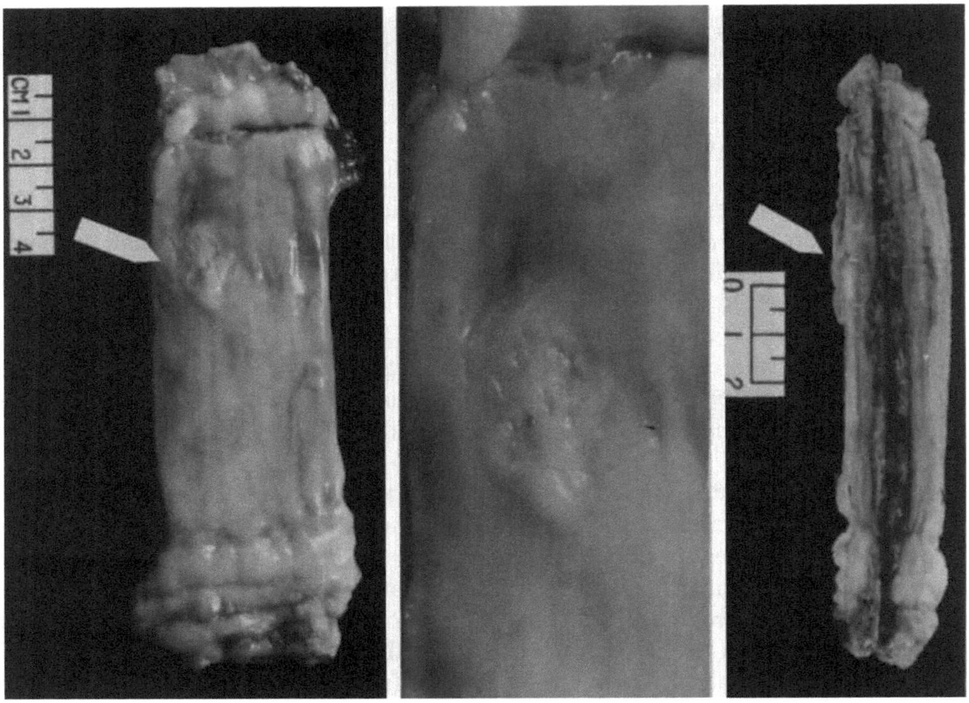

Fig. 9.3. A 55-year-old man (FW Hosp. No. 95363) had retrosternal pain on swallowing food for 6 months. Three barium studies were all negative. Esophagoscopy revealed a 1.5-cm roughening and papillary appearance of mucosa at 31 cm, and biopsy was positive for carcinoma. Resection was carried out in December 1963. Pathological examination showed early infiltrative (stage I) squamous cell carcinoma. *Left:* Resected specimen showing localized thickening and shallow ulceration of the mucosa. *Middle:* Magnified view of the lesion. *Right:* Cut surface of the esophagus showing invasion of tumor only to the submucosa. (Courtesy of Fuwai Hospital)

lesion and rapidly attain a great size. The average survival period without effective treatment in two series of 74 and 23 cases of esophageal carcinoma [2, 1] was only 9.4–9.7 months from the first appearance of symptoms. The operability and prognosis after surgical treatment are fair for stage II lesions but much less favorable in stage III, although a certain degree of palliation is still feasible in a good number of cases.

Terminal Phase. The final phase of esophageal carcinoma is usually very short. The cancer is extensive and inoperable and/or has distant metastases, being stage IV in clinical classification. The average life expectancy of a patient in this stage is only about 3 months without treatment [2].

Analysis of the natural history of an esophageal malignancy is of value in considering prevention and treatment. Prevention should be stressed in the initial phase, and for cases in the developing phase (stage I), the emphasis is on early detection and early surgical treatment. For esophageal carcinoma in the overt phase (stages II and III), careful evaluation and choice of treatment may still bring about a 5-year survival rate of 20%–40%. For those in the terminal phase, only limited palliation can be expected at best [10].

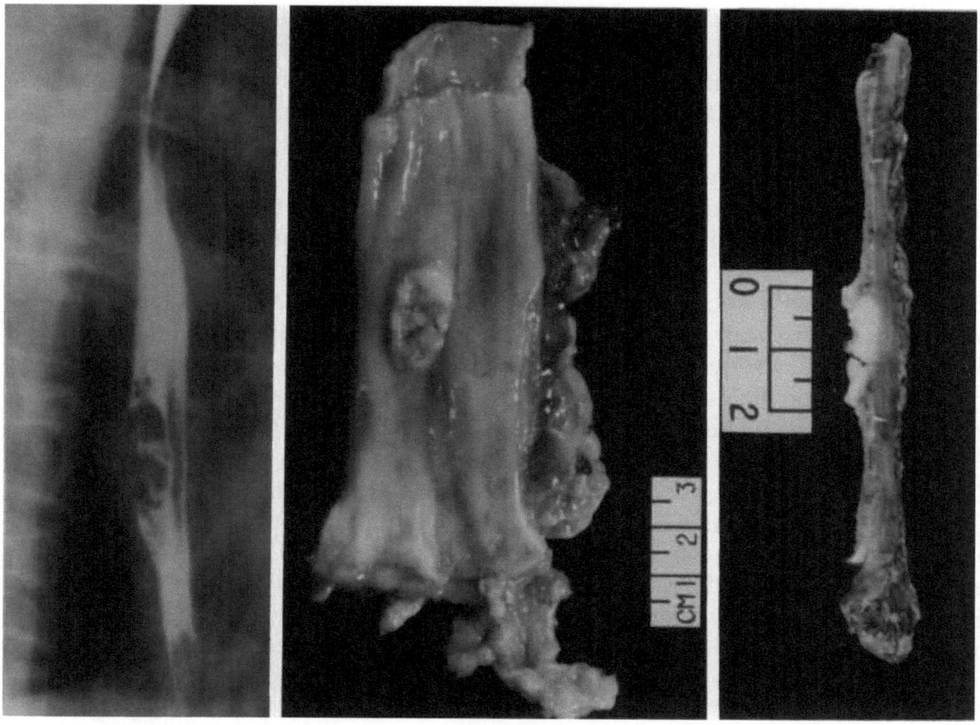

Fig. 9.4. Stage II esophageal carcinoma. A 43-year-old man (FW Hosp. No. 97443) had retrosternal pain on swallowing for 3 months. Barium esophagography revealed a localized filling defect of the lower thoracic esophagus *(left)*. Resection with supra-aortic esophagogastrostomy was performed in November 1963, and the specimen showed a fungating lesion with shallow ulceration *(middle)*. The cut surface showed tumor invasion of part of the muscle coat *(right)*. Pathology: squamous cell carcinoma with no evidence of lymph node metastasis. (Courtesy of Fuwai Hospital)

1.6 Differential Diagnosis

The differential diagnosis of carcinoma of the esophagus depends largely upon careful X-ray and esophagoscopic examination (For details see Chaps 7, 8). Based on clinical history, symptoms, and signs, clinicians should keep several conditions in mind.

Functional Dysphagia. The swallowing mechanism and peristalsis of the esophagus are complex and effected by the central nervous system through different nerve supplies. Motor fibers of the glossopharyngeal nerves and the vagal nerves originate partly from the dorsal vagoglossopharyngeal nucleus and partly from the ambiguous nucleus. Consequently, difficulty in swallowing may be one of the manifestations of disease of the medulla oblongata or may be caused by injury to the supranuclear cortical innervation, usually as a result of arteriosclerosis. Under such circumstances barium swallow frequently shows barium aspiration into the trachea, retention of barium in the pharynx, epiglottic vallecula, and bilateral piriform sinuses, and sluggishness of barium passage through the esophagus. The patients usually have other nervous disturbances of the pharynx and larynx.

Myasthenia Gravis. Patients with myasthenia gravis may present difficulty in swallowing together with other manifestations such as ptosis, blurring of vision or diplopia, weakness in muscular activity, mumbling of words, difficulty in chewing, or even problems in breathing. Muscular weakness may have been present for a long time before dysphagia sets in. In about half of the patients with myasthenia gravis there is enlargement or tumor of the thymus, which may or may not be shown on X-ray examination or CT scan. A test dose of Prostigmin (neostigmine) subcutaneously may bring about marked relief of myasthenic symptoms. Barium swallow, of course, will rule out carcinoma.

Functional Spasm. Functional spasm of the esophagus may cause difficulty in swallowing which is characteristically intermittent and may be relieved by antispasmodic drugs. The filling on barium swallow may show a typical corkscrew or beaded appearance, but the mucosal lining of the esophagus is smooth. In case of doubt, balloon cytology and esophagoscopy should be carried out to rule out carcinoma.

Dysphagia of Extraesophageal Origin. Conditions outside the esophagus may cause dysphagia of varying severity and may require differentiation from esophageal carcinoma. Dysphagia lusoria is the name assigned to difficulty in swallowing due to compression of the esophagus as a result of developmental anomalies, such as double aortic arches, aberrant right subclavian artery, or right-sided aortic arch with left descending aorta (Figs. 9.5, 9.6). In elderly people with advanced arteriosclerotic changes of the aorta, compression on the

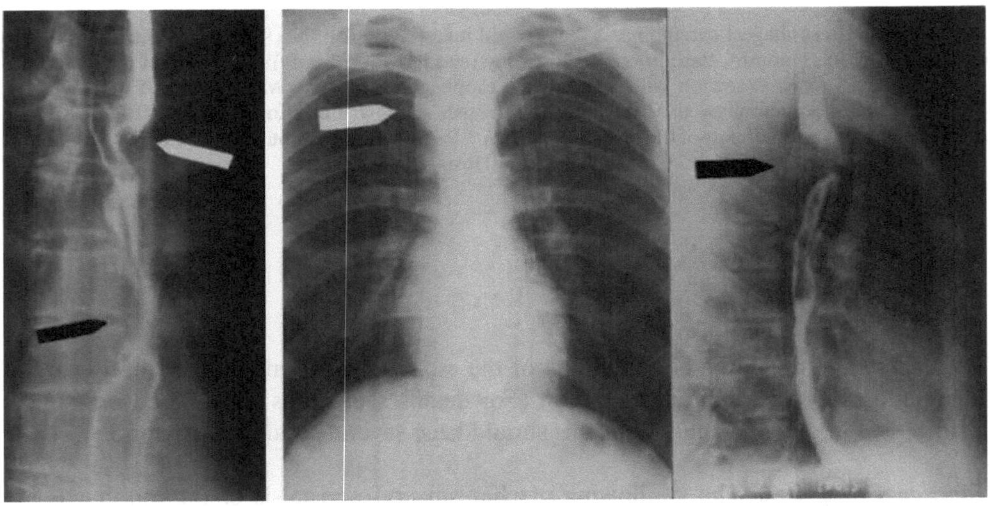

Fig. 9.5 (left). Carcinoma of the esophagus with concomitant aberrant right subclavian artery. A 64-year-old woman (CI Hosp. No. 303 331) had foreign body sensation on swallowing for 3 years and progressive dysphagia for 10 months. Esophagography showed a filling defect of about 6 cm below the tracheal bifurcation *(lower arrow)* and an oblique compression of the esophagus just above the aortic arch *(upper arrow)*. Esophagoscopy revealed an extramural pulsating ridge situated posteriorly at level of aortic arch and tumor growth at 28 cm from the upper incisors. The carcinoma was resected in July 1979 with confirmation of the aberrant right subclavian artery, which was not treated. The patient died 1 year later of metastases

Fig. 9.6 (middle, right). A 32-year-old man (CI Hosp. No. 181 737) complained of sluggishness of food passage on eating and mild shortness of breath for about a year. Roentgenography showed a right-sided aortic arch *(middle)* causing compression of the esophagus *(right)*. No operation was undertaken esophagus by aneurysm should always be borne in mind, and X-ray examination, including aortography, are indicated. Diffuse elongation and tortuosity of the thoracic descending aorta may also lead to dysphagia, which is usually mild but requires examination to rule out concomitant esophageal carcinoma. A prominent rigid left main bronchus in old age may be a cause of esophageal compression and mild dysphagia. Mediastinal tumor, lymph node enlargement, and intrathoracic goiter may also occasionally compress the esophagus. In all these conditions, dysphagia is usually mild, long-standing, and stable and no mucosal destruction is revealed on barium swallow examination. Lung cancer adjacent to the esophagus (or less commonly its metastatic lymph modes) may compress or invade the esophagus with destruction of the wall, simulating or being mistaken for esophageal carcinoma.

*1.7 **Other Diseases of the Esophagus***

Benign Stricture. The most commom benign stricture of the esophagus is that resulting from accidental swallowing of acid, alkali, or other corrosive agents by children. Cicatricial stricture due to chronic reflux esophagitis, rather rare in China, usually occurs in the lower segment of the esophagus and is frequently accompanied by hiatal hernia or congenital short esophagus, with a history of chronic esophagitis and other related symptoms. Benign strictures may not be easy to differentiate from carcinoma of the esophagus on X-ray. On rare occasions carcinoma may develop from the lesion of an old benign stricture, a fact that must be borne in mind by clinicians. Endoscopy and biopsy are usually necessary in differential diagnosis.

Achalasia. The main symptom in patients with achalasia is dysphagia, usually long-standing with periods of remission but overall slow progression. The average age of the patients

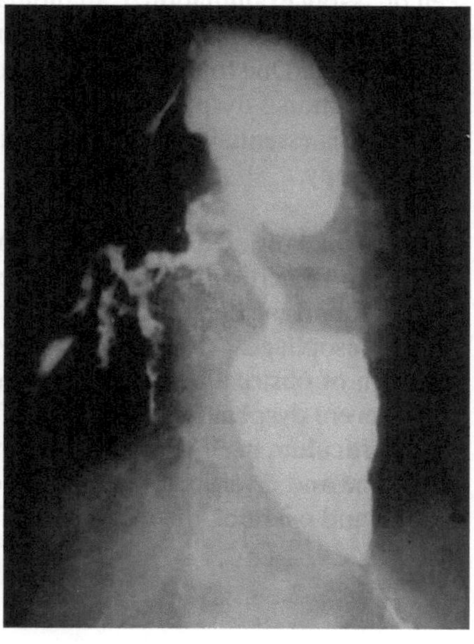

Fig. 9.7. A 50-year-old woman (CI Hosp. No. 334803) had a 16-year history of achalasia with dysphagia which had been aggravated and accompanied by cough and purulent sputum for 4 months. Barium study showed typical achalasia with a marked constricting filling defect at the midesophagus and an esophagopulmonary fistula. Esophagoscopic biopsy revealed squamous cell carcinoma. No operation was performed and the patient died 2 months later

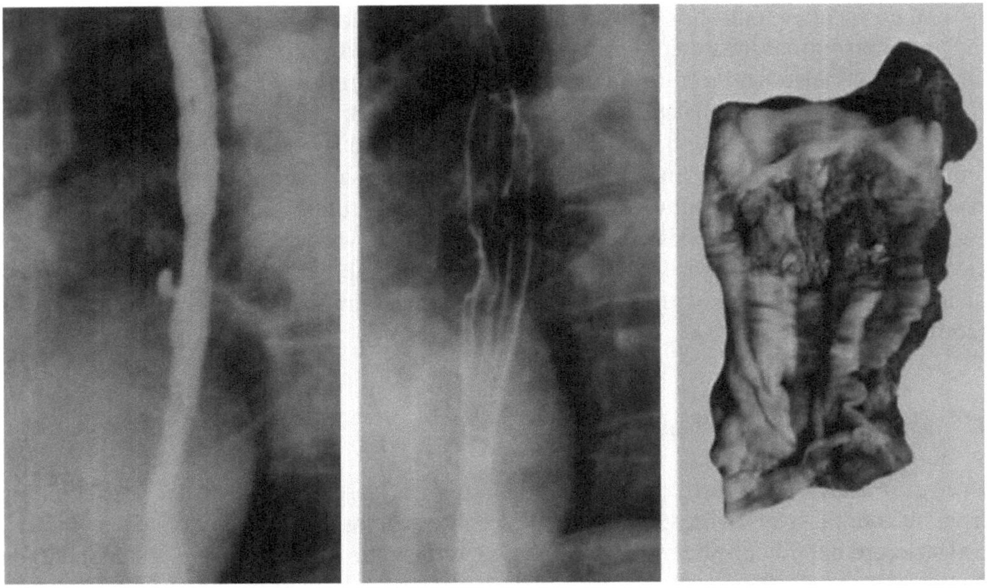

Fig. 9.8. Esophageal carcinoma at the site of a diverticulum. A 51-year-old man (FW Hosp. No. 7470), discovered to have an esophageal diverticulum in 1957 *(left)*, was followed up yearly with no change until 1961, when a filling defect was found at the site of the previous diverticulum *(middle)*. Resection was then carried out, and the specimen *(right)* showed squamous cell carcinoma on pathological examination. The patient is alive and well 21 years after operation. (Courtesy of Fuwai Hospital)

is lower than in carcinoma of the esophagus. In spite of the prolonged dysphagia the nutritional status of the patient is usually fairly well maintained. Many achalasia patients have formed the habit of counteracting difficulty in swallowing by drinking a large amount of hot water with their meals. Characteristic features of achalasia can usually be seen on X-ray examination. Carcinoma of the esophagus developed on the basis of achalasia has been reported (Fig. 9.7), and may develop in any part of the esophagus or at the gastric cardia. Due to marked enlargement of the esophageal lumen, there may be no apparent additional dysphagia resulting from cancer development. In order to avoid misdiagnosis, it is essential that the esophagus be thoroughly irrigated before barium swallow or endoscopy.

Diverticulum. Pulsion diverticulum of the pharyngoesophageal junction is very rare in China. Traction diverticuli of the thoracic esophagus are quite common, however, and are frequently found incidentally during barium examination for other purposes. Patients with thoracic esophageal diverticulum may be entirely symptom-free or may complain of a sensation of obstruction on swallowing, retrosternal discomfort, or other symptoms, but rarely severe dysphagia. Carcinoma of the esophagus may develop at any site, including the diverticulum itself (Fig. 9.8). However, it is not infrequent to find a patient with both carcinoma and diverticulum, and in such a case clinicians may be distracted by the diverticulum and overlook the carcinoma (Fig. 9.9).

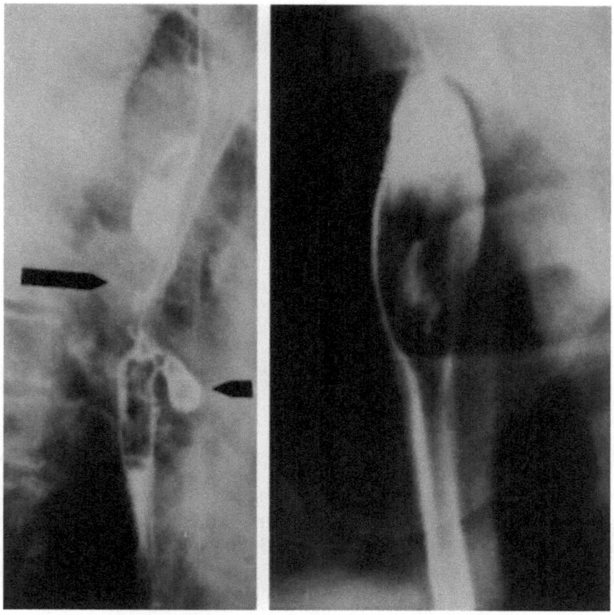

Fig. 9.9 (left). Simultaneous esophageal carcinoma and diverticulum. A 58-year-old man (CI Hosp. No. 237698) had progressive dysphagia for a month. Barium study revealed esophageal carcinoma *(upper arrow)* just above the site of a traction diverticulum *(lower arrow)*; both were confirmed at operation in 1975. The patient died 5 years later of liver metastases

Fig. 9.10 (right). Tuberculosis of the cervical esophagus. A 44-year-old woman (CI Hosp. No. 290204) had mild dysphagia for 2 months. Balloon cytology was negative for carcinoma. Barium study showed filling defect and ulceration, which disappeared completely after a 3-month course of antituberculosis therapy

Tuberculosis. Primary tuberculosis of the esophagus is rare but may occur in younger patients, causing regional destruction of the esophageal mucosa. On X-ray examination it may be extremely difficult to differentiate from carcinoma of the esophagus (Fig. 9.10). Most patients are young adults, usually with tuberculosis of the lung or mediastinal lymph nodes. Dysphagia is usually mild with no marked progression. Balloon cytology and endoscopic biopsy are negative for carcinoma. Antituberculosis treatment is usually effective within a relatively short period of time, and this may be the only means of differential diagnosis.

Leiomyoma. Leiomyoma is the most common benign neoplasm of the esophagus. It is an extramucosal tumor which grows slowly, causing no symptoms or only a slight sensation of obstruction on swallowing solid food. In cases where the tumor is very irregular in configuration or there is ulceration of the overlying esophageal mucosa, carcinoma may be simulated on X-ray. In the majority of patients, however, accurate differential diagnosis is not difficult, based on lower age, milder symptoms, and typical roentgenologic findings. Esophagoscopy may be done if necessary. In case where the mucosa appears normal under endoscopy, deep biopsy is to be avoided as this may cause adhesion between tumor and mucosa, increasing the risk of perforation of the mucosa on subsequent enucleation of the tumor. One must be aware of the possibility of coexistent carcinoma in a case of esophageal leiomyoma.

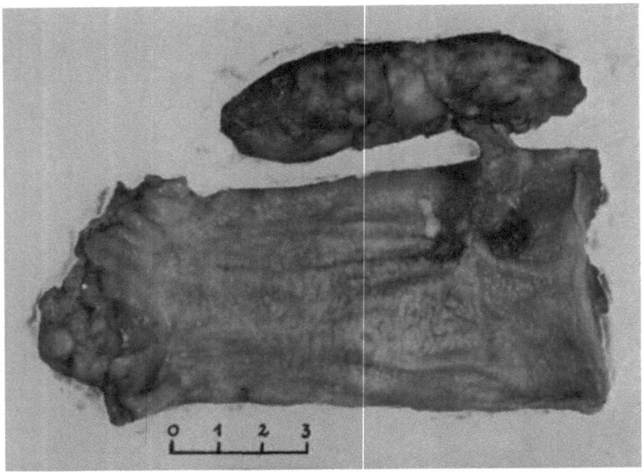

Fig. 9.11. Carcinosarcoma of the esophagus. A 61-year-old man (CI Hosp. No. 173164) had dysphagia for a month. Barium study revealed a filling defect of 13×4.8 cm at the midthoracic esophagus. The resected specimen showed a polypoid intraluminal growth with a thin stalk. Pathological study showed carcinosarcoma of the esophagus

Other Tumors. Leiomyosarcoma, sarcoma, and carcinosarcoma are rare malignant tumors of the esophagus which clinically are not readily distinguishable from esophageal carcinoma. However, *leiomyosarcoma* usually retains its extramucosal character, with relatively mild destruction of the mucosa even when the tumor attains a great size. *Sarcoma* and *carcinosarcoma,* on the other hand, frequently appear as a polypoid intraluminal growth on a thin pedicle or stalk, which may be long enough to allow part of the tumor mass to protrude into the mouth (Fig. 9.11). Differential diagnosis of these tumors depends chiefly on roentgenography and endoscopic biopsy.

2 Carcinoma of the Gastric Cardia

Statistics from various clinical centers show that the ratio between cases of carcinoma of the gastric cardia and of carcinoma of the esophagus is approximately 1:2 [11, 14], although a few centers report a ratio of nearly 1:1 [12, 13].

Carcinoma of the gastric cardia and of the lower esophagus may have similar clinical manifestations. Carcinoma of the gastric cardia frequently encroaches upon the lower esophagus in its advanced stages, as carcinoma of the lower esophagus occasionally does upon the gastric cardia. Distinguishing carcinoma of the gastric cardia from that of the esophagus may then be quite difficult even on X-ray examination. Indeed, it is sometimes quite impossible to determine the exact site of origin. Adenocarcinoma may develop from the esophageal epithelium, and an epidermoid carcinoma may appear to involve mainly the gastric cardia. For these reasons, we have adopted a practical classification for these junctional carcinomas; we designate all squamous cell tumors as carcinoma of the esophagus and all adenocarcinomas as carcinoma of the gastric cardia. Experience has shown this classification to be correct in the vast majority of cases.

Carcinoma of the gastric cardia is even more silent in its early stage than carcinoma of the esophagus. Its early manifestations may merely be some upper abdominal or epigastric discomfort, vague pain, or a burning sensation, which are also common symptoms of peptic ulcer. Dysphagia is a late symptom and is usually not as severe and rapidly progressing as in esophageal carcinoma. It is not infrequent to see patients with terminal carcinoma of the gastric cardia who have never had marked dysphagia.

Bleeding from the tumor is a common sign of carcinoma of the gastric cardia. It is usually occult and small in amount, but may be frank and severe, causing hematemesis or giving rise to tarry stools. In a series of 170 cases, Sun and associates [15] reported massive bleeding as the major symptom in 10 cases (5.9%). Anemia and its sequelae are much more common in carcinoma of the gastric cardia than in carcinoma of the esophagus. It is important to point out that severe hemorrhage may occasionally occur in the early stages perhaps even being the first symptom and fortunately leading to early diagnosis.

Persistent dull aching or pain in the upper abdomen or the back is a late symptom of cardiac carcinoma, usually indicating extensive involvement of the retroperitoneal organs, and is often a sign of unresectability.

In early cases, both physical and laboratory examinations may show nothing noteworthy. In patients with more advanced disease, anemia, hypoproteinemia, edema, and various degrees of cachexia are common findings. Dehydration is uncommon, as most patients do not have severe dysphagia. In extremely advanced cases, upper abdominal tenderness and mass, ascites, and extensive intraperitoneal metastases may be found. Physical examination should include a digital rectal examination to rule out pelvic tumor implantations, which can be distinguished from scybala by their nonpitting consistency on digital pressure.

Balloon cytology, although rather efficient in the detection of early esophageal carcinoma in high-incidence areas, is not very effective for early detection of cancer of the gastric cardia, probably because of the relatively small size of the balloon, which cannot obtain good contact with the surface of the cardiac tumor. In recent years larger balloons have been used, with better preliminary results being reported.

X-ray examination is an important means of diagnosis in carcinoma of the gastric cardia. In advanced cases the tumor mass may be visible through the air-filled fundus. Barium contrasted with air can further outline the margins of the tumor mass and show mucosal destruction, these being the two cardinal X-ray findings in the diagnosis of advanced cases. However, the accuracy of X-ray examination in the determination of the extent of tumor involvement of the gastric wall along the lesser curvature is much lower than in esophageal carcinoma.

In early carcinoma of the gastric cardia, routine roentgenography may not reveal the lesion. Use of the double-contrast technique with barium and air may reveal a crater with elevated edges in the vicinity of the cardiac orifice, which is likely to be an early appearance of carcinoma of the gastric cardia, but the diagnosis has to be confirmed by endoscopic biopsy. Just as one should not overlook the gastric cardia during X-ray of the esophagus, so must the esophagus be inspected in an examination of the gastric cardia, in order to reveal any concomitant disease.

The fiberesophagoscope has recently become one of the indispensable diagnostic tools for early carcinoma of the gastric cardia. In suspected cases of tumor of the gastric cardia where X-ray cannot establish the diagnosis, balloon cytology and fiberesophagoscopy with biopsy should be performed. If no definite diagnosis can be made, it is advisable to repeat the appropriate examinations 3–4 weeks later.

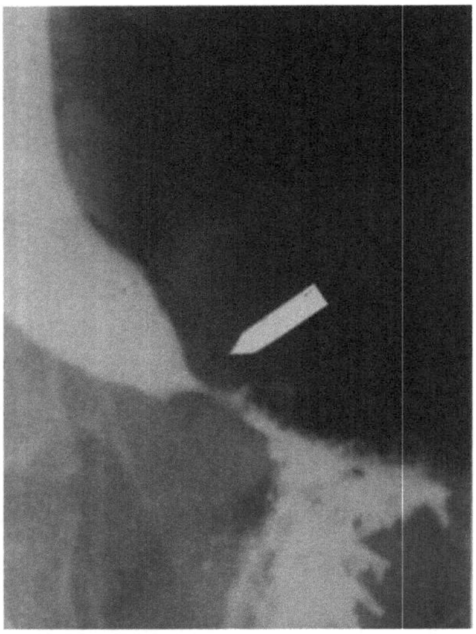

Fig. 9.12. Functional spasm of the cardiac end of the esophagus misdiagnosed as carcinoma. A 43-year-old man (CI Hosp. No. 85432) had dysphagia for 2 months. Narrowing at the esophagogastric junction *(arrow)* was shown on barium study, and a diagnosis of carcinoma of the gastric cardia was made. Exploratory laparotomy was performed in 1965 and no tumor was found. The patient was well on follow-up in 1980

It may sometimes be necessary to differentiate carcinoma of the gastric cardia from achalasia, esophagitis, and benign stricture of the lower esophagus. Patients with achalasia usually have a longer history, more marked dysphagia, a lower average age, and better general condition. Belching of copious quantities of ingested food material is more common in achalasia. On X-ray examination the esophagus is usually found to be tortuous and markedly dilated, with a smooth, symmetrical, funnel-shaped constriction about 2 cm above the cardiac orifice; the diagnosis of achalasia is easily established with such typical findings.

The most common cause of esophagitis is peptic gastric reflux as a result of hiatal hernia, which is rather rare in China. Its major symptoms are heartburn and epigastric discomfort or pain, which may be aggravated in a recumbent position. Roentgenography usually shows thickening and irregularity of the mucosal folds of the lower esophagus and a varying degree of spasm. Further differentiation by esophagoscopy and biopsy may be necessary.

Benign stricture of the lower esophagus is frequently a sequela of long-standing esophagitis. X-ray examination often shows an irregular stricture with filling defects which may not be easily distinguishable from carcinoma of the esophagus or gastric cardia. Most of the patients have a long history of esophagitis, with or without accompanying hiatal hernia. More reliable diagnosis, however, depends on esophagoscopy and biopsy.

In a period of 22 years from 1958 to 1979, 880 patients underwent surgical treatment after diagnosis of carcinoma of the gastric cardia at the authors' institution. At operation, seven of these patients were found in fact to have no tumor in the cardia (Fig. 9.12). Analysis of the preoperative roentgenograms revealed that despite various irregularities in the gastric cardia, none of these cases showed either mucosal destruction or soft tissue mass shadow. It was hence concluded that in the absence of these two findings, positive balloon cytology or positive endoscopic biopsy must be obtained before a diagnosis of carcinoma of the gastric cardia can be made [16].

References

1. Pei YH, Zhang YD, Hou J, Du XQ, Fu WX (1982) Natural evolution and follow up study of early esophageal carcinoma (in Chinese). Cancer Res Prev Treat 9: 75
2. Wu YK (1959) Neoplasm of the esophagus (in Chinese), In Wu YK (ed) Disease of the chest. People's Medical Publishing House, Beijing
3. Huang GJ (1981) Early detection and surgical treatment of esophageal carcinoma. Jpn J Surg 11: 399–405
4. Zhang GL, Wang XT, Guo YL (1980) Multicentric carcinoma of the esophagus and multiple primary carcinoma of the esophagus and upper alimentary tract (in Chinese). Chin J Oncol 2: 112–115
5. Wang GQ, Chang FB, Tien ZJ, Tsng J (1980) Clinical application of intraluminal staining with toluidine blue in the diagnosis of early esophageal carcinoma (in Chinese). Natl Med J China 60: 93–95
6. Harmer MH (1978) TNM classification of malignant tumors. International Union Against Cancer, Geneva
7. Shao LF, Huang GJ (KC) (1981) Detection and surgical treatment of early esophageal carcinoma. In: Proceedings of Beijing Symposium on Cardiothoracic Surgery. Chinese Academic Publishers, Beijing, pp 168–171
8. Wu YK, Liu Y, Hu MH, et al. (1958) The classification of types of carcinoma of the esophagus (in Chinese). Chin Med J 76: 213–228
9. Huang GJ, Ku XZ, Liu FS, et al. (1981) Intraluminal type of cancer of the esophagus (in Chinese). Chin J Oncol 3: 110–112
10. Wu YK, Huang GJ, Shao LF, Zhang YD, Lin XS (1982) Progress in the study and surgical treatment of cancer of the esophagus in China, 1940–1980. J Thorac Cardiovasc Surg 84: 325–333
11. Shao LF, Li ZC, Liu SX, Wang MF, et al. (1980) Results of surgery in 3155 cases of carcinoma of the esophagus and gastric cardia (in Chinese). Chin J Surg 20: 19–22
12. Zhang YD, Du XQ, Zhang W, Yen CS, et al. (1982) Surgical treatment of 4310 cases of carcinoma of the esophagus and gastric cardia (in Chinese) Chin J Oncol 4: 1–4
13. Li CL (1980) Surgical treatment of carcinoma of the esophagus and gastric cardia: clinical evaluation of 327 cases (in Chinese). Chin J Oncol 2: 116–117
14. Surgical Department of Cancer Institute of Chinese Academy of Medical Sciences (1975) Surgical treatment of carcinoma of the esophagus and gastric cardia: an analysis of 1432 cases. Chin Med J 88: 60–63
15. Sun CF, Wang YL, Xu LT, Wu LH (1982) Diagnosis and management of massive bleeding from cancer of the gastric cardia (in Chinese) Chin J Surg 20: 165–167
16. Wang GQ, Huang GJ (1975) Analysis of 7 cases falsely diagnosed as carcinoma of cardia of the stomach (in Chinese) Cancer Res Prev Treat 2: 54–55

Chapter 10
Radiotherapy for Carcinoma of the Esophagus

Xian Zhi Gu

---

1 Introduction

Surgery and radiotherapy are the two chief methods of treatment for carcinoma of the esophagus. As most patients are found to have already advanced lesions when first seen in the clinic, they are not eligible for operation, but can only be treated by irradiation or other palliative measures. Among 9104 patients admitted for treatment from 1958 to 1980 to the Cancer Institute of the Chinese Academy of Medical Sciences, Beijing, only 1798 (19.8%) were operated upon; 947 were treated by surgery alone, 692 by preoperative irradiation and surgery, and 159 by surgery and postoperative irradiation. Of the remaining patients, 6501 (71.4%) were treated by irradiation and 805 (8.8%) by chemotherapy and/or other palliative measures. These figures show that a considerable proportion of patients are at some time irradiated; consequently, the importance of improving the techniques and results of radiotherapy cannot be overemphasized.

2 Principles

Radiotherapy is a local treatment modality whose fundamental principle is the eradication of the cancer without undue damage to the surrounding normal tissues. The primary objective is to leave the patient not only alive and tumor-free, but also to work and to lead a normal, creative life; he should at least be able to take care of himself in his everyday activities. If this objective is beyond our reach, then the patient's chief symptoms should be relieved and his life expectancy prolonged. If good results are to be achieved with radiotherapy, it is of prime importance that the tumor possess at least a certain degree of radiosensitivity, which is determined by the tissue from which it arises, the degree of differentiation, the clinical type, the stage, and the location. Carcinoma of the esophagus is usually of the squamous cell type with differentiation such that it is moderately radiosensitive. Lesions in the early stage respond better to irradiation because they have a better blood supply and are hence well oxygenated. In addition, the volume of normal tissue subjected to irradiation is comparatively limited. In more advanced lesions, such factors as the preponderance of hypoxic cells, the invasion by the tumor of neighboring organs, the poor general condition of the patient due to dysphagia, and the larger volume of tissue to be covered by the beam contribute to a marked radiation reaction on the part of the patient and a poor response on the part of the tumor. Moreover, metastasis via both lymphatics and bloodstream, added to the adverse factors mentioned above, would lead to nothing but failure. For these patients it is usually only possible to offer palliation. As far as clinical type is concerned, the intraluminal and fungating types are relatively more sensitive than the medullary type, and the scirrhous and ulcerative types are radioresistant. The destruction of the muscular layer of the esophagus and the unavoidable damage to the tumor bed as the tumor becomes advanced reduce the tumor's blood supply and hence its radiosensitivity. At the same time, the repair of the normal tissues is impeded. The net result is inevitably failure.

The esophagus is surrounded by a number of organs, e.g., spinal cord, trachea, and lungs. Among these the spinal cord is the most vulnerable to radiation, generally not tolerating any dose beyond 4000 rads over 5–6 weeks. Higher doses are likely to cause radiation myelitis and paraplegia. The volume of tissue irradiated should be strictly limited to avoid acute radiation pneumonitis and severe pulmonary fibrosis. In properly designed and performed radiotherapy with a curative dose, the trachea and spine are usually spared from injury and do not develop any serious sequelae. To guard against complications, it is advisable to employ CT and a computed treatment planning system (CTPS) in designing therapy and simulation in checking it. It is also important to adopt a proper regime of fractionation so as to facilitate repair of normal tissue and reoxygenation of tumor cells, both of which can be expected to increase radiosensitivity and improve results.

3 Selection of Patients

The criteria for patient selection should depend on the equipment available and on clinical experience. Generally, curative radiotherapy is advised for patients with early and moderately advanced lesions in the middle and lower thoracic esophagus when they refuse operation or when there are contraindications for surgery such as inadequate cardiopulmonary reserve or severe pleural or pleuropulmonary disease. The results obtained from radiotherapy in such patients are comparable to those from surgery. For early and moderately advanced lesions of the cervical and upper thoracic esophagus, radiotherapy yields satisfactory results and may be considered the treatment of choice [1].

For advanced lesions, energetic curative or palliative treatment should be given according to the local and general condition of the patient. As a rule, relief of symptoms and prolongation of life can be obtained in about 80% of cases [2]. The fact that a small proportion of patients undergoing palliative radiation are in fact ultimately cured has led to the rationale of giving palliative radiation at a radical dose. It has been reported that a

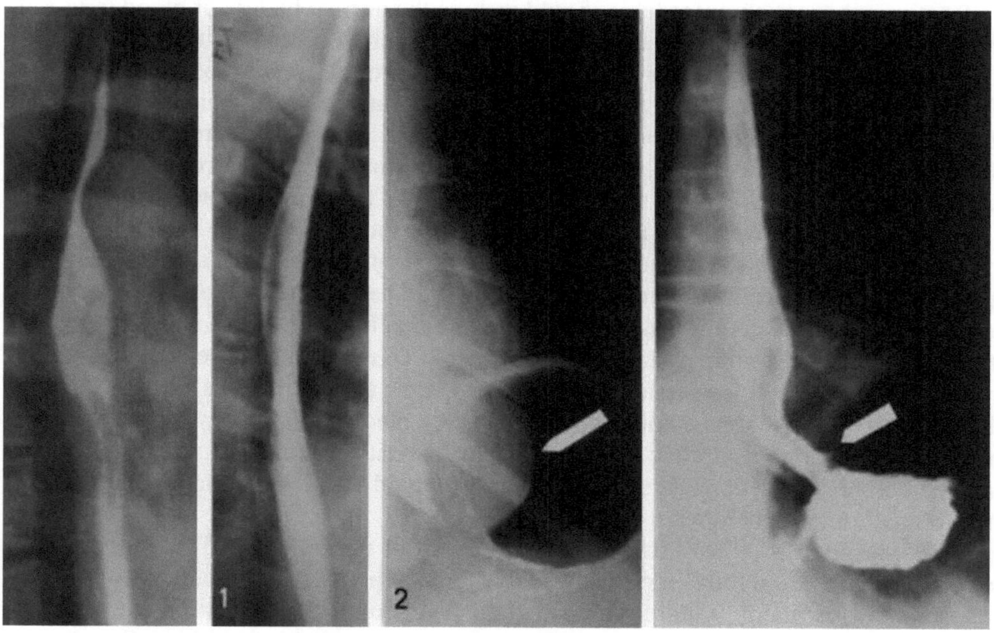

Fig. 10.1. Case 1, 39-year-old man (CI Hosp. No. 36050). *Left:* Carcinoma of midthoracic esophagus, 3 cm, with supraclavicular node metastasis. *Middle 1:* Esophagogram after 7000 rads. *Middle 2:* Left gastric lymph node metastasis 1½ years after irradiation. *Right:* Left gastric area after 6000 rads. Patient died of metastases in liver, abdominal lymph nodes, and abdominal wall 7½ years after first course of irradiation

small number of patients with supraclavicular lymph node metastasis and/or vocal cord paralysis survive for over 5 years after radiotherapy (Fig. 10.1) [3].

When the lesion is far advanced, with either perforation or distant metastasis, e.g., involving intra-abdominal lymph nodes, lung, bone, or liver, radiotherapy, bein a local treatment, has nothing to offer. Indeed, such conditions are to be taken as contraindications. Severe persistent and localized pain in the chest is generally a sign of aortic involvement, and if excruciating is usually the prodromal symptom of perforation of the aorta and is taken as a contraindication. When this type of disease must be treated, irradiation should begin with small doses and be supplemented by generous doses of antibiotics. Improvement can be expected in some of these patients. Complete obstruction of the esophagus is not a contraindication, as radiotherapy can be given after palliative prosthetic intubation.

4 Techniques

4.1 General Management

All effort should be made in order to gain the full cooperation of the patient and relatives, including reassurance and detailed explanation of the aims and methods of radiotherapy, the possible discomfort to be met with, and the precautionary measures to be taken during the course of treatment. Points concerning the prognosis should be explained to the family members preferably without the knowledge of the patient, so as to relieve the latter of undue worry. The patient should be encouraged to participate in proper activities, and attention to oral hygiene and avoidance of common colds should be stressed.

Routine examination procedures should include the normal battery of blood tests, kidney function tests, roentgenograms of the esophagus, chest X-ray or fluoroscopy, ECG, and esophageal cytology or biopsy. Other procedures should be added as indicated by the findings obtained, by the history, and by physical examination. Anemia has adverse effects on the patient's general condition and appetite and should therefore be corrected before radiotherapy. Leukopenia and thrombocytopenia must also be corrected and an adequate status maintained during radiation, with counts of preferably not less than 4000 and 100000 respectively. Weekly routine blood tests are essential.

Energetic treatment should be given to any concurrent diseases such as hepatitis, active pulmonary tuberculosis, cardiac dysfunction, and diabetes. Severe hepatitis and cardiac dysfunction must be compensated before radiotherapy is commenced, and proper maintenance should be continued during the course of treatment. When the beam has to traverse an active tuberculosis lesion in the lung, systemic antituberculous treatment should be given. Hyperthyroidism should be controlled by medication, as it will otherwise give rise to both local and systemic reactions of such severity that treatment is usually interrupted before completion. Due attention must be paid to all these factors before commencement of radiotherapy.

Good nutrition is critical for a satisfactory result of radiotherapy. The importance of adequate calories and fluids should always be borne in mind, and the patient's diet is supplemented with vitamins and proteins in copious amounts. Strong condiments, e.g., hot pepper, are not permitted, smoking is discouraged, and alcohol is forbidden. Supplementary infusion is indicated for patients who rely solely on a liquid diet. For those with complete esophageal obstruction, dilatation and maintenance of nutrition by indwelling gastric tube or prosthetic intubation is advised.

Whenever there is any clinical manifestation of esophagitis or periesophagitis, such as low-grade fever, leukocytosis, or pain in chest or back, radical doses of antibiotics are indicated. Steroids may be necessary in severe cases.

4.2 Treatment Procedure

Curative radiotherapy for patients with cancer of the esophagus not complicated by any of the contraindications mentioned above should be given, as a minority of them can be cured. The plan of treatment should be individualized, but generally the portal should extend 3–4 cm beyond the margin of the tumor. It is advisable that the contour of the lesion and the body outline be delineated by a CT scan and optimum treatment designed with the help of a CTPS. The lesion should on average receive over 90% of the dose and the spinal cord under 50%. The proportion of the lung receiving 50% of dose should be kept below 25% of total lung volume. The treatment plan is checked on a simulator before it is executed (see Figs. 10.2–10.4 for specimen designs).

Fluoroscopic screening of the lesion is carried out at every 2000 rads during the treatment to observe the dynamic response of the tumor. Roentgenograms are taken at 4000 rads for permanent record and for decision on the second half of the plan, and again at 6000–7000 rads before radiotherapy is concluded. Checking with the simulator should be carried out at least once during treatment, and adverse deviation in either size and position of the field or angulation of the beam should be promptly corrected. Should any serious deviation occur, treatment must be replanned.

Based on analysis of 1136 patients who survived for over 5 years after radiotherapy, the optimum dose lies between 6000 and 7000 rads over 6–7 weeks, i.e., 1759–1944 ret (rad equivalent therapy) [4].

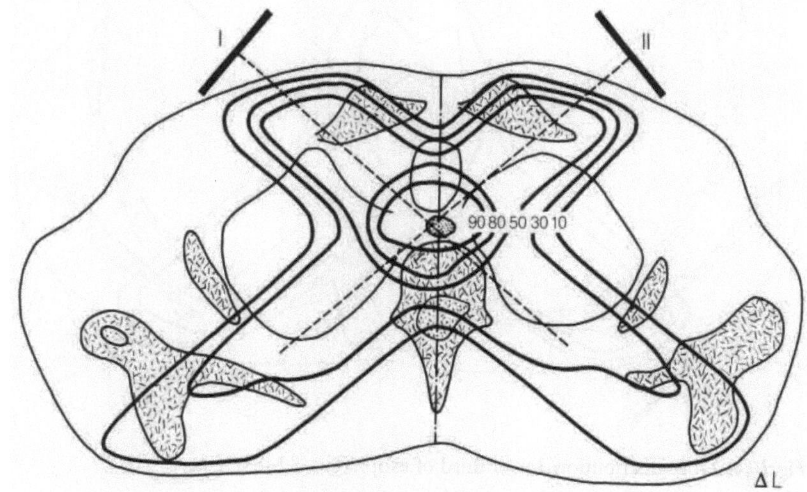

Fig. 10.2. Dose distribution, upper third of esophagus, 8 MeV X-ray

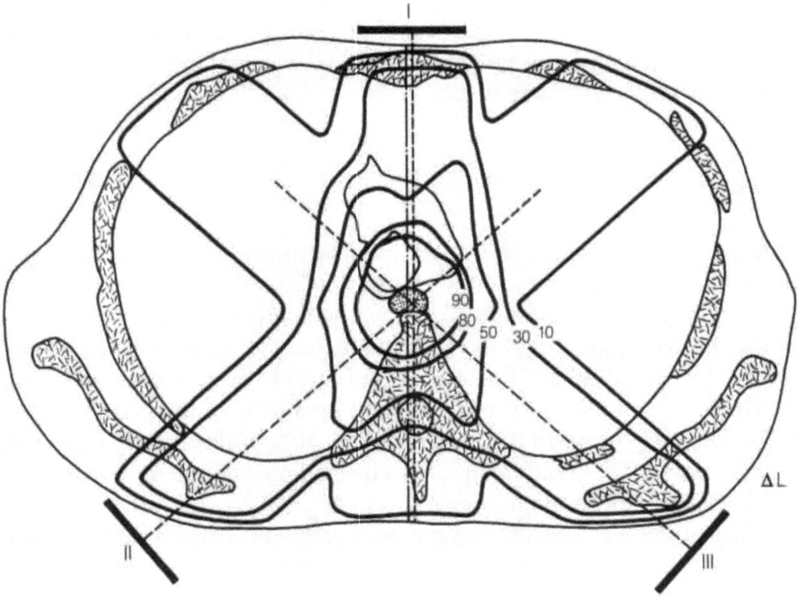

Fig. 10.3. Dose distribution, middle third of esophagus, 8 MeV X-ray

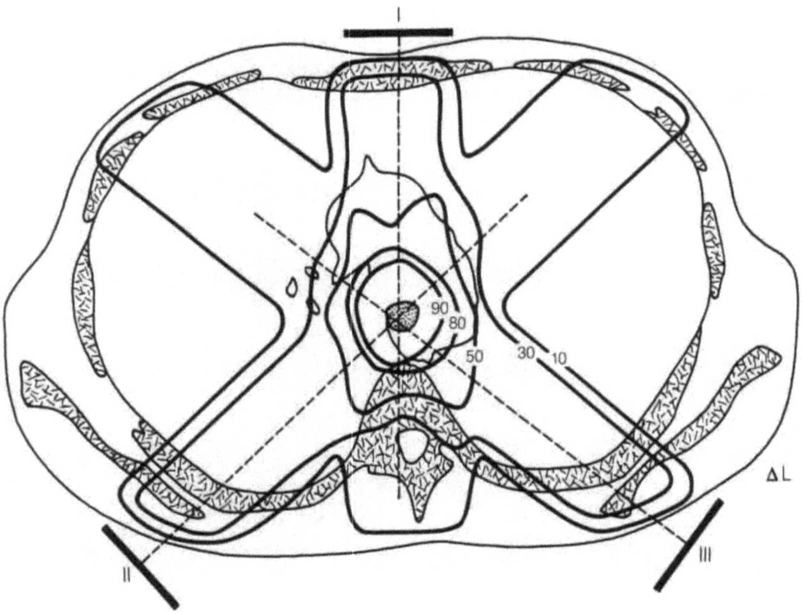

Fig. 10.4. Dose distribution, lower third of esophagus, 8 MeV X-ray

4.3 Cervical and Abdominal Lymph Node Metastases and Vocal Cord Paralysis

In our experience, if vocal cord paralysis or cervical or abdominal lymph node metastasis is shown on X-ray to persist in its original form when the dose has reached 4000 rads, it is futile to go any further and treatment may be discontinued. If there is metastasis in the upper abdominal lymphatics – as proved by clinical examination or CT scan – restriction of treatment to palliation should be considered. With supraclavicular lymph node metastasis or vocal cord paralysis, some patients can be permenently cured if the lesion in the esophagus is not very advanced [3]. For metastatic lesions in the supraclavicular fossa, 4000–5000 rads is given through a large portal covering the whole of the supraclavicular area on the same side and a further 2000–3000 rads through a reduced portal covering only the enlarged lymph node. The other side is left untreated but under close observation. In the case of vocal cord paralysis, if the mediastinal course of the recurrent laryngeal nerve is already included in the portal, no further adjustment is necessary. If not, a separate field should be given for vocal cord paralysis.

4.4 Recurrent Lesions

More than 60% of patients suffer recurrence of the tumor after radiotherapy; local recurrence in 29% of the cases may occur as late as 5–10 years after treatment (Figs. 10.5, 10.6) [5]. As differentiation between local recurrence and radiation reaction is sometimes very difficult, clinically and roentgenolocally, some lesions initially thought to be recurrences

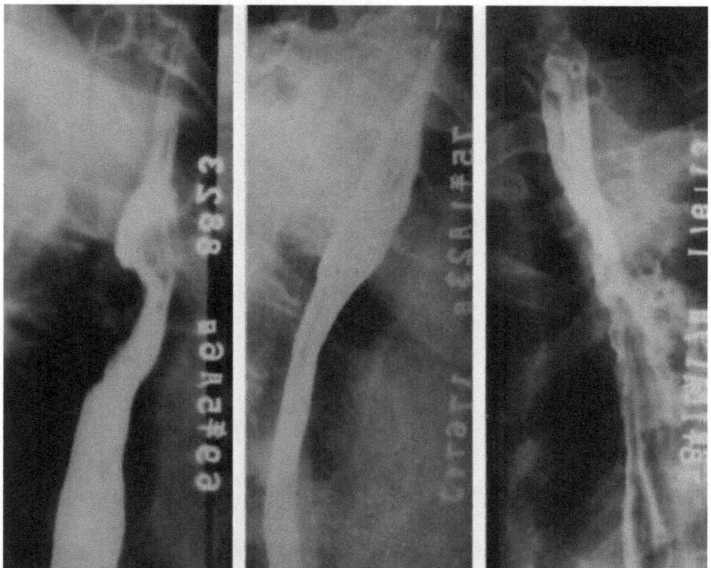

Fig. 10.5. Case 2, 47-year-old man (CI Hosp. Nr. 176173). *Left:* Carcinoma of upper third of esophagus, 4 cm, before irradiation. *Middle:* Six months after 7000 rads. *Right:* Perforation 9 years after treatment, just before patient's death. Endoscopic biopsy proved recurrence 1 year previously, but patient refused further treatment

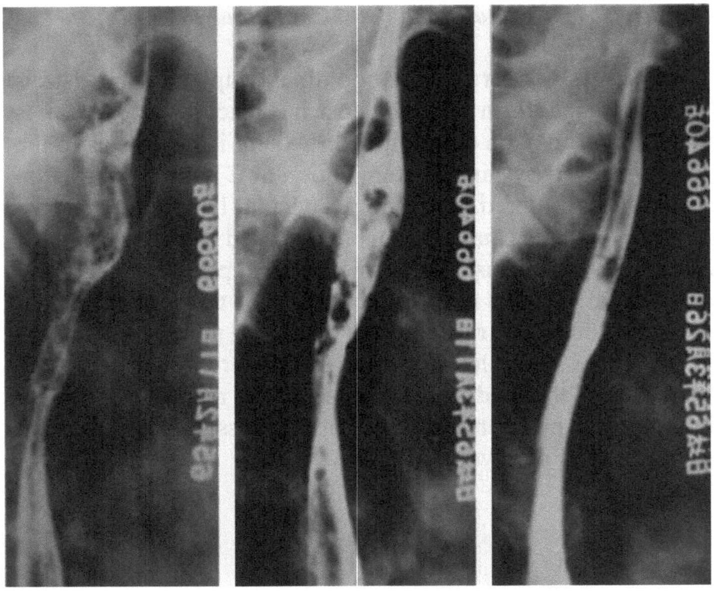

Fig. 10.6. Case 3, 46-year-old man (CI Hosp. No. 66640). *Left:* Carcinoma of upper third of esophagus, 10 cm. *Middle:* Esophagogram after 4000 rads over 4 weeks. *Right:* After 6200 rads over 7 weeks. Patient alive and well 17 years after treatment

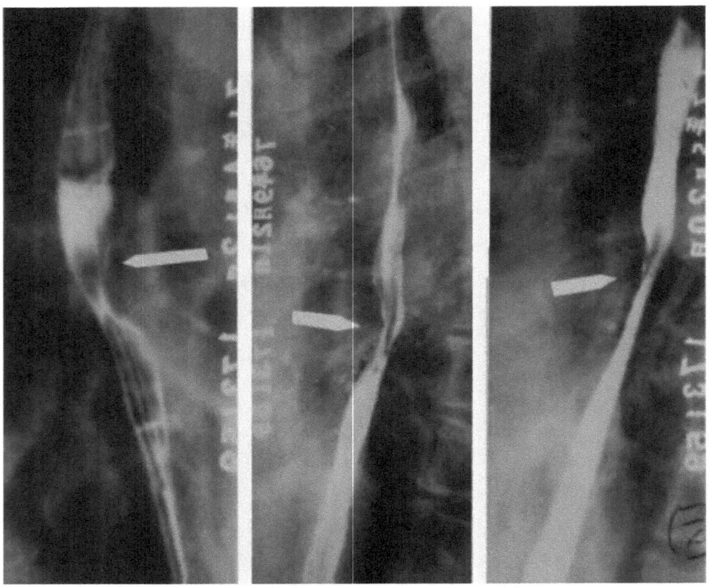

Fig. 10.7. Case 4, 40-year-old man (CI Hosp. No. 173159). *Left:* Carcinoma of middle third of esophagus, 3 cm, before irradiation. *Middle:* Five years after irradiation (4000 rads external and 3000 rads intracavitary). *Right:* Six years after irradiation, suspicion of local recurrence. Granulation tissue found on esophagoscopy and inflammatory tissue obtained by biopsy. Patient alive and well 11 years after treatment

turn out to be radiation reactions, and therefore cytologic or pathological proof should be obtained in doubtful cases. If the nature of the lesion still cannot be established, close observation is necessary; radiation reaction usually decreases or disappears after a period of conservative management (Fig. 10.7). If recurrence is established beyond doubt, surgery should be resorted to whenever possible, as a considerable number of cures can be effected by resection [6]. Irradiation of recurrences improves life expectancy by an average of 6 months compared with untreated patients [7]. Surgery may give satisfactory results in doubtful lesions which do not improve after prolonged observation [6].

4.5 *Primary Lesions*

New cancerous lesions may arise in other parts of the esophagus after radiotherapy (Fig. 10.8) [4, 5]. If the new lesion is located some distance from the previous one, the portals should be so designed that overlapping is at most only minimal. Small limited portals are used when there is considerable overlapping. Routine is undertaken and a curative dose is given.

4.6 *Intracavitary Radiotherapy*

Intracavitary radiotherapy for cancer of the esophagus has largely fallen into disuse since the extensive application and great improvement of external supravoltage irradiation, but in remote rural districts where access to external irradiation is difficult it is still valuable.

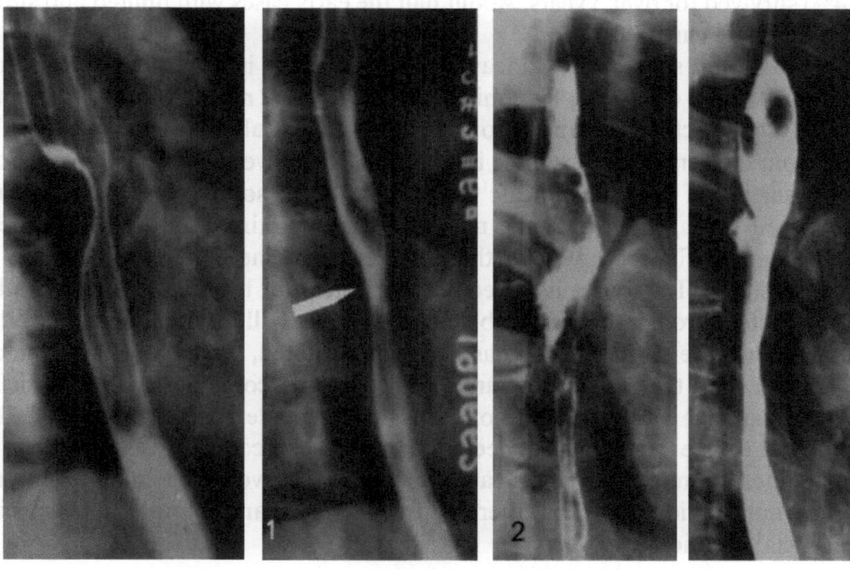

Fig. 10.8. Case 5, 33-year-old woman (CI Hosp. No. 190662). *Left:* Carcinoma of middle third of esophagus, 4 cm. *Middle 1:* Esophagogram 3 months after irradiation. *Middle 2:* New lesion in upper third 7 years after irradation of the middle third lesion. *Right:* Esophagogram of upper third segment after 6000 rads over 6 weeks. Patient died of performation of upper third lesion a year after second course of irradiation

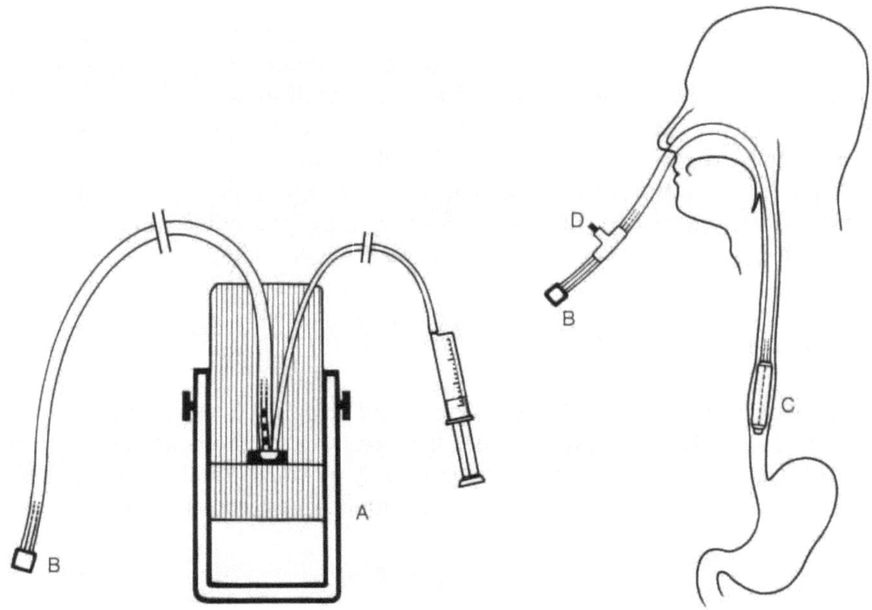

Fig. 10.9. Intracavitary treatment. *A*, Radiation source container; *B*, connector; *C*, radiation source in position; *D*, side tube for air or water injection

For instance, of 203 esophageal carcinoma patients treated by this method in Yaocun commune in Linxian county, Henan province, 88% showed marked improvement and 17 (8.4%) survived for over 5 years. About half the early cases with limited and superficial lesions could be cured [8].

The radiation source for intracavitary radiotherapy is a ^{60}Co capsule with an active length of either 6 cm (83 mg Ra equivalent) or 7 cm (112 mg Ra equivalent) contained in a double tube which carries an appropriate thin rubber balloon on the outside. The dose at 1 cm from the center of the source is 3000–4000 rads over 8–10 h. Two metallic markings on the surface of the tube indicate the position of the source (Fig. 10.9). The tube is first introduced through the patient's nose until the markings coincide with the lesion as checked under fluoroscopy, and then connected to the container in which the cobalt source is stored. The source is forced into the inner tube by compressed air, and air or water is injected through the outer tube into the rubber balloon until it attains a diameter of 1.0 cm. When the required dose has been administered, the balloon is deflated, the tube pulled out, and the radiation source restored to its container. For superficial lesions, 8–10 h treatment is carried out in one session; for moderately or extremely advanced lesion, three to five treatments are needed. In the case of complete obstruction, dilatation is done under fluorescopy before irradiation. Patients have only a mild general reaction to intracavitary radiotherapy, but there is usually very marked local pain, especially in the superficial of lesion.

5 Combination Therapy

5.1 Preoperative Radiotherapy

Preoperative irradiation has two aims:

1. To render inoperable tumors operable. Cancerous infiltration of the surrounding tissues or organs can be eradicated or reduced and the bulk of the tumor decreased, thereby increasing resectability.
2. To reduce the likelihood of local seeding and distant dissemination resulting from the operative maneuvers, thereby promoting the result of surgery.

The value of preoperative irradiation has already been well proved in squamous cell carcinoma of the head and neck. It has also been shown that the rational dose used neither causes any untoward difficulty for the surgeon nor increases the incidence of postoperative complications. In about 10% of the patients who underwent surgical exploration, the lesion could not be resected due to peritumoral infiltration [9, 10]. In addition, mediastinal recurrence ranks first among early failures after radical operation for esophageal cancer [9]. Consequently, preoperative radiotherapy should be considered logical and beneficial in patients with moderately advanced lesions when surgery is not contraindicated.

If the above-mentioned aims are to be achieved, adequate adjustment of dose, size of portal, and length of interval between completion of radiation and surgery are crucial. Cancer of the esophagus is usually moderately radiosensitive. To reduce the main body of the tumor and eradicate the peripheral microfoci, the total dose required should not be less than two-thirds of the curative dose, i. e., 4000 rads in 20 doses over 4 weeks. The portal should preferably be 6 cm in width, covering the lesion and the adjacent mediastinal and the left gastric lymphatic drainage areas, which are frequently involved by tumor metastasis. The left gastric area is usually located at the level of T_{11} and T_{12}.

Operation should be performed at the time of maximum tumor inhibition and minimum radiation reactions; after a preoperative dose of 4000 rads, an interval of 2 weeks is suitable.

Important Points. The question of optimum radiation dose and interval before operation is still unsettled. Analysis carried out at the Cancer Institute of the Chinese Academy of Medical Sciences on dose and prognosis as related to the pathological changes in resected specimens showed that the more marked the changes (i. e., the more radiation damage), the better the prognosis. The differences are statistically significant (Table 10.1) [11]. The severity of the changes is in direct proportion to the dose given and to the response observed in roentgenograms. Lack of response as shown on X-ray usually corresponds to a pathological reaction of grade I in the specimen, obvious improvement to grade II, and complete disappearance to grade III (see Chap. 4, Sect. 8.4). It is thus desirable to give preoperative irradiation in such a dose that a conspicuous improvement is observed in the X-ray films. According to our observations, there is great variation (2000–7000 rads) in the dose giving grade II or III reaction.

The interval before surgery should depend on the individualized preoperative dose. For a dose of over 5000 rads, it should preferably be prolonged to 3–4 weeks.

It is not yet clear whether a curative dose could be adverse to subsequent surgery. It also remains to be investigated whether preoperative irradiation can improve the long-term re-

Table 10.1. Radiation dose in relation to pathological changes

Dose (rads)	Changes						Total
	Grade I		Grade II		Grade III		
	(*n*)	(%)	(*n*)	(%)	(*n*)	(%)	
< 1500	22	100	0		0		22
> 1500	28	75.6	7	18.9	2	5.4	37
> 3000	84	55.6	40	26.4	27	17.8	150
> 5000	3	17.6	6	35.3	8	47.0	17
⩾ 7000	3	12.6	9	37.5	12	50.0	24
Total	140		62		49		250

Five-year survival rates: grade I 22.3%, grade II 32.4%, grade III 37.8%

sults in cases with relatively early cancer of the esophagus (e.g., superficial lesions less than 3 cm length).

5.2 Postoperative Radiotherapy

Postoperative irradiation is indicated when there are partially removed or unremoved metastatic lymph nodes, possible residual tumor invasion deposits, cancerous adhesions to the neighboring structures, or residual cancer tissue observed microscopically at the esophageal stump, Metallic markers (e.g., silver clips) should be placed at the suspicious sites during operation to facilitate localization afterward. Radiotherapy should be commenced about 2 weeks after operation; it is always advisable to start as early as possible, even if the patient's condition is not satisfactory. The portals should be limited to include only the suspected or confirmed cancer tissue, and the dose should be curative.

Metastases and Locally Recurrent Lesions

A number of postresection patients develop local recurrences and/or metastases of the supraclavicular or mediastinal lymph nodes with or without vocal cord paralysis, the intra-abdominal lymph nodes, etc. Some patients may develop hematogenous metastasis of liver, lung and bone. Recurrence at the anastomotic site is not common at this author's institution. Except in hematogenous and intra-abdominal metastasis, curative radiotherapy should be attempted, as some of the lesions can be effectively controlled for long periods.

5.3 Radiotherapy and Hyperthermia

Raising the temperature to a certain level can have a harmful effect on the tumor cells in the S phase, and undernourished (including hypoxic) cells are also damaged, whereas in ordinary radiotherapy they are all radioresistant. By combining hyperthermia and radiotherapy, the local control rate can be increased without harming the normal tissues. It is generally recognized that for superficial cancers, local hyperthermia at 43°–45 °C for

30–60 min before irradiation can conspicuously increase the local control rate. For deep-seated tumors like esophageal carcinoma, however, problems of equipment, technique, and temperature monitoring remain to be solved. The Hyperthermia Collaborating Group of Henan province [12] used a 2450-MH_2 intracavitary heating devise (surface temperature 43°–56 °C) with concurrent external irradiation to treat esophageal carcinoma. Heat treatment was carried out in sessions of 30 min three times a week, up to a maximum of eight sessions, and radiotherapy was given at a dose of 4000 rads in 20 doses over 4 weeks. The immediate results in 103 patients so treated were not inferior to the results in those treated by radiotherapy alone with 6000–7000 rads in 30–35 doses over 6–7 weeks. Some of the patients were subsequently operated upon, and pathological investigation of the resected specimens revealed a more marked response to combined radiotherapy and hyperthermia than to radiotherapy alone. However, a high incidence of recurrence was noted during follow-up, and the recurring lesions were usually resistant to both radiotherapy and hyperthermia. Despite these discouraging results, the combined use of radiotherapy and hyperthermia warrants further investigation, especially in regard to heating technique and the shortcomings in the monitoring of temperature distribution and variation within the tumor.

5.4 Radiotherapy and Chemotherapy

Advanced cancer of the esophagus has been treated with many drugs, e.g., 5-FU, thiotepa, bleomycin, Endoxan, Adriamycin, and *cis*-platinum, with unsatisfactory results. Some authors have used radiotherapy in combination with chemotherapy, but due to the lack of strict control and the preponderance of patients with far advanced lesions have not yet arrived at any definite conclusions. At the Oncologic Department of the First Hospital of Xi'an Medical College [13], 40 patients with cancer of the esophagus were treated with radiotherapy (5000–6000 rads in 25 doses over 6 weeks) and bleomycin (15 mg intramuscularly or intravenously three times a week to a total dose of 300 mg). The 1-, 2-, and 3-year survival rates were 68%, 30%, and 23% respectively. However, there was no control group in this study, and the long-term results of this combined treatment await further evaluation.

6 Results, Prognostic Factors, and Complications

6.1 Results

Most of the results reported in China are from advanced cases; results in early lesions can only be obtained from the high-incidence areas where the patients are discovered in the course of mass screening. The data accumulated are listed in Table 10.2.

6.2 Prognostic Factors

Many factors have been found to have a bearing on the outcome of radiotherapy in esophageal cancer, among the most important being stage, clinical type, location of primary lesion, age of patient, and technique of irradiation.

Table 10.2. Results of radiotherapy reported in China

Institution	Year	Radiation source	(*n*)	Five-year survival (%)
Field station, Linxian county (unpublished material)	1981	^{60}Co	79[a]	61 (83)[b]
Cancer Institute [3]	1980	^{60}Co, B	3798	8.4
Loyang 3rd Hospital [14]	1978	X-ray	266	12
Anyang Prefecture Hospital [15]	1978	^{60}Co	3033	10
Shanghai Cancer Hospital [16]	1978	^{60}Co	1034	16.8
Jiangsu Provincial Cancer Hospital [17]	1978	^{60}Co	331	13.3
Xi'an Central Hospital [18]	1975	^{60}Co	426	9.1
Dept. Oncology, Xi'an Medical College [19]	1974	^{60}Co	2310	9.3
Linxian County Hospital [20]	1981	^{60}Co, X-ray	1081	16.4
Hobei Medical College [2]	1981	^{60}Co	1245	8.3
Field station, Linxian county [8]	1982	Intracavitary	203	8.4

[a] Early lesion, less than 3 cm, superficial
[b] Early lesion, inconspicuous on X-ray film

Table 10.3. Relationship of development of lesion to results of treatment

Development	Five-year survival		(*p*)
	(*n*)	(%)	
Length of lesion (cm)			
<5	63/ 411	15.3	
5.1–7.0	108/1167	9.3	<0.005
7.1–9.0	80/1177	6.8	
>9.1	30/ 584	5.2	
Obstruction			
Marked	37/ 627	5.9	
Moderate	168/1991	8.4	<0.001
Mild	65/ 600	10.8	
Supraclavicular lymph node metastasis			
Positive	14/ 446	3.8	<0.01
Negative	262/2893	9.2	

Stage. It can be seen from Table 10.2 that the 5-year survival rate after radiotherapy for patients with early esophageal carcinoma is as high as 60%. In some the lesions were so early that they could hardly be visualized on the X-ray films and diagnosis was established by cytology and/or pathology with the help of esophagoscopy; radiotherapy in such cases yielded a 5-year survival of more than 80%. The relationship of treatment results to stage can be seen in Table 10.3.

Clinical Type. In the clinicopathological classification of esophageal carcinoma there is a preponderance of medullary and fungating lesions. These two types have different outcomes after radiotherapy. Among the medullary lesions, the prognosis is much better when the contour on esophagography is straight and smooth (benevolent type) than when

Table 10.4. Relationship of clinical type to prognosis

Type	Five-year survival		(*p*)
	(*n*)	(%)	
Medullary	246/2960	8.3	
Fungating	26/ 180	14.4	<0.01
Benevolent	161/1615	10.0	
Malicious	29/ 387	7.5	<0.0001

Table 10.5. Relationship of location of tumor to prognosis

Location	Five-year survival		(*p*)
	(*n*)	(%)	
Cervical	10/ 31	32.3	
Upper thoracic	24/153	15.7	<0.01
Midthoracic	46/469	9.8	
Lower thoracic	3/ 58	5.2	

Table 10.6. Relationship of age to prognosis

Age (years)	Five-year survival		(*p*)
	(*n*)	(%)	
Below 40	18/ 203	8.9	
40–49	71/ 666	10.7	
50–59	123/1280	9.6	<0.01
60–69	63/1000	6.3	
Over 70	6/ 190	3.2	

it is tortuous (malicious type). The tortuosity is caused by infiltration and cancerous adhesions to the surrounding organs, as shown at operation (Table 10.4) [21].

Location. Experience has shown that the higher the location of the lesion, the better the result of radiotherapy. However, this might be because surgeons prefer operating on tumors located in the middle and lower segments of the esophagus, radiotherapists therefore having more opportunity to treat earlier lesions situated high in the esophagus. In contrast, most of the lower lesions referred for radiotherapy are advanced. To show the comparable results in relation to location, we have selected lesions between 5 and 7.9 cm long without metastasis to the supraclavicular fossa or the para-aortic lymphatics which were treated with a nominal standard dose (NSD) of 1800–2099 ret (Table 10.5). There is still a worsening prognosis from the cervical segment toward the distal end of the esophagus.

Age. The treatment results are better in the 40–59 years age-group, rather poor for patients over 60, and least favorable of all when the patients are over 70 (Table 10.6).

Technique. It can be observed from Tables 10.2 and 10.7 that the choice of source is not significantly related to the change in the lesion as observed by roentgenography during radiotherapy. The barium meal response is predetermined by the clinical type, stage, and location of the tumor. According to our analysis, if no change in the tumor is observed on barium study at 4000 rads, it would never disappear completely even if the dose were increased to more than 7000 rads. It is also observed that the three-field technique is superior to the four- to six-field techniques, which corresponds to the experience of the team at Shanghai Cancer Hospital. This is probably because in four- to six-field irradiation, beam direction was not accurate enough without checking by simulator. As to the optimum total dose, although our data do not show any difference in the range of 5000–8000 rads, the results are better at 6000 rads in 30 doses over 6 weeks, as seen from the analysis of 1136 patients surviving for over 5 years after radiotherapy [4] and as reported by workers at Xi'an Medical College [19].

X-Ray Appearance. The appearance of esophageal carcinoma on barium study at the end of radiotherapy may bear some relation to prognosis, which is much better in patients with complete disappearance of barium filling defect than in those with residual tumor or no improvement (Table 10.8).

Table 10.7. Relationship of technique to prognosis

	Five-year survival		*(p)*
	(n)	(%)	
Source			
^{60}Co	230/2613	8.8	>0.05
35-MeV electron	49/ 642	7.6	
NSD			
Below 1600	11/ 343	3.2	
1600–1699	16/ 209	7.7	
1700–1799	30/ 387	7.8	
1800–1899	55/ 781	7.0	
1900–1999	75/ 795	9.4	
2000–2099	35/ 417	8.4	
Over 2100	29/ 407	7.1	
No. of fields			
3	32/ 244	13.1	
6	156/1815	8.6	<0.001

Table 10.8. X-ray appearance of tumor at end of radiotherapy in relation to prognosis

Appearance	Five-year survival		*(p)*
	(n)	(%)	
Disappeared	72/ 402	19.7	
Mostly eradicated	76/ 755	10.0	
Obvious residual tumor	126/1732	7.3	<0.01
No improvement, deterioration	4/ 335	1.2	

Table 10.9. Failure and complications

	(n)	(%)
Local uncontrol	641	48.0
Local recurrence	491	36.8
Postirradiation supraclavicular metastasis	75	5.6
Distant metastasis	60	4.5
Perforation	43	3.2
Fatal hemorrhage	11	0.8
Postirradiation second esophageal primary	6	0.5
Radiation myelitis	5	0.4
Others	2	0.2
Total	1334	100.0

6.3 Causes of Failure and Complications

Local uncontrol (residual tumor at end of therapy shown by X-ray) and local recurrence after radiotherapy are the main causes of failure. Among 1334 patients known cause of death, local recurrence, perforation, and massive hemorrhage accounted for 85%. Distant metastases, including supraclavicular lymph node metastases, made up only 10% of the deaths (Table 10.9).

Complications of radiotherapy for esophageal carcinoma include radiation myelitis (paraplegia), esophagitis, radiation pneumonitis, and mediastinal fibrosis. Radiation myelitis commonly occurs several years after treatment in patients whose spinal cords have received more than 4000 rads in 30–35 doses over 6–7 weeks, and is incurable. Hence extensive irradiation of the spinal cord must be avoided. The chief symptom of esophagitis is severe local pain, sometimes so distressing that the patient refrains from taking any food. Management includes temporary suspension of radiation, antibiotics, corticosteroids, and maintenance of nutrition. Radiation esophagitis usually occurs after the dose has reached 4000 rads or after the end of radiation. It varies greatly in severity and is difficult to predict. Radiation pneumonitis is not a risk when the three-field technique is used and each field has a width of no more than 6 cm, but is apt to occur in ^{60}Co rotation therapy or in the multiple-field technique (18 or more fields) with orthovoltage X-ray. Supravoltage irradiation causes mild mediastinal fibrosis, which appears as haziness in the mediastinal silhouette without giving rise to any complaint by the patient.

References

1. Yu ZH (1979) Radiotherapy of esophageal carcinoma (in Chinese). In: Editorial Committee of "A Practice in Oncology" (ed) A practice in oncology, vol III. The People's Medical Publishing House, Beijing, p 30
2. Wan J, Zhang DA, Guo BZ, Feng SY (1981) ^{60}Co teletherapy for esophageal carcinoma: analysis of 1245 cases (in Chinese). In: Monograph of Third National Symposium on Radiology, p 236
3. Yin WB, Zhang LJ, Yang ZY, Miao YJ, Yu ZH, Zhang ZX, Zhuang CH, Wang M, Li GH, Fan LZ, Zhang LN, Liu YY, Jia YQ, Gu XZ (1980) Radiation therapy of cancer of the esophagus: analysis of 3798 patients (in Chinese). Chin J Oncol 2: 216–221
4. The National Cooperative Group on Radiotherapy of Esophageal Cancer (1981) Analysis of 1136 patients surviving for more than 5 years after radiation for cancer of the esophagus (in Chinese). In: Monograph of Third National Symposium on Radiology, Beijing, p 236
5. Yu ZH (1982) The fate of patients surviving long after radiotherapy for cancer of the esophagus (in Chinese). Chin J Roentgenol 16: 139–141
6. Zhang DW, Huang GJ, Zhu ZB (1981) Surgical treatment of postradiation recurrence of esophageal carcinoma (in Chinese). Chin J Surg 19: 268–270
7. Yu ZH (1979) Radiotherapy of esophageal carcinoma (in Chinese). In: Editorial Committee of "A Practice in Oncology" (ed) A practice in oncology, vol III. The People's Publishing House, Beijing, p 309
8. Miao YJ, Gu XZ, Hu YM, Zhang GF, Gu DZ, Zhang GH, Yang DY, Yui WM, Zhang CL (1982) The intracavitary radiation of esophageal cancer (in Chinese). Chin J Oncol 4: 45–47
9. Li RM, Li YK, Chen HY, Gu YZ, Yang J, Hu JQ (1981) Late results of surgical treatment in esophageal carcinoma and factors influencing prognosis. Chin Med J 94: 729–732
10. Huang GJ, Gu XZ, Zhang RG, Zhang LJ, Zhang DW, Miao YJ, Wang LJ, Liu J, Wang GQ, Xiao QL (1981) Combined preoperative irradiation and surgery in esophageal carcinoma: report of 408 cases. Chin Med J 94: 73–76
11. Liu FS (1977) Pathologic studies of esophageal carcinoma: analysis of 858 cases (in Chinese). Cancer Res Prev Treat 4: 13–17
12. Li DJ, Wang CQ, Wiu ZL, Shao LF (1980) Intracavitery microwave hyperthermia (IMH) in the treatment of esophageal cancer. In: The Third International Symposium on Cancer Therapy by Hyperthermia, Drugs and Radiation, Colorado State University, Fort Collins, Colorado, p 131
13. Zhang ZF (1980) Combined use of bleomycin and radiation in the treatment of cancer of the esophagus: report on 40 cases. In: Text on esophageal carcinoma (in Chinese). Henan Medical College Press, Henan, p 769
14. Li DJ, Yui JL, Liu XP (1980) Orthovoltage X-ray therapy for esophageal carcinoma: report on 266 cases (in Chinese). Chin J Roentgenol 14: 128–130
15. Section of Radiotherapy, Anyang Prefecture Hospital (1979) ^{60}Co teletherapy for esophageal cancer: analysis of 3033 cases (in Chinese). Henan Med 4: 33–39
16. Department of Radiation Oncology, Shanghai Cancer Hospital (1978) Radiotherapy of esophageal carcinoma: report on 1034 cases (in Chinese). Cancer Res Prev Treat 4: 46–49
17. Jiangsu Cancer Prevention and Treatment Institute (1978) Concentric oblique portal irradiation for cancer of the esophagus (in Chinese). Chin J Roentgenol 12: 105–107
18. Section of Radiotherapy, Central Hospital, Xi'an City (1975) ^{60}Co teletherapy for esophageal carcinoma: analysis of 426 cases (in Chinese). Cancer Res Prev Treat 1: 28–31
19. Department of Oncology, Xi'an Medical College Hospital (1974) Radiotherapy for cancer of the esophagus: analysis of 2310 cases (in Chinese). Cancer Res Prev Treat 3: 83–86
20. Hou FX, Xui YJ, Ping SJ, Sha YH (1981) Radiotherapy of cancer of the esophagus in Linxian county: report on 1081 cases (in Chinese). In: Symposium on Radiology in Henan, pp 84–88
21. Gu XZ, Zhang ZF, Zhang DW, Sun SQ (1964) Further typing of medullary type of carcinoma of the esophagus (in Chinese). Tienjing Med [Cancer Suppl] 2: 286–287

Chapter 11
Surgical Treatment

Wu Ying K'ai and Guo Jun Huang

1 Historical Review

Surgeons have striven for over 100 years to achieve curative or palliative results with surgical treatment of carcinoma of the esophagus and gastric cardia. The first recorded survival after resection of cancer of the esophagus was reported by Czerny in 1887 [1], the patient being a 51-year-old woman who lived for a year following resection of a tumor in the cervical segment. In 1909 Evans [2] combined resection of a cervical esophageal carcinoma with pharyngolaryngectomy and the patient lived for 24 years after operation. In 1911 Lane [quoted in 3] related his experience of esophagoplasty with a cervical skin flap following resection of cancer of the cervical esophagus. In 1913 Torek [4] reported the first successful resection of a carcinoma of the thoracic esophagus and Zaaiger [5] announced the first successful esophagogastrectomy for carcinoma of the gastric cardia. Ohsawa, in 1932 [6], reported his experience in resection of cancer of the lower end of the esophagus or gastric cardia via an abdominal approach. In 1938, Marshall [7] and Adams and Phemister [8] independently related their successes in resection of carcinoma of the esophagus and intrathoracic esophagogastrostomy in one intervention. Sweet [9], Garlock [10], and others further developed this type of operation during the next decade. In 1949, Brewer [11] employed a combined thoracocervical approach for resection of a carcinoma of the upper esophagus and performed an esophagogastrostomy at the cervical level.

In China, where carcinoma of the esophagus is prevalent, the first successful esophageal resection and intrathoratic esophagogastrostomy was performed in 1940 by Wu and associates [12]. Extensive clinical and surgical experience has been accumulated in the intervening 40 years [13, 14], and surgical treatment of carcinoma of the esophagus and gastric cardia is practised in a large number of hospitals of all levels. Since the end of the 1950s the technique of abrasive cytologic examination by means of a balloon catheter has yielded gratifying results in the detection of early esophageal carcinoma in high-incidence areas [15], and as a result more and more early cases are being admitted for operation. The risks of surgical treatment are no longer serious and the early and long-term results are as good as in carcinoma at any other site. We strongly believe that the once-widespread doubts about the value of surgery in carcinoma of the esophagus and gastric cardia are no longer justified. We also believe that even better results will be achieved in the future with continued effort by surgeons in collaboration with cancer epidemiologists, pathologists, radiologists, radiotherapists, and others.

2 Selection of Esophageal Carcinoma Cases for Operation

The scope of surgical treatment, in the form of curative or palliative resection, has been extended progressively in the past two to three decades, during which time more and more relatively early cases have been seen. Accumulated clinical and surgical experience has shown that carefully selected radical surgery for esophageal cancer is quite safe and rewarding under modern conditions. In the early and relatively early stages (stages I, II), adequate resection will effect lasting cures in about half the cases, and even in the relatively late stage (stage III), a 5-year survival rate of 25% is feasible and an operation such as esophagectomy and esophagogastrostomy is well worthwhile for the patient in terms of the palliation gained. Time has shown that in carcinoma of the esophagus the best form of treatment is surgery, all other therapeutic modalities being of auxiliary and complementary value. Several factors are important in the selection of patients for surgical treatment.

Table 11.1. Resectability rate in relation to site of cancer of the esophagus [23]

Site of cancer	No. of explorations	No. of resections	Resectability rate (%)
Upper third	66	52	78.8
Middle third	1051	859	81.7
Lower third	530	462	87.2
Total	1647	1373	83.4

2.1 *Site*

We have only limited experience in surgery for cancer in the upper third of the esophagus, as most such cases are treated by radiotherapy. Among 719 esophageal resections reported by our group in 1979, in only 43 cases (6%) was the cancer in the upper third [16]. In these high resections at least a 2- to 3-cm stump was left and cervical esophagogastrostomy or esophagocolonogastrostomy was performed following the resection. In cases of postcricoid carcinoma involving the pharyngoesophageal wall or infiltrating the wall of the larynx, radical resection including laryngectomy and permanent tracheostomy with inversion extraction of the remaining esophagus and pharyngogastrostomy may be carried out, although radiotherapy is often more acceptable to the patient.

Cancer of the upper and middle thirds of the esophagus has the lowest resectability rate, since the growth is often fixed to the tracheobronchial tree or the aorta. Cancer in the lower third of the esophagus offers the best chance for resection (Table 11.1).

2.2 *Gross Size*

Estimation of the gross size of an esophageal carcinoma is made from the roentgenograms. When the lesion is under 5 cm in length, the resectability rate is high, in the range of 80%–90%, especially in the lower third of the esophagus. The chance of resection decreases in direct proportion to the length of the tumor, with the exception of the comparatively infrequent intraluminal type. When the lesion is over 7 cm, the resectability rate is much lower.

2.3 *Clinicopathological Type*

Of the five clinicopathological types of esophageal carcinoma, intraluminal and fungating lesions have the highest resectability rates, the medullary, scirrhous, and ulcerative types offering less favorable prospects. This is, of course, relative and must be considered together with other factors.

2.4 *Roentgenologic Manifestations*

Besides the gross size of the tumor, the general configuration of the filling defect and luminal changes, the soft tissue shadow of the cancer mass when shown, and fistulous extension of the growth are all very significant parameters of extraesophageal invasion and are therefore important in the assessment of resectability. In their study of the "esophageal axis" in in 82 patients, Akiyama et al. [17] reported that when esophageal cancer showed marked infiltration through the adventitia and/or into the surrounding tissue, esophageal axis abnormalities such as tortuosity on the proximal side of the tumor and angulation and deviation of the axis were observed. These are also useful criteria. We found that in addition to axis deviation, other common indications of low resectability or nonresectability are tortuosity and irregularity of the filling defect, with large or deep niches, and the presence of soft tissue shadow on RAO projections. They are also signs of poor radiotherapeutic response and in some cases may even be contraindications to radiotherapy. Preoperative irradiation in such cases will not improve resectability.

2.5 *Effect of Preoperative Irradiation*

In patients who receive planned preoperative irradiation to a total of about 4000 rads in 20 doses, current practice at the Cancer Institute of the Chinese Academy of Medical Sciences, Beijing, a good therapeutic effect on the tumor as shown roentgenologically at the completion of irradiation usually indicates good resectability. In such cases it is not infrequent to find at operation – usually about 3 weeks after irradiation – that the tumor has become much smaller and is soft, with inconspicuous margins. Tissue planes between the tumor and the surrounding structures are easily developed by dissection and so the tumor can be resected without difficulty. In cases with resectability judged roentgenologically as borderline, preoperative irradiation is often recommended as a means of promoting resectability.

2.6 *Clinical Manifestations*

Sex and age do not seem to influence resectability; indeed, some past statistics have even shown higher rates of resectability in persons of advanced age. It is true that older people have a higher operative risk, but only those with severe reduction of cardiopulmonary functions should be deprived of the benefit of surgery. Likewise, duration of illness is only relative in consideration of surgical treatment. Deep-seated pains in the back or epigastric region may indicate compression of the regional nerves by the primary cancer or by lymph node metastases, and should receive serious attention from the surgeon. Other signs of distant metastasis, e.g., in supraclavicular nodes, liver, lung, or pelvic peritoneum, should of course be sought and given due consideration.

3 Resectability Rate and Operative Mortality in Esophageal Carcinoma

The resectability rate in esophageal carcinoma depends largely upon the type of patients and the stage of the lesions. In operative mortality, an important additional factor is the experience of the surgeon. In recent years, the resectability rate has increased greatly and operative mortality has sunk considerably (Table 11.2).

Operative mortality may be calculated in one of two ways. The old method was to count all deaths related to the operation; in recent reports, however, all deaths within 30 days of operation are included. The difference is in fact not very great in large series, as most operation-linked deaths do occur within 30 days.

Table 11.2. Resectability rate statistics from representative clinics in China (1940–1980)

Source	Period	Operations	Resectability rate (%)
Collected data from 13 clinics	1940–1961	3553	59.5
Fuwai Hospital, Beijing	1962–1968	669	69.2
Hebei Medical College Hospital	1952–1976	2226	78.8
Beijing Medical College Hospital	1953–1973	818	81.2
Shanghai Chest Hospital	1957–1978	3309	81.8
Cancer Institute, Chinese Academy of Medical Sciences	1958–1979	1647	83.4
Linxian County Hospital, Henan province (high-incidence area)	1964–1974	1228	94.1

Table 11.3. Operative mortality of resection

Source	Period	Resections	Operative deaths	Operative mortality rate (%)
Wu and associates[a]	1940–1949	56	14	25.0
	1950–1965	603	38	6.3
	1966–1968	92	2	2.2
Hebei Medical College Fourth Hospital[b]	1952–1958	41	9	22.0
	1959–1965	494	72	14.6
	1966–1976	2242	66	2.9
Beijing Medical College Hospital[a]	1953–1973	664	37	5.6
Shanghai Chest Hospital[a]	1957–1978	2706	171	6.4
Cancer Institute, Chinese Academy of Medical Sciences[b]	1958–1979	1264	41	3.2

[a] Including all hospital deaths following resection
[b] Including all deaths within 30 days of operation

Our operative mortality in esophageal resection for carcinoma has changed tremendously over the past 40 years. In the early years of our experience (1940–1950) it was 30%–40%, but by 1950–1960 it had dropped to around 15%, and in recent years has been around 3%–5% (Table 11.3). The lowest rate has been reported by Akiyama [18], with two deaths out of 279 esophageal resections, a mortality of 0.7%.

The common causes of operation-linked death include cardiopulmonary complications and leakage of the anastomosis. With current anesthetic management and proper surgical technique, it is quite possible to keep operative mortality within reasonable limits. However, if one is dealing with a large proportion of relatively advanced cases, radical surgical treatment of esophageal carcinoma will still be associated with comparatively high operative mortality.

4 Long-Term Results in Esophageal Carcinoma

The long-term results of surgical treatment of esophageal carcinoma have been discouraging in the past, but recent statistics from a number of clinics in China have been more encouraging (Table 11.4).

In a series of cases from Linxian county (an especially high incidence area in Henan province) in which a high proportion of stage I carcinomas were resected the 5-year survival rate was as great as 44.0% [19]. In 1981, Shao et al. [20] reported a series of 253 resections of stage I esophageal carcinoma with a 5-year survival rate of 89.9% and a 10-year survival rate of 60.0%. Pei et al. [21] studied the natural course of 23 cases of untreated stage I carcinoma of the esophagus from the time of discovery of the disease to the death of the patients and reported an average life span of 43.6 months (range 20–78 months). Evidently, prompt surgical treatment is also necessary in early carcinoma of the esophagus, and the earlier the stage at the time of intervention, the better the long-term results after resection.

Two parallel series of long-term results reported by Wu et al. [22] in 1965 and Huang et al. [23] in 1981 showed better survival figures for the more recent group at every stage of follow-up, particularly after 5 and 10 years (Table 11.5). The improvement is possibly due to an increase in the proportion of earlier cases and to more clinical experience. In the more recent series, the 5-year survival rate also increased with time, being 28.8% in 1958–1964, 29.1% in 1965–1969, and 33.0% in 1970–1974. The authors of the second series also analyzed their results according to the stage of the cancer at the time of operation, finding a 5-year survival rate of 83.3% (5/6) in stage I, 46.3% (101/218) in stage II, 26.4% (187/707) in stage III, and 6.7% (3/45) in stage IV [23].

Follow-up analysis in a series of 358 late deaths revealed that 90% were related to the original cancer (Table 11.6) [16]. This shows the need for the extension of surgical extirpation to the limits of technical feasibility and for the more effective use of multidisciplinary therapy in carcinoma of the esophagus.

The factors affecting the long-term results of resection of carcinoma of the esophagus are many and interrelated. The best results are seen after adequate resection of a limited primary growth without lymph node metastasis. The following important factors were highlighted in a 1980 analysis of our own statistics from 719 cases [16].

Table 11.4. Five-year survival rate after resection

Source	Operation period	Resections	Patients surviving 5 years	Five-year survival rate (%)
Wu and associates	1956–1973	719	177	24.6
Hebei Medical College Fourth Hospital	1952–1973	1290	303	23.5
Beijing Medical College Hospital	1957–1973	664	164	24.7
Shanghai Chest Hospital	1957–1973	1040	276	26.6
Cancer Institute, Chinese Academy of Medical Sciences [23]	1958–1974	976	296	30.3
Linxian County Hospital, Henan province [19]	1964–1974	250	110	44.0
Shao et al. [20]	1965–1975	159[a]	143	89.9

[a] Stage I cases

Table 11.5. Long-term survival rates after resection

Years since resection	1		2		3		4		5		10	
	A	B	A	B	A	B	A	B	A	B	A	B
Resections	311	1293	232	1206	193	1123	134	1060	97	976	55	652
Survivors	219	955	105	588	65	440	38	345	22	296	6	138
Survival rate (%)	70.4	73.9	45.3	48.8	33.7	39.2	28.4	32.5	22.7	30.3	10.9	21.2

A, Wu et al. [22], operations carried out between 1940 and 1961; *B*, Huang et al. [23], operations carried out between 1958 and 1974

Table 11.6. Causes of late death after resection (Wu et al. [16])

Cause	Time of death (years after resection)					Total	
	⩽1	1–3	3–5	5–10	⩾10	*n*	%
Local recurrence	40	52	5	6	1	104	29.1
Metastasis	70	117	18	10	1	216	60.3
Not cancer-related	8	10	1	4	15	38	10.6
Total	118	179	24	20	17	358	100.0

Site. Cancers in the lower third of the esophagus are best suited for surgical treatment, for the reason that the anatomic situation allows more adequate excision, including the surrounding tissue and the segment of the esophagus proximal to the cancer. In a series which we analyzed in 1965, the 5-year survival rate after resection of cancer of the lower third was 31.3%, that for the upper and middle thirds only 14.3%. The corresponding 10-year rates were 17.9% and 3.7% [22].

Gross Size. The gross size of the lesion has a certain value for prognosis. Among our 719 cases, the 70 involving cancers 3 cm or less in length displayed a 5-year survival rate of 27.1%, while in the 159 with cancers over 7 cm in length the figure was 22.6%. In the 368 cases with no gross involvement outside the esophagus the 5-year survival rate was 28.9%, and in the 351 cases in which the cancer had already infiltrated the surrounding tissue it was 20.2%.

Regional Lymph Node Metastasis. The presence or absence of metastasis in the regional lymph nodes as shown by pathological study of the surgical specimen is a very important prognostic parameter. In the 436 cases where the regional lymph nodes showed no metastasis the 5-year survival rate was 32.1%, while in the 283 cases where metastasis was evident it was only 13.6%.

Adequacy of Resection. In earlier years we used to take a 5-cm "normal" margin above the palpable edge of the cancer at operation. Microscopic study of the upper margin of the surgical specimen revealed cancerous changes in as many as 20% of cases, indicating inadequate resection. The 5-year survival rate in the 616 cases with no cancer tissue at the margins was 26.5%, that in the 103 cases with cancer tissue at the margins only 13.6%. In recent years, we have been practising extensive resection, removing the esophagus to as high a level as technically feasible. No infra-aortic esophagogastrostomy is now performed for carcinoma of the esophagus; more and more, esophagogastrostomy is performed at the level of the dome of the pleural cavity or at the cervical level. All accessible lymph nodes in the mediastinum and those in the celiac region should be included in the resection.

Preoperative Radiotherapy. The rationales for the combination of preoperative irradiation and surgery in the treatment of carcinoma of the esophagus are now well accepted. Iatrogenic tumor cell dissemination at operation, with the possibility of metastasis and tumor implantation, is a well-known phenomenon. The cancer cells most easily disseminated during surgery are those in areas with a richer vascular supply which are better oxygenated and much more radiosensitive. Preoperative irradiation can sterilize or devitalize the cancer cells in these areas and thus eliminate or reduce the risk of dissemination. The two common causes of surgical failure, microscopic deposits of tumor cells not accessible to surgical resection and tumor invasion into adjacent vital organs, are best controlled by preoperative irradiation. Bulky primary tumors usually contain large numbers of poorly oxygenated tumor cells which are radioresistant and are often the source of local recurrence after radiotherapy. Surgery subsequent to radiotherapy removes the primary tumor, not only eliminating the source of local recurrence but also rendering a high dose of irradiation unnecessary. It is therefore logical that better results can be achieved by radiotherapy and surgery in combination than by either alone.

In a series of 408 cases of esophageal cancer with borderline resectability treated with a planned combined regime of irradiation and subsequent surgery [24], the resectability rate was 81.9% and the 5-year survival rate 31.6%. We are convinced that a combined regime does improve the resectability and long-term result in esophageal cancers, especially in those of borderline resectability.

5 Carcinoma of the Gastric Cardia

Carcinoma of the gastric cardia may simulate carcinoma of the lower esophagus clinically and roentgenologically. The lesion may involve both the cardia and the lower esophagus in its late stage. Pathologically, cancer of the gastric cardia is usually adenocarcinoma. Although regional lymph node metastasis may develop early, the disease may remain asymptomatic for longer than esophageal carcinoma, with the result that early diagnosis is even more infrequent. In Linxian county, for example, where balloon cytology is frequently used in mass screening for carcinoma of the esophagus and gastric cardia, from 1964 to 1979, there were 2047 cases of carcinoma of the esophagus and 874 cases of carcinoma of the gastric cardia seen at the County Hospital, a ratio of 2.3:1. Among these cases were 154 early carcinomas of the esophagus and 23 early carcinomas of the gastric cardia, a ratio of 6.7:1. The early carcinomas of the esophagus formed 7.5% of the total (154/2047), the early carcinomas of the gastric cardia only 2.6% (23/874).

Huang and associates at the Cancer Institute, Chinese Academy of Medical Sciences, analyzed a series of 880 cases of carcinoma of the gastric cardia operated on during a 21-year period, 1958–1979. There were 1647 esophageal cancers operated on during the same period at the same institute [23], a ratio of 1:1.87.

Among the 880 patients operated on for carcinoma of the gastric cardia, 612 (69.5%) had resections. The resectability rate increased steadily with time, being 60.5% in 1958–1964, 64.6% in 1965–1969, 74.5% in 1970–1974, and 79.5% in 1975–1979. Thirty-day operative mortality was 1.6% (10/612). The 5- and 10-year survival rates, at 19.5% (92/472) and 12.7% (39/308) respectively, were distinctly inferior to those for esophageal carcinoma during the same period at the same institute. Pathological examination of the surgical specimens revealed gross cancer extension out of the cardia in 36.1% of cases, and regional lymph node metastasis was present in 75.5% of cases.

The long-term results of surgical treatment of cancer of the gastric cardia are far from satisfactory. Better results may be achieved in the future through earlier diagnosis, more extensive resection, and the adjunct use of other forms of therapy, but this can only be tested in comparable series.

References

1. Czerny J (1877) Neue Operationen – Resektion des Oesophagus. Zentralbl Chir 4: 433–434
2. Evans A (1933) Rubber esophagus. Br J Surg 20: 388
3. Ogilvie H (1960) The surgery of the esophagus. Br J Surg 47: 457
4. Torek F (1913) The first successful case of resection of the thoracic portion of the esophagus for carcinoma. Surg Gynecol Obstet 16: 614
5. Zaaiger TH (1913) Erfolgreiche transpleurale Resektion eines Kardiakarzinoms. Beitr Klin Chir 83: 419
6. Ohsawa T (1933) Esophageal surgery. J Jpn Surg Soc 34: 1318
7. Marshall SR (1938) Carcinoma of the esophagus. Surg Clinic North Am 18: 643
8. Adams WE, Phemister DB (1938) Carcinoma of the lower thoracic esophagus: report of a successful resection and esophagogastrostomy. J Thorac Surg 7: 621–632
9. Sweet RH (1945) Transthoracic resection of the esophagus and stomach for carcinoma. Ann Surg 121: 272–284
10. Garlock JH (1944) Re-establishment of esophagogastric continuity following resection of esophagus for carcinoma of middle third. Surg Gynecol Obstet 78: 23
11. Brewer LA (1949) One stage resection of carcinoma of the cervical esophagus with sub-pharyngeal esophagogastrostomy. Ann Surg 130: 9–20
12. Wu YK, Loucks HH (1941) Surgical treatment of carcinoma of the esophagus. Chin Med J 60: 1–33
13. Wu YK, Huang GJ (1979) Chinese experience in the surgical treatment of carcinoma of the esophagus. Ann Surg 190: 361–365
14. Wu YK, Huang GJ, Shao LF, Zhang YD, Lin XS (1982) Progress in the study and surgical treatment of cancer of the esophagus in China (1940–1980). J Thorac Cardiovasc Surg 84: 325–333
15. Huang GJ (1981) Early detection and surgical treatment of esophageal carcinoma. Jpn J Surg 11: 399–405
16. Wu YK, Chen PT, Fang JP, Lin SS (1980) Surgical treatment of esophageal carcinoma. Am J Surg 139: 805–809
17. Akiyama H, Kogure T, Itai Y (1972) The esophageal axis and its relationship to the resectability of carcinoma of the esophagus. Ann Surg 176: 30–36
18. Akiyama H (1980) Surgery for carcinoma of the esophagus. Curr Probl Surg 17: 55–120
19. Collaborating Group for Research on Esophageal Cancer, Linxian, Henan (1976) Early diagnosis and surgical treatment of esophageal cancer under rural conditions. Chin Med J 2: 113–116
20. Shao LF, Huang GJ, Zhang DW et al. (1981) Detection and surgical treatment of early esophageal carcinoma. In: Proceedings of Beijing Symposium on Cardiothoracic Surgery, China Academic Publishers, Beijing, pp 168–171
21. Pei YH, Zhang YD, Hou J, Du XQ, Fu WX (1982) Natural evolution and follow up study of early esophageal carcinoma (in Chinese) Cancer Res Prev Treat 9: 75
22. Wu YK, Huang GJ, Chang W (1965) Cancer of the esophagus and gastric cardia (in Chinese) Shanghai Science and Technology Publishers, Shanghai, p 258

23. Huang GJ, Zhang DW, Wang GQ, et al. (1981) Surgical treatment of carcinoma of the esophagus: report of 1647 cases. Chin Med J 94: 305–307
24. Huang GJ, Gu XZ, Zhang RG et al. (1981) Combined preoperative irradiation and surgery in esophageal carcinoma. Chin Med J 94: 73–76

Chapter 12
Preoperative and Postoperative Care and Management of Postoperative Complications

Guo Jun Huang

1 Introduction

Surgical treatment for carcinoma of the esophagus and gastric cardia always involves major operations bearing considerable risk, and the patients are usually elderly and in poor general condition. There is high operative mortality if the patients are not properly cared for. It is for these reasons that preoperative and postoperative care and the prevention and management of postoperative complications are just as important as the handling of surgical indications and operative techniques. Doctors and nurses in charge of surgical patients should be fully conversant with the relevant principles and techniques of management and apply them to the best of their knowledge with regard to the individual condition of the patient. It is only through meticulous attention to the details of preoperative, intraoperative, and postoperative management that morbidity and mortality can be reduced.

2 Preparation of Patient

2.1 Care of Airway

It is common to find that most of the patients are heavy smokers, and many have chronic bronchitis. Coughing and expectoration of sputum are frequent symptoms, and if they and chronic airway infections are not brought under control or reduced to a minimum, postoperative respiratory complications are prone to occur, increasing the severity and duration of suffering and possibly even being fatal. It is absolutely necessary, therefore, that the patient stops smoking from the day surgery is decided on. A short-term course of antibiotics may be given to patients with more marked respiratory infection.

2.2 Oral Hygiene

Poor oral hygiene increases the chance of postoperative infection of the respiratory tract, the anastomotic suture line, and the pleural cavity, which is usually contaminated by the esophageal and gastric contents when the open technique is used in anastomosis. Patients are advised to brush their teeth well and to use medicated gargles if necessary. Dental caries, pyorrhea alveolaris, and periodontitis, if present, should be treated.

2.3 Investigations

It is essential to compile a comprehensive and detailed medical record, to carry out a careful physical examination, and to perform the routine laboratory tests which should include plasma proteins, serum electrolytes, platelet count, and urinalysis. Pulmonary function studies, blood gas analysis, chest X-ray, and ECG are needed to evaluate cardiopulmonary reserves.

In general, a barium swallow study of the esophagus and/or the stomach must be done within 2 weeks before the operation. It is our custom to have the patient fluoroscoped by the resident surgeon after admission, with barium swallow if indicated, so that the state of the heart and lungs, the excursion of the diaphragm, and any existing abnormalities can be carefully observed. This in combination with the routine chest films will provide the surgeons with all the information they need on the patient's chest condition to enable them to decide on the best operative procedure.

If indicated, CT scan of the liver and of the mediastinum are carried out to detect metastases. CT scan of the esophageal or cardiac tumor may show the extent of invasion to the surrounding structures, thus contributing to the assessment of resectability.

2.4 *Correction of Nutritional, Liquid, and Electrolyte Deficiencies*

The degree of dysphagia and the nutritional status of patients with carcinoma of the esophagus or gastric cardia vary greatly. In general, however, most are in a state of malnutrition with water and electrolyte deficiencies which must be corrected as completely as possible before surgical intervention.

Patients in whom dysphagia is mild are given special soft diets containing 70–150 g protein and 100–200 g sugar or carbohydrates to supply a daily intake of 3000 cal. Egg-milk preparations or cocoa milk and sufficient vitamins B and C or multivitamins are to be added. Fresh and pureed vegetables and fruit juices are given liberally.

For patients with marked dysphagia, a specially prepared liquid diet is given every 2–3 h, providing a daily intake of over 2000 cal. It is desirable to increase the intake of milk and egg products in order to provide a daily protein intake of over 50 g and to give plenty of sugar (100–200 g), vitamins, vegetable puree, and fresh fruit juices.

In patients with severe dysphagia and in those who cannot take even liquids, dehydration, emaciation, and marked disturbances in electrolyte balance are always present. Intravenous infusion with an adequate supply of electrolytes, glucose, proteins, vitamins, etc, should be given according to blood analyses and the degree of hemoconcentration. Esophageal intubation may be indicated in some of these patients as a preoperative preparation to combat and minimize nocturnal aspiration. Short-term nasogastric tube feeding may be appropriate in some other patients. An elemental diet may be administered in this way to provide an adequate daily intake of proteins and calories and possibly obtain a positive nitrogen balance. Parenteral nutrition may also be practised in some cases, but in our experience is rarely necessary. The occasiaonal patient may have had a gastrostomy performed previously in another clinic. Feeding by this route is certainly convenient, but is not good preoperative practise because it does not solve the problem of airway aspiration due to esophageal obstruction, and the presence of a gastrostomy wound with its inevitable local infection may handicap subsequent surgical intervention.

In marked anemia, which is more often seen in patients with carcinoma of the gastric cardia, multiple small blood transfusions are very helpful. It is good practise to raise the blood hemoglobin concentration to over 10 g% before surgery is undertaken.

2.5 *Esophageal Lavage*

In patients with severe dysphagia, retention and putrefaction of food material in the esophagus usually gives rise to inflammation, infection, and edema of the tumor and the esophageal wall, resulting in a vicious circle of more obstruction and more infection. It must be emphasized that infection of the esophagus is one of the unfavorable factors in the healing of the anastomosis, and should therefore be eliminated as thoroughly as possible. In such cases the esophagus should be lavaged every evening shortly before bedtime for 3 days prior to day of operation. Warm saline solution is introduced for this purpose through a temporary large-caliber nasal tube into the esophagus just above the obstruction. The patient is put in a sitting or semi-Fowler's position and esophageal lavage is accomplished by successively instilling and aspirating 20–30 ml warm saline repeatedly until the returning fluid is clear. Topical antibiotics such as streptomycin may be given before withdrawal of the nasal tube.

2.6 *In-Bed Training*

Before operation the patient must be trained in deep breathing exercises and in effective coughing with the help of a nurse and must practice passing urine while lying and sitting in bed. These exercises are of benefit in the prevention of pulmonary complications and avoidance of urethral catheterization after operation.

2.7 *Explanation of Procedure*

It is unwise to operate until the patient has full understanding of and confidence in the procedure. An elective operation should not be scheduled for only 1 or 2 days after admission; on the contrary, at least 3 or 4 days in the ward should be allowed for preoperative assessment and preparation and for the patient to adapt to his situation and his surroundings. During this time he gets acquainted with the doctors and nurses and makes friends with other patients who have successfully undergone operation. Such an experience per se answers many of his questions and is of tremendous help in building up his confidence, which is essential in getting him in the right frame of mind for surgery.

It is our policy to let most patients know the nature of their illness, but not necessarily the prognosis. Carcinoma of the esophagus and gastric cardia are so well known in China that it is often useless or even harmful to try to conceal the true diagnosis. It is not necessary to give the patient details of the surgical procedure, as this may be subject to change depending on operative findings, but it is absolutely essential to inform him of the problems and the pain, albeit temporary, that he will probably have after operation. The purpose of this explanation is to get the patient mentally prepared to overcome any postoperative hardship. The importance of breathing exercises and coughing up of phlegm in prevention of postoperative respiratory infection is emphasized. If not well informed beforehand, many patients would instead try to inhibit coughing and limit movements of the chest for fear of a harmful effect on the wound. In fact disruption of the chest wound due to coughing has never occurred in our experience, and the patient must be reassured on this point.

2.8 *Preparations Within One Day of Operation*

Certain preparations must be carried out the day before operation:

1. Skin preparation to the extent required for the planned operative procedure, followed by a shower or tub bath

2. Antibiotic therapy, repeated the next morning before the patient is taken to the operating room
3. A soapsuds enema in the evening
4. No food by mouth after 9 p.m., no water after midnight

These measures may be quite tiring for a weak patient and should therefore be spaced out so that the patient can rest. It is unwise to interfere more on this day, and visiting should be limited or even forbidden in order to conserve the patient's energy, which is very important in postoperative recovery.
Measures to be taken on the day of operation include:

1. Insertion of a nasogastric tube in the morning before sending the patient to the operating room
2. Initiation of a special nursing chart
3. Premedication as ordered by the anesthetist who saw the patient the day before, usually given by injection when the patient is called to the operating room

2.9 Preparation for Colon Interposition

The necessary steps in preparation for colon interposition are as follows:

1. Careful inquiry is made to ascertain whether the patient has a history of colonic diseases, e.g., dysentery, bloody stool, or evacuation of mucous material, or any unexplained abdominal pain. Roentgenography with barium enema is done to see if there is any evidence of polyposis or other colonic abnormality and to help assess the length and shape of the colon. Angiography of the colonic arteries is of great help in the precise determination of which vascular pedicle to use for optimal interposition, and can save spending a lot of intraoperative time in making such a decision.
2. A low-residue diet is initiated 3–5 days before operation.
3. A soapsuds enema is given every evening for 3 successive days, followed by a cleansing enema the evening before operation.
4. Enteric antibiotic therapy, e.g., neomycin 0.5–0.75 g b.i.d., is started 3 days before operation, accompanied by a sufficient dose of vitamin K.

Belsey [1] claimed that the best preparation of the colon is to make it as empty and dry as possible, and advocated a low-residue diet for 2 weeks and a limited fluid intake for 24 h immediately prior to surgery. The scybalae can then be squeezed out of the colon during the operation without soiling or contaminating the operative field. Belsey even abandoned the use of enteric antibiotics in order to prevent any colitis without increasing the chance of postoperative infection.

3 Postoperative Management

The principles of postoperative management of patients with carcinoma of the esophagus or gastric cardia are largely identical with those for intrathoracic operations in general. However, since many patients with cancer of these sites have had dysphagia and nutritional deficiencies before surgery and are still forbidden to take adequate nutrition by mouth for varying periods of time after the operation, they need much more meticulous care than any other chest surgery patients. The principles of management described here are applicable equally to patients in whom the tumor is resected and to those in whom only a bypass operation is performed.

3.1 General Immediate Postoperative Observation

Most patients are kept in the recovery room for 3–4 days after operation, only those few in critical condition being taken to the intensive care unit.

Vital signs are checked once every 15 min for the first 6 h after surgery and then gradually less frequently until the next day. Temperature is taken every 6 h to check for postoperative fever.

3.2 Position, Coughing, and Breathing

After regaining consciousness and if the vital signs are within normal limits, the patient is put in a low Fowler's position to facilitate respiratory ventilation and chest drainage. Such a position is recommended in order to lower the position of the diaphragm and increase its respiratory excursions. The chest binder, if applied, must not be so tight as to act like a splint; it is not uncommon to find a patient displaying or complaining of shortness of breath due to a tight binder. The patient is encouraged to do deep-breathing exercises every 2–4 h and is helped to cough efficiently and to bring up any sputum. These movements serve to promote lung expansion, which is important in the prevention of atelectasis and respiratory infection. Oxygen may be administered intermittently through a nasal tube if indicated.

Beginning from the 1st postoperative (PO) day, steam inhalation or airway humidification by ultrasonic nebulizer is carried out for 20 min twice a day. Mucolytic agents may be added to the aerosol if the sputum is thick and difficult to cough up, and aerosol antibiotics may also be used if there is evidence of respiratory infection. Steam inhalation is commonly favored by patients, especially on winter days when the weather is dry in the northern part of China. Chinese herbs (*Mentha arvensis* L. 30 g and *Chrysanthemum indicum* Linn. 30 g) are added to the boiling water to produce a medicated steam, which is fragrant and may have an expectorant effect.

The main handicap to coughing is chest pain, which should be alleviated by appropriate doses of analgesics.

Beginning on the 1st PO day, the patient is helped to sit up in bed and to do coughing and deep-breathing exercises 2–4 times daily. Most patients can be out of bed for brief periods from the 3rd or 4th PO day.

3.3 Chest Drainage

Closed chest drainage not only helps to drain fluid and air from the pleural cavity, thus promoting lung expansion and decreasing the risk of pleural infection, but also provides valuable information on intrathoracic physiopathology, which may change from time to time. The chest tube must always be kept patent, all kinking and obstruction being avoided. Nurses and doctors must be able to recognize any intrathoracic abnormality as evidenced by the height and fluctuation of the water column, the amount and character of the fluid aspirated, etc., so that the necessary care can be instituted in time [2]. Abnormally high intrathoracic negative pressure as evidenced by a high water column may indicate pulmonary atelectasis, while excessive fluctuation of the water column is always a sign of increased resistance or even obstruction of the airway. It is important to be aware of intrathoracic hemorrhage in the immediate PO period. An abnormally large amount of chest fluid which rapidly becomes less and less blood-tinged is often evidence of chylothorax.

The chest tube is usually removed on the 2nd PO day, when the amount of drainage is minimal. The drainage wound is closed by tying the open skin ligature laid during the operation.

3.4 Gastrointestinal Decompression

After the patient's return to the recovery room, continuous gentle suction is maintained through the gastric tube which is irrigated every 4 h with about 20 ml warm saline or water to maintain its patency. Gastrointestinal decompression is maintained until 48 h after operation if the gastric fluid is normal in amount and color. An excessive amount of dark-colored gastric fluid during the early PO days, or frequent regurgitation of such fluid in spite of tube decompression, may indicate pyloric obstruction from torsion of the transplanted stomach, rarely from postvagotomy pylorospasm, or from other conditions, such as preexisting peritoneal adhesions.

3.5 Prophylactic Antibiotic Therapy

Routine prophylactic administration of appropriate antibiotics, such as penicillin in combination with streptomycin, is kept up for 7–10 days after operation or until the temperature has been normal for 2–3 days.

3.6 Oral Hygiene

The teeth are brushed every morning and evening. Dobell's solution or saline is gargled gently 3–4 times a day, the patient being warned each time not to swallow the solution.

3.7 Intravenous Fluid Administration and Nutrition

Nothing is allowed by mouth for the first 3 PO days, during which time IV infusion is given. Total fluid intake is adjusted to the total output, which includes gastric drainage, chest drainage, urine, and the estimated insensible loss through perspiration and respiration. In general, 2000–2500 ml 10% glucose and 500–1000 ml 5% glucose in normal saline to a total of 2500–3000 ml is given every 24 h, with the addition of 10–20 ml 10% potassium chloride and 2–3 g vitamin C.

If a duodenal tube has not been inserted, oral feeding is usually started on the 4th PO day in the absence of evident problems in the healing of the anastomosis. A liquid diet of 50 ml q2h 7 times a day is prescribed on the 1st day of oral feeding, with doubling the amount q2h each day until the 7th PO day, when 400 ml q2h is given. During this period 50 ml of plain water or fruit juice may be given between meals. Beginning on the 8th PO day the patient is allowed to have liquids ad lib. A semiliquid diet is started on the 10th–12th PO day, and a soft diet on the 14th PO day. Hereafter a greater variety of food with high protein and calorie content is encouraged as much as the patient's digestion warrants.

It is important that the patient be instructed to follow this feeding regime strictly. He should be encouraged to eat up to the limit of his allowance but warned that extra oral intake may be dangerous to the healing of the anastomosis.

In most of our patients a fine soft plastic nasoduodenal tube is installed at the time of resection or bypass. The tube is practically nonirritant, does not interfere with coughing, and can be tolerated for a considerable length of time. In these patients 1500 ml nutrient fluid can be given on the 3rd PO day by gravity drip, the amount of IV drip being reduced accordingly. Usually each 1000 ml nutrient fluid contains 80 g glucose, 3 g table salt, 1 g potassium chloride, 50 mg vitamin C, and 10 mg vitamin B_1. The formula may of course be modified, and supplements may be added.

With this tube feeding, IV drip can be discontinued on the 4th PO day. A total amount of 3000 ml of nutrient fluid is then usually given each day, with short breaks during which the patient can move around. If the patient shows good tolerance to this regime, half the nutrient fluid may be substituted by a one-tenth strength solution of elemental diet, every 100 g of which contains approximately 70 g carbohydrates, 18 g proteins, 8 g fat, and certain amounts of sodium, potassium, and other trace elements, providing altogether about 420 calories.

Strict aseptic technique is followed in the preparation of tube feeding. The solutions are made up each day and stored in sterile bottles in the refrigerator until needed in order to prevent bacterial overgrowth. If the patient prefers, the fluid may be warmed by immersing the terminal segment of the tube in a thermos containing hot water.

Duodenal feeding of elemental diet should be started with small amounts in low concentrations. If the patient tolerates the diet well, a daily total of 3000 ml at one-tenth strength may be given through the nasoduodenal tube by gravity drip from the 5th–6th PO day. In such cases oral feeding is postponed until the 7th PO day, starting from 200 ml q2h

Table 12.1. Nutritional regime after resection

PO day	IV infusion	Duodenal tube feeding	Oral feeding
1	3000 ml		
2	3000 ml		
3	1500 ml	Nutrient fluid 1500 ml	
4		Nutrient fluid 1500 ml Elemental diet 1500 ml (150 g)	
5		Elemental diet 3000 ml (300 g)	
6		Elemental diet 3000 ml (300 g)	
7		Elemental diet 2000 ml (200 g)	Liquid diet 100 ml q2h (7/day) Water or juice 50 ml between meals
8			Liquid diet 200 ml q2h (7/day) Water or juice ad lib
9			Liquid diet 400 ml q2h (7/day)
10			Semiliquid diet
11			Soft diet

6–7 times daily and doubling the amount each day, with concomitant reduction in tube feeding. When the oral feeding reaches 3000 ml on the 8th–9th PO day, tube feeding is discontinued and the nasoduodenal tube is removed. A semiliquid diet is allowed on the 10th–12th PO day and a soft diet on the 14th PO day.
Table 12.1 summarizes the nutritional regime.

Nasoduodenal tube feeding of elemental diet as postoperative nutritional support may provide not only a sufficient calorie intake, but also a positive nitrogen balance, thus minimizing weight loss, promoting general condition, and speeding up recovery. The delay in oral feeding made possible by tube feeding may also reduce the incidence of anastomotic leakage.

In patients with severe malnutrition, multiple small blood transfusions and IV infusion of plasma or albumin are of benefit.

3.8 Routine Examinations

Bedside chest X-rays are taken if necessary. Fluoroscopy of the chest is routinely carried out 4–5 days after surgery to check for chest fluid and the site of thoracentesis if indicated. A barium swallow examination is performed 2 weeks after operation to review the condition of the anastomosis and the functional status of the stomach. With a smooth recovery the patient is discharged from the hospital 2–3 weeks after the operation. A special service takes care of all follow-up.

3.9 Adjuvant Therapy

A weekly joint conference on thoracic oncology is held, bringing together members of the departments of surgery, radiotherapy, chemotherapy, diagnostic radiology, immunology, and pathology to discuss, among other subjects of common interest, adjuvant treatment plans for every postsurgical patient. Decisions are based on the clinical and operative findings, the results of pathological examination of the resected specimen, the patient's recovery, etc. The plan is carried out meticulously for each patient.

4 Postoperative Complications

Although the morbidity and mortality associated with surgery for carcinoma of the esophagus and gastric cardia have shown a slow decline during the past three decades, there is still much potential for further reduction.

Among 1373 resections for carcinoma of the esophagus at the author's institution from 1958 to 1979, a wide range of postoperative complications occurred for an incidence of 28.6% (392 times). Thirteen of the complications had an incidence of over 0.5% and were considered common, occurring altogether 342 times for an incidence of 24.9% (Table 12.2). During the same period, 612 carcinomas of the gastric cardia were resected with a lower postoperative complication rate of 16.0% (Table 12.3). The occurrence of the individual complications also differed in the two diseases.

The major problems (incidence over 1.5%) were, in decreasing order of frequency, pulmonary complications, leakage of anastomosis, empyema, wound infection, and cardio-

Table 12.2. Incidence and hospital mortality of postoperative complications in 1373 resections for carcinoma of the esophagus (1958–1979)

Complications	Cases	Incidence (%)	Deaths	Mortality (%)
Pulmonary	68	5.0	19	27.9
Anastomotic leakage	62	4.5	22	35.5
Empyema	35	2.6	6	17.1
Wound infection	29	2.1	–	–
Cardiovascular	26	1.9	8	30.8
Vocal cord paralysis	19	1.4	–	–
Shock	14	1.0	2	14.3
Pleural effusion	13	1.0	–	–
Anastomotic stricture	12	0.9	–	–
Chylothorax	12	0.9	3	25.0
Internal bleeding	12	0.9	4	33.3
Pneumothorax	11	0.8	–	–
Pseudomembranous colitis	9	0.7	1	11.1
Miscellaneous	50	3.6	6	12.0
Total	372	27.1	71	19.1

Table 12.3. Incidence and hospital mortality of postoperative complications in 612 resections for carcinoma of the gastric cardia (1958–1979)

Complications	Cases	Incidence (%)	Deaths	Mortality (%)
Anastomotic leakage	18	2.9	9	50.0
Anastomotic stricture	15	2.5	–	–
Empyema	13	2.1	3	23.1
Pulmonary	12	2.0	2	16.7
Cardiovascular	7	1.1	2	28.6
Pneumothorax	7	1.1	1	14.3
Wound infection	6	1.0	–	–
Pseudomembranous colitis	5	0.8	–	–
Subphrenic abscess	3	0.5	1	33.3
Pleural effusion	3	0.5	–	–
Miscellaneous	9	1.5	–	–
Total	98	16.0	18	18.4

vascular complications in esophageal carcinoma, and leakage of anastomosis, stricture of anastomosis, empyema, and pulmonary complications in carcinoma of the gastric cardia. The incidences and mortalities of these major postoperative complications are similar to those in large Chinese series reported by Shao et al. [3] and Zhang et al. [4] (Table 12.4).

It must be noted that in calculating mortality from any given complication, all deaths attributable to the complication should be counted, irrespective of the number of days after operation. In other words, one must not use 30-day mortality as an index of frequency.

Table 12.4. Incidence and mortality of several common postoperative complications following resection reported in China

Authors	Total resec-tions	Pulmonary		Anast. leakage		Empyema		Cardiovasc.		Chylothorax	
		Incid. (%)	Mort. (%)	Incid. (%)	Mort. (%)	Incid. (%)	Mort. (%)	Incid. (%)	Mort. (%)	Incid. (%)	Mort. (%)
Zhang et al. [4]	3321	2.9	20.0[a]	4.8	25.2[a]	4.2	13.6[a]	1.2	34.1[a]	0.8	22.2[a]
Shao et al. [3]	2890	2.1	45.9[a]	3.4	44.9[a]	1.9	5.5[a]	1.0	64.3[a]	0.6	18.8[a]
Huang et al. [20]	1985	4.0	26.3	4.0	38.8	2.4	18.8	1.7	30.3	0.6	25.0

[a] Thirty-day mortality

4.1 Pulmonary

The most commonly encountered complications after resection for carcinoma of the esophagus are respiratory, e.g., tracheobronchitis, bronchopneumonia, pneumonia, and atelectasis. Akiyama et al. [5] also reported pulmonary complications as the most common postoperative problems (13.3%) in 210 cases of esophageal carcinoma treated by resection. Nakayama and Kakegawa [6] reported that among 3426 resections for cancer of the esophagus at 75 leading institutions in Japan from 1974 to 1978, pulmonary complications occurred in 601 cases (17.5%). At the author's institute, pulmonary complications also had the highest incidence, occurring after 5.0% of the 1373 resections for carcinoma of the esophagus from 1958 to 1979.

The incidence of pulmonary complications is lower after resection for carcinoma of the gastric cardia. It was 2.0% among 612 resections for carcinoma of this site at the author's institute from 1958 to 1979, ranking fourth.

The reasons for the frequency of pulmonary complications after surgery for carcinoma of the esophagus are many. The basic factors are that most of the patients are elderly with preexisting emphysema and chronic respiratory infections and that the operation is lengthy with the patient in a fixed position, which tends to cause accumulation of bronchial secretion. Another important but often underemphasized factor is excessive intraoperative traumatization of the trachea, bronchi, and pulmonary hili due to the difficulties in dissection of the esophagus, the tumor, and the mediastinal lymph nodes. Not infrequently, in gaining exposure for these procedures the surgeon pays little respect to the lung, casually exposing it to prolonged mechanical pressure and excessive manipulation. This results in the development of multiple (diffuse) microatelectases, increased bronchial secretion, and bronchopulmonary infection. Furthermore, partial paralysis of the hemidiaphragm as a result of the transthoracic approach and postoperative pain from the chest wound are both major obstacles to the patient's clearance of secretion and sputum from the airway and thus increase the likelihood of pulmonary infection and atelectasis.

Statistics show that the higher the location of the carcinoma, the higher is the incidence of postoperative pulmonary complications. This can easily be explained on the basis of operative magnitude and trauma; the lower incidence of pulmonary complications after resections for carcinoma of the lower esophagus and gastric cardia is obviously due to the shorter operating time and, more crucially, to the lesser degree of trauma to the lung and mediastinum.

The mortality associated with pulmonary complications after surgery for carcinoma of the esophagus and gastric cardia has been rather high. Ong et al. [7] reported a 41.7% incidence with mortality of 40% in 88 resections. The mortality observed by Nakayama and Kakegawa [6] was 17%, and the 30-day mortality reported by Shao et al. [3] and Zhang et al. [4] was 46% and 20% respectively. In the author's series, mortality was 27.9% in esophageal carcinoma and 16.7% in carcinoma of the gastric cardia.

In the 601 cases involving pulmonary complications after resection for carcinoma of the esophagus reported by Nakayama and Kakegawa, atelectasis, pneumonia, and bronchopneumonia were the most common, constituting 91.6% of the total, and acute respiratory distress syndrome and pulmonary edema made up the remaining 8.4%. In the author's series of 68 cases with pulmonary complications after resection for esophageal carcinoma, bronchopneumonia, atelectasis, and pneumonia were also the most frequent, comprising a total of 90%. In fact these three varieties often occurred concomitantly in different degrees and were sometimes difficult to differentiate.

Death in pulmonary complications is most commonly from cardiopulmonary failure due to hypoxia as a result of retention of and difficulty in clearance of bronchial secretions. The amount and nature of these secretions are influenced by the presence or absence of preexisting pulmonary diseases, the degree of intraoperative trauma, the kind of anesthetics used, the number and virulence of pathogenic organisms that might have been introduced through instrumentation of the tracheobronchial tree during anesthesia, the patient's pulmonary and circulatory functions, etc. It is therefore of prime importance in the prevention of pulmonary complications that effective measures be taken to minimize preexisting pulmonary infections, the production and retention of bronchial secretion during and after anesthesia, and intraoperative trauma to the tracheobronchial tree and lung tissue.

It must be emphasized that preventive measures are initiated at the moment when surgical treatment is decided on and that extreme gentleness must be exercised to reduce trauma to any tissue to a minimum. It is also important to avoid overloading of fluid infusion during and after operation and to guarantee the quality of whole blood transfusion, e. g., by filtration of microaggregates of blood cells.

The clinical manifestations of pulmonary infection vary according to pathogenesis and site. Excessive mechanical trauma with exogenic bacterial infection as a result of faulty endotracheal anesthesia may cause early postoperative purulent tracheobronchitis, with the production of copious purulent sputum. Diffuse retention of bronchial secretion peripheral to segmental bronchi may give rise to bronchopneumonia. Retention of secretion with obstruction of the lobar bronchus may cause lobar atelectasis. More than one pathologic condition may occur together, with the result of widespread infection and collapse of the lung. Atelectasis of one or more lobes of the lung, once present, is hard to correct by mere coughing, because no air can enter the distal part of the collapsed lung to blow out the obstruction. In such cases aspiration by means of a fiberbronchoscope with a wide suction channel may be employed. The procedure can be performed at the bedside at frequent intervals and is very effective in clearing the bronchial obstruction and reexpanding the lung.

It is very important to help the patient perform deep-breathing exercises and cough up sputum during the early postoperative period. Since the patient has been informed of the significance of these measures and has received preoperative training, effective cooperation is usually forthcoming. Proper administration of analgesics, preferably in smaller and more frequent doses than usual, is helpful in alleviating postoperative pain and facilitating coughing.

Pulmonary complications usually develop 24–72 h after operation. The usual signs are elevation of temperature and pulse rate, shortness of breath or progressive dyspnea, mild cyanosis, restlessness, and sweating. Moist rales and tubular breathing sounds may be detected by auscultation over the affected lung. In cases of lobar or massive atelectasis, there is restriction of the respiratory movements of the chest wall, with a sucked-in appearance of the intercostal spaces and the supraclavicular fossa on the diseased side. Shifting of the trachea and mediastinum to the affected side and other signs of consolidation of the lung may be evident. As a rule there is marked leukocytosis. The patient may have difficulty in coughing up the sputum, which is often thick and purulent. Careful clinical observation and physical examination and timely bedside X-ray of the chest are usually sufficient to arrive at the diagnosis.

Treatment of pulmonary complications consists chiefly of care of the respiratory tract, aid in expectorating sputum, and adequate antibiotic therapy (see also Sect. 3.2).

In patient who have copious sputum but cannot breathe deeply or are too weak to cough effectively, tracheal suction by means of a clean 18-F catheter introduced through the nose and into the trachea as the patient takes a deep breath while facing forward is usually helpful in clearing the bronchial tree and preventing atelectasis. However, this procedure may not be successful in some patients and it has the drawback of being blind – it cannot be aimed at a specific location. Fiberbronchoscopić aspiration has the advantages of providing a clear internal view of the tracheobronchial tree and accurately aspirating any desired bronchus, and is also less traumatizing. It has consequently become indispensable in the postoperative management of pulmonary complications. Under light topical anesthesia the aspiration can be done at the bedside every 2–3 h as desired. Because of its reliability in relieving obstructive atelectasis and retention of bronchial secretion and its relative noninvasiveness, it has in many instances replaced tracheostomy, the indications for which have been reduced to those patients who need mechanical respiratory support.

Nakayama and Kakegawa [6], reviewing pulmonary complications following esophageal cancer surgery, pointed out that protracted hypoxemia is the result of intrapulmonary shunt, which cannot be treated simply by removal of airway secretions, and suggested the use of mechanical respiratory support in the hope of reducing the shunt. Prophylactic mechanical respiratory support for short periods after operation has been advocated by Schmidt et al. [8].

The proper use of specific antibiotics is of benefit in both prevention and treatment of pulmonary infections. The choice of drugs depends on the nature of the chief offending microflora and their antibiotic sensitivities and on the antibiotic history of the patient, including allergic reactions. Specific antibiotics may be used singly or in combination, but overuse, particularly of those with wide-spectrum activities, is to be avoided, as suprainfections such as staphylococcal pseudomembranous colitis may occur.

4.2 Anastomotic

Anastomotic complications, i.e., leakage, fistula to the aorta, or bleeding are a serious problem after resection or bypass for carcinoma of the esophagus or gastric cardia, and constitute one of the major causes of operative mortality.

4.2.1 Leakage

Huang [9] reported in 1963 that among 1503 resections for carcinoma of the esophagus or gastric cardia in nine leading hospitals in China there was an incidence of anastomotic leakage of 4.8% (73/1503), with mortality of 57.5% (42/73), or 28.4% of all operation-linked deaths (42/148). More recent statistics [3, 4, 10–12] show that the incicende of anastomotic leakage is still 3%–5%, although the mortality displays a slow decrease. Leakage thus remains a problem, and its prevention and appropriate management are of great significance.

A small number of cases are missed due to difficulty in diagnosis, and therefore discrepancies exist between actual occurrence and reported incidence. For instance, leakage may sometimes be misdiagnosed as acute empyema or mediastinal abscess. On the other hand, perforation of the transplanted intrathoracic stomach may well be mistaken for anastomotic leakage if additional evidence is lacking. Further, a small encapsulated anastomotic leakage may escape notice altogether in the absence of obvious symptoms and signs.

In the author's series of 1373 resections for carcinoma of the esophagus (at the Cancer Institute of the Chinese Academy of Medical Sciences during the period 1958–1979) esophagogastric anastomotic leakage occurred in 52 cases and cervical esophagocolonic anastomotic leakage in 10 cases, with an overall incidence of 4.5% (62/1373). Of these 62 patients, a total of 40 recovered after intensive treatment and 22 eventually died, a mortality of 35.5%. The 10 cases of cervical esophagocolonic leakage occurred among 25 colonic interpositions, giving a leakage rate of 40%. All these 10 patients recovered after local drainage. Counting only those cases involving resection of esophageal carcinoma and esophagogastric anastomosis, there were 52 leakages among 1348 resections, an esophagogastrostomy leakage rate of 3.9%. All 22 deaths were in this group, a mortality of 42.3% [10]. The incidence of leakage in relation to site of esophagogastric anastomosis is shown in Table 12.5.

During the same period of time (1958–1979), 612 resections for carcinoma of the gastric cardia with low intrathoracic esophagogastrostomy were performed at the Cancer Institute. Leakage occurred in 18 cases (2.9%), with nine deaths (50.0%).

Most anastomotic leakages occurred between 2 and 7 days after operation, with a peak at 4–6 days. Huang [9] found that 16 of 17 leakage occurred between 1 and 10 days after operation, with an average of 4.5 days. Zhang and Huang [13] judged the time of occurrence of leakage clinically in 61 cases and found that in 80.3% it was between 2 and 8 days after operation, with a peak at 5–6 days (Fig. 12.1).

Early leakages (developing within 3 days of operation) are probably due to technical

Table 12.5. Incidence of esophagogastric anastomotic leakage following resection for carcinoma of the esophagus according to site of anastomosis (1958–1979)

Site of anastomosis	Resections	Leaks	Incidence (%)
Cervical	43	6	14.0
Intrathoracic supra-aortic	1056	36	3.4
Intrathoracic infra-aortic	249	10	4.0
Total	1348	52	3.9

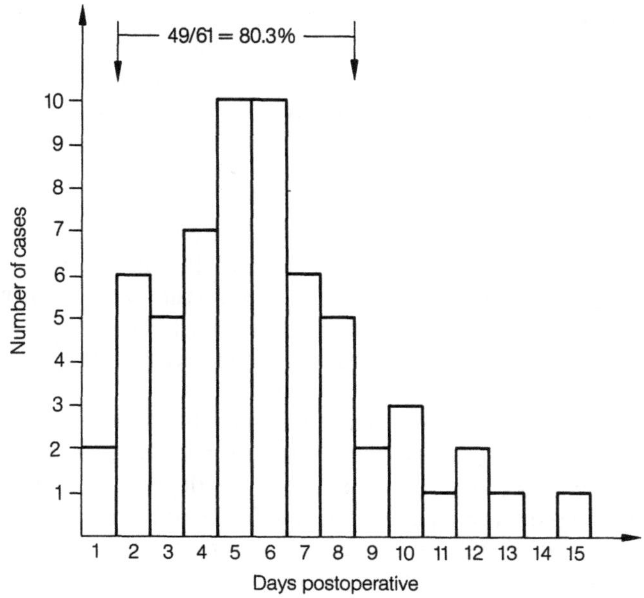

Fig. 12.1. Days of occurrence of 61 anastomotic leakages as judged on clinical grounds

defects, while late leakages (over 7 days after operation) are most likely caused by healing defects. The earlier the leakage occurs, the more severe are the resulting derangements to body physiology, and hence the poorer the prognosis.

Clinical manifestations vary according to the site of anastomosis. Small leakages from cervical anastomoses usually cause only local congestion and tenderness, with or without subcutaneous crepitation but without constitutional symptoms, and may be difficult to differentiate from localized infection. Diagnosis can often be verified, however, on incision of the wound, and spontaneous healing usually takes place after drainage. With more extensive leakage there is more marked local infection and the patient may have low-grade or moderate fever with leukocytosis. There may be spontaneous rupture of the wound with discharge of foul purulent material, possibly containing saliva or gastric or intestinal fluid. Upon incision of the wound the leakage may be seen.

Intrathoracic leakage during the early postoperative period may cause acute tension pneumopyothorax, high fever, dyspnea, or even shock and death, whereas leakage developing after 4–5 days usually gives rise to more localized empyema of pyopneumothorax. The patient may have chest pain followed quickly by fever, tachycardia, and general intoxication. Roentgenography usually shows pleural effusions with one or more fluid levels confined to the operated side, occasionally on the opposite side if the contralateral mediastinal pleura was opened during the operation, or sometimes on both sides. Chest X-rays usually show marked changes over a short period. Chest aspiration usually yields turbid foul fluid in which mucous material or food particles may be found.

Sometimes a late-developing or very small leakage may resemble an encapsulated intrapleural or mediastinal abscess close to the site of anastomosis. The patient may have persistently high or moderate fever, aching in the chest or back, and some degree of dysphagia. Roentgenography may show encapsulated effusion with or without fluid level close to the site of anastomosis, or what appears to be localized heavy pleural reaction. Depending on the intracavitary pressure gradient, which may be high enough to prevent inflow of barium, barium swallow may or may not show a fine fistula leading from the anastomosis to the encapsulated cavity; once the cavity is drained or aspirated, however, the fistula is usually obvious on barium examination. The possibility of a localized anastomotic leakage must be kept in mind in cases of persistent fever and general weakness after the operation or of unexplained heavy pleural reaction or encapsulated effusion with or without fluid level.

Leakage from an infra-aortic or low mediastinal anastomosis may give rise to symptoms and signs of peritonitis, which is usually confined to the upper abdomen but can be located in the right lower quadrant, and thus may even be mistaken for acute appendicitis. The infection apparently arises when the fluid leaking from the anastomosis in the posterior mediastinum drains into the peritoneal cavity.

The diagnosis of leakage is usually straightforward in cervical anastomosis, but may be quite difficult in intrathoracic anastomoses. Among the 1373 resections for esophageal carcinoma at the Cancer Institute, only about one-third of the intrathoracic leakages were promptly recognized by typical symptoms and signs. In another third of the cases the diagnosis was established later, the delay depending on the type of clinical manifestations and on the efforts made by the medical staff. An average delay of 4 days was reported by Huang [9] in 1963. In Zhang and Huang's report of 61 cases with leakage [13], the diagnosis was made promptly in 12 cases (19.7%), delayed by 1–3 days in 20 cases (32.8%), delayed by 4–7 days in 21 cases (34.4%), and delayed by over 7 days in eight cases (13.1%). The average delay in diagnosis was also 4 days in this series of cases.

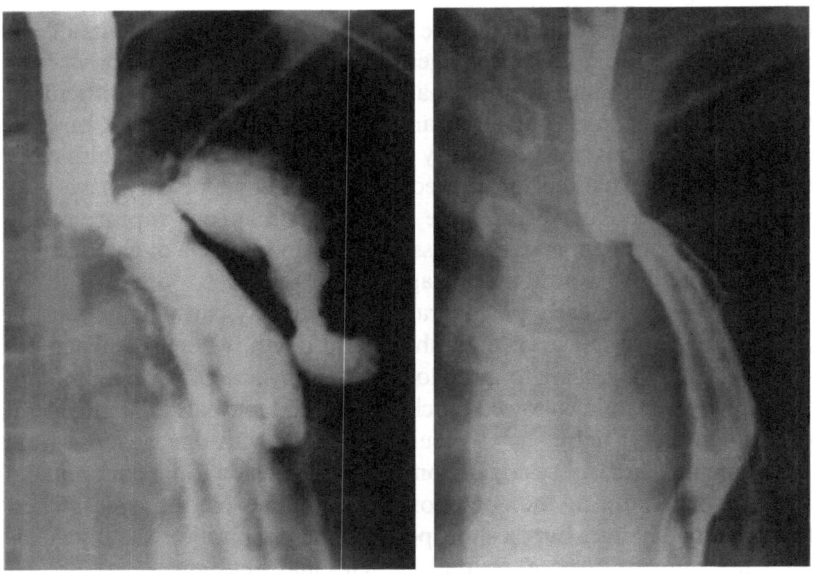

Fig. 12.2. Postoperative anastomotic leakage healed after conservative treatment. A 43-year-old woman (Fuwai Hosp. Nr. 11765) underwent resection of carcinoma of the midthoracic segment of the esophagus and intrathoracic supra-aortic esophagogastrostomy. On the 4th PO day she had high fever, and fluoroscopy and thoracentesis revealed empyema of the left chest. Barium swallow on the 6th PO day showed anastomotic leakage *(left)*. Treatment was conservative: closed chest drainage and jejunostomy feeding. Barium swallow 3 weeks later showed complete healing of the leakage *(right)*. The patient was alive and well 4 years after operation. (Courtesy of Fuwai Hospital)

In X-ray examination of leakage with contrast medium (either iodized oil or thin barium), if the leakage cannot be demonstrated with the patient in the upright position, then the patient must be put in the recumbent position and turned from side to side while swallowing the contrast medium, a maneuver which enables detection of even a small fistula. Further films are taken to prove the diagnosis and assess the size and location of the fistula (Fig. 12.2). The presence of floating mucous substance or food particles in the chest fluid is often diagnostic for anastomotic leakage or perforation of the intrathoracic stomach. In tapping the chest care must be taken not to puncture the intrathoracic stomach, which is usually situated along the paravertebral gutter but may be markedly dilated, in order to avoid misleading findings. Methylene blue taken by mouth is a simple and efficient diagnostic test for anastomotic leakage, but a patient may be upset on seeing the blue chest fluid.

The management of anastomotic leakage is by no means easy, as most of the patients are in poor general condition and have postoperative physiologic disorders aggravated by the acute infetion due to the leakage and by the rapid loss of body fluids and electrolytes. Further circulatory and respiratory disturbances often put the patient into a critical condition. Even if the patient's condition stabilizes after intensive treatment, the existence of a fistula precludes feeding by mouth and makes nutrition a difficult problem. Malnutrition will in turn retard spontaneous healing of the leak. It is a real challenge, therefore, to solve these problems, break the vicious circle, and promote recovery.

When deciding on the form of treatment, the time of occurrence of the leakage, the site of the anastomosis, the size of the leak, and the general condition of the patient must all be taken into consideration. In small or late-developing leakages, there is generally a rather good chance of healing by conservative treatment, i.e., drainage, antibiotics, and nutrition, but in larger or early-developing leakages, conservative treatment is likely to fail. On secondary thoracotomy the leak is occasionally found to involve one-third or more of the circumference of the anastomosis with everting mucosal margins, a situation which precludes spontaneous healing.

As already mentioned, small cervical leakages usually heal spontaneously after incision and drainage of the wound. In the case of extensive necrosis of the transplanted bowel, however, excision of the necrotic bowel and subsequent reconstruction to establish alimentary continuity are necessary. For promptly recognized early anastomotic leakages, the choice of treatment may be between the following:

1. Immediate secondary thoracotomy with excision of the primary anastomosis and construction of a new one. This offers an excellent chance of success if pleural infection has not yet taken hold and if adequate lengths of both esophagus and stomach remain to allow reanastomosis without tension. At the author's institution, about two-thirds of a limited number of patients so treated recovered smoothly after the second operation. Former experience in secondary thoracotomy with repair of the leak was discouraging, as in most cases leakage recurred.
2. Immediate secondary thoracotomy with excision of the primary anastomosis, exteriorization of the esophageal stump in the neck, closure of the gastric stoma and reduction of the stomach into the abdomen, and construction of a feeding gastrostomy or jejunostomy. A subcutaneous or retrosternal colon interposition is performed later to reestablish alimentary continuity.
3. Conservative treatment if the patient's condition does not allow reoperation. In such cases adequate, efficient, closed-chest drainage of the pneumopyothorax is very impor-

tant. Pleural infection is controlled by sufficient antibiotic coverage. Adequate nutrition is maintained chiefly by feeding through the duodenal tube inserted during the operation or through the newly created gastrostomy or jejunostomy. It has been proved that tube feeding with elemental diet is appropriate and can provide sufficient calorie and nitrogen intakes. If all these measures go smoothly and the leak is reasonably small, the chance of spontaneous healing of both the fistula and the empyema is good, although the process usually takes about 1.5–3 months.

In cases in which leakage occurs or is first recognized late in the postoperative period, secondary thoracotomy is not advisable because of active infection and pleural adhesions. For such cases conservative management is indicated.

It is clear that prevention of anastomotic leakage is of prime importance. Since many factors can combine to cause a leak, prevention must have a broad foundation based on the different aspects of every individual patient's condition and must be initiated prior to surgery. Attention is paid to the patient's nutritional status, which is invaluable to tissue healing, and dietary supplements are given when indicated. Preoperative treatment of oral and/or esophageal infections is also important.

Meticulous care is taken in performing the anastomosis. Great refinement and skill are needed, as the esophagus lacks a serosa and its muscular coat has little tensile strength. Every stitch of the anastomosis must be placed accurately and securely, yet overtension must be avoided to prevent pressure necrosis or cutting into the tissue. The corresponding tissue planes of the esophagus and of the transplanted stomach or intestine must be accurately approximated to facilitate primary healing. An invagination of 2.5–3 cm of the distal esophagus into the stomach or colon at the anastomosis is desirable in order to increase the mechanical strength of the anastomosis and reduce postoperative reflux. To obtain an invagination of this length the anastomosis is made at a higher level so that the length of esophageal resection is not diminished. Ease of exposure and convenience of manipulation are prerequisites for a good anastomosis, and for this reason the supra-aortic site is often preferred to the high infra-aortic; similarly, the cervical site is often preferred to the apex of the thoracic cavity [9, 14].

Two general principles of anastomosis construction are maximal preservation of blood supply to the organs and minimal tension at the anastomosis. Excessive freeing of the esophageal stump is to be avoided, and in mobilizing the stomach as a substitute for the resected esophagus, great care must be taken to preserve its blood supply from the right gastric and right gastroepiploic arteries and their communicating branches with the left gastric, left gastroepiploic, and short gastric arteries, which are to be divided. The stomach must be manipulated very gently to prevent trauma to the gastric wall, e.g., pressure contusion and abrasion, which may result in focal ischemia or even necrosis. Overtension at the esophagogastric anastomosis may be encountered in cases involving concomitant partial or subtotal gastrectomy, as in resection for carcinoma of the gastric cardia, and in high anastomosis with a small stomach. This should be borne in mind in the planning of surgical procedures and avoided at operation.

Gastric decompression for at least 36–48 h after operation and avoidance of oral feeding sooner than ordinarily allowed are also of importance in the prevention of leakage. Every postoperative routine should be strictly followed.

The lack of strong tissue coverage around the intrathoracic anastomosis is one of the problems in the prevention of leakage, and is especially significant in the presence of postoperative atelectasis, pneumothorax, or profuse pleural effusion. It is therefore advisable to use available surrounding tissues, such as mediastinal pleura or omentum, to cover and thus strengthen the anastomosis. Prevention or timely treatment of postoperative pulmonary and intrapleural complications helps to lessen the risk of anastomotic leaks.

The increasing use of a stapler for esophagogastric anastomosis during the past decade has been reported to reduce the incidence of anastomotic leakage [15], but the incidence of stricture at the anastomosis has increased. Further refinement of the device seems necessary.

The advances in microsurgery have made possible the interposition of an isolated free graft of a segment of bowel [16]. This technique of small blood vessel anastomosis may also be used to reinforce the blood supply of an ordinary transplant of colon or jejunum with a blood vessel pedicle, providing a double blood supply to this segment of the bowel. Further clinical trials are under way.

4.2.2 Aortoanastomotic Fistula

On rare occasions leakage at the anastomosis or perforation of an intrathoracic gastric ulcer results in erosion of the adjacent adherent aorta, forming a fistula and leading to fatal hemorrhage [17]. This usually occurs about 2–3 weeks after operation. Prodromal symptoms such as discomfort or pain in the chest and low-grade fever may be present for a short time before massive fatal hematemesis occurs. Sometimes bleeding is temporarily halted by formation of a clot at the fistula; intermittent hematemeses may then persist for 2–3 days, only to be followed by dislodgement of the clot and fatal hemorrhage.

The avoidance of aortoanastomotic fistula apparently depends on the prevention of leakage from the anastomosis and ulcer formation in the transplanted stomach, which may result from operative trauma. It is advisable not to have the anastomosis in direct contact with the aorta. For that reason, anastomosis performed lateral to or at the level of the aortic arch should be raised to the supra-aortic region, and that below the aortic arch should be separated from the descending aorta by a pedicle of omentum, usually available on the wall of the thoracic stomach.

Aortoanastomotic fistula is practically always fatal. Salvage could be possible if thoracotomy were performed immediately with occlusion of the bleeding segment of the aorta followed by excision of the fistula and anastomoses of both aorta and alimentary tract, but this has not been reported in the literature.

4.2.3 Stricture

The reported incidence of stricture of the anastomosis varies with different authors and different techniques. In the author's institution, stricture of the esophagogastrostomy stoma has occurred in 0.9% of the cases of carcinoma of the esophagus and 2.5% of cases of carcinoma of the gastric cardia.

Dysphagia within a month or so after operation is often due at least in part to swelling or congestion of the anastomosis as a result of general hypoproteinemia or inflammation, and will therefore slowly improve as these conditions subside.

An occasional patient way have severe obstruction at the anastomosis in the early postoperative period as a result of errors in surgery. For instance the author has encountered a case in which a silk stitch had passed from the anterior to the posterior wall of the esophagus, closing the lumen almost completely; the stitch was removed under esophagoscopy with immediate relief of the obstruction.

Anastomotic stenosis appearing late after surgery is not infrequently due to recurrence of tumor, but in the majority of cases it is cicatricial and benign in nature. In rare instances a second primary carcinoma of the remaining segment of the esophagus may be the cause.

Use of excessive sutures at the anastomosis, poor approximation of the mucosal layers, local infection, granulation formation, and reflux esophagitis are some of the many causes of cicatricial stricture. The etiology of late cicatricial stenosis is not always certain; it is our impression that reflux esophagitis is not a common factor. The use of certain staplers for anastomosis may lead to eventual cicatricial stenosis through excessive crush injury of both esophageal and gastric walls at the anastomosis.

Stricture of the anastomosis should be examined by barium swallow. The contour and distensibility of the esophageal wall above the anastomosis as shown on roentgenograms may help differentiate cicatricial from cancerous stenosis. Esophagoscopy and biopsy are usually needed to determine the precise nature of the stricture.

Benign cicatricial strictures are usually treated by endoscopic dilatation repeated at intervals until a reasonable improvement of dysphagia is obtained, but can also be dealt with by dilatation and intubation, the tube then serving both as a passage for food and as an indwelling dilator. Benign strictures of cervical anastomoses may sometimes be treated by local plastic operations to enlarge the lumen.

In strictures due to local recurrence of cancer, dilatation can only afford a temporary improvement of dysphagia. Local radiotherapy may offer some palliation as the tumor tissue recedes, but in some cases subsequent scar formation may further aggravate the stenosis. In some cases with no evidence of metastasis, a secondary operation with esophageal reconstruction may be carried out.

4.3 Cardiovascular

The incidence of cardiovascular complications after resection for carcinoma of the esophagus or gastric cardia is generally reported in China as about 1%–2%. Mortality, however, is high; it was reported as 64.3% by Shao et al. [3] and 34.1% by Zhang et al. [4], both referring to deaths within 30 days of operation. In the author's series of 1373 resections for carcinoma of the esophagus and 612 resections for carcinoma of the gastric cardia, the hospital mortality for cardiovascular complications is 30.8% and 28.6% respectively.

The most common cardiovascular complications are myocardial infarction, heart failure, cardiac arrest, cardiac arrhythmia, and pulmonary embolism. Most of the problems arise from the action of intra- and postoperative hypoxemia or other serious complications on a preexisting coronary insufficiency. Hence thorough preoperative assessment of the patient's cardiac function and ECG manifestations, detailed evaluation of the preexisting insufficiency and its possible manifestation during and after the operation, meticulous intra- and postoperative monitoring of the cardiopulmonary functions, and proper prevention of hypoxia, blood pressure fluctuations, pulmonary complications, etc., are all important in the prevention of cardiovascular complications. Early movements and changes of position in bed and early ambulation are also significant in the prevention of pulmonary embolism.

Elderly patients and those with poor or borderline cardiopulmonary reserves are preferably kept in the intensive care unit for careful monitoring and treatment after operation.

4.4 Empyema

Empyema as a postoperative complication includes only pleural infections that are due neither to anastomotic leakage nor to perforation of the alimentary tract. However, such differentiation is sometimes difficult, and in practise a small number of borderline cases are wrongly classified.

The incidence of empyema following surgery for carcinoma of the esophagus and gastric cardia is about 2%–4% (Table 12.4), but mortality is as high as 15%, which indicates the danger posed by empyema following major operations. In the author's series of 1373 resections for carcinoma of the esophagus the incidence of postoperative empyema was 2.6% (35 cases) with mortality of 17.1% (six cases), and in 612 resections for carcinoma of the gastric cardia there was an incidence of 2.1% (13 cases) and mortality of 23.1% (three cases). In 472 exploratory thoracotomies in nonresectable carcinoma of the esophagus or gastric cardia, there was only one case of postoperative empyema, which healed after treatment. It is clear that the risk of pleural infection is significantly greater in intrathoracic open anastomosis of the esophagus than in simple exploration.

The empyema often occurs about a week after operation. Clinically, there are signs of suppuration of the pleural cavity. X-ray may reveal generalized or loculated pleural effusion which usually shows no fluid level before tapping, and the change in the roentgenographic picture is not as rapid and marked as in anastomotic leakage. Thoracentesis usually yields relatively clear purulent fluid which may have a foul odor but contains none of the floating mucous material that is usually present in leakage. In case of doubt, a barium swallow examination should be carried out.

The classical treatment for postoperative empyema is closed chest drainage, either with resection of a small segment of rib or by means of intercostal intubation. Despite the usually good final results, its time-consuming nature and the necessity of changing from closed to open drainage before the tube can finally be removed make this method unattractive. Furthermore, in emaciated patients the drainage wound frequently becomes eroded and enlarged by the pressure of the chest tube and is then no longer airtight. The premature open drainage results in collapse of the lung and widening of the empyema cavity.

During the past two decades, most cases of postoperative empyema at the author's institution have been treated with daily needle aspiration and local instillation of antibiotics. The empyema fluid is aspirated as completely as possible and the empyema cavity is gently irrigated with saline and an effective antibiotic is instilled. The fever will usually go down in 2–3 days. As the empyema cavity becomes smaller and the amount of purulent fluid decreases, aspiration may be done every other day until no more fluid can be withdrawn and X-rays show no evidence of fluid collection. The results of this treatment are usually gratifying, especially in early and localized cases where the wall of the cavity is not greatly thickened. In a few cases, however, the condition may recur in 2–3 months and treatment by aspiration or tube drainage may again be necessary.

Care must be taken to avoid perforation of the intrathoracic stomach by either necrosis resulting from pressure exerted by the tube or puncture by the aspirating needle.

There are two crucial points in the prevention of postoperative empyema: (a) strict isolation of the operative field and the surgical instruments used, to reduce bacterial contamination to a minimum, and (b) maintenance of effective chest drainage after operation so that the lung is reexpanded promptly and collection of pleural fluid is prevented. Any significant collection of pleural fluid after the chest tube is removed should be aspirated by thoracentesis.

4.5 Chylothorax

Because of its close anatomic relationship to the esophagus, the thoracic duct, which has a very thin wall and usually contains clear fluid at the time of operation, may suffer unnoticed injury during dissection of the carcinoma or construction of the anastomosis, resulting in chylothorax.

Huang and Zhang [18] reported 15 cases of postoperative chylothorax among 903 esophageal carcinomas operated upon from 1947 to 1963, an incidence of 1.7%, whereas none developed in 337 cases of carcinoma of the gastric cardia operated upon during the same period. One case (0.3%) occurred in one of the 366 patients who underwent exploratory thoracotomy, the remaining 14 (2.6%) among the 537 resection cases. The incidence varied according to site of tumor (Table 12.6). Eleven of the patients recovered after treatment and four died (26.7%).

In the author's series of 1373 resections for carcinoma of the esophagus, 12 cases (0.9%) were complicated by postoperative chylothorax and three of the patients died (25.0%). During the same period, no postoperative chylothorax occurred in 204 exploratory thoracotomies and 70 bypass operations for carcinoma of the esophagus or in 880 operations for carcinoma of the gastric cardia. Combining the figures for carcinoma of the esophagus and gastric cardia, Zhang et al. [4] and Shao et al. [3] reported incidence of 0.8% and 0.6% and 30-day mortality of 22.2% and 18.8% respectively.

Postoperative chylothorax occurs most frequently after resection for carcinoma of the upper and midthoracic esophagus, in anastomosis above the aortic arch, and in more marked extraesophageal tumor invasion. Thus the cause is apparently intraoperative injury of the thoracic duct at, below, or above the aortic arch in the course of dissection of the tumor or construction of the anastomosis.

In the majority of cases the chylothorax develops within 4 days of surgery. In a few cases it manifests itself on the day of operation or on the 1st PO day, and occasionally it shows up as late as 2 weeks or more after operation. The diagnosis of postoperative chylothorax is relatively simple in the early postoperative stage, but may be more difficult later, when differentiation from empyema or anastomotic leakage needs to be made.

Table 12.6. Incidence of chylothorax following resection for carcinoma of the esophagus according to location of tumor

Segment	Resections	Chylothorax	Incidence (%)
Upper	46	2	4.3
Middle	283	9	3.2
Lower	208	3	1.4
Total	537	14	2.6

The characteristic signs of early postoperative chylothorax are exceptionally copious drainage of chest fluid from the chest tube, rapid pulse, and low blood pressure. If the chest tube has been removed the large collection of chest fluid in the pleural cavity usually causes shortness of breath, palpitation, and signs of pleural effusion with deviation of the mediastinum. Shock may manifest itself in severe cases. The chylous chest fluid is usually bloodstained in the early postoperative period due to oozing of blood from the operative fields, and also contains fat droplets as a result of tissue dissection, but will gradually become serous and slightly turbid. When oral feeding starts the intrapleural fluid soon becomes typically chylous and rapidly increases in amount, reaching levels varying from a few hundred to as much as 3000 ml/day.

The intrapleural chylous fluid is alkaline, with a specific gravity of about 1.006–1.020. Protein content is 1.3–7.0 g% depending on how long the fluid has been in the pleural cavity, where the protein may coagulate and separate out. Microscopically the cell count may vary from 400 to 4000, with a vast predominance of lymphocytes. In about half the cases fat droplets can be found on staining with Sudan III.

If a right thoracotomy approach is used, postoperative chylothorax is usually on the right. In cases involving a left thoracotomy approach and opening of the contralateral mediastinal pleura, one may see a right chylothorax if the injury of the thoracic duct is below the aortic arch and a left-sided or bilateral chylothorax if the injury is above the arch. This is because when the patient is in a supine position the descending thoracic aorta acts as a dam, diverting the chyle extravasated from below the aortic arch through the opened mediastinal pleura into the right chest. If the contralateral mediastinal pleura is not opened, the chylothorax after a left thoracotomy approach is usually on the left.

Treatment for chylothorax following surgery for carcinoma of the esophagus should be energetic and comprehensive. Besides adequate antibiotics and vitamins, sufficient amounts of whole blood, plasma, or their substitutes, and glucose, electrolytes, and water should be given to compensate the losses. When the patient is allowed to eat, a low-fat, high-protein, high-carbohydrate diet should be given. If the patient is in a good nutritional state, temporary abstention from oral feeding may be of benefit in decreasing the outflow of chyle and in favoring spontaneous closure of the thoracic duct.

Chest fluid should be evacuated in order to reexpand the lung and prevent infection. Repeated chest tappings are usually needed. When accumulation of chest fluid is rapid with severe compression and cannot be managed by thoracenteses, closed chest tube drainage may be instituted. Under aseptic precautions the aspirated chylous fluid may be given to the patient through the gastric tube or duodenal tube, but not by IV infusion.

Conservative treatment leads to slow recovery with spontaneous healing of the chylothorax in a few cases, but most patients eventually succumb as a result of rapid depletion of water, electrolytes, and nutrition. The long-term use of total parenteral nutrition may prolong life but is costly and may in some cases never effect spontaneous healing of the thoracic duct.

During the past two decades many authors have adopted surgical treatment for postoperative chylothorax, with a marked reduction in mortality.

In the 15 cases reported by Huang and Zhang [18], there were three deaths (33.3%) among the nine patients treated conservatively, but only one (16.7%) among the six treated surgically.

It is our opinion that only a few patients should be treated conservatively, i.e., those in whom doubt exists about the diagnosis or the course of the complication is slow and the outflow of chyle is limited. Surgical treatment should be chosen in the majority of patients in whom the diagnosis is clear and the complication appears early and runs a rapid course. The results of surgery are often most rewarding.

The patient must be properly prepared for surgery. To facilitate location of the site of thoracic duct injury, 400–600 ml milk fortified with butter or cream is given by mouth or through the gastric or duodenal tube about 3 h prior to induction of anesthesia. Chest fluid is aspirated as completely as possible to increase pulmonary ventilation.

As regards choice of thoracotomy approach, it is advisable to use the original one again if the second operation is not later than a week after the first, in order to preserve lung function on the contralateral side. If surgery is more than 10 days after the initial operation, it is wise always to operate on the side of the chylothorax, or on the side contralateral to the primary operation, in order to avoid difficulties due to postoperative pleural adhesions.

After the chest is opened the collected fluid is quickly evacuated and the original esophageal bed is exposed. Careful inspection will usually locate the thoracic duct injury, from which milky chylous fluid oozes. The duct is gently dissected and double ligations are made above and below the leak. If no further leakage of chyle is found upon careful inspection, closed tube drainage is inserted and the chest wound is closed. If the thoracic duct injury cannot be found, usually a result of poor filling of the duct, double ligation is performed at a short distance above the hiatus of the diaphragm.

The secret of prevention of postoperative chylothorax lies in careful avoidance of injury to the thoracic duct during exploration, resection, and anastomosis. Meticulous care must be taken in dissection of the esophagus above the aortic arch, where the duct, obliquely crossing the left aspect of the esophagus upward and anteriorly, is particularly vulnerable. The thoracic duct may be resected and ligated if it is invaded by tumor, and is also ligated in case of known or suspected injury. Routine prophylactic ligation may not be advisable in esophageal surgery, as ligation per se may cause inadvertent injury.

4.6 Injury of Recurrent Laryngeal Nerve

The recurrent laryngeal nerves are anatomically closely related to the esophagus in the superior mediastinum and the neck, and are prone to injury in surgery for carcinoma of the upper and middle segments of the esophagus, with the result of vocal cord paralysis. They may also be damaged by excessive traction on the left vagal trunk during surgery for carcinoma of the lower esophagus. A similar injury may result from removal of the esophagus in "esophagectomy without thoracotomy" by means of inversion extraction, where considerable traction is often exerted on both vagal trunks.

Although injury of the recurrent laryngeal nerve in surgery for carcinoma of the esophagus is usually unilateral and is rarely a direct cause of death, the resulting cord paralysis and hoarseness are real handicaps to recovery because they deprive the patient of his ability to cough effectively and increase the risk of pulmonary infection due to aspiration.

In surgery of the cervical esophagus, good exposure and meticulous attention to the recurrent nerves are crucial in the prevention of cord paralysis. A left-sided approach is usually preferred, as differences in anatomic relations lead to a lower incidence of cord paralysis on that side than on the right.

4.7 Prepyloric Obstruction Due to Torsion of Transplanted Stomach

Postoperative prepyloric obstruction due to torsion of the transplanted stomach is a rare but serious complication which is entirely preventable. It occurs mostly in high esophagogastrostomies and is a result of inadvertent rotation of the stomach through 360° counterclockwise as viewed from below. This may escape the surgeon's notice because the lesser and greater curvatures of the stomach remain in the "normal" position intrathoracically, the twisting taking place in the prepyloric segment under cover of the diaphragm. This condition inevitably causes obstruction and retention, but apparently does not interfere with the stomach's blood supply.

In the author's series of 1373 resections for carcinoma of the esophagus there were four occurrences of torsion of the stomach. In two cases the condition was recognized at the completion of the anastomosis, which then had to be excised and reconstructed after correction of the torsion. In the other two patients it was not discovered until the 3rd PO day, when severe gastric retention developed with abdominal pain, nausea, and vomiting of copious sour, dark-colored material. X-ray examination revealed a markedly dilated intrathoracic stomach and retention of fluid. Barium could not pass into the duodenum. A diagnosis of pyloric obstruction was made but conservative treatment, including gastric decompression, failed to relieve the obstruction. Exploratory celiotomy was done, in one case on the 7th and in the other on the 8th PO day. Torsion of the antrum of the stomach was found and a gastrojejunostomy bypass was carried out in each case. Both patients recovered smoothly after the second operation [19].

This complication cannot occur if the surgeon is aware of the risk and places the transplanted stomach carefully in the correct position before constructing the anastomosis.

4.8 Diaphragmatic Hernia

Postoperative diaphragmatic hernia occurs mostly in cases involving left thoracotomy with transplantation of the stomach through an incision on the left hemidiaphragm. The chief causes are defects in suturing or healing of the diaphragm, and severe cough after operation and high intra-abdominal pressure may be contributory factors.

The hernia may occur early or late after operation. In severe cases there may be symptoms and signs of complete intestinal obstruction and lung compression. Intrathoracic rupture of the herniated intestine may occur, resulting in acute pleural infection. Shock and death may ensue if appropriate treatment is not instituted immediately. In cases with no or only mild symptoms the condition may pass unnoticed, so the true incidence of this complication is probably higher than is commonly recognized.

The usual site of the hernia is the anterior part of the diaphragmatic incision. The part most commonly herniating into the chest is the left colon, sometimes accompanied by a length of small intestine. In occasional cases the rupture is at the posterior angle of the diaphragmatic incision, and loops of colon or jejunum may enter the right pleural cavity.

The diagnosis of postoperative diaphragmatic hernia can be verified by the finding of a loop of intestine in the chest (Fig. 12.3). Barium enema examination may be necessary.

In general, postoperative diaphragmatic hernia should be treated surgically, with reduction of the herniated intestine and repair of the diaphragmatic defect. In early cases this may be done through an abdoinal incision. In late cases, however, the herniated intestine

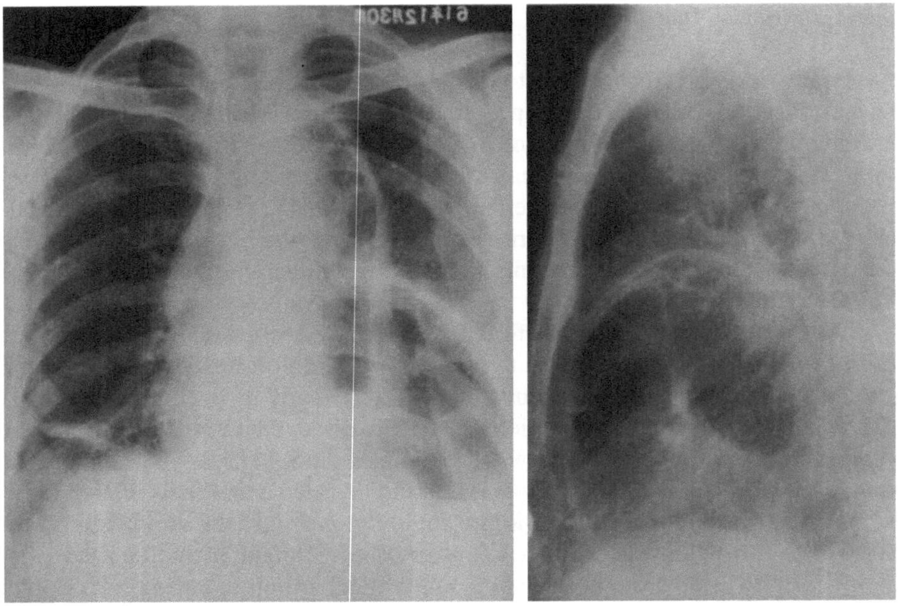

Fig. 12.3. X-ray manifestation of postoperative diaphragmatic hernia. A 51-year-old man (CI Hosp. No. 27711) had symptoms and signs of intestinal obstruction 9 days after resection of midthoracic esophageal carcinoma. X-ray showed an air-filled loop of colon in the left lower chest, anterior and lateral to the intrathoracic stomach

is often adherent to the intrathoracic organs, making reduction difficult and dangerous through an abdominal incision, so a thoracotomy approach is usually needed.

It is clear that careful suturing of the diaphragmatic incision at operation and avoidance of a severe postoperative increase of intra-abdominal pressure are important in the prevention of this complication.

References

1. Belsey R (1981) Esophageal reconstruction with colon for benign disease. In: Stipa S, Belsey R, Moraldi A (eds) Medical and surgical problems of the esophagus. Academic, London New York, Serono symposium no 43, p 195
2. Huang GJ (1966) Clinical application of closed chest drainage (in Chinese). Chin J Surg 14: 44–47
3. Shao LF, Li ZC, Liu SX, et al. (1982) Results of surgery for 3155 cases of carcinoma of the esophagus and gastric cardia (in Chinese). Chin J Surg 20: 19–22
4. Zhang YD, Du XQ, Zhang W, et al. (1982) Experience in surgical treatment of 4310 cases of carcinoma of the esophagus and gastric cardia (in Chinese). Chin J Oncol 4: 1–4
5. Akiyama H, Tsurumaru M, Kawamura T, Ono Y (1981) Principles of surgical treatment for carcinoma of the esophagus: analysis of lymph node involvement. Ann Surg 194: 438–446
6. Nakayama K, Kakegawa T (1981) Latest management of pulmonary complications following esophageal cancer surgery in Japan. Int Adv Surg Oncol 4: 111–125
7. Ong GB, Lam KH, Wong J, Lim TK (1978) Factors influencing morbidity and mortality in esophageal carcinoma. J Thorac Cardiovasc Surg 76: 745–754
8. Schmidt GB, O'Neil WW, Kotb, et al. (1976) Continuous positive airway pressure in the prophylaxis of the adult respiratory distress syndrome. Surg Gynecol Obstet 143: 613

9. Huang GJ (1963) Leakage of esophagogastric anastomosis following resection of carcinoma of the esophagus and gastric cardia (in Chinese). Chin J Surg 11: 859–862
10. Huang GJ, Zhang DW, Wang GQ, Lin H, Wang LJ, et al. (1981) Early detection and surgical treatment of esophageal carcinoma. Jpn J Surg 11: 399–405
11. Akiyama H (1973) Esophageal anastomosis. Arch Surg 107: 512–514
12. Kasai M, Mori S, Watanabe T (1978) Follow up results after resection of thoracic esophageal carcinoma. World J Surg 2: 543–551
13. Zhang DW, Huang GJ, Zhang RG (1980) Early secondary thoracotomy in the treatment of anastomotic leakage following resection for carcinoma of the esophagus and gastric cardia: a report of 7 cases (in Chinese). Chin J Oncol 2: 231–234
14. Huang GJ (1973) Certain preventive and therapeutic measures for anastomotic leakage after resection for carcinoma of the esophagus and gastric cardia (in Chinese). Chin Med J 53: 670–672
15. Wu WJ, Chen FT, Chou HK, et al. (1978) Esophagogastrostomic anastomosis instrument (in Chinese). Chin Med J 4: 204–211
16. Zhang DS, Huang OL, Wang W, Guan WX, Sun DK (1979) The use of microsurgery in jejunum transplantation for esophageal defect (in Chinese). Chin J Surg 17: 154–159
17. Huang GJ (1963) Aorto-esophagogastro-anastomotic leakage as a complication after resection for esophageal carcinoma (in Chinese). Chin J Surg 11: 401–402
18. Huang GJ, Zhang W (1965) Diagnosis and management of chylothorax following resection for carcinoma of the esophagus (in Chinese). Chin J Surg 13: 130–132
19. Wang GQ, Huang GJ (1979) Volvulus of the transplanted stomach: a complication of surgery for esophageal carcinoma (in Chinese). Chin Med J 59: 234–235
20. Huang GJ, Zhang DW, Zhang RG, et al. (1982) Surgery for carcinoma of the esophagus: results and problems. Proceedings of Symposium Sino-Francais de Chirurgie, Kunming, p 35

Chapter 13
Operative Technique for Carcinoma of the Esophagus

Guo Jun Huang and Wu Ying K'ai

---

1 Choice of Approach

Because the esophagus is a median organ situated in the posterior mediastinum in front of the vertebral column, a number of surgical approaches are possible. In choosing the optimal approach for carcinoma of the esophagus, many factors must be considered, e.g., the size, location, and clinicopathological type of the tumor; the specific treatments received previously; the surgical procedure and site of anastomosis planned; the patient's general build and condition; the shape of the thoracic cage; the presence or absence of special intrathoracic features such as elongation and tortuosity of the aorta, old lesions of the lung, and pleural thickening and adhesions; the patient's cardiopulmonary reserves; and the surgeon's specialities and preferences. These factors will be discussed in detail in connection with each individual approach.

It must be pointed out that the surgeon's specialities and preferences may play an important role in the choice of approach as well as in the type of surgical procedure, as they are derived from years of practical experience. The surgeon can use his strong points to help make the operation a success, this being closely related to the ultimate overall results of treatment. This does not mean, however, that the surgeon may overlook the advantages of one approach over another under certain given conditions or ignore the principle of individualization in selecting the optimal approach for a particular patient.

1.1 Left Posterolateral Thoracotomy

Left posterolateral thoracotomy is the approach most frequently used for carcinoma of the esophagus by thoracic surgeons in China. It provides the best exposure and convenient access to lesions of the lower thoracic esophagus and gastric cardia, and is a good approach to the midthoracic esophagus below the aortic arch. It can also be used, but less conveniently, for thoracic esophageal lesions situated at or above the level of the aortic arch.

The excellent exposure of the lower thoracic esophagus and the gastric cardia and fundus gives easy access to the cancer and means that relations to the aorta, the left main bronchus, and other adjacent structures, and thus resectability, can be determined at an early stage of the exploration. It also allows easy transplantation of the stomach through an incision of the left hemidiaphragm to any level in the thorax or to the neck for anastomosis with the esophagus. Dissection of the paracardiac and left gastric groups of lymph nodes is facilitated, which is important as they are the most common sites of metastasis in carcinoma of the lower esophagus and the gastric cardia. There is no need to change the position of the patient during operation, which means that time is saved. If necessary, the incision can easily be extended to form a combined thoracoabdominal, which gives excellent exposure for an extended resection of carcinoma of the gastric cardia that may involve excision of the spleen and part of the pancreas, or other retroperitoneal structures, and also for jejunal transplantation or colon interposition. When tumor involvement of the aorta necessitates dissection or excision of the adventitial layer or injury of the aorta or its branches needs repair, left posterolateral thoracotomy offers unparalleled exposure, enabling these procedures to be carried out very safely under direct vision. If the tumor is not resectable and esophagogastric bypass is needed, the same incision still affords the most convenient approach. The relative simplicity of surgical procedure, the minimal tissue trauma, and the shorter operating time provided by left posterolateral thoracotomy may all contribute to decreasing the incidence of postoperative complications and operative mortality.

Left posterolateral thoracotomy does have certain shortcomings. In carcinoma situated above the midthoracic esophagus, exposure is not as good as that provided by the right-sided approach. Carcinoma at this level may invade the azygos vein, which is hard to dissect from the left, and dissection of the superior mediastinal and subcarinal lymph nodes is not as convenient as from the right. For exposure of the left gastric vessels and performance of pyloroplasty, left thoracotomy is of course much inferior to the abdominal approach.

Furthermore, the incision of the left hemidiaphragm which is involved in gaining access to the abdomen causes partial paralysis of the hemidiaphragm, with resulting impairment of pulmonary ventilation and the patient's ability to cough.

The level of the left thoracotomy depends upon the location of the tumor, the build of the patient, the level of the diaphragm, the particular features of the operation, and the expected site of anastomosis. In general, an incision at the level of the seventh rib is suitable in carcinoma of the lower esophagus or gastric cardia, with metastasis to the paracardiac and left gastric lymph nodes necessitating more extensive dissection of these regions. Thoracotomy at this level provides good exposure of the left upper abdomen, the paraphrenic region, and the lower esophagus, and may be readily extended downward and anteriorly to form a combined thoracoabdominal incision when indicated. If necessary a small segment of the posterior portion of the sixth rib may be resected to further enlarge the operative field.

If an intrathoracic supra-aortic anastomosis is expected, a left thoracotomy at the level of the sixth rib may be employed. This approach gives satisfactory exposure to the esophagus both above and below the aortic arch, but is not as good for anastomosis at the apex of the thoracic cage, especially in patients with a prominent and elongated aorta or a narrow chest. Under such circumstances, a portion of the posterior segment of the fifth rib may be resected to improve exposure.

For left posterolateral thoracotomy the patient is put in the right lateral position with a cushion under the right chest below the axilla to minimize pressure on the right shoulder. Both upper limbs are flexed at the elbow joint and put in front of the patient's face. The left arm is not fixed, so as to allow free mobility of the left scapula. The right lower limb is straightened, the left flexed mildly with a sand bag under the knee to maintain body stability. A binder is applied to the hip and fixed to the operating table (Fig. 13.1).

When cervical anastomosis is planned, the position is as above, but the area of skin disinfection should include the neck and chest and also the left shoulder and left upper arm. The left upper limb is then wrapped in a sterile towel and placed in the operative field (Fig. 13.2).

1.2 Right Posterolateral Thoracotomy

Right posterolateral thoracotomy provides the best exposure to the thoracic esophagus because of the slight deviation to the right of the upper thoracic segment of the esophagus and the left-sided location of the arch and descending portion of the aorta. Dissection of the superior mediastinal, subcarinal, and paraesophageal lymph nodes draining the esophagus is also convenient. Ligation or resection of the arch of the azygos vein and ligation of the thoracic duct, when indicated, are easily accomplished.

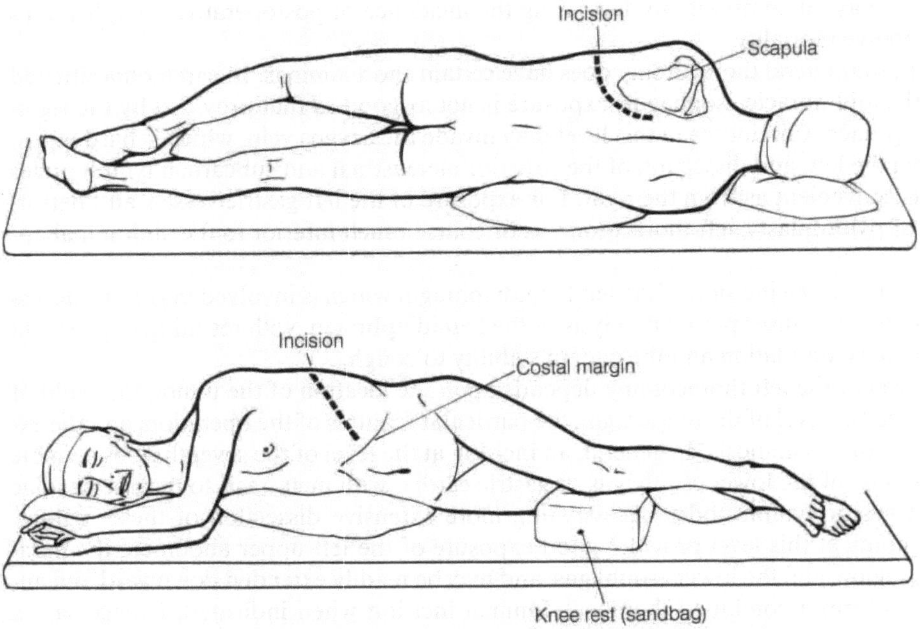

Fig. 13.1. Position for left posterolateral thoracotomy approach in carcinoma of the esophagus or gastric cardia. *Above:* Back view; *below:* front view

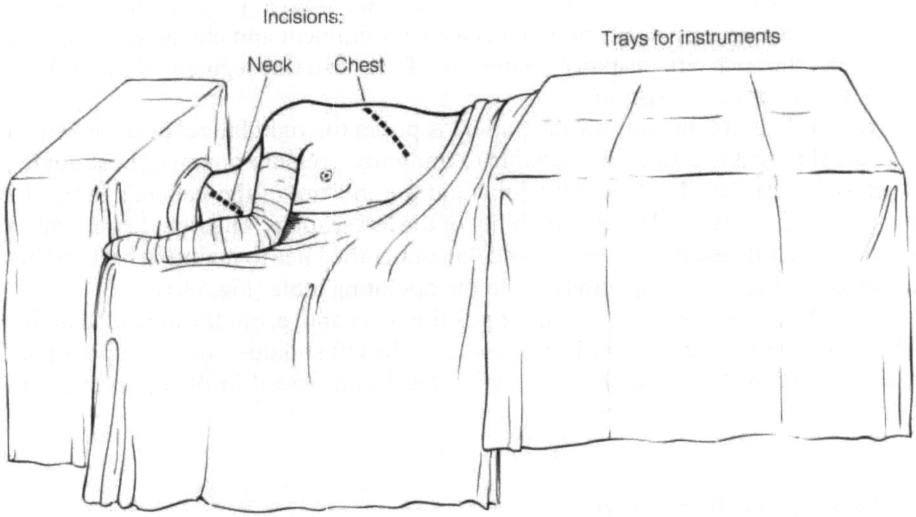

Fig. 13.2. Position for left thoracotomy with cervical incision for anastomosis, the left upper limb being wrapped in a sterile towel and placed in the operative field

Before going ahead with the right posterolateral thoracotomy, some surgeons prefer to make a small pilot upper abdominal incision for exploration and assessment of intra-abdominal metastasis. In the absence of widespread metastases a right posterolateral thoracotomy incision is then made (usually through the fifth or the sixth rib) to explore and resect the esophageal carcinoma and the abdominal incision is enlarged to allow mobilization of the stomach for anastomosis with the esophageal stump in the thorax or neck. If exploration of the abdomen reveals widespread metastases contraindicating resection of the esophageal tumor, thoracotomy may be omitted, thus avoiding unnecessary open chest surgery.

The shortcoming of this approach is that the position of the patient has to be changed, either from a left lateral position for thoracotomy to a supine position for abdominal and cervical procedures or vice versa, thus prolonging operative time. Furthermore, this approach usually requires two or three incisions, abdominal, thoracic, and cervical, which obviously means more extensive surgery and more trauma to the patient. Clearly, the exposure of the fundus of the stomach through an abdominal incision, be it vertical, oblique, or transverse, is usually not adequate, particularly in obese patients. In cases of midthoracic esophageal carcinoma, despite the right thoracotomy's good exposure of the esophagus, considerable dissection of the tumor must usually be performed before its relations to the left main bronchus and the aorta, and thus its resectability, can be assessed. Further, when there is tumor invasion or injury of the aorta, management is much less convenient and safe than through left thoracotomy. Finally, if exploration via the right thoracotomy approach reveals that the tumor is unresectable, esophagogastric bypass is impossible without an additional abdominal incision.

The right posterolateral thoracotomy incision may be made through either the fifth or sixth rib, depending on the location of the tumor and the anticipated site of anastomosis. The concomitant abdominal incision may be median or paramedian, running from below the costal arch left of the xiphoid process, which may be resected if necessary, to the level of the umbilicus. A bilateral transverse incision at about the midpoint between the costal angle and the umbilicus may also be used.

In thin patients, a semilateral position with the patient's back at an angle of about 45°–60° to the operating table may sometimes be used, avoiding the need to change the position during operation. A posterolateral thoracotomy incision is made along the fifth or the sixth rib, and if the tumor is resectable, then the choice is between making a separate abdominal incision and extending the chest incision obliquely downward to the left side of the abdominal wall to make it a thoracoabdominal incision, with division of the right costal arch and the anterior part of the right hemidiaphragm.

1.3 Exclusive Right Thoracic Approach

In 1974, Belsey and Hiebert [1] reported experience of an exclusive right thoracic approach for cancer of the middle third of the esophagus, with operative mortality of 28%. This approach provides good exposure of the thoracic esophagus and necessitates no change of the patient's position during operation. It does, however, entail mobilization of the stomach and division of the related vessels through the esophageal hiatus, which may be difficult and dangerous. Assessment of intra-abdominal metastasis and dissection of intra-abdominal lymph nodes are impossible. Serious intra-abdominal bleeding may result if vessels are inadvertently torn or vascular ligatures slip. If there are heavy peritoneal adhesions, mobilization of the stomach may be difficult or even impossible. It is probably for these reasons that this approach has not been widely accepted.

1.4 Right Anterolateral Thoracotomy

For carcinoma of the middle and upper segments of the esophagus in which cervical anastomosis is anticipated, a right anterolateral approach through the fourth interspace may be employed, with the patient supine. If the tumor is resectable, an abdominal incision is then made for mobilization of the stomach or colon and a cervical incision, usually on the left side along the anterior border of the sternocleidomastoideus muscle, for anastomosis (Fig. 13.3). This approach has the advantages of causing less trauma and being easy to perform. The supine position affords less cardiorespiratory disturbance and better exposure to the upper intra-abdominal organs than the lateral position. Mobilization of the stomach is greatly facilitated after the lower end of the esophagus is divided through the chest incision. This position is also the most suitable for colon interposition via either the subcutaneous or the retrosternal route.

The most serious shortcoming of this approach is its inadequate exposure of the esophagus, especially the part behind and below the hilus of the lung. Dissection of the esophagus cannot be done entirely under direct vision and thus may well be oncologically imperfect, and dissection of the lymph nodes in the region of the thoracic inlet and under the tracheal bifurcation is difficult. When the aorta or the left bronchus has been invaded by the cancer, dissection is difficult or even dangerous, and resection of the cancer may have to be abandoned because of inadequate exposure. The poor exposure can lead to excessive traction of the esophagus and excessive pressure on the lung, with resulting trauma to these organs.

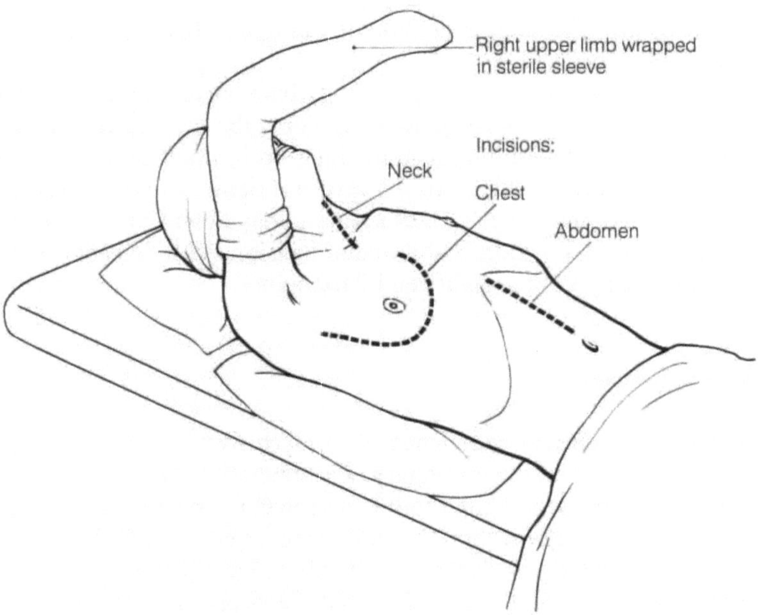

Fig. 13.3. Position for right anterolateral thoracotomy with three incisions for resection of carcinoma of the middle and upper segments of the esophagus (arm rest for right upper limb omitted for simplicity)

When the right anterolateral thoracotomy approach is used, the surgical team may be divided into two groups working simultaneously on the chest and the abdomen in order to minimize operating time.

1.5 Combined Cervicosternoabdominal Incision

A combined median cervicosternoabdominal incision may be used for upper thoracic or cervical esophageal carcinoma, affording excellent exposure (Fig. 13.4) [2]. The advantages are that the patient lies in the comfortable and physiologic supine position, that the trachea is very well exposed, so that the two recurrent laryngeal nerves can easily be seen and protected, and that it provides better access than any other approach to the tumor and to lymph nodes at the thoracic inlet. There is also excellent exposure for anastomosis of the esophagus or hypopharynx to the colon or stomach. The median sternotomy renders the heart and other mediastinal structures more displaceable in the forward direction, thus facilitating insertion of the fingers or even the whole hand for blunt dissection of the entire thoracic esophagus, from behind the trachea above and through the esophageal hiatus below. After being divided at its lower end, the entire esophagus can be extracted from the posterior mediastinum without the pleural cavities being opened.

However, the lack of direct vision in this approach does not allow dissection of the subcarinal and paraesophageal lymph nodes, which are often involved by the tumor and can ordinarily be removed through any posterolateral thoracic approach. Another drawback is the excessive trauma and bleeding during operation.

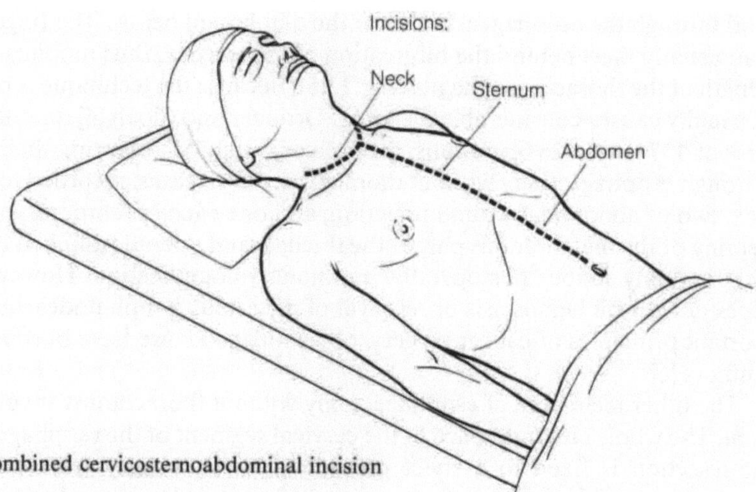

Fig. 13.4. Position for combined cervicosternoabdominal incision

1.6 Esophagectomy Without Thoracotomy

The esophagus may be extracted through cervical and abdominal incisions without opening the chest. Such a procedure is sometimes used in patients with inadequate pulmonary reserve or in whom the pleural cavities are densely adherent and cannot be entered.

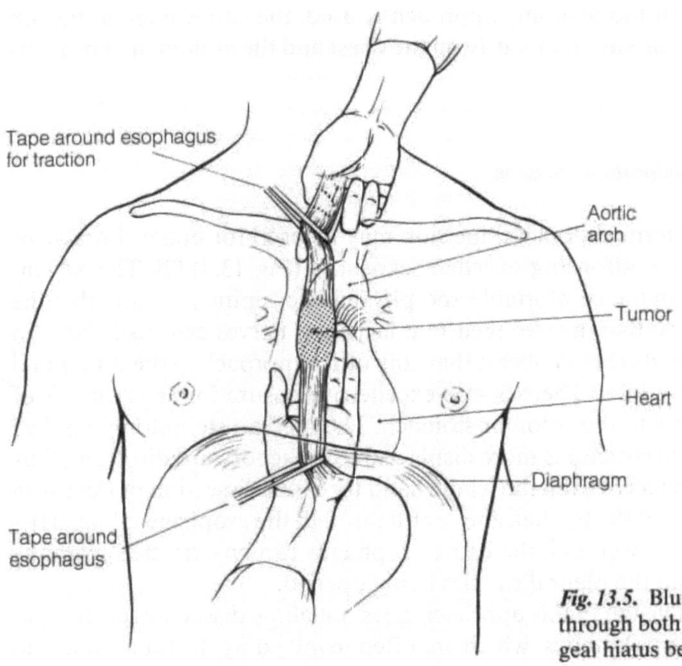

Fig. 13.5. Blunt finger dissection of esophagus through both neck incision above and esophageal hiatus below

There are two methods of removing the esophagus [3]. One is *pull-through esophagectomy,* by means of blunt finger dissection simultaneously through the thoracic inlet above and through the esophageal hiatus of the diaphragm below. The fingers of the two hands can usually meet behind the bifurcation of the trachea, thus mobilizing blindly the entire length of the thoracic esophagus (Fig. 13.5). Because the technique is both blunt and blind, it usually causes considerable bleeding. Orringer and Sloan [4] reported an average blood loss of 1370 ml in 26 operations. Szentpetery et al. [5], reporting their experience of pull-through esophagectomy without thoracotomy in 17 cases, recorded ten cases of hemothorax, two of abdominal wound infection, and one each of temporary vocal cord paralysis, tearing of the membranous part of the trachea, and operation-linked death. Neither group reported any serious postoperative pulmonary complication. However, as the technique does not permit hemostasis or removal of metastatic lymph nodes, thus going against important principles of cancer surgery, objections to its use have been raised by some other authors [6].

The other technique of esophagectomy without thoracotomy involves *inversion extraction.* The whole circumference of the cervical segment of the esophagus just below the line of resection is fixed to a stylet passed up intraluminally from below the diaphragm through a small incision in the lower end of the esophagus or the fundus of the stomach. The stylet is then pulled gently but firmly downward and the esophagus, divided above the point of fixation, is turned inside out and gradually extracted (Fig. 13.6). The extraction may also be done from above, depending on the location of the tumor, but as the nutrient vessels and nerve fibers to and from the esophagus almost all converge on it from above, downward extraction seems more efficient in detaching these structures.

The chief indications for inversion extraction of the esophagus are carcinoma of the upper cervical esophagus and less extensive carcinoma of the gastric cardia, in both of

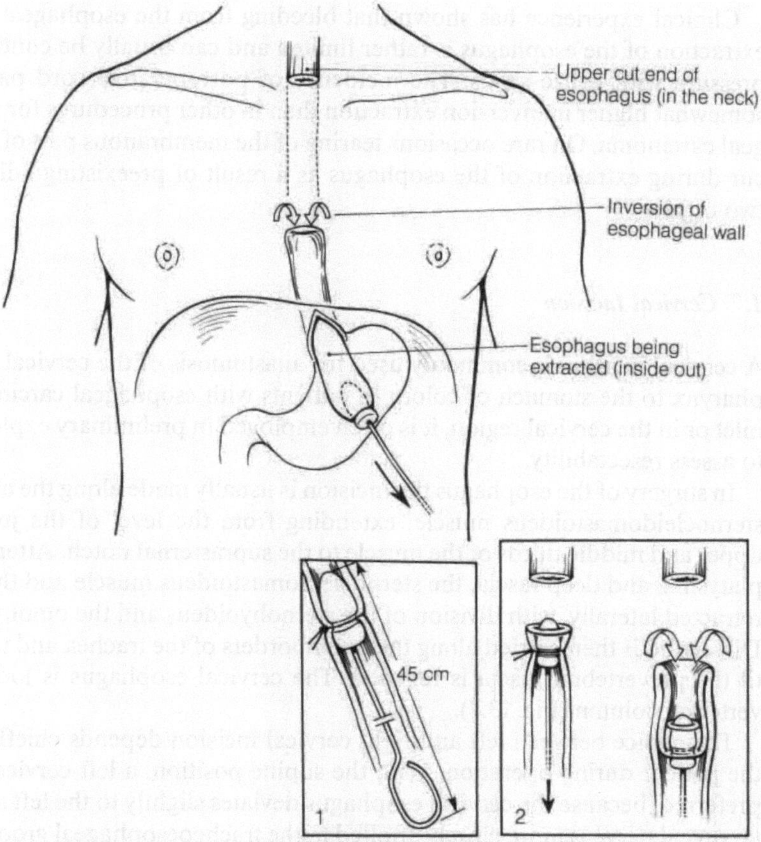

Fig. 13.6. Inversion extraction of the esophagus through an opening at the cardiac end. *1* The extractor is passed to the cervical esophagus, which is ligated from outside the wall to the groove of the extractor head. *2* The esophagus is divided above the ligature and its lower portion is then inverted and gradually removed by pulling downward on the extractor

which the thoracic esophagus is practically normal [7]. It may also be indicated in early (stage I) carcinoma of the thoracic esophagus in which the lesion is confined to the mucosa or submucosa with normal muscular coat and no lymph node metastasis [8]. After the esophagus is extracted the stomach or the colon can be brought up through the former esophageal bed into the neck for anastomosis with the esophageal stump or the hypopharynx.

Inversion extraction has the advantages that the patient is in the supine position and the chest is not opened, thus minimizing cardiopulmonary stress. Transplantation of the stomach or colon through the former esophageal bed is more direct than via the retrosternal, subcutaneous, or intrapleural route.

One shortcoming, however, is the limited indication in cases where the tumor is relatively localized. In carcinoma of the gastric cardia, the performance of a cervical esophagogastric anastomosis entails limitation in gastric resection in order to conserve an adequate length of stomach. This seems unsound both surgically and oncologically, as an unnecessary total esophagectomy is performed without eliminating the risk of inadequate tumor resection.

Clinical experience has shown that bleeding from the esophageal bed after inversion extraction of the esophagus is rather limited and can usually be controlled by temporary pressure with gauze strips. The incidence of postoperative cord paralysis seems to be somewhat higher in inversion extraction than in other procedures for resection of esophageal carcinoma. On rare occasions tearing of the membranous part of the trachea may occur during extraction of the esophagus as a result of preexisting adhesions between the two organs.

1.7 *Cervical Incision*

A cervical incision is commonly used for anastomosis of the cervical esophagus or hypopharynx to the stomach or colon. In patients with esophageal carcinoma at the thoracic inlet or in the cervical region, it is often employed in preliminary exploration of the tumor to assess resectability.

In surgery of the esophagus the incision is usually made along the anterior border of the sternocleidomastoideus muscle, extending from the level of the junction between the upper and middle thirds of the muscle to the suprasternal notch. After division of the skin, platysma, and deep fascia, the sternocleidomastoideus muscle and the carotid sheath are retracted laterally, with division of the sternohyoideus and the omohyoideus if necessary. Dissection is then carried along the outer borders of the trachea and the thyroid gland until the prevertebral fascia is reached. The cervical esophagus is located in front of the vertebral column (Fig. 13.7).

The choice between left and right cervical incision depends chiefly on the position of the patient during operation. With the supine position, a left cervical incision is usually preferred, because the cervical esophagus deviates slightly to the left and the left recurrent laryngeal nerve is more closely applied to the tracheoesophageal groove and less susceptible to injury than its counterpart on the right.

The ipsilateral thyroid lobe may be removed to improve exposure in high cervical anastomosis of the esophagus. In colonic interposition via the retrosternal route, a portion of the manubrium sterni together with the head of the clavicle may be excised to enlarge the tunnel and avoid pressure on the bowel.

When mobilization of the trachea and wide dissection of lymph nodes are needed in cervical esophageal carcinoma, a low cervical U-shaped incision or a low collar incision may be used to gain access to both sides of the neck. These incisions can be extended at the midline to form a combined median cervicosternoabdominal incision, as already described.

2 Exploration

The object of exploration in carcinoma of the esophagus, as at other sites, is not only assessment of resectability, but also determination of the size and location of the cancer, the extent of invasion, and the sites and extents of metastases and/or implantation. It is only with this information that accurate postsurgical histopathological staging, evaluation of prognosis, and planning of further treatment can be made.

In order to obtain as much information as possible on oncologic and surgical conditions, a complete and systematic exploration of every accessible related organ should be

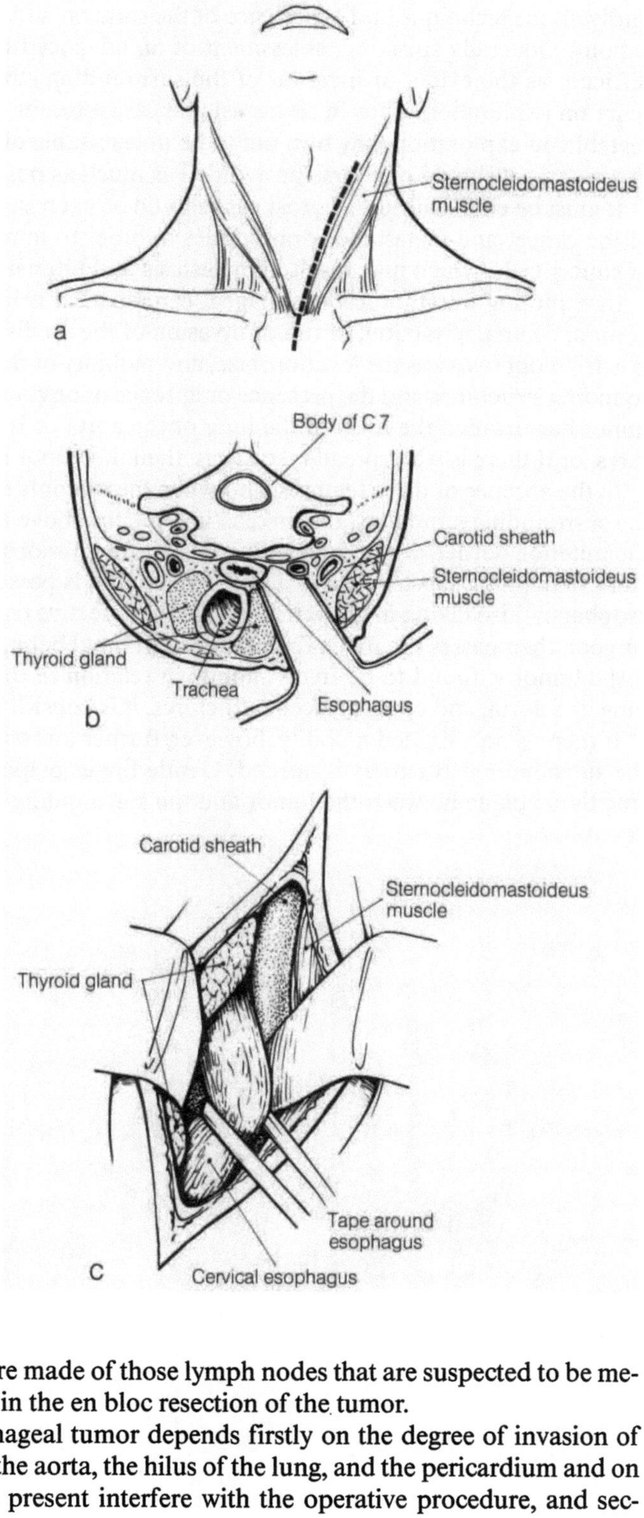

Fig. 13.7. ***a*** Cervical incision; ***b*** approach to cervical esophagus; ***c*** exposure

carried out. Excision biopsies are made of those lymph nodes that are suspected to be metastatic but cannot be included in the en bloc resection of the tumor.

The resectability of an esophageal tumor depends firstly on the degree of invasion of surrounding structures such as the aorta, the hilus of the lung, and the pericardium and on whether any metastatic lesions present interfere with the operative procedure, and secondly on the technique and experience of the surgeon and his assessment of surgical indications. Generally speaking, assessment of an advanced midthoracic tumor is relatively difficult, as the extent of invasion of the surrounding structures may sometimes be obscure on exploration. Thus in an occasional case a tumor which had been considered resectable on exploration may turn out to be unresectable on actual dissection. Such errors in assessment should of course be avoided as much as possible.

It must be emphasized that great care should be exercised in exploration and dissection of the cancer and metastatic lymph nodes in order to minimize iatrogenic dissemination of cancer cells, which may result in metastasis and ultimate treatment failure.

In exploring intrathoracic esophageal carcinoma it is important first to note any congestion, edema, retraction, or tumor invasion of the mediastinal pleura. Gentle palpation is carried out to assess the location, size, and mobility of the tumor, its relations to the surrounding structures, and the presence or absence of obvious lymph node metastasis. If the tumor has invaded the hilus of the lung or the aorta or is "frozen" to neighboring structures, or if there is widespread metastasis, then the tumor is considered unresectable.

In the absence of these features, and when the tumor is reasonably mobile in relation to the surrounding structures, the mediastinal pleura above the diaphragm is opened along the anterior border of the descending aorta, the inferior pulmonary ligament is divided close to the lung substance, and a tape for traction is passed around the lower end of the esophagus, also taking in the periesophageal connective tissue and the vagi (Fig. 13.8). The surgeon then passes the index finger of his left hand behind the tumor to assess mobility; if the tumor is found to be freely mobile in relation to the pericardium, the hilus of the lung, the aorta, and other adjacent structures, it is considered resectable (Fig. 13.9).

If there is only limited mobility, however, further assessment of the tumor's relations to the surrounding structures is needed. Gentle finger palpation reveals whether there is a fine tissue plane between the tumor and the surrounding structures, and if not, indicates

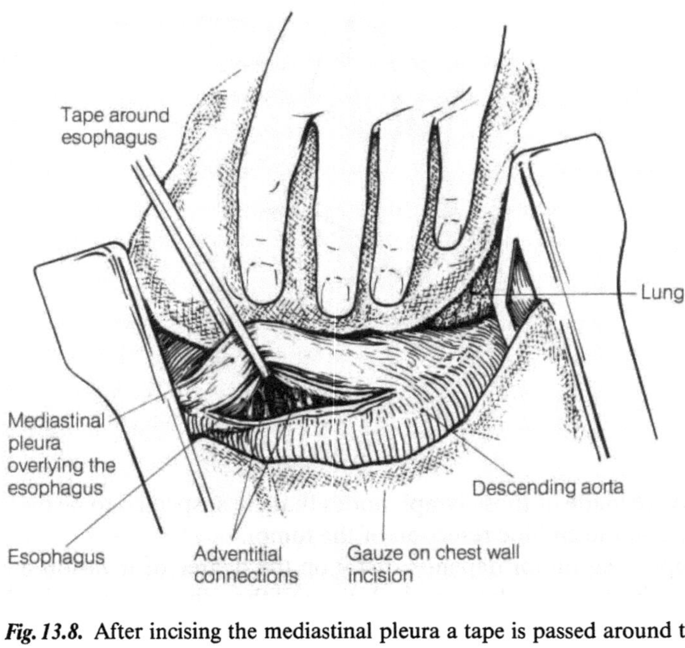

Fig. 13.8. After incising the mediastinal pleura a tape is passed around the esophagus for traction

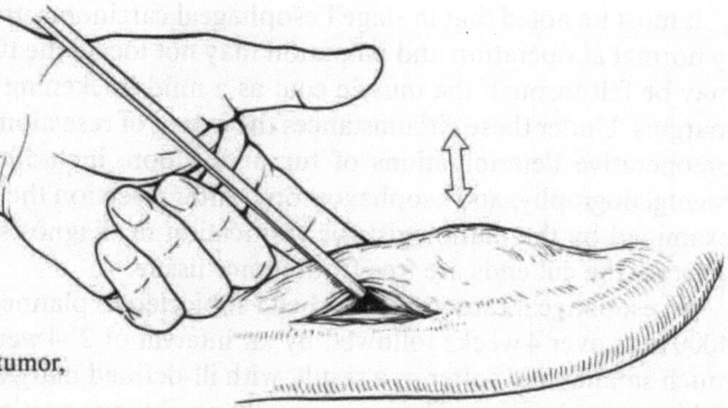

Fig. 13.9. Testing for mobility of the tumor, a good sign of resectability

the thickness, extent, and consistency of the interposing tissue, which usually determines resectability. Additional palpation of a midthoracic esophageal tumor may be done through the tissue spaces normally existing behind the inferior pulmonary vein, the left main bronchus, and the left pulmonary artery. In the absence of severe invasion of surrounding structures, resection is still regarded as possible.

In case of borderline resectability, it is often necessary to perform partial dissection of the tumor before a final decision can be made. This "pilot" dissection gives useful additional information but should be as limited as possible in extent for the following reasons:

(a) extensive pilot dissection would be of no benefit to the patient, and possibly even harmful, if the tumor is finally proved to be unresectable because of severe local invasion;

(b) if a pilot dissection is carried out with the esophagus in situ, and exposure is hence inadequate, it may carry the risk of fragmenting the tumor;

(c) excessive pilot dissection with poor exposure may lead to rupture of the contralateral mediastinal pleura, which at this early stage may handicap the patient's respiration during the subsequent intraoperative period.

If the cancer is shown to be resectable, intrathoracic exploration is ended and the surgeon proceeds to intra-abdominal exploration. At this point the lung is released from retraction and reexpanded.

When a left thoracotomy approach is used, the abdominal exploration and subsequent operative procedures are carried out through an incision of the left hemidiaphragm, which is made between the left lobe of the liver and the spleen, from the hiatus outward and anteriorly, making the medial flap of the incised diaphragm as wide as possible with intact innervation by the phrenic nerve. A circumferential incision of the diaphragm may sometimes by useful for maximal conservation of innervation and therefore motor function of the hemidiaphragm. The hiatus may not be opened until resection has been decided on.

Intra-abdominal exploration should include the stomach with its two curvatures, the celiac region, the abdominal aorta, the liver, the spleen, the lesser omentum, and the pelvic cavity. Special attention is paid to the paracardiac and left gastric lymph nodes, particularly in carcinoma of the lower esophagus. The greater omentum should be opened to gain access to the lesser peritoneal sac for exploration of the retrogastric organs. The final decision can then be made as to the resectability of the tumor and the mode of resection, palliative or radical.

It must be noted that in stage I esophageal carcinoma, the esophagus appears practically normal at operation and palpation may not locate the tumor, although in some cases it may be felt through the muscle coat as a mild thickening of the mucosa with ill-defined margins. Under these circumstances the extent of resection of the esophagus is decided by preoperative determinations of tumor location, including segmental balloon cytology, roentgenography, and esophagoscopy. After resection the specimen must be immediately examined by the pathologist for verification of diagnosis and extent and assessment of whether the cut ends are free from tumor tissue.

An esophageal tumor that has been subjected to planned preoperative irradiation, e.g., 4000 rads over 4 weeks followed by an interval of 2–4 weeks before operation, is usually much smaller and softer as a result, with ill-defined margins, and may even be hardly palpable on exploration. There are usually no obvious postirradiation changes of the neighboring structures.

In cases of recurrence or stricture after previous curative radiotherapy (e.g., 6000–7000 rads) the irradiated esophagus and neighboring structures are found at operation to be markedly shrunken, indurated, and adherent, with loss of the intervening tissue planes. In most such cases resection of the irradiated part of the esophagus is difficult and can often only be accomplished with sharp dissection. Our experience is that in 28% of 54 such cases the resected specimens showed no residual tumor tissue on pathological examination [9]. It seems reasonable, therefore, that postirradiation esophageal carcinomas with dense scar adhesions may be resected palliatively, as in cases of benign strictures.

If careful exploration shows radical resection of the esophageal cancer to be impossible, it is advisable to do a palliative resection if feasible, so that oral feeding can be assured. Adjuvant therapy such as postoperative radiotherapy or chemotherapy may be of benefit in prolonging survival.

3 Resection

Resection for esophageal carcinoma should include not only a certain length of normal esophagus above and below the tumor, but also all resectable paraesophageal tissues which are rich in lymphatics, together with the accessible draining lymph nodes; it is unwise to emphasize only one of these points at the expense of the other. The principle of extensive excision of both the tumor-bearing esophagus and the draining lymph nodes is even more important in relatively early esophageal carcinoma, in which there is an excellent chance of cure. In advanced cases displaying marked tumor invasion of the surrounding structures and widespread lymph node metastasis, with no apparent hope of surgical cure, it would be of no benefit to overresect the esophagus and subject the patient to the risk of a long and extensive operation. In this situation, adjuvant postoperative radiotherapy is recommended; local recurrence at the anastomosis has not been a significant problem in our experience of this policy.

It is well known that submucosal infiltration in carcinoma of the esophagus may extend 3–5 cm or occasionally even further from the gross tumor substance. Different clinicopathological types of esophageal cancer show different patterns of submucosal infiltration, but in the majority of cases resection for a minimum of 5 cm from the margins of the tumor will be sufficient for there to be no tumor tissue at the cut edge, although more extensive resection is encouraged if feasible. With the increasing use of preoperative irradiation which covers the entire mediastinum and has the particular property of sterilizing microfoci of tumor dissemination, the extent of esophageal resection becomes less problematic. Our experience in about 600 surgical cases of esophageal carcinoma treated with preoperative irradiation also shows that with the radiation dose used, there was no ill effect on the healing of the anastomosis between the irradiated esophageal stump and the stomach or colon.

Resection of carcinoma of the lower esophagus should include the cardia and part of the adjacent stomach. In resection of carcinoma in the midesophagus or higher, the esophagus may be divided at its junction with the gastric cardia, together with dissection of the paracardiac group of lymph nodes and adipose tissues; there is no need to excise part of the adjacent stomach unless it is involved by metastasis.

In the absence of other contraindication for surgical resection, localized invasion of esophageal cancer into the pericardium, the contralateral mediastinal pleura, the thoracic duct, the azygos vein, etc., may be treated by en bloc local excision of the invaded tissue or organs. Ong and Kwong [10] reported the management of malignant esophagobronchial fistula by resection of both the esophagus and the affected lobe of lung, with reasonably good palliation. Occasionally, when the tumor invades a limited part of the trachea, the tracheal segment involved may be resected with the esophagus, followed by end-to-end tracheal anastomosis. In one case in our experience in which the midthoracic esophageal carcinoma invaded a small segment of the descending aorta, the affected portion was resected for a length of 5 cm with the esophageal cancer and replaced with a length of vascular prosthesis. The patient did well in the early postoperative period but died suddenly a month later on rupture of the aortic anastomosis due to infection.

It is obvious that in resection of esophageal carcinoma and its metastatic lymph nodes sharp dissection is preferred to blunt finger dissection, which is prone to lead to fragmentation and therefore incomplete excision of the cancer.

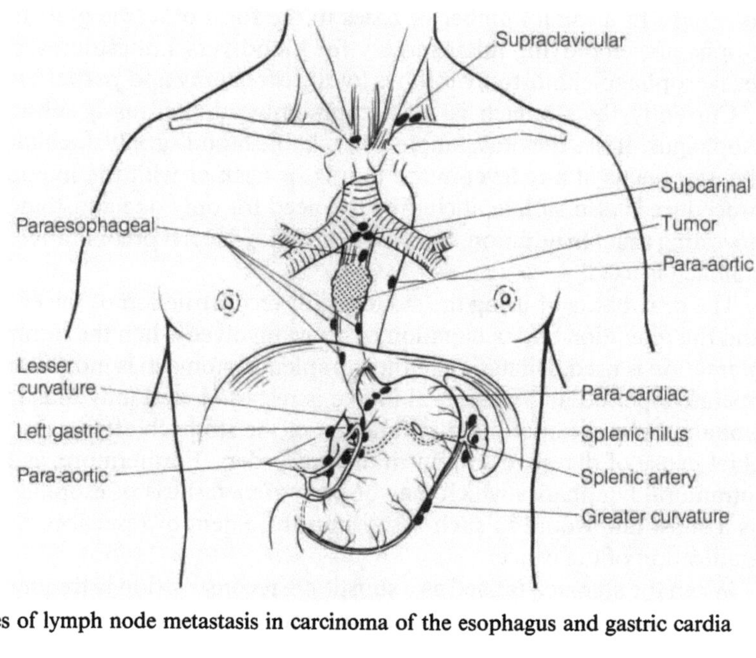

Fig. 13.10. Common sites of lymph node metastasis in carcinoma of the esophagus and gastric cardia

In carcinoma of the esophagus of any location, lymphatic spread and lymph node metastasis take place both upward and downward along the esophagus, downward more frequently and further than upward (Fig. 13.10). In carcinoma of the midthoracic esophagus, for example, metastasis to the lower paraesophageal and paracardiac lymph nodes may be even more frequent than to the subcarinal and superior mediastinal nodes. In carcinoma of the lower esophagus, there is a strong tendency toward metastasis to the paracardiac, lesser curvature, left gastric, and even the celiac nodes, although metastasis to the subcarinal and higher mediastinal nodes is also not infrequent. Akiyama et al. [11] showed in their study of the rate of lymph node metastasis in resections that besides other groups, the rate of metastasis to the superior gastric group alone, including the paracardiac, lesser curvature, and left gastric nodes, was 31.8% in 24 cases of upper esophageal carcinoma, 32.8% in 116 cases of midesophageal carcinoma, and 61.5% in 65 cases of lower esophageal carcinoma. In the cases of lower esophageal carcinoma there was a 9.8% rate of lymph node metastasis to the superior mediastinum. In some cases lymph node metastasis may "jump," involving a distant group while sparing a nearer group. Due to difficulty in verifying at operation whether a lymph node is mestastatic, all draining nodes and suspected metastatic nodes should be removed, identified by site, and sent for pathological examination.

4 Reconstruction of the Esophagus

4.1 Choice of Organ

The choice of organ for reconstruction of the resected esophagus has for many years been a subject of clinical study. The early practise of using a skin tube has been abandoned. Due to difficulties in obtaining a sufficient blood supply and an adequate length of organ, the use of the jejunum for high-level esophagoplasty has frequently resulted in failure. It is now used in a small number of cases in the form of a free graft for replacement of the esophagus, employing microsurgery for blood vessel anastomosis, and sometimes low-level esophagojejunostomy follows total gastrectomy and partial esophagectomy.

Currently the stomach is most commonly adopted as a substitute for the resected esophagus. It has the most ample and reliable blood supply, facilitating anastomosis with the esophagus at any level in the thorax or neck or with the hypopharynx. The surgical procedure is also simple, including the need for only one anastomosis, which minimizes operating time. In addition, there is no need for special preoperative preparation when the stomach is used.

The drawbacks of using the stomach for reconstruction of the esophagus are its atonia and the dilatation and occupation of space involved when the intrapleural route of transplantation is used. Dilatation of the intrapleural stomach is more marked in the early postoperative period and when oral intake is restarted, and may thus give rise to respiratory embarrassment. Impairment in function of the stomach after transplantation is often the chief cause of digestive and nutritional disorders. Furthermore, as the stomach is rich in intramural lymphatics which may be sites of metastasis of esophageal carcinoma, its use as a substitute would in such cases limit the extent of resection, resulting in incomplete eradication of the cancer.

When the stomach is used as a substitute, reconstruction is frequently performed via the very convenient intrapleural route, but may also be done via the posterior mediastinal route with esophagogastric anastomosis above the aortic arch or in the neck. In cervical anastomosis, the intrapleural route is also the most commonly employed, but the posterior mediastinal and the retrosternal routes may also be used. The posterior mediastinal route involves the shortest distance for reconstruction and the most natural alignment with the esophagus.

Colon interposition is another common method of reconstruction, with the advantage that a sufficient length of bowel can be made available for even the highest level of esophageal replacement, thus facilitating extensive resection. The marginal vascular arcades of the colon approximate the bowel in length and possess relatively abundant and constant collateral anastomoses favorable for transplantation. Study of their anatomic distribution shows that the middle colic vessels alone can usually provide a sufficient supply of blood to the segment from the cecum to the descending colon, and that with preservation of the left colic vessels alone an isoperistaltic interposition of the left colon can be accomplished to replace the esophagus at any level [12]. This can also be done quite conveniently through a left thoracoabdominal approach. The left colon is very similar in caliber to the esophagus and is more capable than any other segment of the colon of performing the esophagus' task of propelling semisolid materials.

Isoperistaltic reconstruction is preferred in colon interposition because of the difficulty in swallowing and regurgitation of food which may be the result of antiperistaltic reconstruction.

Progress in microsurgery has made possible the interposition of an isolated segment of colon (or jejunum) through small vessel anastomosis; however, interposition with a vascular pedicle remains the routine procedure.

The drawbacks of colon interposition include the need for (a) preoperative bowel preparation to minimize intraoperative contamination, which may burden the patient; (b) performance of three anastomoses at operation, which is time consuming; and (c) thorough preoperative examination to rule out preexisting diseases of the colon, the incidence of which is relatively high.

The use of a reversed gastric tube for reconstruction of the esophagus was strongly advocated and indeed practised by Gavriliu and Heimlich in the 1950s [13]. The tube consists of the greater curvature of the stomach with its base at the fundus, using the left gastroepiploic vessels for blood supply. The tube is turned in an antiperistaltic direction for anastomosis with the esophagus. An isoperistaltic gastric tube may also be made, using the right gastroepiploic vessels for blood supply (Fig. 13.11).

The advantage of using a gastric tube to replace the esophagus is that a considerable part of the stomach remains in situ, part of the gastric function thus being preserved. However, the tedious and time-consuming tailoring and suturing and the considerable blood loss involved in fashioning the tube preclude its routine use.

4.2 Choice of Anastomotic Site

In selecting the site for anastomosis a number of factors should be considered, such as completeness of tumor resection, technical feasibility, and operative risk. Our policy is to resect the esophagus at least 5–7 cm from the gross margin of the tumor. The use of preoperative irradiation is of great benefit in minimizing the risk of residual tumor at the cut edge. Assessment of the gross extent of tumor involvement of the mucosa by direct observation through an esophagotomy, as advocated by Akiyama et al. [14], may also be benefi-

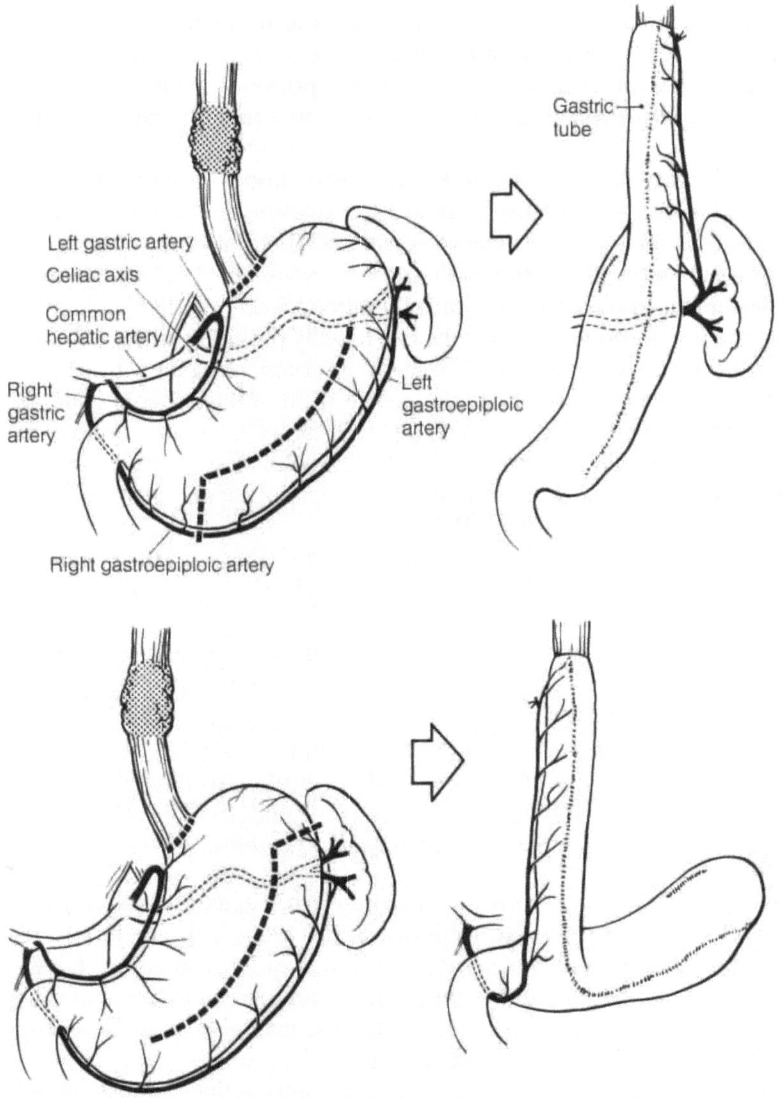

Fig. 13.11. Tailoring of a reverse gastric tube *(above)* and an isoperistaltic gastric tube *(below)*, *heavy broken lines* indicating sites of division

cial. In the majority of cases, however, routine total esophagectomy does not seem to be justified and may add to the risk of the operation.

Technically speaking, a high infra-aortic anastomosis is more difficult than a supra-aortic one, and an anastomosis done at the apex of the pleural cavity is not as easy as one performed in the neck. Leakage from an intrathoracic anastomosis is life threatening, whereas a leak from a cervical anastomosis as a rule carries no additional risk to the patient and usually heals spontaneously after drainage.

In general, with the exception of cases involving localized cancer at the lower end of the esophagus, when reconstruction after resection may be by means of infra-aortic anastomosis, reconstruction must be by anastomosis at supra-aortic level or at the apex of the thorax. In cases of high midthoracic esophageal carcinoma in which the upper end of the tumor reaches the level of the aortic arch or higher, the anastomosis should usually be made in the cervical region.

It should be borne in mind in the selection of anastomotic site that with increasing age and sclerotic change of the aorta, the aortic arch becomes elongated and higher in position. As a result, access to the supra-aortic region becomes more difficult, and problems may be encountered in performing anastomosis in this region.

4.3 Technique of Anastomosis

In recent years staplers for esophagogastric anastomosis have been widely used in China and in many other countries with broadly satisfactory results (Fig. 13.12). The incidence of postoperative leakage has been reduced, but there has been a 10% incidence of anastomotic stricture [15]. In addition, it may not be possible to employ the stapling apparatus at certain sites with limited space, such as the cervical region. For the present, manual anastomosis remains a fundamental technique.

As the esophagus does not hold sutures well, due to its lack of a serosa and to the friability of its muscular coat, meticulous care and great skill are needed in performing anastomosis. The prevention of anastomotic leakage has been a subject of continous investigation. Authors with different experiences have developed different techniques with different points of emphasis in esophageal anastomosis, and most of them have reported good results with their own methods. The consensus, however, is that the nature of suture material and the method of suturing are of relatively minor importance, while enhancement of or at least minimal interference with tissue healing are of greater significance. This means stress is laid on things such as preservation of a good blood supply to the site of anastomosis; avoidance of undue tension; good apposition of tissue layers, especially of mucosal layers; avoidance of defects in the anastomotic line; minimization of tissue trauma and tissue strangulation from instrumentation, manipulation, or excessive suturing; prevention of infection at the anastomosis; and prevention and effective management of intrathoracic complications.

Despite the segmental pattern of blood supply to the esophagus, the ample intramural vascular network allows mobilization of a considerable length of the organ without obvious ischemia. Nevertheless, excessive mobilization of the esophageal stump should be avoided.

The stomach has an abundant intramural vascular network which allows mobilization of the whole organ and permits it to be brought right up to the neck for anastomosis, provided the right gastric and right gastroepiploic arteries are well preserved. This makes the stomach one of the most commonly used organs for esophageal reconstruction. However, the blood supply to the site of anastomosis must be meticulously preserved. In making the incision in the fundus for anastomosis, care must be taken that it is not too close to the suture line of the stomach where the vascular network has been cut. In handling the stomach, great gentleness should be exercised to avoid contusion of the wall, which may result in focal ischemia. Damage to intramural venous channels is especially prone to occur if the stomach is not manipulated delicately.

Postoperative gastric perforation, sometimes multiple, may result from focal necrosis due to traumatic ischemia.

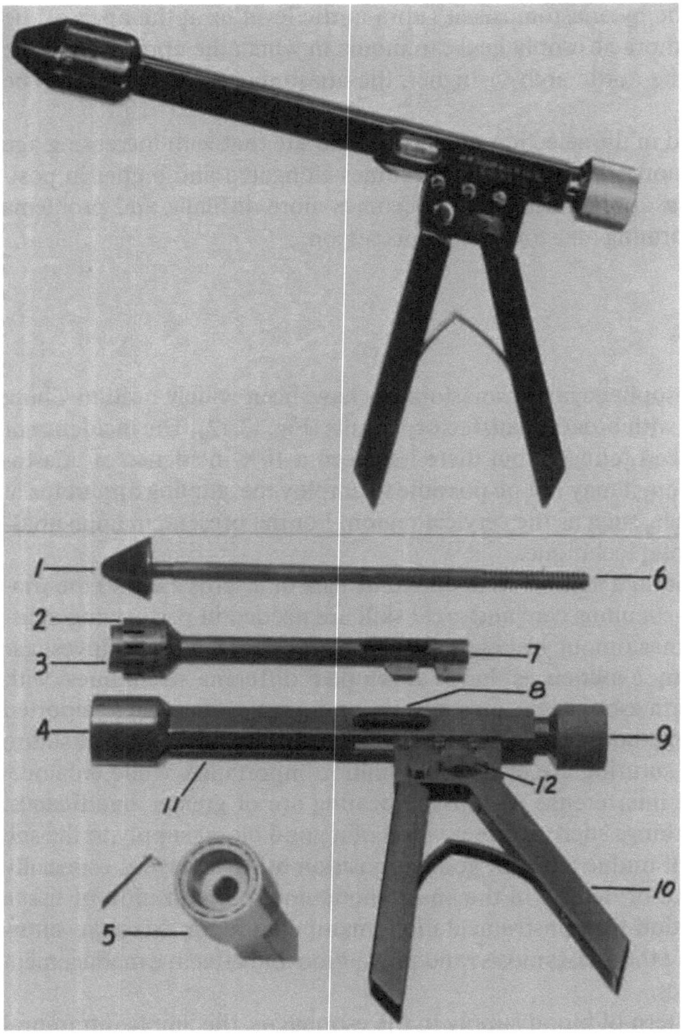

Fig. 13.12. A stapling device for esophagogastric anastomosis and its parts (designed by WJ Wu and associates). *1* Conical head; *2* staple feeder; *3* circular blade; *4* shell; *5* staple holder; *6* central shaft for clamping the head; *7* tube shaft for pushing the staples and the circular blade forward; *8* scale; *9* screw bolt; *10* handle; *11* outer case; *12* release lever. (Courtesy of Dr. WJ Wu)

Nonirritating monofilament synthetic suture material is preferred to conventional silk sutures because of its minimal interference with tissue healing, even in the presence of local infection.

We use a double-row suturing technique in which the first or inner row consists of single whole-layer interrupted sutures bringing together the esophageal and gastric stomas in accurate apposition and without tissue strangulation. Care is taken to approximate the mucosal layers precisely and intimately with no eversion or interposition. The second or outer row telescopes the anastomosis into the fundus of the stomach in much the same manner as fundoplication in Nissen's operation for hiatal hernia. This is accomplished by

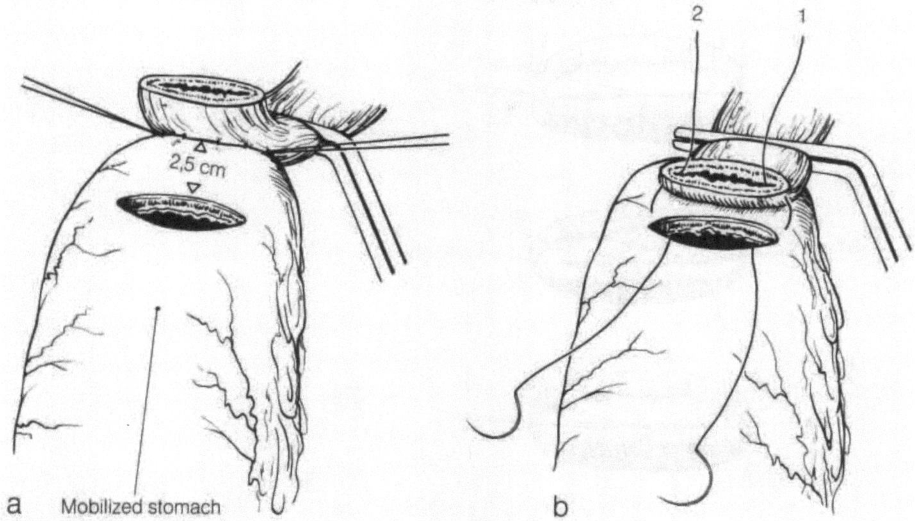

Fig. 13.13a–g. Technique of end-to-side esophagogastrostomy. ***a*** Placing of sutures to anchor the gastric fundus to the esophagus 2.5 cm above the line of resection. Note that a soft clamp is applied to the esophagus for temporary hemostasis. ***b*** Placing the first two sutures for anastomosis. ***c–g*** see pp. 334–335

anchoring the gastric wall to the esophagus at a distance of about 2.5 cm above the anastomotic line (Fig. 13.13). The telescoping serves to minimize tension on the anastomotic line from the weight of the transplant itself or from gastric distension and creates a valvular mechanism for the prevention of postoperative gastroesophageal reflux.

An end-to-side esophagogastrostomy is usually preferred if all or most of the stomach is available. The gastric stoma is made either on the anterior wall of the fundus 3–4 cm below the greater curvature or at the highest point of the fundus, in the form of either a linear incision or a circular fenestration with a circumference approximating that of the esophageal stump. Excessive gastric mucosa may be trimmed off to prevent its eversion.

In performing end-to-end esophagogastrostomy there is usually a sufficient width of the fundus to allow fundoplication around the lower segment of the esophageal stump. This is preferred to a purse-string type invagination of the anastomotic line, in which a dead space is created inside the "purse" where fluid may collect and infection may occur (Fig. 13.14). End-to-end esophagogastrostomy is more commonly employed in resection of carcinoma of the gastric cardia (for discussion see Chap. 14).

It is essential to have a good exposure of the esophagus for laying sutures. This is especially true when anastomosis is done in the narrow supra-aortic region, where the right side of the esophagus is hard to expose for this purpose. To overcome this difficulty we have used a simple esophageal retractor made of malleable wire (Fig. 13.15) to lift the mobilized esophagus at right angles to its bed so that sutures can without difficulty be laid on the right aspect of the esophageal wall.

When four or five anchoring sutures have been laid between the fundus of the stomach and the right esophageal wall, an opening is made on the wall of the fundus 2.5 cm below the anchoring sutures for anastomosis. The sutures are then tied and the esophageal retractor removed.

To facilitate anastomotic suturing, a soft, noncrushing auricular clamp or other suitable nontraumatizing clamp is applied to the esophagus just above the anchoring sutures. This

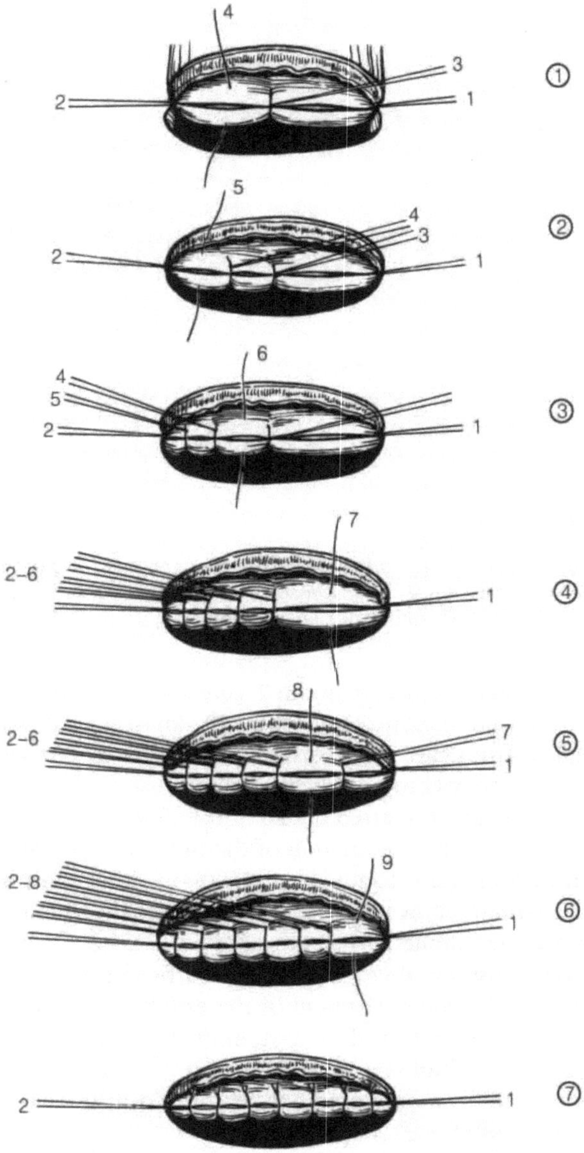

Fig. 13.13. ***c*** Order of laying sutures on the far half of the stoma, leaving knots inside the lumen

serves to prevent spillage of the esophageal contents and excessive bleeding from the esophageal stump, thus providing a bloodless field with minimal contamination (Fig. 13.13). The esophagus is now divided at the level 2.5 cm below the anchoring sutures.

The esophagogastric anastomosis is made with single-layer whole-thickness interrupted suturing. The right half of the anastomosis (so named when a left posterolateral thoracotomy approach is used) is started by putting the first and the second stitches at the two ends. Gentle traction on these two stitches in opposite directions will bring the edges of the sto-

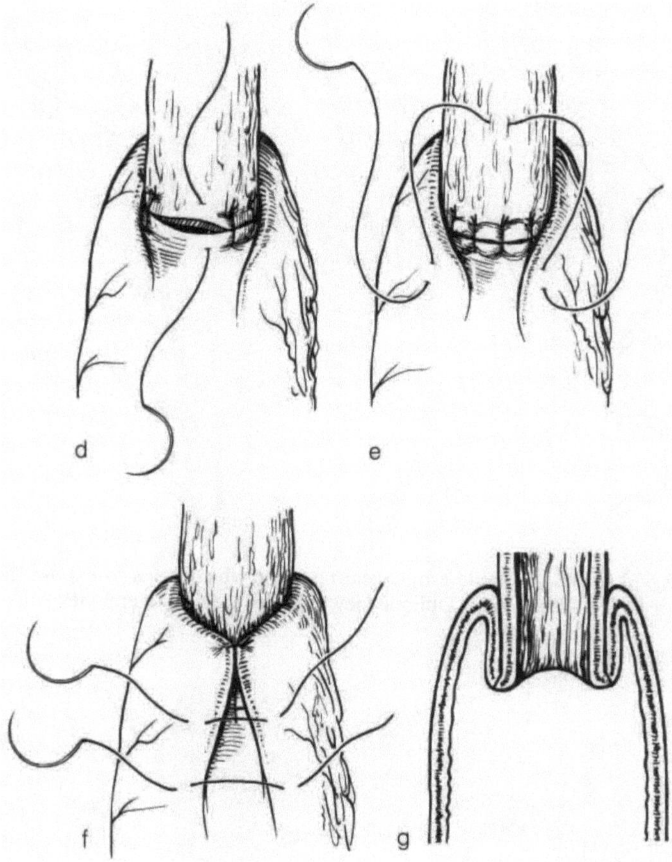

Fig. 13.13. ***d*** Suturing the near half of the stoma, with knots tied outside the lumen. ***e*** After completion of anastomosis fundoplication is accomplished by placing external sutures in continuation with the anchoring sutures. ***f*** Fundoplication completed. ***g*** Longitudinal section of fundoplication

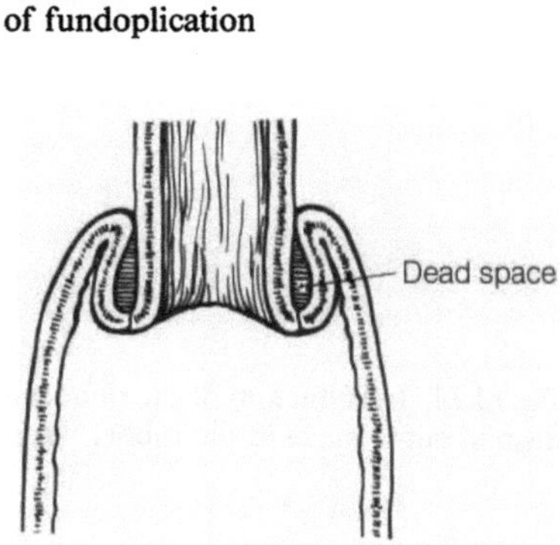

Fig. 13.14. The dead space after purse-string suture where fluid may collect and infection arise

ma into alignment with good approximation of tissue layers. The third stitch is laid halfway between the first two. The next two stitches are laid at the midpoints, followed by a further four laid in similar fashion to give a total of nine stitches evenly spaced out along the right half of the anastomotic line, with knots tied inside the lumen. Care is taken to ensure good approximation of the mucosal and muscular layers (Fig. 13.13).

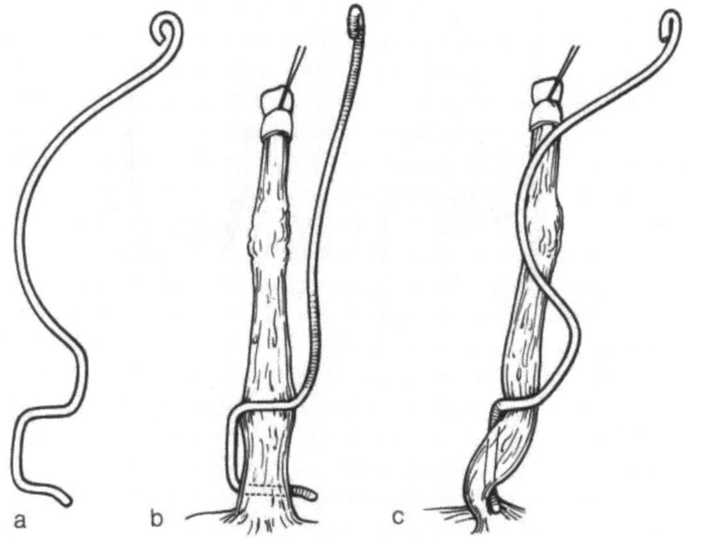

Fig. 13.15 a–c. A simple esophageal retractor which helps to expose the undersurface of the esophagus for laying of sutures. ***a*** Oblique view; ***b*** front view; ***c*** lateral view

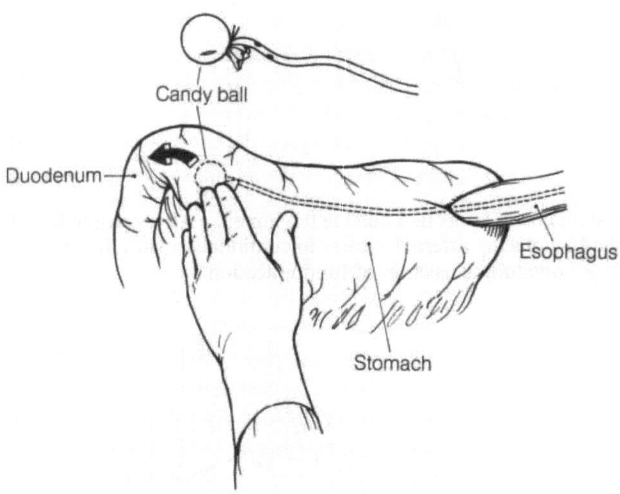

Fig. 13.16. Introduction of the duodenal tube into the duodenum from outside the gastric wall. Note that a small cut is made in the rubber wrapping of the ball to allow the candy to dissolve

The left half (often erroneously called the anterior half) of the anastomotic line is sutured from the two ends inwards, with knots tied preferably outside the lumen to avoid interposing them in the anastomotic line.

Before the completion of anastomotic suturing, the auricular clamp on the esophagus is opened and the nasogastric tube inserted before the operation is drawn out from the esophageal stump and connected to a gastric tube and a duodenal tube available at the operating table. The upper ends of these two tubes are then drawn out of the nostril by the anesthetist, using the original nasogastric tube as a guide, and the lower ends are inserted into the gastric transplant. The gastric decompression tube is properly positioned and fixed to the nose by the anesthetist, while the duodenal feeding tube will be inserted into the duodenum after completion of the anastomosis (Fig. 13.16).

The duodenal feeding tube is a fine Silastic or plastic tube about 1.5 mm in outer diameter and 1.2 m in length with one or two side holes at the distal end, to which is attached a candy ball about 1.2 cm in diameter wrapped in a rubber glove finger (Fig. 13.16). The ball serves as a pilot to bring the feeding tube into the duodenum when the surgeon exerts pressure from outside the gastric wall. Both tube and ball are previously disinfected by soaking in alcohol. A small cut is made in the rubber wrapping before the ball is inserted into the stomach and subsequently the duodenum to allow the candy to slowly dissolve.

The suturing of the anastomosis is completed by adding a few final stitches to close the stoma (Fig. 13.13 d). Fundoplication, which has been started by the anchoring sutures on the right half of the esophagus, is finished on the left half as shown in Fig. 13.13 e–g.

A similar single-layer whole-thickness anastomosis technique is used in esophagocolostomy and esophagojejunostomy. End-to-end anastomosis is usually used in esophagocolostomy, end-to-side anastomosis in esophagojejunostomy. Here too the anastomotic line is telescoped into the transplant to produce a plication of 1–2 cm. As both colon and jejunum are larger in caliber than the esophagus, care is taken in spacing the sutures of the two cut ends in proportion to their circumferences when an end-to-end anastomosis is constructed.

In the above open technique of anastomosis, isolation precautions are taken to minimize bacterial contamination. The operative field is reduced to as small an area as possible by walling it off from the rest of the wound with gauze pads. All instruments used should be isolated. After completion of the open procedure all contaminated materials are removed and the surgical team's gloves are changed. Finally, the duodenal tube in the stomach is introduced into the duodenum by pushing or milking the candy ball through the pylorus (Fig. 13.16).

5 Some Important Intraoperative Considerations

5.1 *Protection of the Lung*

Pulmonary infection, atelectasis, and acute respiratory distress are common complications following resection of carcinoma of the esophagus or gastric cardia, and are sometimes life threatening. Although their possible causes are many, e.g., preexisting chronic pulmonary infection, pulmonary emphysema, smoking-related bronchitis, postoperative chest pain, and difficulty in evacuation of sputum, their close relation to traumatization from excessive compression and squeezing of the lungs during surgery cannot be overlooked. It must be stressed that the lungs are delicate organs which must be fully respected by the surgeons during operation. Trauma to the lung substance is often not fully appreciated and may be hardly noticeable from outside the lung, but may result in contusion of the pulmonary parenchyma, inflammation, microatelectases, or pneumonitis. The lung should therefore be handled very gently and should be periodically moistened, reexpanded, and ventilated during the operation. All these measures are of importance in reducing postoperative complications and operative risk related to the lungs.

5.2 Management of Bleeding from Aorta and Left Gastric Artery

Injury to the aorta, with resulting active hemorrhage, may occur in dissection of thoracic esophageal carcinoma which invades the aorta, or in attempted ligation of the intercostal or bronchial arteries from close to the aorta. Direct repair by suturing may be successful in a certain number of cases where the bleeding point is relatively small and the adjacent aortic wall is normal, but may sometimes be difficult, especially when the aortic wall is weakened as a result of dissection or tumor invasion, or may cause further damage to the aorta if the sutures cut through the wall. In some other cases an aortic clamp can be applied and the injury repaired with padded sutures, but this may not be practicable if the injury is on the concealed side of the aorta. When all these measures are of no avail, or in case of a large tear of the aorta, then the simple and reliable method of controlling the hemorrhage shown in Fig. 13.17 may be used. The bleeding is first temporarily halted by finger pressure. The relevant segment of aorta is freed from its surrounding tissues and then wrapped with either a tube of vascular prosthesis cut open longitudinally or a strip of Dacron or cotton. The wrapping is then closed with sutures under slight tension so as to exert a certain pressure on the aortic wall. Bleeding will then stop. We have employed this method successfully in a number of cases.

The left gastric artery may be damaged in resection of carcinoma of the esophagus or gastric cardia, during dissection of enlarged metastatic lymph nodes or as a result of crushing by clamps or slipping of ligatures, giving rise to copious hemorrhage. In managing such an accident, good exposure of the celiac region is of prime importance and must be provided by the assistant. Attempts to control the bleeding by massive tissue clamping or massive gauze packing must be avoided. Left hand finger pressure is applied by the surgeon to the site of bleeding and the extravasated blood is swiftly removed by suction. In

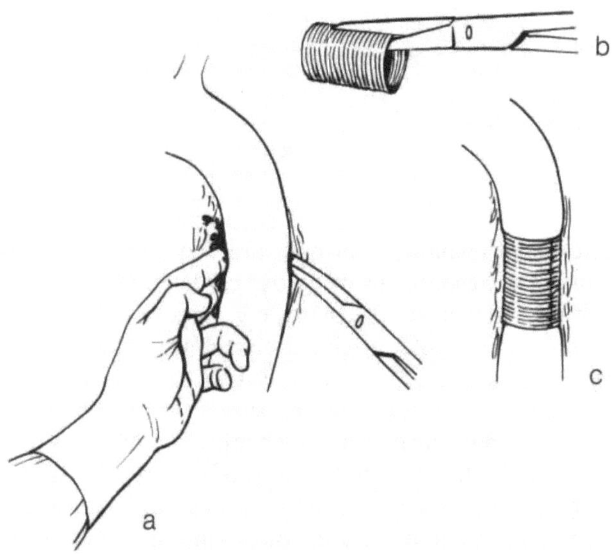

Fig. 13.17a–c. Method of halting hemorrhage from an injured aorta. ***a*** Controlling bleeding temporarily by finger pressure and freeing the affected segment of the aorta with a curved hemostatic clamp. ***b*** Cutting open a segment of vascular prosthesis. ***c*** Wrapping the injured segment of aorta

case of severe bleeding the lower part of the thoracic descending aorta may be temporarily occluded between the fingers of an assistant. When the site of bleeding has been located it is gently and accurately grasped with two or three Allis forceps applied one after the other and then carefully transfixed.

5.3 Prevention and Management of Thoracic Duct Injury

Anatomically the thoracic duct is closely related to the thoracic esophagus. It may occasionally be injured during resection of the esophageal carcinoma, resulting in postoperative chylothorax.

There are two common sites of injury [16]: (a) at the tumor bed of a midthoracic esophageal cancer invading the thoracic duct, which is prone to damage during dissection of the cancer, and (b) in the left superior mediastinum above the aortic arch, where the duct crosses the left aspect of the esophagus upward and anteriorly to enter the root of the neck (Fig. 13.18) and can easily be injured during dissection of the esophagus for excision of the tumor or construction of the anastomosis. In incising the mediastinal pleura of this region for dissection of the esophagus through a left thoracic approach, it is advisable to insert the index finger of the left hand from below the aortic arch along the paraesophageal plane to the superior mediastinum, where the subpleural tissue, including the thoracic duct, is gently swept forward by the finger. Using the finger tip pressing against the mediastinal pleura as a guide, a small oblique incision is made on the posterior part of the superior mediastinal pleura (Fig. 13.19) and then enlarged bluntly to allow identification of the thoracic duct, which is anterior to the incision.

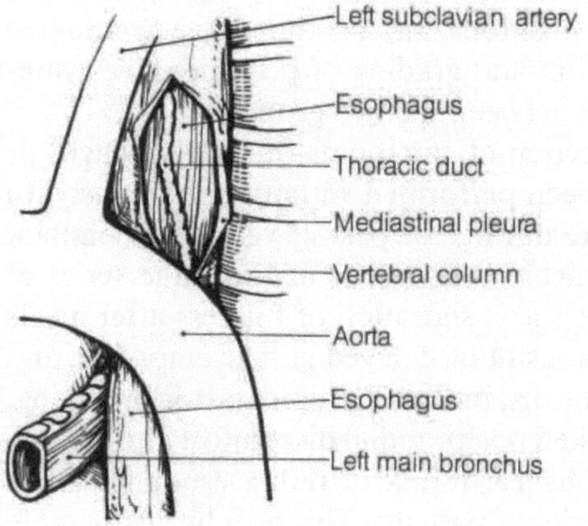

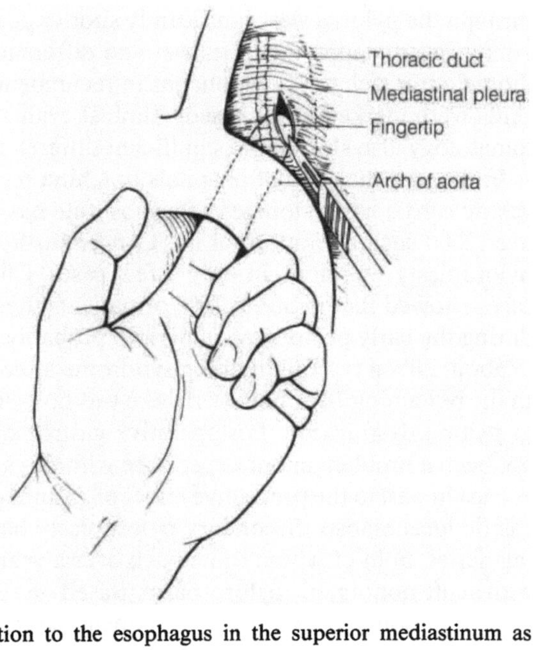

Fig. 13.18 (left). The thoracic duct and its relation to the esophagus in the superior mediastinum as viewed from the left side

Fig. 13.19 (right). Method of protecting the thoracic duct during incision of the left mediastinal pleura above the aortic arch

After dissection of the tumor and opening of the left superior mediastinal pleura, care is taken to ascertain whether the thoracic duct is injured or collapsed as a result of being ruptured, or there is any outflow of clear or milky chyle. In case of confirmed injury, the duct must be ligated both above and below the site. If injury is suspected but the site cannot be identified, it is recommended that the duct be ligated at a short distance above the diaphragm as a preventive measure. Routine ligation of the thoracic duct during resection of esophageal carcinoma seems unnecessary, as ligation per se may occasionally cause injury of the duct leading to chylothorax.

Below the aortic arch the thoracic duct lies between the azygos vein and the descending aorta anterior to the prevertebral fascia. Since the duct has a very thin wall which is prone to rupture if left unprotected, it is wise during its ligation to preserve the periductal connective tissue carefully and use a noncutting heavy silk ligature.

5.4 The Question of Pyloroplasty

Pylorospasm and gastric retention occur only occasionally after intrathoracic or cervical esophagogastrostomy. Roentgenologic study of the upper gastrointestinal tract at different periods after resection of carcinoma of the esophagus or gastric cardia without pyloroplasty revealed that in the majority of patients there was hyperperistalsis of the abdominal stomach and rapid passage of barium through the pylorus [17]. A comparative study of gastric function following use of the stomach as a substitute after resection of carcinoma of the esophagus with and without concomitant pyloroplasty, recently carried out at the Cancer Institute of the Chinese Academy of Medical Sciences [18], showed that in both groups the interval between the ingestion of barium and the first passage of barium through the pylorus was significantly shorter postoperatively than preoperatively, postoperative gastric emptying times were no different, there was no reflux of barium from the thoracic stomach to the esophagus in recumbent positions, and postoperative gastric free acids were markedly decreased. Clinical evaluation and grading of postoperative symptomatology also showed no significant difference between the two groups.

In the vast majority of hospitals in China resection of carcinoma of the esophagus or gastric cardia using stomach as a substitute has been performed without pyloroplasty. In over 2000 such operations at the Cancer Institute during the past 25 years, concomitant pyloroplasty was done in only a few cases. Clinical observations of this large series of cases showed that in about 10% of patients there was a sensation of fullness after meals during the early postoperative period, probably a result of delayed gastric emptying, and in about 20% a typical dumping syndrome after meals, indicating rapid gastric emptying. In the remaining 70%, however, there was no marked postprandial discomfort attributable to pyloric dysfunction. Postoperative gastroesophageal reflux or reflux esophagitis has not been a problem in our experience with this series of patients. This may be attributable at least in part to the preventive effect of a fundoplication incorporated into the esophagogastric anastomosis. Secondary pyloroplasty has only been necessary in two patients in this series, both of whom came back over a year after resection of esophageal carcinoma with acute nonorganic pylorospasm. Based on very wide clinical experience, including the study mentioned above, it may be concluded that routine pyloroplasty is not necessary in the resection of carcinoma of the esophagus and gastric cardia using stomach as a substitute. However, when adequate exposure is provided by an abdominal approach, pyloroplasty, being a simple procedure, may be justified.

6 Resection and Intrathoracic Esophagogastrostomy Via Left Thoracotomy

Much has been written about general principles in the resection of esophageal carcinoma; only surgical techniques will be discussed here.

The patient is placed in a right lateral position with his back close to and parallel with the edge of the operative table, in order to facilitate manipulation by the surgeon. With the exception of carcinoma located at the lower end of the esophagus, for which the incision may be made along the seventh rib, a posterolateral thoracotomy is made through the sixth interspace or through the sixth rib with resection of its entire length. After the chest is opened the wound is protected with thick gauze pads and a rib spreader is placed and widened gradually in two or three steps, in order to allow compliance of the chest wall and to avoid rib fracture, which is apt to occur in elderly patients.

Any pleural adhesions present are separated, with hemostasis as necessary. Adhesions in the anterior mediastinum and the apex may not be touched unless interfering with the operative procedure. The assistant, using his left hand, gently retracts the left lung to expose the posterior mediastinum, and the surgeon then proceeds to exploration of the cancer.

When thoracic and abdominal exploration proves the tumor to be resectable, the following procedure is gone through. The diaphragmatic incision is extended to involve the hiatus, and in the process the subdiaphragmatic artery is divided and transfixed. Two or three sutures on each edge of the diaphragm are retained for traction. The assistant lifts the stomach, which is mobilized by dividing the greater omentum and the short gastric vessels at a short distance from the greater curvature, care being taken to preserve the right gastroepiploic vessels, which together with the right gastric vessels constitute the sole blood supply to the mobilized stomach. The extent of mobilization of the greater curvature depends on the size of the stomach and the level of anastomosis. In general it should reach the pyloric antrum, in order to free a sufficient length of the stomach for transplantation and release the connection between the stomach and the transverse colon, which otherwise would be under traction after the stomach is brought up to the chest. All divided vessels along the cut edges of the greater omentum and the gastrosplenic ligament should be securely ligated.

The esophagogastric junction is freed from the hiatus, and the lesser omentum and the gastrohepatic ligament are divided, the latter possibly containing a small artery which should be ligated with it. The stomach is then raised from its bed by the assistant and the location of the left gastric artery is palpated between the upper border of the pancreas and the lesser curvature. All accessible celiac lymph nodes are dissected and the left gastric vessels are freed to their proximal parts, where three clamps are applied as shown in Fig. 13.20. The vessels are divided between the second and the third clamps, leaving two clamps proximally for safety. The first clamp is released when a ligature with heavy silk is tied on the proximal stump and the second clamp is released after transfixion.

Management of the left gastric vessels is one of the important points in resection of carcinoma of the esophagus and gastric cardia. Adequate exposure and careful manipulation are essential in the prevention of accidental bleeding from the vessels. It is also of importance that the gastrohepatic ligament and the lesser omentum be divided prior to division of the left gastric vessels, so that any bleeding from the vascular stump can be handled more easily, with the stomach retracted away from the operative field.

In carcinoma of the lower esophagus, it is advisable also to resect part of the cardiac portion of the stomach in order to extirpate any intramural tumor infiltration and metastatic paracardiac lymph nodes. This can readily be done with a stapler.

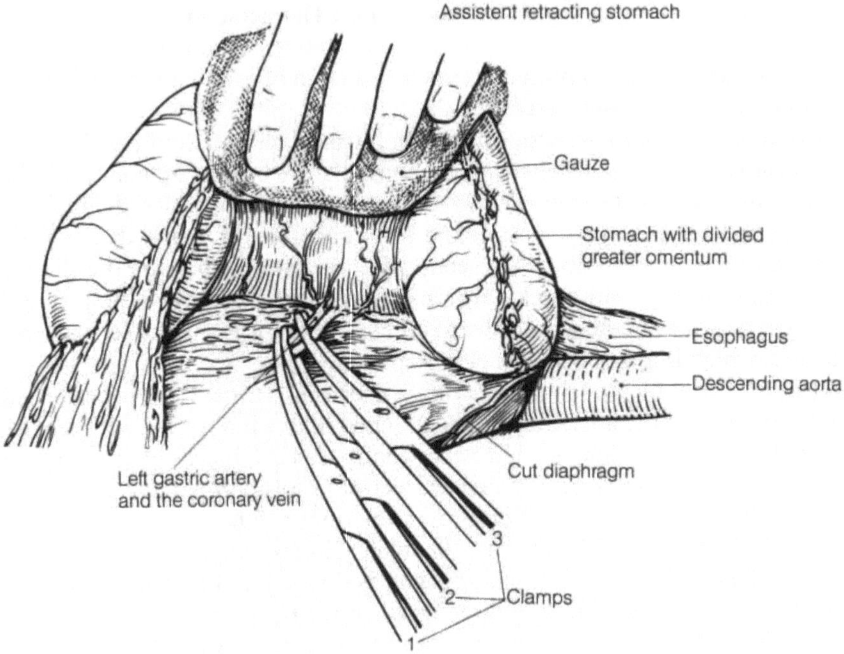

Fig. 13.20. Application of three long curved Kelly clamps to the left gastric vessels before their division between the second and third clamps

In carcinoma of the midthoracic esophagus or of higher sites, the distal esophagus may be divided at the cardiac junction. The paracardiac adipose tissue with its possibly metastatic lymph nodes should routinely be removed along with the esophagus. The divided distal end of the esophagus is ligated with heavy silk and covered by a rubber sheath to avoid contamination. The cut end of the gastric cardia may be closed with two or three mattress sutures, which are then buried with Lambert sutures or a purse-string suture.

Dissection of the cancer-bearing esophagus is best carried out from below upward with gentle traction applied to the distal end. All the paraesophageal connective tissues and lymph nodes should be included in the resection. In dissecting the esophagus at the level of the tracheal bifurcation, the upper end of the descending aorta is retracted laterally to give better exposure of the subcarinal lymph nodes, which are to be removed. Dissection is then continued up to the level of the aortic arch, where care is taken to avoid injury to the azygos vein to the right of the esophagus and the thoracic duct to the left.

The surgeon slides the index finger of his left hand along the paraesophageal tissue plane to the superior mediastinum to serve as a guide for incision of the mediastinal pleura and to protect the thoracic duct from accidental injury, as already described. The aortic arch may be mobilized by dividing its posterior attachments, which contain intercostal arteries, if better exposure of this part of the esophagus is needed or when injury to the arch of the azygos vein requires repair. The esophagus is further dissected to its superior mediastinal portion and is then drawn out of this region for a supra-aortic anastomosis with the stomach.

In bringing up the mobilized stomach to the supra-aortic region for anastomosis, care is taken to avoid a 360° rotation, which would result in postoperative gastric obstruction. In performing esophagogastrostomy, twisting of the esophageal stump must also be avoided, as a rotation of over 90° is likely to cause severe dysphagia.

Intrathoracic esophagogastrostomy is most frequently done at the supra-aortic region, the stomach being transplanted either intrapleurally or via the posterior mediastinal route. Intrapleural transplantation of the stomach has the advantage of affording easy anastomosis with the esophagus, but the disadvantage of filling part of the space normally occupied by the lung, thus diminishing its ventilatory function.

The stomach can be transplanted through the posterior mediastinal route created by resection and anastomosed intrathoracically or in the cervical region with the remaining esophagus. This route has the advantages of not depriving the lung of any space and of having good alignment with the esophagus. A major shortcoming, however, is the inconvenience in performing the intrathoracic anastomosis when a left thoracotomy approach is used, especially in an elderly patient with an enlarged and elongated aortic arch. Furthermore, a large stomach with its plication at the anastomotic site may compress the membranous part of the trachea, possibly even causing dyspnea.

When the anastomosis is complete, all the contaminated materials are removed or changed and the duodenal tube is introduced into the duodenum from outside the gastric wall as already described (Sect. 4.3).

In supra-aortic anastomosis, the intrapleural stomach is fixed by a few stitches to the mediastinal pleura. When the anastomosis is infra-aortic, the stomach is simply put into the esophageal bed without fixation.

The number of gauzes and instruments used is checked and the abdominal and pleural cavities are inspected to rule out retention of any foreign body. The diaphragm is closed around the gastric transplant with interrupted sutures so spaced as to admit only the fingertip between them. Any redundant part of the intrathoracic transplant is reduced into the abdomen. The rest of the diaphragmatic incision is securely closed with figure-of-eight sutures to prevent postoperative herniation.

A chest tube is inserted through the seventh or eighth interspace just behind the midaxillary line for closed drainage, and the chest wound is closed in layers. If the contralateral mediastinal pleura has been opened, intermittent positive pressure through the endotracheal tube is supplied by the anesthetist to reexpand the lung and to expel the air from both pleural cavities before the patient is turned flat.

7 Resection and Cervical Esophagogastrostomy Via Left Thoracotomy

Resection of carcinoma of the middle and upper segments of the esophagus usually necessitates anastomosis at the cervical region in order to minimize the risk of residual tumor and local recurrence. This can often be done using the left thoracic approach, with procedures much the same as those already described for intrathoracic anastomosis. Only some special points need be mentioned here.

For cervical anastomosis, the whole stomach must be mobilized to gain free access to the neck. Particular care is paid to preservation of the vascular supply to the stomach and avoidance of trauma to the gastric wall.

After the entire thoracic esophagus has been dissected free, the cervical esophagus can be mobilized by blunt finger dissection from inside the left chest. The dissecting finger may also go between tissue planes to reach the subcutaneous layer anterior to the sternocleidomastoideus muscle, where an oblique skin incision is made for neck dissection.

The stomach may be transplanted via the convenient intrapleural route, which is the most commonly used, or via the mediastinal route, which has the merits of being the shortest and having the best alignment with the esophagus.

Three or four traction sutures are placed at the highest point of the fundus and used to bring it up to the base of the neck through the thoracocervical tunnel just created and enlarged, care being taken to avoid injury and rotation of the stomach.

The surgical team may now be divided into two groups, one dealing with the cervical esophagogastrostomy and the other with the thoracic procedures, which include anchorage of the gastric transplant to the apex of the thorax, closure of the diaphragmatic incision, insertion of a chest tube, and closure of the chest wound.

Cervical esophagogastrostomy is performed in much the same manner as intrathoracic esophagogastrostomy. Great care is taken in cervical dissection to avoid injury to the left recurrent laryngeal nerve.

After completion of the anastomosis, a cigarette drain or rubber tissue drain is inserted through a stab wound posterior to the neck incision, to be removed 48 h later. Precautions are taken to prevent air entering the pleural cavity through the drainage wound.

8 Resection with Colon Interposition

The vascular supply of the colon, from the ascending to the descending sections, consists of four arteries, the ileocecal, the right colic, the middle colic (deriving from the superior mesenteric), and the left colic (deriving from the inferior mesenteric), which are linked by collateral anastomoses. Their common pattern of distribution is shown in Fig. 13.21. Sonneland and associates [19], in a study of 600 autopsy specimens, found that the ileocecal artery was the most constant, being present in all 600 cases. In 12.6% of cases the right

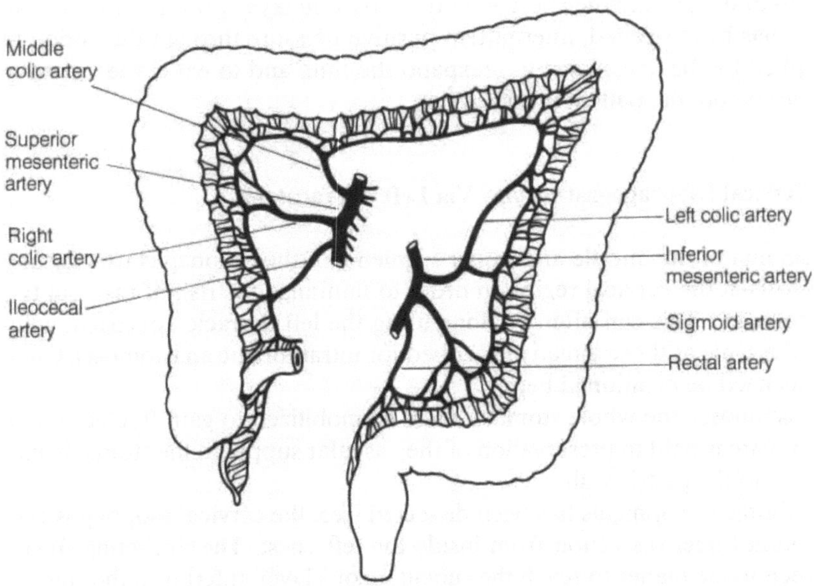

Fig. 13.21. The most common pattern of blood supply to the colon

colic artery was missing, in 3.6% the middle colic artery. In a small number of cases there was no or only feeble collateral anastomosis between the middle colic and right colic arteries. The pattern of arterial supply to the colon can be demonstrated by preoperative arteriography, and must be carefully assessed during operation.

Right Colon Interposition. The ascending colon together with a small segment of the terminal ileum is used for isoperistaltic interposition with the middle colic vessels as vascular pedicle (Fig. 13.22a). It has an ample length for interposition, and the segment of terminal ileum may be used for anastomosis with the esophagus, with the advantage that the ileocecal valve then serves to prevent reflux. The shortcomings of this technique are that the cecum is often too voluminous to be transplanted into the neck and that anatomic variations of vascular supply are relatively common.

Transverse Colon Interposition. The length of transverse colon used for interposition may include part of the right or left colon, with the middle colic artery as the vascular pedicle. The transverse colon has the advantage over other sections of the colon of ease of mobilization, but because of the frequent deviation of the middle colic artery to the right segment of the transverse colon, isoperistaltic interposition is often not feasible, and the surgeon may frequently be compelled to fashion an antiperistaltic interposition, which may interfere with the passage of food (Figl 13.22b).

Left Colon Interposition. Using the left colic vessels as vascular pedicle, an isoperistaltic left colon interposition is almost always successful (Fig. 13.22c). This is the reconstruction of choice and may be done using the same left combined thoracoabdominal approach employed for resection of the esophageal carcinoma, with the patient in the right lateral posi-

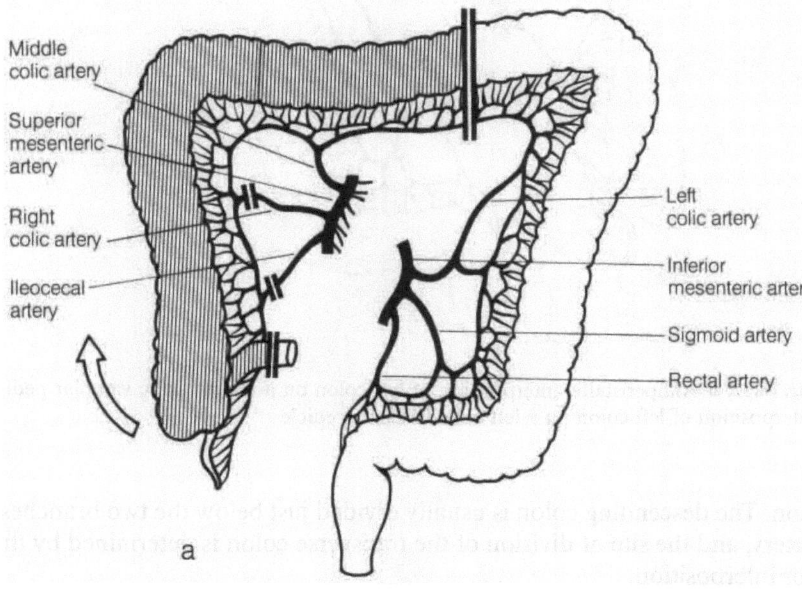

Fig. 13.22a–c. Various modes of colon interposition. ***a*** Isoperistaltic interposition of right colon on a middle colic vascular pedicle. ***b, c*** see p. 346

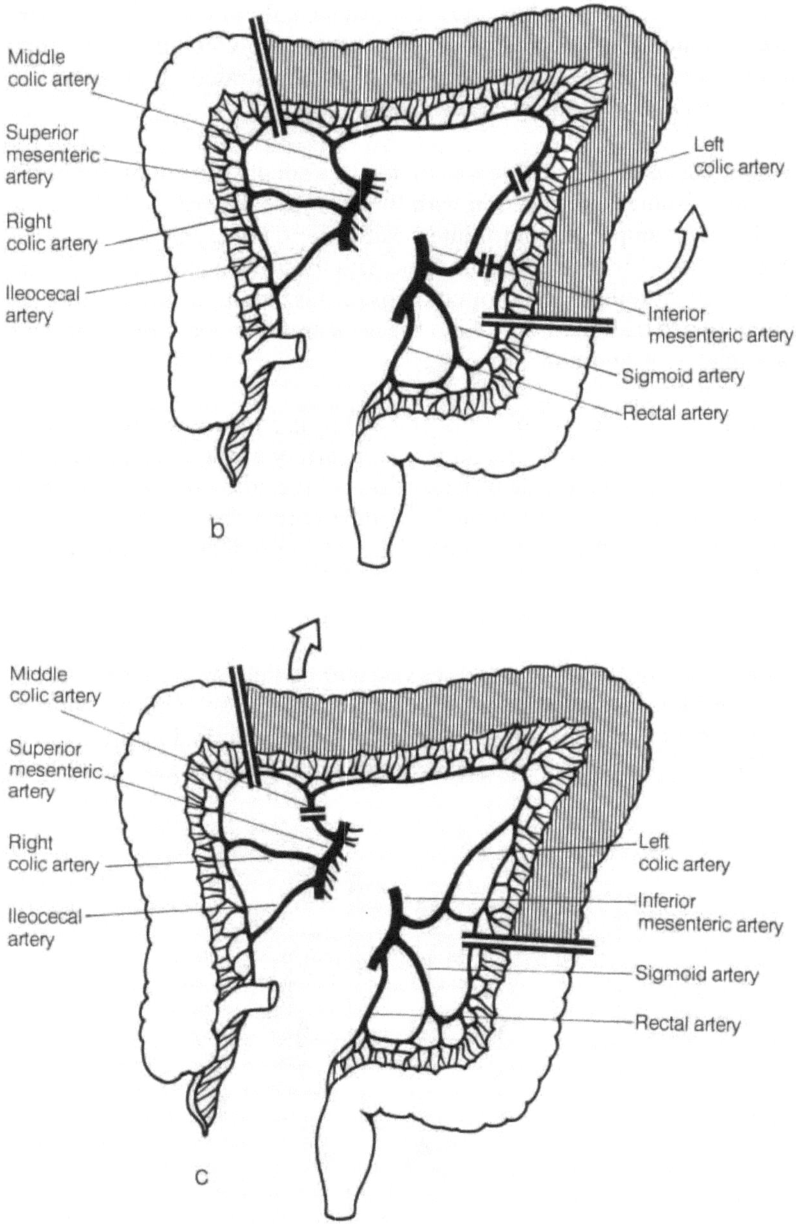

Fig. 13.22. ***b*** Antiperistaltic interposition of left colon on a middle colic vascular pedicle. ***c*** Isoperistaltic interposition of left colon on a left colic vascular pedicle

tion. The descending colon is usually divided just below the two branches of the left colic artery, and the site of division of the transverse colon is determined by the length needed for interposition.

Three routes may be used for colon interposition: subcutaneous, retrosternal, or mediastinal. The *subcutaneous* (antethoracic) is the safest and most easily fashioned, and in in-

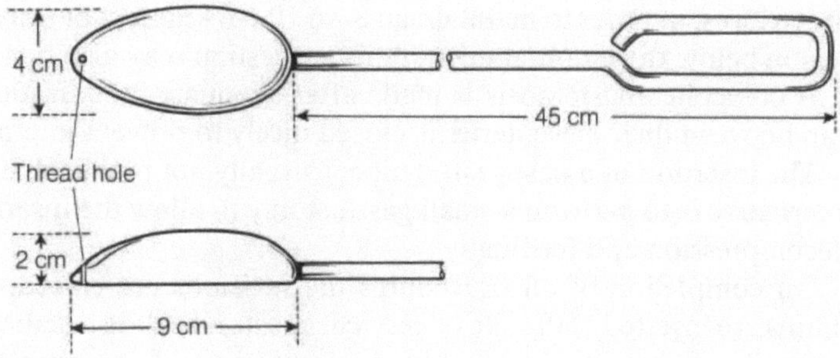

Fig. 13.23. Retrosternal tunnel opener

fection or necrosis of the colon provides easy access for management. However, it is the longest route and the least satisfactory cosmetically. The *posterior mediastinal* route has the advantages of being the shortest and of being in alignment with the esophagus, but is the most inaccessible for treatment in the case of complications with the intrathoracic colon. The *retrosternal* route, the most commonly used, is perhaps intermediate in both merits and shortcomings.

When exploration confirms colon interposition as feasible, it is wise to divide the surgical team into two groups, one working on the chest and neck and the other on the abdomen.

The selected length of colon is mobilized and divided at the appropriate sites. Its upper end is closed temporarily with sutures, which are subsequently used for drawing the transplant up to the neck. Simultaneously, the thoracic procedures are completed and the divided esophagus is delivered into the cervical incision for anastomosis. The retrosternal tunnel is started by excising the xiphoid process and opening the retrosternal space from both upper and lower ends. A tunnel opener (Fig. 13.23) is then applied with the flat surface against the inner surface of the sternum and gently pushed upward along the midline until its tip reaches the suprasternal notch. A heavy silk suture is threaded through the tip hole and the opener is withdrawn from the lower end of the tunnel, taking the suture with it. The upper aperture of the tunnel is enlarged with the fingers or by excising part of the manubrium sterni and the left sternoclavicular joint to avoid their compression on the transplant. In developing the tunnel, care is taken not to rupture the mediastinal pleurae.

The colon transplant is then brought up via an opening made in the lesser omentum through the retrosternal tunnel to the neck for anastomosis with the esophageal stump. In bringing the colon through the tunnel care must be exercised to avoid rotation of the transplant and injury to its blood supply, especially the venous return.

End-to-end esophagocolostomy is performed in much the same manner as end-to-end esophagogastrostomy. If the diameter of the colon is much greater than that of the esophagus, the excess may be closed with sutures. If end-to-end esophagocolostomy is carried out, the opening of the colon should be made transversely at the antimesenteric side. It is essential that no part of the transplant is allowed to overlap the anterior wall of the trachea, to avoid interference in case tracheostomy is necessary postoperatively.

The cologastrostomy may be made on the anterior wall of the stomach near the midline of the body, and redundancy of the colon is avoided so that no kinking can result. Belsey [20] advocated forming an antireflux cologastric anastomosis on the posterior aspect of the stomach near the greater curvature, one-third of the distance from the closed cardia to the pylorus, in order to maintain an 8- to 10-cm segment of transplant in the high-pressure region below the diaphragm, and this suggestion may also be followed.

A colocolic anastomosis is made after adequate mobilization of the two stumps. The gap between their mesenteries is closed nicely to prevent internal hernia.

The insertion of a nasogastric tube is usually not practicable in colon interposition. An alternative is to perform a small gastrostomy to allow the insertion of a fine tube for both decompression and feeding.

On completion of all procedures the incisions are closed. One or two rubber tissue drains are inserted at the site of cervical anastomosis via a stab wound, and one or two cigarette drains may be inserted in the lower part of the retrosternal tunnel via a similar wound on the abdominal wall. If the mediastinal pleura has been ruptured, it is advisable to insert a chest tube for closed drainage.

References

1. Belsey R, Hiebert CA (1974) An exclusive right thoracic approach for cancer of the middle third of the esophagus. Ann Thorac Surg 18: 1–15
2. Ong GB, Lam KH, Lam HN, Wong J (1978) Resection for carcinoma of the superior mediastinal segment of the esophagus. World J Surg 2: 497–504
3. Akiyama H (1981) Esophagectomy without thoracotomy. Surg Annu 13: 109–121
4. Orringer MB, Sloan H (1978) Esophagectomy without thoracotomy. J Thorac Cardiovasc Surg 76: 643–654
5. Szentpetery S, Wolfgang T, Lower RR (1979) Pull-through esophagectomy without thoracotomy for esophageal carcinoma. Ann Thorac Surg 27: 399–403
6. Postlethwait RW (1979) Esophagectomy without thoracotomy (editorial). Ann Thorac Surg 27: 395–396
7. Wu TQ, Jiang XM (1979) Treatment of carcinoma of the gastric cardia by inversion esophagectomy without thoracotomy (in Chinese). Chin Med J 59: 358–360
8. Huang GJ, Zhang DW, Lin H, Wang LJ, Zhang RG, Wang GQ (1979) Treatment of early esophageal carcinoma by inversion esophagectomy without thoracotomy (in Chinese). Chin J Oncol 1: 245–248
9. Zhang DW, Huang GJ, Zhu ZB (1981) Surgical treatment of recurrent esophageal carcinoma after curative radiotherapy: report of 54 cases (in Chinese). Chin J Surg 19: 268–270
10. Ong GB, Kwong KH (1970) Management of malignant esophagobronchial fistula. Surgery 67: 293–301
11. Akiyama H, Tsurumaru M, Kawamura T, Ono Y (1981) Principles of surgical treatment for carcinoma of the esophagus. Ann Surg 194: 438–445
12. Belsey R (1981) Esophageal reconstruction with colon for benign disease. In: Stipa S, Belsey RHR, Moraldi A (eds) Medical and surgical problems of the esophagus. Academic, London New York (Serono symposium no 43, p 195)
13. Heimlich HJ, Winfield JM (1955) Use of gastric tube to replace or by-pass esophagus. Surgery 37: 549
14. Akiyama, H, Kogure T, Itai Y (1974) Role of esophagotomy in the surgical treatment of esophageal cancer. Int Surg 59: 478–482
15. Wu WJ, Chen FC, Chou HK, et al. (1978) An esophagogastrostomic instrument. Chin Med J 4: 204–211
16. Huang GJ, Zhang W (1965) Diagnosis and management of chylothorax following resection of carcinoma of the esophagus (in Chinese). Chin J Surg 13: 130–132
17. Su JH (1978) Roentgenological study of gastrointestinal function following resection of carcinoma of the esophagus and gastric cardia (in Chinese). Cancer Res Prev Treat 1: 9–13
18. Zhang DC, Huang GJ, Zhang DW (1983) A comparative study of resection of esophageal carcinoma using stomach as a stubstitute with and without pyloroplasty (in Chinese). Chin J Surg 21: 455–457
19. Sonneland J, Anson BJ, Beaton LE (1958) Surgical anatomy of arterial supply to the colon from the superior mesenteric artery based upon a study of 600 specimens. Surg Gynecol Obstet 106: 385–398
20. Belsey RHR (1980) Palliative menagement of esophageal carcinoma. Am J Surg 139: 789–794

Chapter 14
Operative Technique for Carcinoma of the Gastric Cardia

Guo Jun Huang and Wu Ying K'ai

---

1 Choice of Approach and Operation

The principles of surgical treatment of carcinoma of the gastric cardia are in general similar to those in carcinoma of the esophagus, but a number of technical details differ. As the lower segment of the esophagus is often involved in carcinoma of the gastric cardia, surgical resection invariably includes the adjacent portion of the esophagus. Whether gastrectomy is partial or total depends upon the extent of the growth (Fig. 14.1). Reconstruction of the food passage following resection is usually accomplished with infra-aortic esophagogastrostomy or esophagojejunostomy via the transpleural route. Other techniques, such as posterior mediastinal esophagogastrostomy through a combined median sternoabdominal approach and cervical esophagogastrostomy following inversion extraction of the thoracic esophagus without thoracotomy, are used comparatively rarely. End-to-side or Roux-en-Y esophagojejunostomy is usually performed after total gastrectomy.

1.1 Left Posterolateral Thoracotomy

Left posterolateral thoracotomy through the bed of the seventh rib is the most frequently employed approach for resection of carcinoma of the gastric cardia, and provides the best exposure for the lower segment of the esophagus, the structures around the esophageal hiatus, and other organs in the left upper quadrant of the abdomen. When total gastrectomy or extensive lymph node dissection in the celiac region is necessary, the left costal margin may be divided with a short downward and anterior extension of the incision, which is then combined thoracoabdominal. This type of approach is adequate not only for intrathoracic esophagogastrostomy, but also for esophagojejunostomy or colon interposition for esophageal reconstruction (Fig. 14.2).

1.2 Upper Abdominal Incision

Cancer of the gastric cardia may be approached through a median, transverse, or oblique upper abdominal incision. This type of incision is usually inadequate for resection of cancer of the gastric cardia, but may be employed for preliminary exploration in cases of doubtful resectability. If extensive metastasis is found in the peritoneal cavity, then the op-

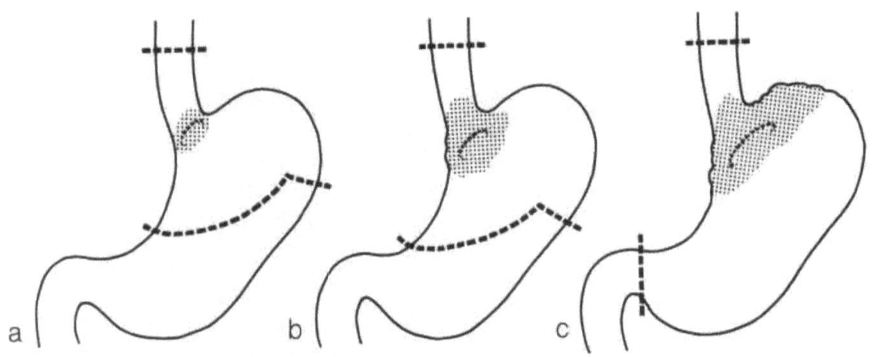

Fig. 14.1 a–c. Gastrectomy for carcinoma of the gastric cardia according to extent of lesion. ***a*** Partial; ***b*** subtotal; ***c*** total

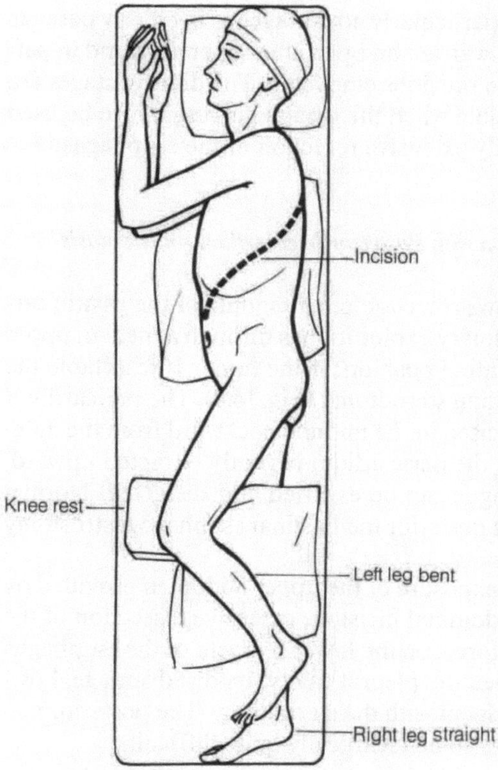

Fig. 14.2. Combined left thoracoabdominal incision

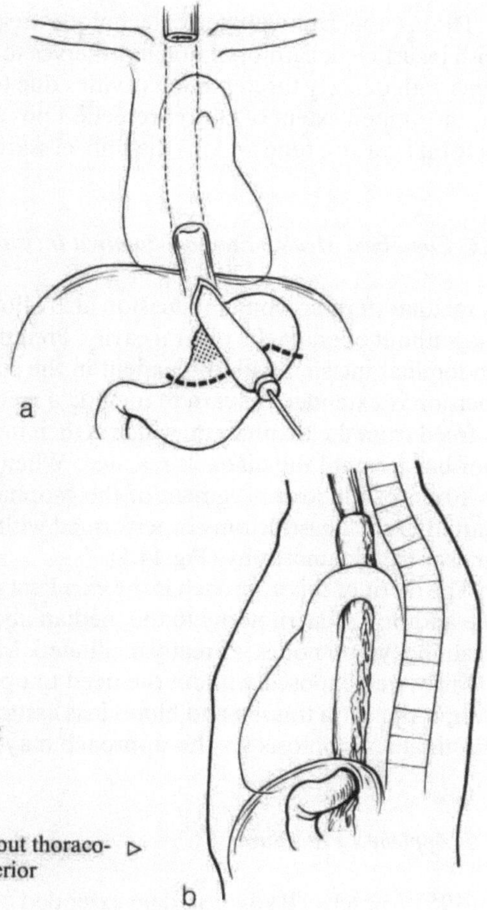

Fig. 14.3. ***a*** Inversion extraction esophagectomy without thoracotomy. ***b*** Cervical esophagogastrostomy through posterior mediastinum ▷

eration may be concluded without thoracotomy. If the cancer is found to be resectable, then the incision is extended upward and laterally to become a combined thoracoabdominal incision.

1.3 Partial Gastrectomy and Inversion Esophagectomy Without Thoracotomy

Preliminary exploration of the cancer of the gastric cardia is via an upper abdominal incision. If the tumor is resectable, the lower esophagus is bluntly dissected through the hiatus and a cervical incision is made for access to the upper esophagus, which is also bluntly dissected down to the superior mediastinum. A longitudinal incision is then made in the abdominal esophagus, an esophageal extractor is inserted intraluminally to the cervical esophagus, and the thoracic esophagus is extracted downward using the technique already described in Chap. 13.1.6. Through the abdominal incision the stomach is mobilized and partly excised with the tumor, leaving most of the greater curvature to form a gastric tube, which is brought up to the neck through the posterior mediastinum and anastomosed with the esophagus (Fig. 14.3) [1].

The approach and operative technique are particularly advantageous in elderly patients with insufficient cardiopulmonary reserves to warrant an open chest operation and in patients with densely fused pleural cavities due to previous empyema. The disadvantages are (a) the limited extent of cancer resection possible when the greater curvature is to be used to form a gastric tube and (b) the unnecessarily extensive resection of the esophagus.

1.4 Combined Median Sternoabdominal Incision with Posterior Mediastinal Anastomosis

A median sternoabdominal incision also allows resection of carcinoma of the gastric cardia without opening the pleural cavity. Preliminary exploration is through a median upper abdominal incision with the patient in the supine position; if the tumor is resectable the incision is extended upward to include a median sternotomy (Fig. 14.4). The pericardium is freed from the diaphargm, which is then incised in the midline backward from the anterior border until the hiatus is reached. When the pericardium is gently retracted upward, 8–10 cm of the lower segment of the esophagus can be exposed and dissected. Normal partial or total gastrectomy is performed with posterior mediastinal esophagogastrostomy or esophagojejunostomy (Fig. 14.5).

The merit of this approach is the excellent exposure of the upper abdomen provided by the addition of sternotomy to the median abdominal incision; extensive dissection of the draining lymph nodes is greatly facilitated. Moreover, the lower segment of the esophagus is fairly well exposed without the need to open the pleural cavity. Its disadvantage, however, is the extra trauma and blood loss associated with the sternotomy. The posterior mediastinal anastomosis via this approach may also be technically quite difficult.

1.5 Appleby's Procedure

In 1953 Appleby [2] advocated an extended operation for gastric carcinoma, to include excision of the celiac axis and its branches, subtotal or total gastrectomy, removal of the spleen, the tail and body of the pancreas, the greater and lesser omenta, and the perito-

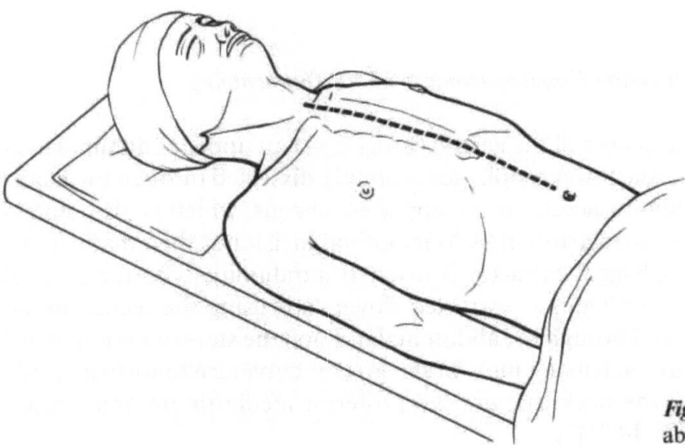

Fig. 14.4. Combined median sternoabdominal incision

neum overlying the lesser sac and dissection of all the lymph nodes along the branches of the celiac artery. This procedure was followed by Wada and associates in treating carcinoma of the gastric cardia, with gratifying results [3, 4].

Appleby's procedure has the advantage of eradicating all draining lymph nodes and may thus be expected to yield better results from surgery for carcinoma of the gastric cardia. It has the drawbacks, however, of increasing the trauma from surgery and adding the risks associated with hepatic artery ligation. In advanced cases involving lymph node metastasis proximal to the root of the celiac artery, this procedure would not achieve radical extirpation of the tumor.

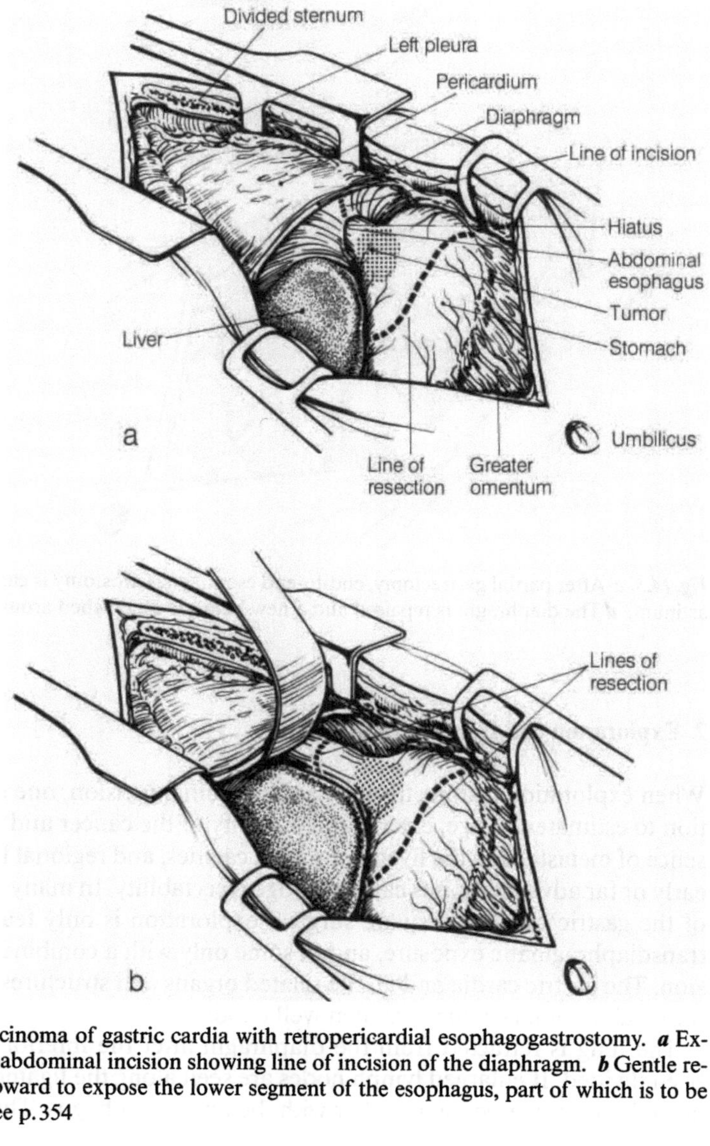

Fig. 14.5 a–d. Resection of carcinoma of gastric cardia with retropericardial esophagogastrostomy. ***a*** Exposure through median sternoabdominal incision showing line of incision of the diaphragm. ***b*** Gentle retraction of the pericardium upward to expose the lower segment of the esophagus, part of which is to be resected with the tumor. ***c, d*** see p. 354

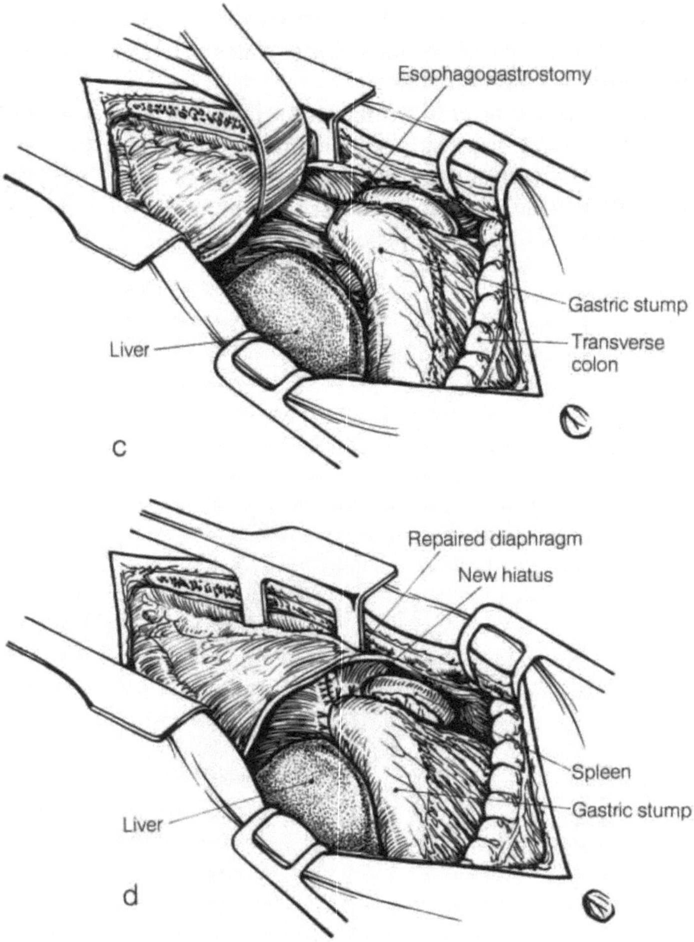

Fig. 14.5. ***c*** After partial gastrectomy, end-to-end esophagogastrostomy is carried out in the posterior mediastinum. ***d*** The diaphragm is repaired and a new hiatus is established around the gastric stump

2 Exploration and Decision on Resection

When exploration is done through an abdominal incision, one depends largely on palpation to estimate the size, extent, and mobility of the cancer and assess the presence or absence of metastasis in the liver, peritoneal cavities, and regional lymph nodes. Only in very early or far advanced cases can one judge resectability. In many cases of borderline cancer of the gastric cardia, adequate surgical exploration is only feasible with a thoracic and transdiaphragmatic exposure, and in some only with a combined thoracoabdominal incision. The gastric cardia and all the related organs and structures in the lower thoracic and upper abdominal cavities are then well exposed.

The lung is retracted from the diaphragm after the inferior pulmonary ligament has been divided. If enlarged lymph nodes are seen along the ligament, they should be left attached for later resection together with the lower esophagus. The dome of the left hemidiaphragm is then opened radially up to a point about a centimeter or so from the margin of the esophageal hiatus, which should be resected with the gastric cardia unless the cancer is limited and grossly distant from the hiatus. By this time the tumor is both visible and palpable, and its size and extent can be ascertained. Before extensive palpation, careful inspection should be carried out to discover whether the cancer has already invaded the overlying peritoneal surface or infiltrated into the diaphragm and whether it extends down to the lesser curvature of the stomach or up to the lower end of the esophagus. Involvement of the posterior aspect of the gastric cardia is usually more extensive than one estimates on palpation from the front, and one may sometimes be misled by apparent mobility on palpation, only to find later that the cancer has already infiltrated the body of the pancreas or the hilum of the spleen. Therefore before the decision on resection is made, the surgeon should always open the omental sac and inspect the relationship of the cancer to the surrounding structures from behind.

The left lobe of the liver is usually well exposed and may be examined for metastases by both inspection and palpation, but the right lobe can only be palpated. Lymph node metastasis should first be checked for in the paracardiac group, then in the groups along the lesser gastric curvature, the left gastric artery, and the upper border of the pancreas toward the splenic hilum. Finally, the nodes around the celiac axis and in the para-aortic regions, must be palpated. The findings from these steps give more information as to resectability.

Gross peritoneal implantation of cancer nodules is sometimes seen in the greater omentum and occasionally in the pelvic peritoneal sac, which should always be palpated during exploration.

Findings on exploration usually place the carcinoma in one of the following three categories:

1. Obviously resectable cancer with good prospects for cure. The criteria of this category include limitation of the primary cancer, without infiltration into the neighboring structures, and either no gross metastasis to the regional lymph nodes or metastasis confined to noedes which can be removed completely along with the primary. Under these circumstances, a radical curative resection should be carried out.
2. A resectable cancer with poor prospects for cure. A tumor in this category is moderately advanced with extension of growth toward the lesser curvature and the fundus of the stomach, and the surrounding portion of the diaphragm or the body of the pancreas may also be involved. However, the primary cancer is still resectable in toto. The regional lymph nodes are grossly involved but may be completely or partially removed by the resection. A few small metastatic nodules may also be found in the liver. Cancer of this description is certainly not curable by operation, but palliative resection is usually still worthwhile.
3. Obviously inoperable cancer. The criteria for inoperability include fixation of the tumor to the surrounding structures in a "frozen" state, massive liver metastasis, and extensive peritoneal implantation. Resection of the cancer is not possible and should not be attempted. If dysphagia is marked and the greater curvature of the stomach is in good condition, a bypass may be fashioned with a side-to-side anastomosis between this curvature and the lower esophagus. It should be pointed out, however, that such a low bypass is prone to cause gastroesophageal reflux, which may distress the patient.

3 Technique of Resection

The extent of resection of carcinoma of the gastric cardia depends upon the size of the tumor and on the presence or absence of infiltration beyond the boundary of the stomach and regional lymph node metastasis. Curative radical resection is to be undertaken when both tumor and regional lymph node metastasis are limited. The gastric resection must be adequate and all the regional lymph nodes should be removed en bloc with the cancer. In a resection aiming rather at palliation, the safety of the patient should be given priority over the completeness of the operation.

As much as possible of the greater curvature is retained, to be used in forming a gastric tube for esophagogastrostomy after resection. The line of division on the stomach should be at least 5 cm away from the margin of the cancer. When the cancer has extended beyond the midpoint of the lesser curvature, total gastrectomy is usually indicated. A combined thoracoabdominal incision is preferable for adequate exposure for such an operation, and is easily made by extending the original thoracotomy incision to the left upper abdomen and dividing the costal margin. Following partial or total gastrectomy, the esophagogastrostomy or esophagojejunostomy is established in the posterior mediastinum at the level of the inferior pulmonary vein or slightly above (Fig. 14.6).

If the cancer has involved the diaphragm in the region of the esophageal hiatus, hilum of the spleen, or body and tail of the pancreas, all the involved tissue, including the overlying peritoneum and ligaments, should be resected in the form of a block excision. The lymph nodes around the left gastric artery are the most frequent site of regional metastasis; the artery and the adjacent part of the stomach should be resected together with the cancer.

When resection of the cancer is decided upon after exploration, the first step is division of the greater omentum along the greater curvature toward the gastric fundus. If the spleen is to be preserved, the line of division continues through the gastrosplenic ligament, dividing the short gastric arteries. If the spleen is to be removed, the peritoneum is divided below and lateral to the lower pole of the spleen and the phrenicocolic ligament is cut.

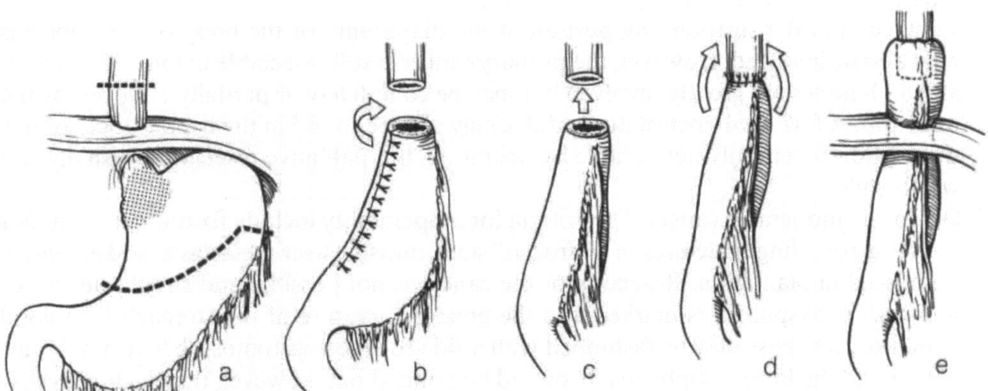

Fig. 14.6a–e. Technique of end-to-end esophagogastrostomy. ***a*** Extent of gastric resection. (broken lines) ***b*** Clockwise rotation of the gastric tube through 90°. ***c*** Bringing up the gastric tube for anastomosis with the esophagus. ***d*** Single-layer esophagogastrostomy completed. ***e*** Telescoping the anastomotic line about 2.5 cm into the gastric tube

The spleen is rotated anteriorly and toward the midline, and the splenic artery and vein are divided following double ligation. In some cases, the tail and part of the body of the pancreas may also be resected along with the tumor. The cut surface of the pancreas requires multiple sutures for hemostasis and measures to prevent postoperative formation of a pancreatic fistula. The left gastroepiploic artery is divided and attention is paid to the vascular arch along the greater curvature all the way to the pyloric region.

The next step is mobilization of the lower segment of the esophagus following division of the inferior pulmonary ligament. All the paraesophageal lymph nodes are removed with the esophagogastric junction. The esophagus is isolated to just above the level of the inferior pulmonary vein, where the subsequent esophagogastrostomy or esophagojejunostomy is to be established. The esophageal hiatus of the diaphragm is removed along with the esophagogastric junction. The gastrohepatic ligament and the lesser omentum are divided as far away from the tumor as possible and are left attached to it for removal.

Dissection and division of the left gastric artery at a proximal level requires great care and skill in eliminating as completely as possible all lymphatic involvement. It is sometimes difficult to isolate the artery because of the enlarged lymph nodes surrounding it, and precautions against injury to the artery should be strictly observed.

3.1 Partial Gastrectomy

On the basis of operative exploration as described above in Sect. 2, a proximal partial gastrectomy is decided upon if the cancer is not too extensive and sufficient normal gastric wall is available along the greater curvature to form a gastric tube for esophagogastrostomy after resection. Division and closure of the stomach is best done with a stapler. When no such device is available, Payr clamps or Kocher forceps may be used, the edges of the gastric tube along the greater curvature being closed with multiple absorbable or nonabsorbable mattress sutures. The inner suture line is buried with a second row of nonabsorbable Lambert sutures. These stitches go through only the seromuscular coats of the gastric wall, ensuring proper approximation of the edges of the gastric wall but without tissue strangulation or puckering. The long gastric tube formed in this manner is used later for esophagogastrostomy. The isolated proximal portion of the stomach bearing the cancer of the cardia is wrapped in a wet pad and lifted upward toward the chest. The posterolateral aspect of the lower segment of the esophagus is then exposed ready for division and esophagogastrostomy.

Our current method of esophagogastrostomy following resection of carcinoma of the gastric cardia is end-to-end anastomosis between the esophageal stump and the gastric tube. The upper tip of the gastric tube is amputated to leave an opening approximately equal in size to that of the esophagus so that the mucosal edges of the esophageal and gastric stomas can be approximated by a single layer of multiple interrupted silk sutures. The next step is to rotate the gastric stump 90° to the right in order to have the sutured lesser curvature side of the gastric tube facing toward the patient's right, coming to the midpoint of the right half of the anastomotic suture line (Fig. 14.6). In this way, the suture line of the gastric tube and the right half of the esophagogastrostomy suture line are both in clear view and approximation and tissue protection in the cirtical area can be optimal.

The technical details of esophagogastrostomy after resection of carcinoma of the gastric cardia are essentially the same as after resection of esophageal carcinoma. After putting in the first row of anchoring sutures for invagination of the anastomotic line, a nontraumatic auricular clamp may be applied just proximal to them to control spilling and bleeding from the esophageal stump during anastomosis.

Just before completion of anastomosis, the gastric decompression tube and the duodenal feeding tube are inserted in the same manner as after resection of esophageal carcinoma (Chap. 13 Sect. 4.3).

When the last anastomotic sutures have been placed, the presenting layer of invagination sutures is inserted in such a way that the line of anastomosis is telescoped into the gastric tube for a distance of about 2.5 cm (Fig. 14.6). The anastomosed esophagus and gastric tube are then placed in the original esophageal bed in the posterior mediastinum.

At this stage all contaminated pads in the operative field are removed, and all members of the team change their gloves. The anesthetist reexpands and ventilates the lungs through the endotracheal tube. The tip of the duodenal feeding tube is pushed into the duodenum. Instruments, pads, gauzes, etc. are checked by the nurses to ensure that no foreign body has been left in the thoracic or abdominal cavity. The diaphragmatic incision is closed with the gastric wall properly attached to the newly reconstructed diaphragmatic hiatus, and the pleural cavity is thoroughly washed with saline solution. A thoracostomy tube is inserted through a small stab wound in the eighth intercostal space just anterior to the posterior axillary line and positioned with its tip toward the posterior costodiaphragmatic gutter. If necessary, a temporary fixation suture of fine absorbable material can be placed to keep the tube properly aligned. Finally, the chest incision is closed in layers.

3.2 Total Gastrectomy

The indications for total gastrectomy in carcinoma of the gastric cardia may vary widely between surgeons, but we have not practised it extensively, although we do perform it in selected cases involving moderately advanced carcinoma of the cardia extending into the lesser curvature or the adjacent posterior aspect of the gastric wall. A proximal partial gastrectomy may be sufficient in relatively more localized cancer of the cardia, and when the cancer is more invasive, with extensive regional lymph node metastasis, even total gastrectomy will not give long-term results good enough to justify operating.

The best exposure for total gastrectomy is obtained with a combined thoracoabdominal incision, usually through the left seventh intercostal space or involving resection of the seventh rib and extending downward and toward the midline to the left upper abdomen. The stomach is dissected and isolated along both greater and lesser curvatures to beyond the pylorus. The greater omentum is always removed in toto together with the stomach, the spleen is included in the majority of cases, and sometimes the tail and part of the body of the pancreas are also resected, depending upon the extent of involvement. After proper isolation of the distal end of the stomach, the proximal duodenum is divided between Kocher forceps just distal to the pyloric ring and the duodenal stump is closed with two layers of sutures. Dissection of the esophagogastric junction and the fundus of the stomach proceeds as in partial gastrectomy. With the entire stomach wrapped in a large pad and rotated upward, the lower esophagus is exposed for division and anastomosis. The usual method is end-to-side esophagojejunostomy, but sometimes Roux-en-Y anastomosis is performed (Fig. 14.7). In both instances, a side-to-side jejunojejunostomy is constructed to prevent emptying complications.

The ligament of Treitz is divided, and the freed proximal jejunum is brought upward through an opening made in the mesocolon to be approximated to the lower esophagus.

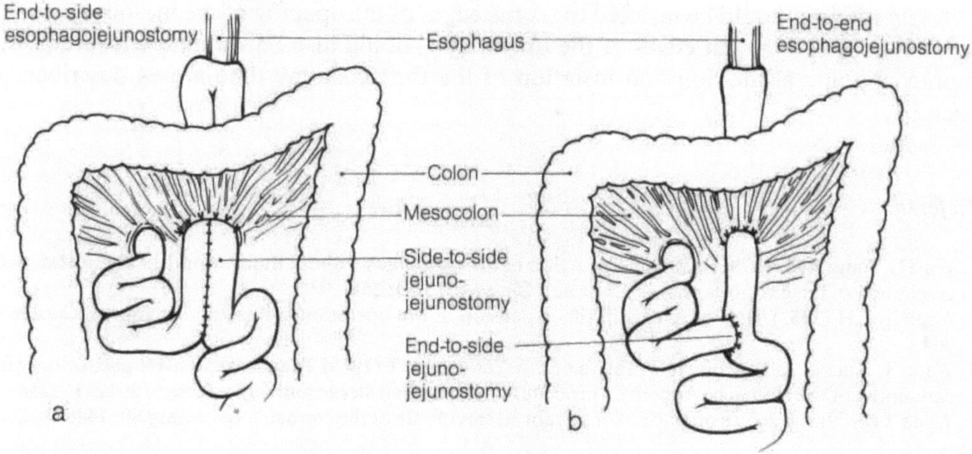

Fig. 14.7. ***a*** Total gastrectomy and end-to-side esophagojejunostomy. ***b*** Total gastrectomy and Roux-en-Y esophagojejunostomy

The proximal limb of the jejunal loop is placed on the right anterior side. The posterior aspect of the distal esophagus is anchored to the anterior aspect of the distal limb of the jejunal loop with multiple seromuscular silk sutures. A nontraumatic esophageal clamp is applied to the esophagus proximal to the anastomosis site for control of spilling and limitation of bleeding during anastomosis. Parallel incisions are made on the posterior aspect of the esophagus and the anterior aspect of the jejunum about 1.5 cm from the posterior suture line of the esophagojejunostomy. The esophageal and jejunal edges are approximated with five or six interrupted silk sutures. A decompression tube and a feeding tube are inserted a sufficient distance into the distal jejunal loop. The esophagus is then completely divided and removed from the operative field with the attached stomach. The clamp on the esophagus is removed and a previously inserted tube is pushed through the esophagostomy opening and tied to the upper ends of the other two tubes in the distal jejunum, which are then drawn upward and out through the nostril for postoperative use. The anterior lips of the esophagojejunostomy are approximated with interrupted silk sutures, due care being taken to avoid puckering and narrowing, and the anterior aspect of the anastomosis is covered with the distal limb of the jenunal loop, secured with seromuscular sutures.

A side-to-side jejunojejunal anastomosis is then established, usually at the level of the duodenojejunal junction. The anastomosis is about 6–8 cm in length and secured with two layers of interrupted silk sutures. This additional procedure is necessary for prevention of bile or food stasis in the proximal duodenojejunal loop.

When Roux-en-Y anastomosis is planned, the jejunum is divided about 20 cm distal to the duodenojejunal junction. One or two branches of the jejunal artery are divided to allow the distal jejunal limb to be brought upward for the end-to-end esophagojejunostomy. Multiple interrupted sutures are used to approximate the mucosal edges of the esophageal stump to the upper end of the jejunal limb, and a second layer of seromuscular sutures is placed so as to cover the first suture line in telescope fashion. The distal end of the proximal jejunal limb is anastomosed to the side of the distal jejunal limb. Roux-en-Y anastomosis is advantageous when the jejunal mesentery is short, but otherwise has no special merit.

A few stitches should be inserted to fix the edges of the opening of the mesocolon to the jejunal loop, and the cut edges of the diaphragm should also be sutured. Closure of the thoracoabdominal incision and insertion of the thoracostomy tube are as described in Sect. 3.1.

References

1. Wu TQ, Jiang XM (1979) Inversion extraction of the esophagus without thoracotomy in the treatment of carcinoma of the gastric cardia (in Chinese). Chin Med J 59: 358–360
2. Appleby LH (1953) The celiac axis in the expansion of the operation for gastric carcinoma. Cancer 6: 704
3. Wada T, Katayama K, Konishi T, Takahama T, Yamamura T (1978) The most extensive gastrectomy for carcinoma of the stomach: Appleby's procedure with median sternotomy. Jpn J Surg 79: 1251–1254
4. Wada T (1979) Appleby's operation for advanced carcinoma of the stomach. Jpn J Surg 80: 1448–1452

Chapter 15
Palliative Treatment

Guo Jun Huang

1 Introduction

It has been estimated that only about 25% of patients with carcinoma of the esophagus or gastric cardia can be considered operable at the time of diagnosis, the remaining 75% of patients being unsuitable for surgery mostly by reason of the advanced stage of their disease, sometimes because of other contraindications. Among patients who have come to operation, the resectability rate has been about 80% in carcinoma of the esophagus and about 65% in carcinoma of the gastric cardia. In about three-fourths of the resectable cases the tumor was in stage III or IV, with tumor invasion of the surrounding structures or lymph node metastasis, and in more than half of these cases the resection was palliative.

When patients come to operation, our policy is to resect the cancer and reconstruct the esophagus whenever technically possible, with cure as the primary objective. When curative resection cannot be accomplished, palliative resection is worthwhile because it enables the patient to eat reasonably normally and prevents many of the complications of tumor obstruction, invasion, and infection, such as aspiration pulmonary infection, fistula formation, bleeding, and pain, which often occur as the disease progresses. It also reduces the tumor burden by eliminating the primary growth; the patient's immunologic defence mechanism may be better able to deal with the cancer that remains. In some cases the residual tumor after palliative resection may be treated by radiotherapy with reasonable prolongation of life.

Other forms of palliative treatment may be needed in patients with the following conditions:

1. Contraindications to surgery or radiotherapy
2. Cancer ascertained unresectable at operation
3. Severe dysphagia during or after radiotherapy
4. Malnutrition due to dysphagia
5. Esophagobronchial or -tracheal fistula
6. Postoperative anastomotic leakage or stricture

The commonly employed palliative treatments other than resection are (a) esophageal intubation, (b) bypass operation, and (c) gastrostomy or jejunostomy. All these measures give only temporary relief from symptoms, but if used properly may improve the quality of the patient's limited span of life. In a number of patients undergoing bypass operations, there may even be a slight prolongation of survival time (Table 15.1) [1]. However, these palliative measures are not without risk to the patient and should therefore only be undertaken when clearly indicated.

Table 15.1. Average survival in months after palliative treatment for nonresectable carcinoma of the esophagus or gastric cardia [1]

Treatment	Cases	From onset of symptoms	From admission to hospital
None	157	9.0	3.1
Gastrostomy/jejunostomy	101	9.2	3.2
Esophagogastric bypass	63	11.8	6.2

2 Esophageal Intubation

Esophageal intubation is one of the oldest methods of relieving dysphagia, and is still used clinically in a limited number of patients. Among various devices designed for this purpose in this century, the Souttar, Mousseau-Barbin, and Celestin tubes have been the most commonly employed.

Souttar, in 1924 [2], designed a tube made of rubber with an external metal coil and a proximal funnel. Intubation was performed under direct vision using a rigid esophagoscope. Satisfactory relief of dysphagia was achieved, but perforation of the esophagus during intubation and subsequent dislocation of the tube were the drawbacks. Numerous other devices have since then come into clinical use. Apart from the peroral approach, intubation has been done transcervically or via thoracotomy.

The risk of esophageal perforation existed as long as intubation was by pulsion. Mousseau and Barbin, in 1956 [3], introduced intubation by traction, with better results. Their tube was plastic with a V-shaped proximal funnel and a long distal pilot catheter, which was used to pull the tube down into position through an opening in the stomach. In spite of the advantages of traction over pulsion, the Mousseau-Barbin tube did have shortcomings. The blind pilot catheter did not always locate the lumen of the tumor, and the tube was of small caliber, permitting only liquids or semiliquids to pass. The tube was frequently displaced upward, and its V-shaped funnel sometimes caused pressure ulceration of the esophageal mucosa, which could become so edematous as to obstruct the funnel.

Prompted by these factors, Celestin designed an improved tube in 1959 [4]. This tube, still in use, is made of latex reinforced by a nylon spiral and has a shaft 25 cm long with an internal diameter of 11 mm and a tulip-shaped head which is nontraumatic to the esophageal wall. The lower end of the shaft is connected to a solid pilot bougie which can always be successfully navigated through the lumen of a tumor. The bougie is recovered from the stomach through a gastrotomy and used to pull the tube down into position. The excess length of tube below the cardia is then removed with a bevelling cut and the tube is anchored to the lesser curve with a braided nylon stitch. This tube is so well designed that it has remained unchanged in over 20 years of clinical use.

More recently, Celestin [5] has designed a pulsion tube based on the long experience of traction tubes. The new tube has a collapsible skirt at the lower end which prevents upward migration during coughing or vomiting but allows extubation by means of a firm steady pull, which everts the skirt. This tube is inserted under fiberendoscopic direct vision by means of an introducer which rides with the tube on the outside of the fiberendoscope and can be disconnected and withdrawn once the tube is in position.

Esophageal intubation has been widely practised and investigated in China since the early 1960s. Most tubes have been of the pulsion type and most have been inserted under direct vision through a rigid esophagoscope after dilatation of the stricture, although intubation has also been done transcervically or during thoracotomy via an esophagotomy above the tumor [6, 7]. Traction intubation devices have also been used via cervical incision and gastrotomy. In some tubes a metallic ring is incorporated into the proximal funnel to prevent collapse of the funnel and to enable visualization on X-ray examination. The outside of the tube incorporates reversed serration to prevent upward displacement.

In many patients with late carcinoma of the esophagus and gastric cardia, intubation may give a certain relief from dysphagia and enable reasonably satisfactory eating and drinking. It can be used in patients destined for radiotherapy who have servere dysphagia (Fig. 15.1), and also to relieve dysphagia and act as an indwelling dilator in patients with

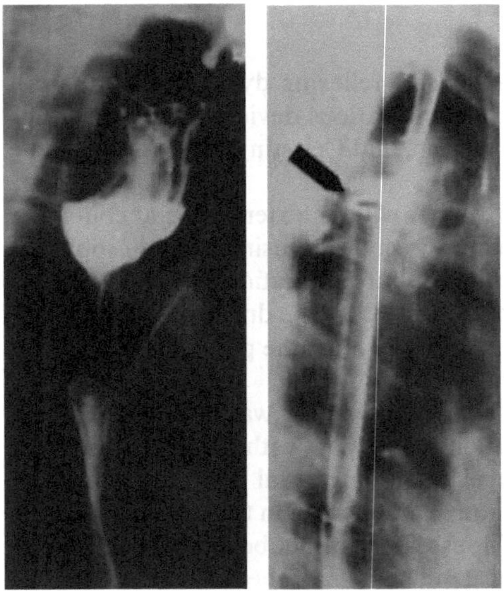

Fig. 15.1. Intubation in a case of esophageal carcinoma with severe dysphagia (CI Hosp. No. 78116). *Left:* Esophagogram showing filling defect at upper thoracic esophagus with marked obstruction. *Right:* Free passage of barium after intubation. Note the metal ring *(arrow)* at the upper end of the tube. The patient received radiotherapy with the tube in position

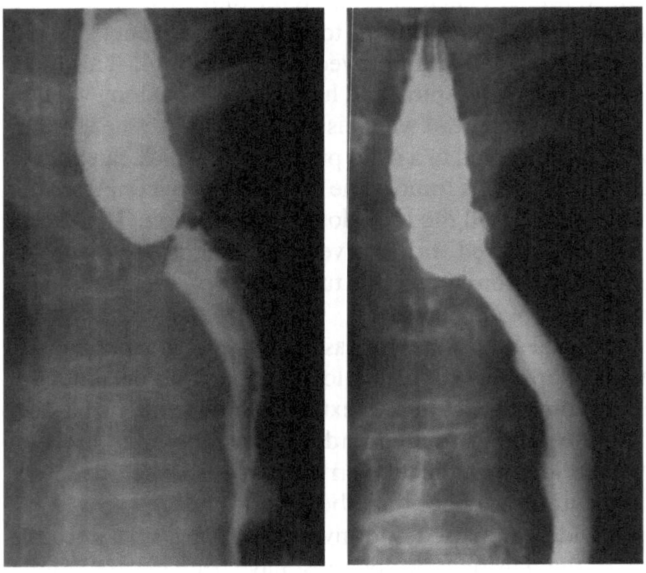

Fig. 15.2 Intubation for anastomotic stricture. A 58-year-old woman (Fu Wai Hosp. No. 50483) with midthoracic esophageal carcinoma was treated by preoperative irradiation and resection and intrathoracic esophagogastrostomy. *Left:* The anastomosis became stenosed 3 months after operation. *Right:* Intubation was carried out and the tube was left in position for 7 months. The patient was able to eat a semiliquid diet for the following 3 years. (Courtesy of Fu Wai Hospital)

postoperative anastomotic stricture (Fig. 15.2). In malignant esophagotracheal fistula, intubation may give temporary relief from continuous aspiration [8].

The shortcomings of intubation are well known. Displacement and food obstruction of the tube are common reasons for failure. Large tubes are rarely tolerated, especially for high lesions, while palliation is usually unsatisfactory with small tubes. In severe, long, and tortuous strictures, intubation is difficult or even dangerous, and perforation of the esophagus, hemorrhage, and mediastinitis are common complications. For all these reasons, the indications for intubation are limited.

3 Esophagogastric Bypass

In recent years, improvement in surgical technique and the wider use of palliative resection and adjuvant therapy such as preoperative irradiation have brought about a marked rise in resectability rates for carcinoma of the esophagus and gastric cardia, with a consequent decrease in the need for bypass operations, which are now indicated chiefly in patients whose tumor is proved unresectable at operation and in whom dysphagia is severe. Esophagogastric bypass may be performed at various intrathoracic levels, depending on the site of the cancer (Fig. 15.3). For cancer of the gastric cardia without extensive involvement of the gastric fundus, and for cancer of the lower segment of the esophagus, bypass can be achieved by mobilizing the fundus and bringing it up to a level slightly above the tumor for side-to-side anastomosis with the esophagus. In midthoracic esophageal carcinoma, the greater part of the stomach and the lower segment of the esophagus are mobilized to allow the fundus to reach the supra-aortic region, where a side-to-side anastomosis is constructed.

Side-to-side anastomosis is normally used in esophagogastric bypass, but if there is a tendency to perforation of the tumor, an end-to-side anastomosis may be fashioned between the divided upper end of the esophagus and the mobilized stomach some distance above the tumor, closing the distal cut end of the esophagus. Such an operation may delay or even prevent the formation of a fistula into the airway, as all food and drink is diverted

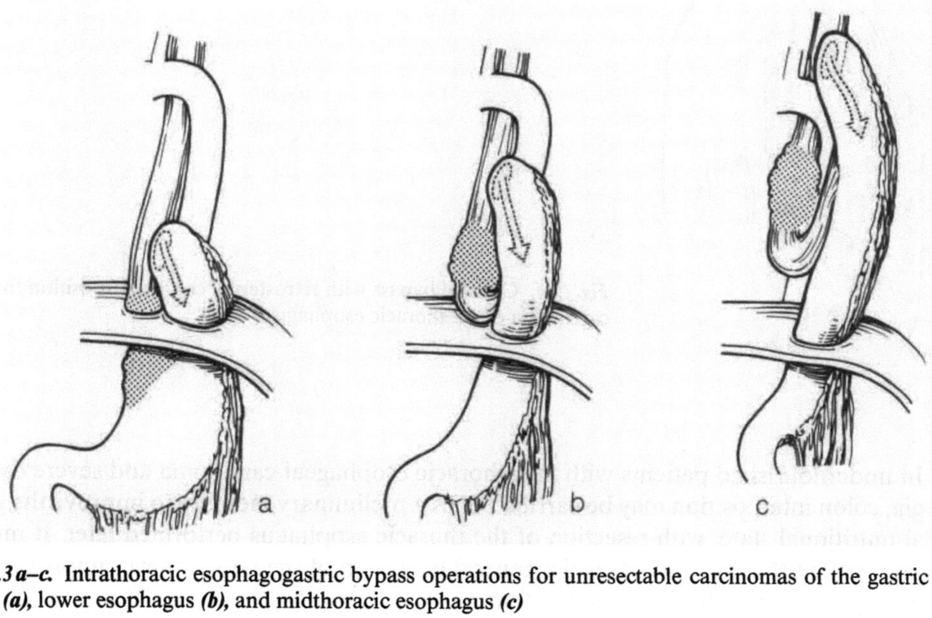

Fig. 15.3 a–c. Intrathoracic esophagogastric bypass operations for unresectable carcinomas of the gastric cardia ***(a)***, lower esophagus ***(b)***, and midthoracic esophagus ***(c)***

away from the tumor. In any cases where postoperative radiotherapy is indicated, metal markers are placed at each end of the tumor during operation for subsequent localization.

A bypass can usually offer good relief of dysphagia, thereby improving the quality of the patient's life. At high levels, however, the intervention is of a magnitude practically equal to that of esophageal resection, and also carries a considerable operative risk. At low levels there is often postoperative gastric reflux and esophagitis, with resulting symptoms of heartburn and pain, possibly even ulceration and hemorrhage.

In the author's series of 106 esophagogastric bypass operations for nonresectable carcinoma of the esophagus, there were five hospital deaths, an operative mortality of 4.7%. The causes of death were anastomotic leakage in two cases and tumor metastases in three. Follow-up study showed that the 6-month survival rate was higher in this group than in those with gastrostomy or without any palliative treatment. However, only 10.9% of the patients survived for 1 year.

4 Esophageal Bypass with Colon Interposition

The technique of colon interposition for esophageal bypass is similar to that of esophageal reconstruction, the only difference being that in the bypass operation only cervical and abdominal incisions are needed, without thoracotomy. The colon is brought up to the neck via the retrosternal or the subcutaneous route (Fig. 15.4). Such an operation is indicated in patients with severe dysphagia whose esophageal cancer is clinically nonresectable or whose cardiopulmonary reserves are not sufficient for a major open chest operation.

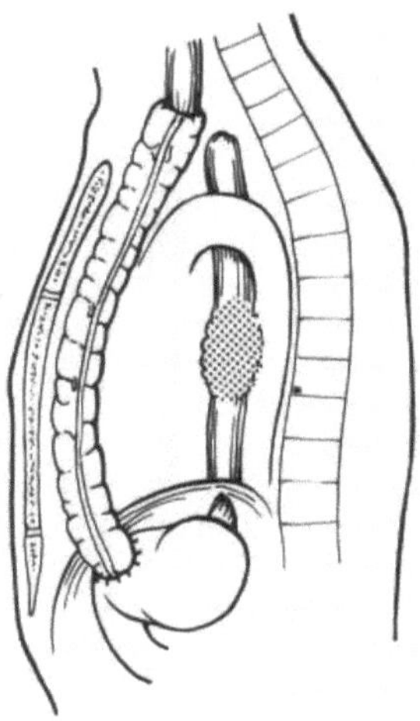

Fig. 15.4. Cervical bypass with retrosternal colon interposition for carcinoma of the thoracic esophagus

In undernourished patients with intrathoracic esophageal carcinoma and severe dysphagia, colon interposition may be carried out as a preliminary measure to improve the general nutritional state, with resection of the thoracic esophagus performed later. It must be pointed out that in some cases the general condition of the patient never improves sufficiently to warrant the second operation.

5 Gastrostomy and Jejunostomy

Experience has shown that in patients with advanced carcinoma of the esophagus or gastric cardia, gastrostomy neither provides any meaningful palliation, because it cannot relived dysphagia or prolong life, nor solves the problem of aspiration pneumonitis. It may even add to the patient's distress through maceration of skin around the gastrostomy tube caused by leakage of chyme from the stomach.

Jejunostomy has similar shortcomings, and is not employed as a palliative treatment for patients with severe dysphagia. It may be used, however, as a means of administering an elemental diet in the preoperative preparation of undernourished patients, or in patients with anastomotic leakage following resection.

References

1. Huang GJ, Zhang W (1965) Palliative treatment for carcinoma of the esophagus and gastric cardia (in Chinese). In Wu YK, Huang GJ (eds) Carcinoma of the esophagus and gastric cardia. Shanghai Science and Technology Publishers, Shanghai, p 328
2. Souttar HS (1924) A method of intubating the esophagus for malignant stricture. Br Med J 1: 782–783
3. Mousseau M, le Forestier J, Barbin J, Hardy M (1956) The indications for permanent intubation in the palliative treatment of carcinoma of the stomach. Arch Mal Appar Dig 45: 208
4. Celestin LR (1959) Permanent intubation in inoperable cancer of the esophagus and cardia. Ann R Coll Sur Engl 25: 165–170
5. Etienne J, Celestin LR (1979) Esophageal intubation: past and present. Acta Endosc 9: 235–243
6. Mei GN (1965) Esophageal intubation via cervical incision for late upper thoracic esophageal carcinoma (in Chinese). Chin J Surg 13: 635–636
7. Zhang YD (1965) Intubation for carcinoma of the esophagus and gastric cardia (in Chinese). Chin J Surg 13: 363–364
8. Mei GN (1975) Esophageal intubation for malignant esophagotracheal fistula: a clinical observation (in Chinese). Chin Med J 55: 196–197

Chapter 16
Medical Treatment

Yan Sun

1 Introduction

In spite of the recent progress in surgery and radiotherapy for carcinoma of the esophagus and gastric cardia, the prognosis remains poor. Although cancer chemotherapy did not establish itself until World War II, subsequent progress has increasingly shown it to be one of the most important treatment modalities in various malignancies. A large number of effective antineoplastic agents have become available, and the strategy in the treatment of hematologic malignancies and solid tumors has become much more refined during the past three decades.

In recent years, it has been firmly established that several types of biologic response modifiers may increase the host antitumor response through augmentation and restoration of effector mechanisms or mediation of host defense. Clinical experience of the cultural legacies of Chinese traditional medicine has also accumulated in the field of carcinoma of the esophagus and gastric cardia.

2 The Role of Medical Treatment

Chemotherapy, as one of the systemic therapeutic modalities currently available, has been used in patients with disseminated disease. It is most effective when the tumor cell population is small, and when used optimally has the potential of eradicating metastatic foci in their early phase. However, it has not yet been successful in carcinoma of the esophagus and gastric cardia because of its less than ideal selectivity and its toxicity to the host.

Certain traditional Chinese medicines are believed to have special merit in enhancing the host defense mechanism or modulating cell-mediated immunity during and after other treatments. They may be of help in relieving certain symptoms and improving the general condition of the patient, but their effect in the local control of the tumor is generally poor. Immunotherapy, or the use of biologic response modifiers, is still under clinical trial, and can only be used as adjuvant therapy to other effective treatments.

The superiority of multimodality treatment over single treatment has been confirmed by the cures obtained in many solid neoplasms, such as Wilms' tumor, bone and soft tissue sarcomas, malignant lymphomas, breast cancer, testicular cancer, small cell lung cancer, and ovarian cancer.

Modern multimodality treatment is based on the following experimental and clinical factors:

1. Most failures following surgery or radiotherapy are the result of clinically undetected micrometastases.
2. Residual tumor may still be present after curative surgery in the form of microscopic extensions.
3. Research in tumor-cell kinetics has shown that some cells in G_0, the resting phase, can be triggered into the cell cycle by resection of the bulky tumor. Proliferative cells are more sensitive to antineoplastic agents, especially cell-cycle-dependent drugs, than are nonproliferative cells.
4. The development of metastatic desease is usually in close relation to the pathological type and size of the primary disease.
5. Curability after surgery decreases with increase in the volume of tumor mass resected.
6. The effect of chemotherapy varies inversely with the total numer of tumor cells present.

The curative potential of chemotherapy can be augmented by surgical or radiotherapeutic reduction in the size of the tumor mass.
7. Immunotherapy can improve cure rates among patients with a low tumor burden.

Experience in multimodality treatment of carcinoma of the esophagus and gastric cardia is still insufficient. The study of tumor markers for esophageal and cardiac cancer has just got under way. There are still no accurate parameters available for the determination of residual tumor volume, making design of a properly effective multimodality protocol difficult. However, a certain amount of clinical experience has been accumulated in the treatment of carcinoma of the esophagus and gastric cardia by the combinations of surgery and radiotherapy, radiotherapy and chemotherapy, and chemotherapy and traditional Chinese herbs.

3 Chemotherapy

3.1 General Principles and Strategy in Cancer

During the past three decades, more than half a million samples of synthetic compounds or natural products have been screened for antitumor activity in animal models, and more than 60 antineoplastic agents are being used clinically. The efficacy of chemotherapy in the treatment of various malignancies has been improved markedly, thanks to tremendous progress in basic cell biology and accumulation of clinical experience. A certain proportion of patients with acute lymphoblastic and myelocytic leukemia, choriocarcionoma, malignant lymphoma, testicular cancer, or skin cancer can now be cured by chemotherapy alone. It is clear that chemotherapy is a rapidly changing discipline capable of improving the overall cure rate in cancer patients [1–3].

Due to lack of ideal selectivity, most antineoplastic agents affect all rapidly growing cells, malignant and normal, particularly in bone marrow, gastrointestinal epithelium, hair roots, and gonads. In general, most patients can tolerate chemotherapy well if the schedule and dosage are adjusted according to their general condition and bone marrow function.

Surgery and radiotherapy are chiefly used to eliminate primary tumors and bulky tumor masses; chemotherapy is most effective against microscopic metastases. Of paramount importance in the strategy of cancer treatment is the proper use of each modality which may play a specific role in achieving cure, according to the stage of the disease at which the patient presents for treatment. "Curative chemotherapy" has been claimed by Zubrod for a decade. It is clearly recognized that chemotherapy is most effective against a small body of tumor cells; the earlier the chemotherapy, the better the results.

Toward the end of the 1950s, tumor cells were detected in the blood or lymph of even early-stage cancer patients during surgical intervention. The importance of adjuvant chemotherapy to eliminate the circulating cancer cells during and after surgery was thus emphasized by many authors. More recently, the existence of micrometastases has provided a definite indication for adjuvant chemotherapy. Chemotherapy is expected to eradicate subclinical metastases that may already be present when curative surgery is attempted [4], and so far the results obtained in breast cancer, osteosarcoma, and testicular cancer have been gratifying. Clinical trials of adjuvant chemotherapy in many solid tumors such as large intestinal cancer, gastric cancer, and small cell lung cancer are now under way.

The great majority of antineoplastic agents, administered alone or in combination, bear a certain degree of toxicity. Physicians must therefore be familiar with the principal adverse effects of each drug before using it, and it is mandatory to have complete blood counts immediately before, during, and after each course of chemotherapy.

3.2 Carcinoma of the Esophagus

3.2.1 Single Agents

There are only a few reports of single-agent chemotherapy for carcinoma of the esophagus. Up to 1980, 141 cases of esophageal carcinoma were treated with various single antineoplastic drugs at the Cancer Institute of the Chinese Academy of Medical Sciences in Beijing and in Linxian county, Henan province. The results are shown in Table 16.1.

a) Thio-TEPA (Triethylenethiophosphoramide, TSPA)

Among 19 patients treated with thio-TEPA in our series, relief of symptoms and measurable lesion reduction on X-ray films were seen in two cases and partial remission in five, with remission periods varying from 4 to 9 months (Fig. 16.1).

Mechanism of Action and Metabolism. Thio-TEPA is a polyfunctional alkylating agent. It acts on DNA as a cell-cycle-nonspecific agent. Most of the drug is cleared from plasma within a few minutes to 2 h, and 85% is excreted in urine within 24–48 h.

Dosage. Usually 0.2 mg/kg IV daily for 5 days and then every other day for a total course of 200–300 mg.

Table 16.1. Results of single-agent chemotherapy in carcinoma of the esophagus

Drug	Cases	Marked improvement[a]	Partial remission[b]	Response rate (%)
Nitrogen mustard	5		1	20
Thio-TEPA	19	2	5	37
Cyclophosphamide	11	2	2	36
Fluorouracil	25	2	3	20
Ftorafur	4		1	25
Bleomycin	30		7	23
Pingyangmycin	28	4	10	50
Methyl GAG	9	1	1	22
Others[c]	10			0
Total	141	11	30	28

[a] Marked improvement or disappearance of dysphagia and other symptoms and total or near-total disappearance of abnormal X-ray findings after treatment, lasting for more than 1 month

[b] Improvement of dysphagia or other symptoms and definite reduction of measurable extent of lesion on X-ray films after treatment, lasting for more than 1 month. (Definitions by the 1972 National Conference on the Management of Esophageal Cancer)

[c] Adriamycin, mitomycin C, N-F, A139

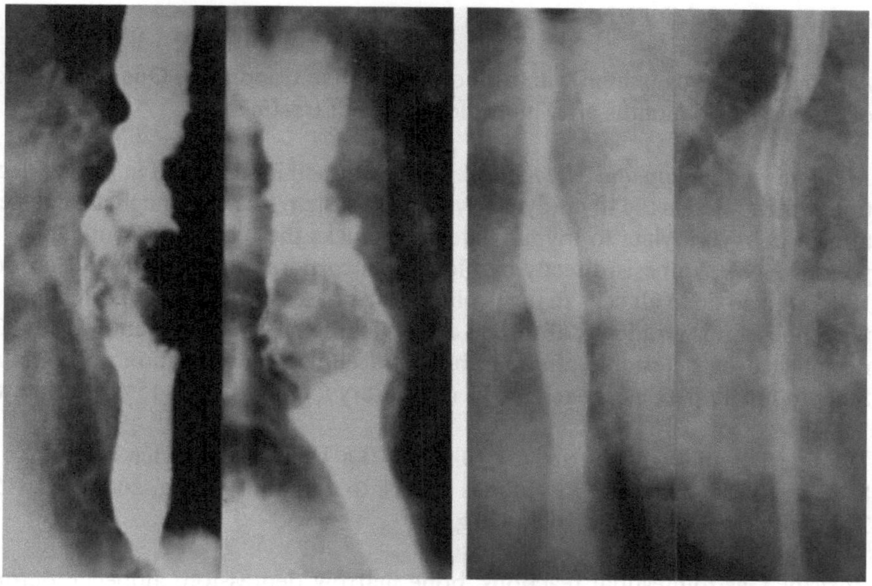

Fig. 16.1. Esophagograms of a 50-year-old man (CI Hosp. No. 180123) with carcinoma of the midthoracic esophagus treated with 400 mg thio-TEPA. *Left:* Before treatment, lesion 10 cm in length. *Right:* After treatment, showing marked improvement. There was a remission of 9 months and the patient survived for 18 months after chemotherapy

Toxicity. Gastrointestinal reactions and bone marrow depression, beginning 5–30 days (median 15 days) after administration.

b) Cyclophosphamide (Cytoxan, Endoxan)

Cyclophosphamide has been widely used in combination chemotherapy for esophageal cancer. Among 11 patients treated in our institution, marked improvement was seen in two cases and partial remission in another two.

Mechanism of Action and Metabolism. Cyclophosphamide must be activated, mainly by liver microsomal enzymes, to have its effect as an alkylating agent. It inhibits DNA synthesis, and belongs to the group of cell-cycle-nonspecific agents, although it is most effective during the S phase. Plasma $T^1/_2$ is 4–6.5 h. Fifty to seventy percent is excreted in urine within 48 h, 68% of this as metabolites and 32% as active drug.

Dosage. Usually 15–20 mg/kg or 600 mg/m^2 IV a week for a total course of 8–12 g; or 2–4 mg/kg PO daily for a total course of 10–15 g.

Toxicity. Gastrointestinal reactions and bone marrow depression. Thrombocytopenia is uncommon. Cystitis may be caused. Alopecia, transverse ridging of nails, and hyperpigmentation are also common. Liver or kidney function may sometimes be impaired.

c) 5-Fluorouracil (5-FU)

Among 25 patients treated with 5-fluorouracil, five responded. One showed no evidence of disease for 15 months after multiple courses of treatment.

Mechanism of Action and Metabolism. 5-Fluorouracil is converted in vivo to deoxynucleotide, which inhibits the thymidylate synthetase system, the enzyme that catalyzes methylation of deoxyuridylate to thymidylate, and blocks the biosynthesis of DNA. It also depresses RNA synthesis directly by blocking incorporation of uracil and orotic acid into RNA. It is toxic to all cells in the proliferating phases of the cycle, particularly to those in the S phase. It is erratically absorbed orally. T½ after IV administration is 10–30 min, with no intact drug detectable after 3 h, but intracellular concentration persist much longer. Sixty to ninety percent is excreted as respiratory CO_2 und 10%–15% in urine within 24 h.

Dosage. Possible courses are (a) 10–12 mg/kg IV infusion twice a week to a total of 8–13 g, (b) 250–500 mg PO 3–5 times a week to a total of 8–13 g, and (c) 250–500 mg PO 3–5 times a week to a total of 15–20 g.

Toxicity. Gastrointestinal reactions, bone marrow depression, alopecia, dermatitis, skin and nail hyperpigmentation.

d) Bleomycin

Bleomycin is a glycopeptide antibiotic isolated from fermentation products of *Streptomyces verticillus,* and can be separated by chromatography into group A und group B, containing altogether 13 peptides. Fraction A2 is the major component, accounting for more than 50% of the clinical preparation. Further analysis by hydrolysis yields seven components. A wide range of responses, from 8% to 75%, has been reported in the treatment of esophageal cancer [5].

Mechanism of Action and Metabolism. Bleomycin inhibits DNA synthesis through binding to DNA, while synthesis of RNA is unimpaired. It causes breaking of single-stranded DNA and inhibits cell DNA repair by a marked inhibition of DNA ligase. Cells in the G_2 phase are especially sensitive to bleomycin, which also acts on cells in the G_1, early S, and M phases. Bleomycin disappears rapidly from plasma after IV administration, T½ being 1.5 h. It is distributed throughout the body, with relatively high concentrations in skin, kidney, peritoneum, and lymph nodes. Inactivation is rapid in all normal tissues except skin and lung. Twenty-five to fifty percent of the administered dose is excreted in urine within 24 h, 20%–40% as active drug.

Dosage. Alternative courses are (a) 15–30 mg IV or IM daily or 2–3 times a week or (b) 15–30 mg IV infusion daily for 4 days a week, with a total dose of 300–400 mg.

Toxicity. Allergic reactions and fever and chills are quite common after injection, and gastrointestinal reaction, skin rash, hyperpigmentation, hyperkeratosis, dyskeratosis, and alopecia are frequent. Direct exposure to sunlight should be avoided during treatment. Pulmonary damage, pneumonitis, and fibrosis, although rare, may be fatal. Special attention should be paid to monitoring possible pulmonary reaction during treatment, which must be discontinued if any such reaction becomes evident.

e) Pingyangmycin (Bleomycin A5)

Pingyangmycin is an antibiotic isolated from fermentation products of *Streptomyces pingyangnensis* sp. nov., which in turn was isolated from a soil sample in Zhejiang province in 1969 by scientists of the Institute of Antibiotics, Chinese Academy of Medical Sciences. Its structure and effective components are those of bleomycin, but are mainly of fraction A5. Laboratory studies have revealed that its activity against some transplantable animal tumors is identical to that of bleomycin, but its toxicity is lower than that of fraction A2 and other components. It inhibits the growth of 91% of mouse transplantable esophageal cancers [6], and the results of clinical trials indicated effectiveness in human esophageal cancer [7, 8]. Among 47 esophageal cancer patients treated with pingyangmycin by a Coordinated Study Group [8] seven exhibited marked improvement and 16 had partial remission, while among the 28 patients treated in our institution, four showed marked improvement and ten had partial remission. Some patients achieved complete remission after a course of pingyangmycin (Figs 16. 2, 16.3).

Mechanism of Action and Metabolism. Pingyangmycin inhibits DNA synthesis in the same way as bleomycin.

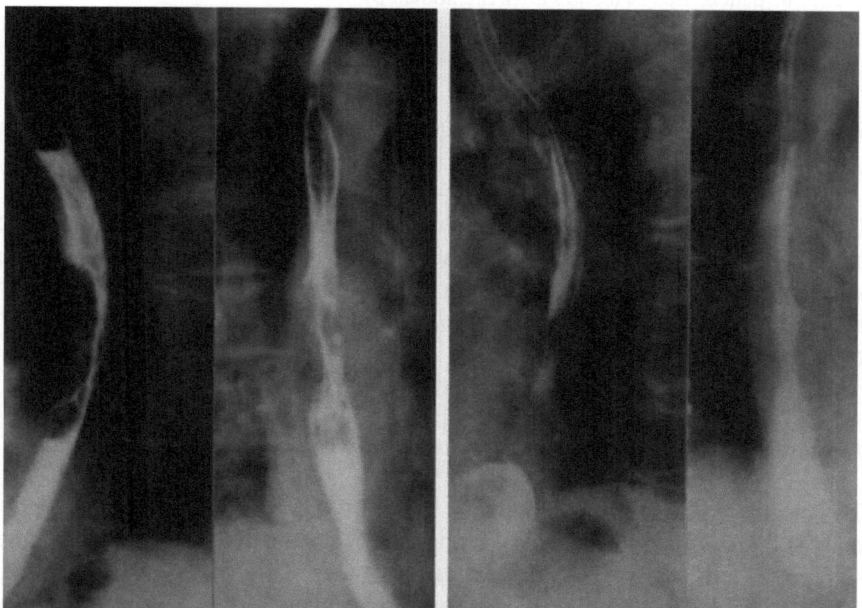

Fig. 16.2. Esophagograms of a 49-year-old man (CI Hosp. No. 272553) with carcinoma of the midthoracic esophagus treated with 285 mg pingyangmycin. *Left:* Before treatment, lesion 6 cm in length. *Right:* After treatment, lesion almost completely disappeared. Radiotherapy was added 2 weeks after chemotherapy for consolidation

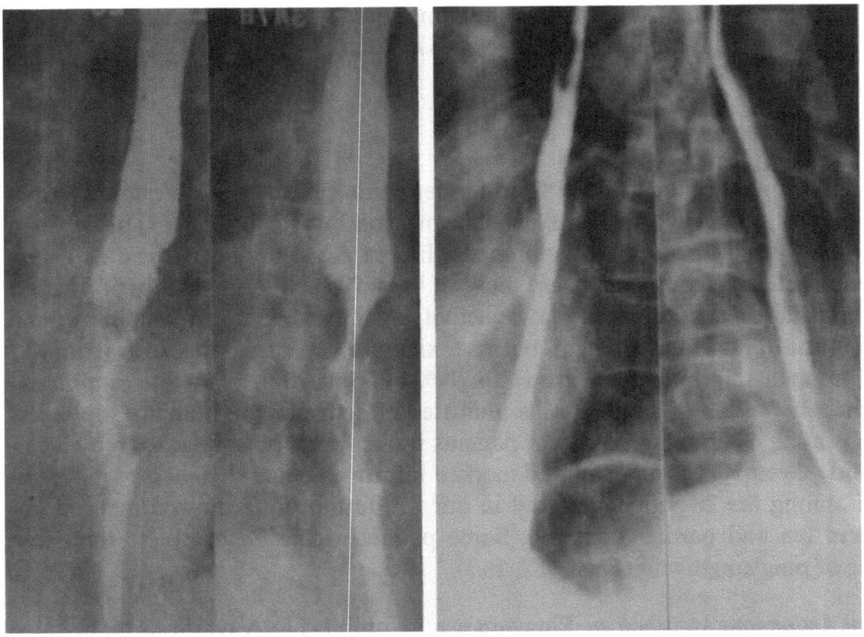

Fig. 16.3. Esophagograms of a 75-year-old man (CI Hosp. No. 262128) with carcinoma of the midesophagus treated with 360 mg pingyangmycin. *Left:* Before treatment, lesion 8 cm in length. *Right:* After treatment, lesion almost completely disappeared. Another course of 120 mg pingyangmycin was given for consolidation, but there was recurrence 3 months later. Further pingyangmycin and irradiation were without effect. The patient died 20 months after chemotherapy

Dosage. A course consists of 10–20 mg dissolved in 4 ml normal saline IM 3 times a week to a total dose of about 300 mg.

Toxicity. Gastrointestinal and allergic reactions are common. Fever usually appears 1½ h after injection and lasts for 3–4 h. The usual skin reactions, such as hyperpigmentation and hyperkeratosis, may occur; a few patients may have rash, alopecia, finger paresthesia, and pain. Bone marrow depression and pulmonary toxicity are reported to be rare, but need to be observed further [8, 9].

f) Methyl GAG (Methylglyoxal Bisguanylhydrazone, Mitoguazone)

The original clinical studies involving methyl GAG demonstrated its activity against human acute leukemia. Falkson [10], using a daily dose schedule, reported five partial remissions in 21 patients with esophageal cancer. Later, Knight et al. [11] observed the clinical efficacy of this drug in solid tumors using a weekly schedule. Carbone and his colleagues (personal communication) now combine methyl GAG with methotrexate, bleomycin, and cisplatin as front-line treatment for carcinoma of the esophagus. Of nine patients treated with this drug in our institution, two showed partial remission. Serious toxictiy limits its clinical use.

Mechanism of Action and Metabolism. The mechanism of action of methyl GAG is not fully understood. There is evidence that it inhibits 5-adenosylmethionine decarboxylase, which catalyzes synthesis of spermidine and spermine. It also bonds to DNA, thereby inhibiting the synthesis of both DNA and RNA, and behaves as a mitochondrial poison in high concentrations. It is rapidly cleared from the blood after IV injection, but only 25% is excreted in urine during the first 24 h. Over 3 weeks, 60% is excreted in urine, less than 20% in the feces.

Dosage. Possible courses are (a) 500–700 mg/m^2 weekly, (b) 150–200 mg/m^2 weekly, or (c) 150–200 mg/m^2 every 2 days, all by IV infusion to a total of 4–6 g. Currently most physicians prefer a weekly schedule.

Toxicity. Gastrointestinal reactions, bone marrow depression, and renal and hepatic damage occur with a daily dose schedule but are minimal or absent with a weekly schedule. Weight loss, malaise, vasculitis, neuromyopathy, balanitis, ileus, and hypoglycemia may occur.

g) Adriamycin (Adriblastina, Doxorubicin)

Adriamycin is an antibiotic extracted from *Streptomyces peucetius* var. *caesius*. It belongs to the anthracycline group with a wide antitumor spectrum. Kolaric et al. [12] reported one complete and five partial remissions among 18 esophageal cancer patients treated by adriamycin. They later treated 15 patients with adriamycin in combination with radiotherapy, obtaining four complete and five partial remissions, duration of remission ranging from 3 to 15 months.

Mechanism of Action and Metabolism. Adriamycin inhibits DNA and RNA synthesis by intercalating between DNA base pairs with inhibition of DNA-dependent RNA synthesis and DNA-dependent DNA synthesis. It is a cell-cycle-nonspecific agent, but is more effective in the S phase. Adriamycin is rapidly metabolized in liver after IV infusion and significantly eliminated in bile, 50% as unchanged drug and 23% as active metabolite (adriamycinol). Five to ten percent of the administered dose is excreted in urine. Adriamycin has a biphasic plasma disappearance, with T½ at 1.1 h and 16.7 h. It is well known that toxicity may be aggravated by hepatic dysfunction, but not by impaired renal function.

Dosage. The alternative courses are (a) 60–75 mg/m^2 IV every 3 weeks or (b) 30 mg/m^2 IV for 2 consecutive days once every 3 weeks. The total dose should be kept below 450 mg/m^2.

Toxicity. Gastrointestinal reactions are usually mild, but can be severe. Bone marrow depression, leukopenia, and thrombocytopenia reach their worst 10–15 days after administration, the counts returning to normal by approximately 21 days. Cardiac toxicity with transient ECG changes may occur 72 h after administration, and congestive cardiac failure, secondary to a diffuse cardiomyopathy, is usually dose dependent. Vitamin E, coenzyme Q10, and persantin should be given during treatment. Alopecia develops between 3 and 4 weeks after the initial dose, but the hair usually regrows within 3–5 months of cessation of therapy.

h) Cisplatin (cis-Diamminedichloroplatinum, cis-Platinum)

Cisplatin is an inorganic platinum compound with a wide antitumor spectrum, and is currently used in combination chemotherapy for solid tumors such as testicular and nasopharyngeal cancers. Ravry et al. [13] reported that it was effective in four of ten esophageal cancer patients. Kelsen et al. [14] combined cisplatin and bleomycin in 37 esophageal cancer patients and found a response in seven. Recently, a new three-drug regimen consisting of bleomycin, cisplatin, and vindesine has appeared to be much more effective [15].

Mechanism of Action and Metabolism. Cisplatin forms bridges between the two strands of DNA and then inhibits DNA synthesis, while RNA and protein synthesis are less affected. It is a cell-cycle-nonspecific drug, but the G_1 phase is more sensitive in vitro. Cisplatin is inactive when administered orally, and is repidly cleared from plasma after IV injection, with only 10% found later. It has a biphasic plasma disappearance, with T½ of 25–50 min and 58–73 h. Twenty-five percent is excreted in urine within 24 h, 43% within 96 h. Platinum is still detectable in the tissue at least 4 months after administration.

Dosage. Alternative courses are (a) 20 mg/m^2 IM or IV infusion daily for 5 days once every 3 weeks or (b) 80–120 mg/m^2 IV every 3 weeks, in either case for 4–5 cycles.

Toxicity. Gastrointestinal tract reactions and nausea and vomiting appear 1–4 h after administration and last for 24 h to 1 week. Bone marrow depression is usually mild; leukopenia reaches its worst 18–23 days after injection, with recovery by day 39. Renal damage is common, and therefore renal function should be monitored before and after treatment. Blood urea nitrogen, serum creatinine, and creatinine clearance should be measured before each dose. For patients with impaired renal function, cisplatin should be used very carefully, with doses kept low. Tinnitus may occur, and peripheral neuropathy, such as sensory impairment and loss of deep tendon reflexes, is usually seen at total doses above 300 mg/m^2.

i) Vindesine (Desacetyl Vinblastine Amide, Eldisine)

Vindesine, a new analogue of vinblastine with a wide antitumor spectrum and lower toxicity, is undergoing extensive clinical trials. Phase I–II studies indicate that it is active in acute leukemia and various solid tumors, and not cross-resistant with vinblastine or vincristine. Kelsen et al. [15, 16] treated 23 cases of esophageal cancer, of whom 18% responded, some of them having previously received irradiation without effect.

Mechanism of Action. Like vinblastine, vindesine bonds to a cytoplasmic precursor of the spindle and inhibits RNA synthesis by effecting the DNA-dependent RNA polymerase system. It causes rearrangement of binding sites in the protein of the microtubular units in the mitotic spindle. It is a phase-specific agent.

Dosage. A course consists of a dose of 3–4 mg/m^2 once every 1–2 weeks by IV injection or infusion, usually for 6–8 weeks, for a total dose of about 20 mg/m^2.

Toxicity. Gastrointestinal reaction, nausea and vomiting, or constipation may occur. There is bone marrow depression; WBC counts are lowest 3–5 days after administration, but usually recover within 6–8 days. Peripheral neuropathy is less severe than with vincristine.

3.2.2 Combination Chemotherapy

Esophageal cancer is one of the tumors with a slow growth rate, its cell cycle lasting about 1 week (5.4–8.1 days), a little longer than that of normal esophageal epithelium (6 days). Theoretically its doubling time is 235–250.7 h, but in fact it is usually much longer. This indicates that in esophageal cancer only a small fraction of the cells are proliferating, the rest being in the G_0 phase. As most drugs act only on proliferating cells, this constitutes one of the main obstacles to the curative treatment of esophageal cancer.

Some cell-cycle-nonspecific agents have been developed which are effective in this setting. It has been shown in animal experiments that reduction of the tumor mass increases the growth fraction of the remaining cells, thus rendering them more sensitive to chemotherapy. Thus in combination chemotherapy for solid tumors with a lower growth rate and less proliferating cells, it is preferable to use a cell-cycle-nonspecific agent first and follow it with cell-cycle-especific drugs. Generally speaking, the drugs should be active against the tumor in question when used alone. Dose-limiting toxicity should not be produced by other agents employed in the combination, making it possible to use three or four antitumor agents at nearly maximum tolerated dosage. The effective combinations for carcinoma of the esophagus are listed in Table 16.2.

In the author's institution, regimens consisting of 5-fluorouracil and bleomycin plus either cyclophosphamide or mitomycin C have been used since 1973. A regimen consisting of cisplatin, vindesine, and bleomycin was recently tested at the Sloan-Kettering Cancer Center in New York [15]. Over 55% of the 53 patients, including those with metastatic disease, had partial or nearly complete remissions. Among patients with localized disease, more than 80% of those who received preoperative chemotherapy were found to have resectable tumors [15]. Gisselbrecht et al. [18] treated eight esophageal cancer patients with a combination of fluorouracil, adriamycin, and cisplatin, and six with cisplatin, bleomycin, and vindesine. Dramatic tumor regression was observed in seven cases.

3.2.3 Chemotherapy with Radiotherapy and/or Surgery

Multimodality treatment can potentially cure a higher proportion of patients with localized carcinoma of the esophagus, and is being studied in many institutions. Franklin et al. [19] reported the results in 54 esophageal cancer patients treated with mitomycin C, 5-fluorouracil, radiotherapy, and surgery. The median survival time for 28 patients with localized tumor was 9+ months, and 14 were still alive 4–32.5 months after treatment; in 26 patients with nonresectable tumors it was 4 months, with eight still alive 3.5–22 months after treatment. Leichman et al. [20] treated nonmetastatic esophageal cancer with combination chemotherapy (cisplatin and 5-fluorouracil) and radiotherapy. Three weeks after the last dose of chemotherapy, a repeat metastatic workup was done. If this was negative, the patients were subjected to celiotomy and esophagectomy. Among 11 patients so treated, seven were found to be tumor-free in the resected esophagus; only one died following surgery. Kolaric et al. [12] treated esophageal cancer patients with chemotherapy and irra-

Table 16.2. Combination chemotherapy courses in carcinoma of the esophagus

Combination	Cases	Response		Author(s)
		(*n*)	(%)	
CFB CTX 600 mg/m² IV 1/week FU 250–500 mg IV 2–3/week BLM 30 mg IM 2–3/week 7–10 days/cycle 4–6 cycles/courses	30	7	23	Cancer Institute, CAMS
MFB MMC 4–6 mg IV 1/week FU 500 mg IV 2/week BLM 30 mg IM 2–3/week 6 weeks/course	9	3	33	Cancer Institute, CAMS
FB FU 500 mg IV 2/week BLM 30 mg IM 2–3/week 6 weeks/course	22	3	14	Cancer Institute, CAMS
MVB MMC 20 mg IV 1/5 weeks VCR 1 mg/m² IV 1/week BLM 10 units/m² IV 1/week	4	4	100	Lod [17]
PMB PDD 100 mg/m² IV infusion for 24 h, days 1, 22 MMC 20 mg/m² IV day 3 BLM 10 units/m² IV 1/week and IV infusion days 24–27	13	7	54	Cancer Institute, CAMS
PVB PDD 3 mg/kg, hydration, and diuresis IV day 1 VDS 3 mg/m² IV days 3,8,15,22 BLM 10 units/m² IV after loading IV infusion for 4 days 28 days repeat cycle	53	29	55	Kelsen et al. [15]
PB PDD dosage as PVB BLM	58	11	19	Kelsen et al. [15]

Abbreviations: CTX, cyclophosphamide; FU, 5-fluorouracil; BLM, bleomycin; MMC, mitomycin C; VCR, vincristine; PDD, cisplatin; VDS, vindesine; CAMS, Chinese Academy of Medical Sciences

diation combined. Among 15 patients treated with adriamycin and irradiation, there were four complete and five partial remissions, mean duration of remission being 8.6 months; among 15 others treated with bleomycin and adriamycin plus irradiation, three complete and six partial remissions were obtained and the median duration of remission was 11 months. Marcial et al. [21] used methotrexate, bleomycin, and vindesine plus irradiation to treat 25 patients with esophageal cancer; 15 complete remissions were obtained, and four patients (16%) survived for over 3 years. Protocols designed by Karlin at M.D. Anderson Hospital and presently being studied involve adriamycin, bleomycin, and cisplatin followed by irradiation, after which cisplatin and adriamycin are used as maintenance. Kubla et al. [22] treated 11 esophageal cancer patients with an aggressive multimodality protocol including staging laparotomy and bronchoscopy, induction chemotherapy (cisplatin, mitomycin C, bleomycin, and prednisone), esophagectomy and pharyngogastrostomy, consolidation chemotherapy, irradiation, and maintenance chemotherapy (mitomycin C, vincristine, and prednisone). Six patients showed objective response to chemotherapy, but five died postoperatively. The conclusion is that although the induction regimen was effective, the pulmonary toxicity caused death. Modifications of the multimodality sequence have been made for ongoing trials.

3.3 Carcinoma of the Gastric Cardia

Many drugs are effective against adenocarcinoma of the gastric cardia, including 5-fluorouracil, mitomycin C, adriamycin, ftorafur, camptothecin, thio-TEPA, and nitrosoureas [23]. In the author's institution, among 42 cardiac cancer patients treated with 5-fluorouracil, six (14%) responded; three of 18 cases (16%) showed partial remission after administration of thio-TEPA.

Some Single Agents

a) Ftorafur

Ftorafur is an analogue of 5-fluorouracil, being transformed to active 5-fluorouracil by liver enzymes after administration. Its therapeutic index is twice as high as that of 5-fluorouracil, its toxicity only 16%–20% as great. Its mechanism of action is similar to that of 5-fluorouracil. It is absorbed rapidly after oral administration, and the concentration of 5-fluorouracil in the serum remains measurable much longer than after IV injection. It is effective against carcinomas of the stomach, colon, pancreas, and breast.

Dosage. One course of 800–1200 mg/day to a total dose of 20–40 g.

Toxicity. Gastrointestinal reactions, anorexia, and nausea and vomiting may occur. Hyperpigmentation of skin somewhat resembles that after 5-fluorouracil, but bone marrow depression is usually relatively mild.

b) Camptothecin

Camptothecin is an alkaloid from *Camptotheca acuminata* Decsne. Which inhibits DNA synthesis by affecting DNA polymerase or binding with DNA. It is a cell-cycle-specific drug, effective in the S phase. Clinical trials have revealed that it is active in gastric and hepatic cancer [24].

Dosage. A course of 5–10 mg/IV or IM a day to a total dose of 140–200 mg.

Toxicity. Sterile hemorrhagic cystitis is common and dose-limiting, but can be prevented by maintaining high fluid intake. Gastrointestinal reactions, bone marrow depression, and alopecia may sometimes occur.

c) Mitomycin C (Ametycin, Mutomucin)

Mitomycin C, an antibiotic isolated from *Streptomyces caespitosus,* is a complex structure with several potentially active groupings, such as the aziridine ring and the aminoquinone and methylurethane moieties. After activation by intracellular reductive enzyme systems, it is a bifunctional or trifunctional alkylating agent, forming a cross-link between the two strands of DNA and inhibiting its replication. Mitomycin C is a cell-cycle-nonspecific agent which acts on all phases of living cells, the late G_1 and early S phases being most sensitive. It is active against gastric carcinoma and adenocarcinomas of the breast, colon, pancreas, and liver.

Table 16.3. Combination chemotherapy courses in carcinoma of the gastric cardia

Combination		Cases	Response rate (%)	Author(s)
MFC				
MMC	0.04–0.08 mg/kg			
FU	10 mg			
Ara-C	0.4–0.8 mg/kg in normal saline or 5% glucose IV twice a week for 2 weeks, then weekly or biweekly, 9–10 weeks/course	44	50	Ota et al. [25]
MF				
MMC	8–10 mg/m^2 IV			
FU	500 mg/m^2 IV for 5 days every 2–3 weeks	140	24	Ogawa [23]
MFV				
MMC	6–8 mg IV 1/week			
FU	500 mg IV 2/week			
VCR	1 mg IV 1–2/weeks 6 weeks/course	27	39	Cancer Institute, CAMS
MF				
MMC	6–8 mg IV 1/week			
FT	200 mg PO 6 weeks/course	14	35	Cancer Institute, CAMS
FAM				
FU	600 mg/m^2 IV 1/week			
ADM	30 mg/m^2 IV days 1,28			
MMC	10 mg/m^2 IV day 1 56 days/course	29	55	MacDonald et al. [26]
FAM II				
FT	1.5 g/m^2 IV days 1–5			
ADM	40 mg/m^2 IV days 1,29			
MMC	10 mg/m^2 IV day 1 8 weeks/course	10	60	Woolley et al. [27]
AF				
ADM	50 mg/m^2 IV day 1			
FU	500 mg/m^2 IV days 1–3 21 days/course	25	12	Friedman et al. [28]

Abbreviations: FT, ftorafur; ADM, adriamycin; see also Table 16.2

Plasma clearance is rapid after IV administration, with a T½ of 10–17 min. Metabolization is primarily in the liver, 20% being excreted unchanged in urine.

Dosage. Alternative courses are (a) 4–6 mg IV twice a week or (b) 20 mg IV once every 3–4 weeks, in either case to a total dose of 30–50 mg.

Toxicity. Bone marrow depression, leukopenia, and thrombocytopenia are usually cumulative and dose limiting, and gastrointestinal reactions, nausea, and vomiting are common. Alopecia and local irritation may occur after subcutaneous injection.

Effective combination chemotherapy regimes are listed in Table 16.3.

3.4 Long-Term Results

Clinical trials of chemotherapy for early-stage carcinoma of the esophagus and gastric cardia were carried carried out in Linxian county, an esophageal cancer high-incidence area. The long-term results from a group of 32 male and 36 female patients aged between 32 and 70 years shown in Table 16.4 and Fig. 16.4. For the esophageal cancer patients, the drugs used were 5-fluorouracil, bleomycin, and lomustine; for those with cardiac cancer, they were 5-fluorouracil, lomustine, and cyclophosphamide. The control groups consisted of concurrent patients with similar disease who for various reasons refused chemotherapy.

Table 16.4. Chemotherapy in early carcinoma of esophagus and gastric cardia

Survival rates Site	Rate (%)		
	1-year	3-year	5-year
Esophagus			
Chemotherapy	100 (21/21)	87 (13/15)	67 (6/9)
Control	91 (20/22)	52 (11/21)	28 (5/18)
Cardia			
Chemotherapy	100 (20/20)	64 (9/14)	25 (1/4)
Control	80 (4/5)	40 (2/5)	0 (0/4)

Diagnostic criteria Site		Cases	
		Chemotherapy	Control
Esophagus			
Stage 0	Cytologically or pathologically positive, no roentgenologic findings	8	7
Stage I	Cytologically or pathologically positive, lesion < 3 cm on roentgenography	13	15
Cardia			
Early stage	Roentgenologic evidence of lesion < 3 cm, including mucosal change and filling defect	20	5

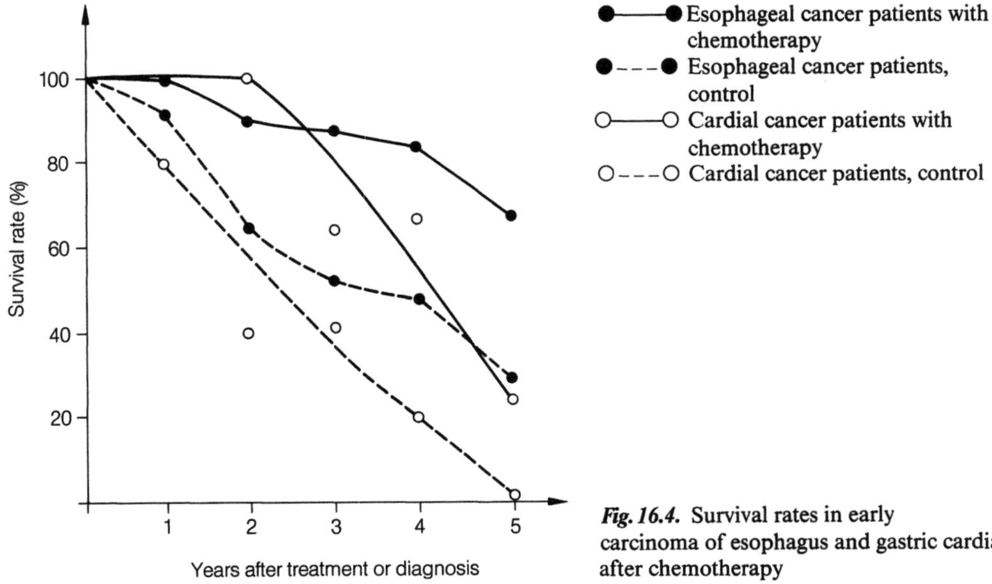

Fig. 16.4. Survival rates in early carcinoma of esophagus and gastric cardia after chemotherapy

The 3-year survival rate for early carcinoma of the esophagus after chemotherapy was 87%, significantly higher than the 52% in the control group ($\chi^2 = 4.63$, $P < 0.05$). The 3-year survival rate for carcinoma of the gastric cardia was 64%, higher than the 40% in the control group but not significantly ($P > 0.05$). Thirteen of the treated patients died within 3 years, ten of obstruction, hemorrhage, or perforation of the esophagus, one of systemic metastasis, and two of cardiovascular diseases. It was our impression that the long-term results could be further improved if local irradiation be added to the treatment protocol.

The long-term results in advanced carcinoma of the esophagus and gastric cardia in the Linxian high-incidence area were also studied. Table 16.5 shows the data from 122 cases treated with combination chemotherapy and 97 controls during the same period. There were seven men and six women (age range 36–84) with esophageal cancer, 51 men and 33 women (age range 48–79) with cardiac cancer.

The results indicate that the survival time was prolonged by chemotherapy in both esophageal cancer and cardiac cancer patients. The 1-year survival rate for esophageal cancer patients was 23% in the treated group, 8% in the control group ($\chi^2 = 4.02$, $P < 0.05$); for the cardiac cancer patients it was 36% in the treated group, 11% in the control group ($\chi^2 = 5.75$, $P < 0.05$).

4 Traditional Chinese Medicine

In records dating from 2000 years ago, the Chinese medical classics described the "dysphagia and belching" among the inhabitants in the northern part of the country. Since then progressive improvement in diagnosis and treatment of esophageal cancer has been described, and during the past 30 years, experience in the management of esophageal cancer has accumulated rapidly.

Table 16.5. Combination chemotherapy in carcinoma of the esophagus and gastric cardia

Site	Cases	Survival rate (%)			Average survival (months)	
		1-year	2-year	3-year	Median	Mean
Esophagus						
Chemotherapy	75	23 (17/75)	6 (4/63)	0 (0/50)	7	9.0
Control	60	8 (5/60)	4 (2/57)	2 (1/55)	3	5.4
Cardia						
Chemotherapy	47	36 (17/47)	11 (4/36)	3 (1/31)	9	12.4
Control	37	11 (4/37)	0 (0/36)	0 (0/31)	5	6.2

Distribution by stages Site	Cases (%)	
	Chemotherapy	Control
Esophagus		
Stage II (lesion 3.1–5 cm)	16 (21)	18 (30)
Stage IIIA (5.1–7 cm)	25 (33)	19 (32)
Stage IIIB (>7 cm)	24 (32)	15 (25)
Stage IV (distant metastasis)	10 (13)	8 (13)
Cardia All cases showed filling defect > 3 cm roentgenologically or presented distant metastasis		

4.1 Forms of Treatment

Treatment regimens depend on the patients' symptoms and signs. For example, at the Taiyuan Hospital of Traditional Medicine, Shanxi province, esophageal cancer was divided into five types – *yang xu* (deficiency of yang), *yin xu* (deficiency of yin), *yin yang liang xu* (deficiency of both), *yin yang liang jie* (exhaustion of both), and intermediate – and patients were treated individually according to their types with Chinese herbs or prescriptions from Chinese medical classics. The average survival time in the 12 patients treated was 11.8 months, two surviving more than 3 years and another two over 1 year [29].

Traditional medicine is now being used in several hospitals in China as adjuvant therapy after surgery, irradiation, or chemotherapy to promote or enhance the recovery of immunity and improve the general condition so as to prolong survival time. Promising preliminary results have been obtained.

4.1.1 Set Prescriptions

There are many set prescriptions used in the management of carcinoma of the esophagus and gastric cardia. Some examples are as follows.

Hui Chun San and *Jin Deng Gao.* In 1972, the Henan Medical College presented the results of *hui chun san* (nux vomica and ocher) and *jin deng gao* (*Tulipa endulis* Baker, *Caulis millettiae, Carthamus tinctorius* L., *Catechy seugambia,* and *Acorus gramineus* Soland) in the treatment of esophageal cancer. The average survival time of patients treated was 17.2 months, while that of untreated controls was 6 months [29].

Zi Nao Sha and *Zi Jin Ding He Ji.* The results of *zi nao sha* (a metal complex of a violet color) and *zi jin ding he ji* in the treatment of esophageal cancer were reported by Beizhen

School of Health Sciences and Hui Min District Hospital in Shangdong province [30]. Among 445 patients with esophageal cancer and 190 with cardiac cancer, marked improvement was obtained in eight cases and significant relief in 452 cases. Some institutions in Hubei province observed the results of *zi nao sha* in esophageal cancer, but found no apparent change of tumor mass in the majority of patients although there was tumor regression after treatement in a few cases.

Prescription for Esophageal Cancer No. 2. The Shuguang Hospital, under Shanghai College of Chinese Traditional Medicine, for many years used a prescription including *Pinellia ternata* (Thunb.) Breit., *Inula japonica* Thunb., *Aristolochia debilis* (Bge. and Zucc., *Syringa vulgaris* L., agalloch (eaglewood), *Amomum cardamomum, Fructus meliae* var. *toosendan, Magnolia officinalis, Glehnia littoralis* Fr. Schmidt, *Asparagus cochinchinensis* (Lour.) Merr., *Asparagus liriopespicata* Lour., *Dendrobium nobile, Impatiens balsamina* L., cockroach, *Angelica sinensis* (Oliv.) Diels, and *Agrimonia pilosa* Ledeb. var. *japonica* (Mig.) Nakai as basic drugs and added other drugs according to the symptoms and signs of individual patients. Definite improvements were achieved in 21 of 69 patients treated [29].

4.1.2 Single Agents

There are some single herbs effective in the treatment of carcinoma of the esophagus and gastric cardia, as shown by clinical and laboratory studies over the past 20 years.

a) Rhabdosia Rubescens (Hamst, 732) Hara

Rhabdosia rubescens, an herb used in the northern part of China for many decades, was investigated recently by a coordinated study group in Henan province. Its roots and leaves contain terpenes, sesquiterpenes, diterpenes, and triterpenes, and two effective components, oridonin and ponicidin, have been isolated (Fig. 16.5).

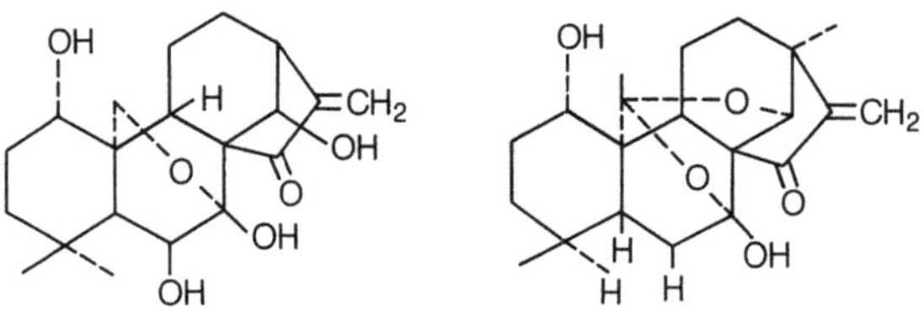

Fig. 16.5. Structures of oridonin *(left)* and ponicidin *(right)*

The water- and alcohol-soluble portion of *Rhabdosia rubescens* inhibited the growth of HeLa cells and an esophageal cell line CaEs-17 in vitro. In transplantable animal tumor models such as Erlich ascitic carcinoma (ascitic and solid forms), S-180 (ascitic and solid forms), liver carcinoma (ascitic and solid forms) and reticulum cell sarcoma, its inhibitory effect was also apparent. It was also able to block the transformation of nitrosamine-induced hyperplasia to carcionoma of esophageal epithelium in rats. The herb has been used in the management of esophageal cancer, with 15 of 43 patients responding; in cardiac cancer, 10 of 25 patients responded. The majority of patients experienced symptom relief and improvement of appetite and general condition. Among the 42 patients followed up after treatment, 25 survived for more than 1 year, and three and one survived for over 2 and over 3 years respectively.

Combination of *Rhabdosia rubescens* with cyclophosphamide and bleomycin was effective in three of nine cases. The side effects of the chemotherapeutic agents were also mild [31].

Dosage. A course consists of five tablets (one tablet contains 3 g rough herb) PO 3 times a day and liquid extract (1 g/ml rough herb) 10–20 ml PO 3 times a day for 1–3 months.

Toxicity. Gastrointestinal reactions, nausea, mild diarrhea, and abdominal pain may occur, and allergic reactions such as skin rash may appear occasionally. There is no apparent toxic effect on the liver, kidney, or bone marrow.

b) *Syrup of Cudrania tricuspidata (Carr.)*

The water-soluble portion of the roots and leaves of *Cudrania tricuspidata* has been used in China for several decades for detoxication, invigoration of the circulation, prevention of excessive phlegm, and as a tonic or nourishing drug. It contains flavanone, β-glutasteroids, alkaloids, phenol, organic acids, and amino acids. Inhibition was observed in cell line U27, S-180, Erlich ascitic carcinoma, and esophageal cancer in vitro or in animals. The syrup is effective in the relief of clinical symptoms of esophageal cancer [32], and also has anti-infection and pain-relief properties.

Dosage. A course consists of 24 ml 3 times a day for several months.

Side Effects. Sometimes the syrup induces liquid stools and increased movement of the bowels.

c) *Cantharidin*

Cantharidin, a terpene from the insect *Myladris sidae,* was tested for its antineoplastic effect in animal tumors and clinically. The effective component is hexahydro-3a, 7a-dimethyl-4,7-epoxy-isobenzofuran-1,3-dione (Fig. 16.6).

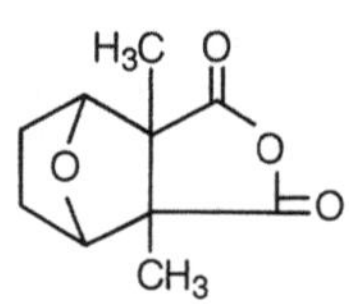

Fig. 16.6. Structure of cantharidin

Inhibitory effects in transplantable animal tumors were observed in liver cancer and reticulum cell sarcoma L2. Prolongation of survival of tumor-bearing animals was also observed in mice when the number of ascitic tumor cells inoculated was comparatively small. The mechanism of action was probably inhibition of protein and nucleic acid synthesis.

Cantharidin can usually be absorbed well by the oral or intraperitoneal route, with a consistent blood level for quite a long period. The concentrations of cantharidin are higher in the intestine, stomach, gall bladder, liver, and tumor tissue, and toxicity is greatest in the heart and kidney [33].

Dosage. A course consists of 0.25–0.5 mg PO 3 times a day for adults (alternatively starting from a low dose and increasing gradually) or between 0.25 mg and a maximum of 2 mg IV a day for 1–3 months.

Other agents under investigation include *Sarcandra glaber* (Thunb) Nakai, *Hericium erinaceus* (Bull. ex Fr.) Pers, *Dioscorea balsamina, Euphoria helioscopia* L., *Engleromyces goetxe* Henn., and gossypol.

References

1. Zhang ZY, Sun Y (1981) Cancer chemotherapy, 1st edn (in Chinese). Shanghai Scientific and Technical Publishers, Shanghai
2. Carter SK, Bakowski MT, Hellmann K (1981) Chemotherapy of cancer, 2nd edn. Wiley Medical, New York
3. Clarysse A, Kenis Y, Mathé G (eds) (1976) Cancer chemotherapy. Springer, Berlin Heidelberg New Yor, pp 173–178 (Recent results in cancer research, vol 53)
4. Valagussa P, Bonadonna G Clinical trials on adjuvant therapies in cancer: short-term and long-term results. – Volterrani F, Sigurta D. Long-term costs of adjuvant therapy. – Weil M, Jacquillat C, Auclerc E, Unger PF, Bernard J. Long-term cost of combined radiotherapy and chemotherapy (1982) In: Mathe G, Bonadonna G, Salmon S (eds) (1982) Adjuvant therapies of cancer. Springer, Berlin Heidelberg New York, pp 303–316 (Recent results of cancer research, Vol 80)
5. Nabeya K (1976) The use of bleomycin in the treatment of carcinoma of the esophagus. Gann 19: 177–186
6. Lin FT, Li DD, Yang XP, et al. (1979) Antitumor activity and preclinical pharmacologic evaluation of pingyangmycin (in Chinese). Chin J Oncol 1: 161–166
7. Xian MS, Wu QG, Bian XX, et al. (1979) Pathologic study of the selective therapeutic effect of pingyangmycin on squamous cell carcinoma (in Chinese). Chin J Oncol 1: 167–171
8. Zhejiang Pingyangmycin Coordinated Study Group (1979) Therapeutic effects of pingyangmycin on malignant tumors (in Chinese). Chin J Oncol 1: 172–175
9. Department of Medical Oncology, Ritan Hospital (1978) Clinical observation on the efficacy of bleomycin A5 on esophageal cancer (in Chinese). In: Collection of Papers for the Twentieth Anniversary of the Cancer Institute and Ritan Hospital, CAMS, pp 446–450
10. Falkson G (1971) Methyl-GAG (NSC-32946) in the treatment of esophagus cancer. Cancer Chemother Rep 55: 209–212
11. Knight WA III, Livingston RB, Fabian C, Costanzi (1979) Phase I–II trial of methyl-GAG: a Southwest Oncology Group pilot study. Cancer Treat Rep 63: 1933–1937
12. Kolaric K, Maricic Z, Bistrovic M, et al. (1980) Controlled clinical trials with a adriamycin in inoperable esophageal cancer. Excerpta Med Int Congr Ser 542: 453–454
13. Ravry MJR, Moore M, The Southeastern Cancer Study Group (1980) A phase II pilot study of cisplatinum (II) (DDP) in advanced squamous cell esophageal cancer. Proc Am Assoc Cancer Res 21: 353
14. Kelsen DP, Cvitkovic E, Bains M, et al. (1978) *cis*-Dichlorodiammine platinum (II) and bleomycin in the treatment of esophageal carcinoma. Cancer Treat Rep 62: 1041–1046
15. Kelsen DP, Bains M, Hilaris B, et al. (1982) Combination chemotherapy of esophageal carcinoma using cisplatinum, vindesine, and bleomycin. Cancer 49: 1174–1177
16. Kelsen DP, Bains M, Cvitkovic E, Golbey R (1979) Vindesine in the treatment of esophageal carcinoma: a phase II study. Cancer Treat Rep 63: 2019–2021
17. Lod TE (1980) Platinum, mitomycin C, and bleomycin chemotherapy of esophageal carcinoma. Proc Am Assoc Cancer Res 21: 419

18. Gisselbrecht C, Belpomme D, Mignot L, Marty M, Boiron M (1982) Chemotherapy of carcinoma of the digestive treact. Springer, Berlin Heidelberg New York, pp 298–302 (Recent results in cancer research, vol 80)
19. Franklin R, Steiger Z, Vaishampayan G, et al. (1980) Combined therapies in esophageal squamous cell cancer. Proc Am Assoc Cancer Res 21: 418
20. Leichman L, Steiger Z, Seydel HG, Haas CD (1981) Potentially curative combined modality therapy for inoperable carcinoma of the esophagus. Proc Am Assoc Cancer Res 22: 458
21. Marcial VA, Vélez-Garcia E, Cintrón J, Yolrach AA (1980) Radiotherapy preceded by multidrug chemotherapy in carcinoma of the esophagus. Cancer Clin Trial 3: 127–130
22. Kubla L, Lad T, McGuire WP, Thomas P (1981) Multimodality therapy of squamous carcinoma of the esophagus. Proc Am Assoc Cancer Res 22: 449
23. Ogawa M (1980) An overview of chemotherapy for advanced gastric cancer. In: Friedman M, Ogawa M, Kisner D (eds) Diagnosis and treatment of upper gastrointestinal tumors. Excerpta Medica Int Congr Ser 542: 357–369
24. Oncology Study Group, Department of Pharmacology, Shanghai Institute of Materia Medica (1975) Laboratory study of antitumor activity of camptothecin (in Chinese). Chin Med J 55: 274–278
25. Ota K, Kurita, S, Nishimura M, et al. (1972) Combination therapy with mitomycin C (NSC 26980), 5-fluorouracil (NSC 19893) and cytosine arabinoside (NSC 63878) for advanced cancer in man. Cancer Chemother Rep 56: 373–385
26. MacDonald J, Schein P, Veno W, Woolley P (1976) 5-fluorouracil (5-FU), mitomycin C (MMC) and adriamycin (ADR) – FAM: a new combination chemotherapy program for advanced gastric carcinoma. Proc Am Assoc Cancer Res 17: 264
27. Woolley P, MacDonald J, Rosenoff S, et al. (1977) Treatment of advanced gastric cancer with combination chemotherapy: 5-fluorouracil (F) or ftorafur (Fur) plus adriamycin (A) and mitomycin C (M) (FAM and FAM II). Proc Am Assoc Cancer Res 18: 304
28. Friedman MA, Ogawa M, Carter SK, Sakurai Y (1981) Chemotherapy of disseminated gastric cancer: USA-Japan Joint Study. Excerpta Med Int Congr Ser 542: 347–356
29. Zhang DZ (1979) Traditional Chinese medicine in carcinoma of the esophagus and gastric cardia (in Chinese). In: Editorial Committe on Practical Oncology (ed) Practical Oncology, vol III, People's Medical Publishing House, Beijing, pp 327–329
30. Oncology Study Group, Beizhen School of Health Sciences and Hui Min District Hospital, Shangone Province (1974) *Zi nao sha* and *zi jin ding he ji* in the treatment of 635 cases of carcinoma of the esophagus and gastric cardia (in Chinese). New Med 5: 110–111
31. Department of Pharmacology and Pharmaceuticochemistry, Institute of Medical Science, Henan Province (1978) A new antitumor substance – rubescensine (in Chinese). Kexue Tongbao 23: 53–56
32. Proc Syrup *Cudrania tricuspidata* (1977) Shanghai (in Chinese)
33. Chen RT, Hua J, Yang JL, et al. (1977) Pharmacological study of cantharidin (in Chinese). Chin Med J 57: 475–477

Subject Index

MIX
Papier aus verantwortungsvollen Quellen
Paper from responsible sources
FSC® C105338

If you have any concerns about our products,
you can contact us on
ProductSafety@springernature.com

In case Publisher is established outside the EU,
the EU authorized representative is:
Springer Nature Customer Service Center GmbH
Europaplatz 3, 69115 Heidelberg, Germany

Printed by Libri Plureos GmbH
in Hamburg, Germany